PEARSON'S
Administrative Medical Assisting

VOLUME I

Administrative Competencies

Nina Beaman, MS, RNC, CMA
Bryant and Stratton College
Richmond, VA

Lorraine Fleming-McPhillips, MS, MT, CMA
Medical Assisting Program Coordinator (retired)
Quinebaug Valley Community College
Danielson, Connecticut

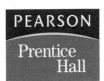

Upper Saddle River, New Jersey 07458

Library of Congress Cataloging-in-Publication Data

Beaman, Nina.
   Pearson's administrative medical assisting / Nina Beaman, Lorraine Fleming-McPhillips.
     v. ; cm.
   Includes index.
   Contents: v. 1. Administrative competencies.
   ISBN 0-13-220904-7 (v. 1)
   1. Medical assistants. 2. Medical secretaries. 3. Medical offices—Management.   I. Fleming-McPhillips, Lorraine. II. Pearson/Prentice Hall. III. Title: Administrative medical assisting.
   [DNLM: 1. Physician Assistants. 2. Medical Secretaries. 3. Practice Management, Medical.   W 21.5 B366p 2006]
   R728.8.B42 2006
   610.73'7—dc22

2005036391

Notice: The authors and the publisher of this volume have taken care that the information and technical recommendations contained herein are based on research and expert consultation, and are accurate and compatible with the standards generally accepted at the time of publication. Nevertheless, as new information becomes available, changes in clinical and technical practices become necessary. The reader is advised to carefully consult manufacturers' instructions and information material for all supplies and equipment before use, and to consult with a healthcare professional as necessary. This advice is especially important when using new supplies or equipment for clinical purposes. The authors and publisher disclaim all responsibility for any liability, loss, injury, or damage incurred as a consequence, directly or indirectly, of the use and application of any of the contents of this volume.

Publisher: Julie Levin Alexander
Publisher's Assistant: Regina Bruno
Executive Editor: Joan Gill
Editorial Assistant: Bronwen Glowacki
Development Editor: Teri Zak
Executive Marketing Manager: Katrin Beacom
Director of Marketing: Karen Allman
Marketing Coordinator: Michael Sirinides
Director of Production and Manufacturing: Bruce Johnson
Media Product Manager: John Jordan
Manager of Media Production: Amy Peltier
New Media Project Manager: Tina Rudowski
Manufacturing Manager: Ilene Sanford
Senior Design Coordinator: Christopher Weigand

Interior Designer: Brigid Kavanagh and Pearson Education Development Group
Cover Designer: Yin Wong, Pearson Education Development Group
Director, Image Resource Center: Melinda Reo
Manager, Rights and Permissions: Zina Arabia
Manager, Visual Research: Beth Brenzel
Manager, Cover Visual Research & Permissions: Karen Sanatar
Image Permission Coordinator: Frances Toepfer
Composition: *The GTS Companies/York*, PA Campus
Printing and Binding: Courier Kendallville
Cover Printer: Phoenix Color Corporation

Pearson Prentice Hall™ is a trademark of Pearson Education, Inc.
Pearson® is a registered trademark of Pearson plc.
Prentice Hall® is a registered trademark of Pearson Education, Inc.

Pearson Education Ltd., *London*
Pearson Education Australia Pty. Limited, *Sydney*
Pearson Education Singapore, Pte. Ltd.
Pearson Education North Asia Ltd., *Hong Kong*
Pearson Education Canada, Ltd., *Toronto*
Pearson Education de Mexico, S.A. de C.V.
Pearson Education—Japan, *Tokyo*
Pearson Education Malaysia, Pte. Ltd.
Pearson Education, Upper Saddle River, New Jersey

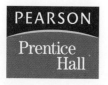

10 9 8 7 6 5 4 3 2 1
ISBN 0-13-220904-7

Brief Contents

Contents

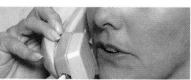

Unit One — Introduction to Health Care 1

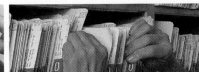

Unit Two **Administrative Medical Assisting** 93

Contents *continued*

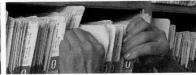

Preface

Pearson's Administrative Medical Assisting

Pearson's Administrative Medical Assisting is a brand new approach to learning the profession of Medical Assisting. It is all about successful skill building to help the student be successful in the classroom and in the physician's office. To help ensure that success, Professional Considerations and Cultural Considerations are also explored. These are skills that will help the medical assistant relate to the workplace: your administrative responsibilities, your patients, your co-workers, and your physicians. It's about making the connection between your skills and your whole profession.

Medical assisting is, after all, a "people helping people" profession. What could be more important than the connections that make the medical assistant the vital link between people and their personal health and well-being? This comprehensive administrative textbook helps the student learn the right skills for becoming the very best and most effective medical assistant through a step-by-step, competency based approach that covers virtually all the facets of the administrative medical assisting profession. Through up to the minute content and careful planning, *Pearson's Administrative Medical Assisting* prepares students to make successful connections in class, in their externships, and in their professional placements.

How does *Pearson's Administrative Medical Assisting* accomplish these goals? A thorough table of contents that covers all the material necessary for student success, a curriculum that follows the AAMA and AMT competencies, a fully developed instructional package that contains everything an instructor needs to successfully connect with students and challenge their skills, and the latest interactive technology that will engage students and instructors alike all foster these goals. The entire package is comprehensive, easily implemented, and completely up to date.

Each chapter in *Pearson's Administrative Medical Assisting* begins with a Role Delineation Chart highlighted with the concepts covered in that chapter. Both students and their instructors easily see which competencies will be covered in the chapter. Learning Objectives underscore the chart, listing the skills and procedures the student will be able to demonstrate after completing the chapter. Terms to Learn are also included so that the student can immediately see the new vocabulary that she will experience. A case study vignette introduces the reader to central concepts and is followed up on later in the chapter with critical thinking questions. Other learning aids in the book include hundreds of color photos and photo sequences; hundreds of full color,

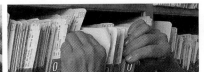

detailed drawings; easy to understand charts and tables; step-by-step procedures; and clear, informative guidelines.

A helpful chapter review allows students to check their knowledge in several ways:
- Competency Review questions test the student's understanding of key chapter concepts.
- Critical Thinking questions relate back to the case study vignette that opens each chapter.
- "On the Job" presents the student with a new scenario with more critical thinking opportunities.
- Certification Exam-style questions help prepare the student for the CMA and RMA exams and review the chapter material.
- An Internet Activity and a MediaLink is also included in each chapter review.

Developed by Pearson Education and Legacy Interactive, Inc., the Medical Assisting Interactive CD-ROM found in the back of the book provides a fascinating journey through the responsibilities, the administrative skills, and the "people skills" of the Administrative Medical Assistant. The CD-ROM opens to the waiting room of a typical Doctor's office. The player can move from room to room in the medical office or, for the more sequentially-minded student, from chapter to chapter. There are medical assisting terminology memory games to play, interactive animations and simulations, tips from professionals, decision-making and critical thinking scenarios, an audio glossary, a Spanish/English glossary, a resource library, and many other wonderful things to do.

Special features throughout the book include segments on *Patient Education*; important *Legal and Ethical* concerns: and *Lifespan Considerations* which focus on the pediatric patient and the geriatric patient. *Preparing for Externship* deals with topics and issues relating to students' participation in an externship program as a capstone to their training. It addresses pertinent issues including student responsibilities, caring attitudes, enthusiasm, grooming/dress, interpersonal skills with patients and colleagues, language skills, poise under pressure and other issues.

Cultural Considerations addresses the medical assistant's encounters with people of different cultural backgrounds, a brief tip, advice, or general guideline on how to deal with a specific cultural or communication issue. Many different cultural issues arise in any physician's office. There may be taboos against certain procedures, removal of clothing, discussion of birth control, showing emotions or feelings, eating certain foods, or taking certain kinds of medication. In our multi-cultural world today, every Medical Assistant will deal with all kinds of people from many different backgrounds. This feature will help the Medical Assistant react with grace, graciousness, and a professional manner.

In the medical office today, the medical assistant must go a step further than mastering a myriad of challenging, detailed, and precise administrative skills. The Medical Assistant must show complete *Professionalism* in the office. This element of each chapter provides a focus on grooming and dress, interpersonal skills, ethical standards, language skills, punctuality, dependability, and a caring attitude. These highly important qualities help the medical assistant maintain a completely professional demeanor at all times. Coupled with mastery of administrative skills, these "soft" skills will guarantee the professional status of the new administrative medical assistant.

Use this book in any of a variety of learning environments and situations including the traditional classroom; the self-paced or individualized course; as a review for those seeking certification and preparing for a certification examination; or in an on-the-job training program in a doctor's office.

The Learning Package:

The Student Package:
- Textbook
- Interactive CD-ROM with exercises, learning games, skills review, medical office simulation for real-life application, skills videos, simulations, animations, resources, Spanish/English glossary.
- Student Workbook that contains chapter-specific assignments; additional procedures and guidelines; review questions; terminology review; skill exercise; vocabulary exercises; forms; other activities designed to reinforce the content of the text.

The Instructional Package:
- Instructor's Resource Guide
- CD-ROM with Test Gen and over 1500 test questions and Classroom Management software.
- Lesson Plans
- Hundreds of PowerPoint slides for daily lessons
- Syllabus, teaching tips, notes, additional exercises, instructional strategies, answers to all text questions and workbook questions.
- Administrative Medical Assisting videos in VHS or DVD format
- Pearson Solutions Medical Assisting Curriculum and Pearson Training Master

Reviewers

The invaluable editorial advice and direction provided by the following educators and health care professionals is deeply appreciated:

Kendra Allen, LPN
Ohio Institute of Health Careers
Columbus, OH

Minda Brown, RMA
Pima Medical Institute
Colorado Springs, CO

Lisa Cook, CMA
Bryman College
Port Orchard, WA

Beverley Giteles, CPC, CMM
Gibbs College
Livingston, NJ

Amy Knight, CMA
Remington College
Largo, FL

Shirley Jelmo, CMA
Pima Medical Institute
Colorado Springs, CO

Tanya Mercer, BS, RN, RMA
KAPLAN Higher Education
Rowell, GA

Kay Nave, CMA, MRT
Hagerstown Business College
Hagerstown, MD

Lynn Slack, CMA
ICM School of Business and
   Medical Careers
Pittsburgh, PA

Janet Sesser, RMA, CMA, BS
High-Tech Institute
Phoenix, AZ

Roberta C. Weiss, Ed.D.
Allied Health Curriculum Specialist
   and Instructional Designer

Authors & Contributors

It is with the greatest appreciation and admiration that we acknowledge the following Health Professions Educators for their contributions to the content of this text. Their dedication to the Medical Assisting profession and to the education of successful Medical Assistants has made this text the premier learning tool.

Authors

Nina Beaman, MS, RNC, CMA
Bryant and Stratton College
Richmond, VA

Lorraine Fleming-McPhillips, MS, MT, CMA
Medical Assisting Program
    Coordinator (retired)
Quinebaug Valley Community College
Danielson, Connecticut

Contributors

Jessica Holtsberry
Ohio Institute of Health Careers
Columbus, OH

Kendra Allen, LPN
Ohio Institute of Health Careers
Columbus, OH

Karen Minchella, Ph.D., CMA
Consulting Management Group
Warren, MI

Christine Malone, BS
Everett Community College
Everett, WA

Susie Huyer, MSN, RN
University of Phoenix Online Affiliate
    Faculty
Heartland Hospice, Administrator

Melanie Sheffield, LPN, AHI
Remington College
Mobile, AL

Roberta C. Weiss, Ed.D.
Allied Health Curriculum Specialist
    and Instructional Designer

Nancy Wright, RN, BS, CNOR
Virginia College
Birmingham, AL

Demetria Jackson
Virginia College
Birmingham, AL

Michelle Buchman, BSN, RN, BC
Springfield College
Springfield, MO

Mary Warren-Oliver, BA
Gibbs College
Vienna, VA

Lynn Slack, CMA
ICM School of Business and
    Medical Careers
Pittsburgh, PA

Innova Inc.
Littleton, Colorado

Acknowledgments

Cover Photo Credits

Photodisc (background); Adam Smith/SuperStock (center); Thinkstock/Age Fotostock (bottom left); Arthur Tilley/Taxi/Getty Images (top left)

Interior Photo Credits

Matthew Brady/National Archives and Records Administration 22; Patrick Clark/Getty Images, Inc./Photodisc 171 (BR); Stewart Cohen/Getty Images, Inc./Stone Allstock 29(TR); Corbis/Stock Market 37; Futura Medical Corporation 102; Getty Images, Inc./Photodisc 159(BR), 247; Michal Heron/Pearson Education/Prentice Hall College 1, 2, 3, 4, 6, 7, 8, 15(BR), 31, 32, 33, 43, 48, 50, 57, 61, 64, 65(TL), 70, 71, 72, 76, 80, 84, 93, 94, 95, 103, 107, 108, 112, 113, 114, 115, 118, 119, 128, 129, 130, 131, 134, 137, 138, 142, 143, 144, 145, 146, 151, 158, 159(TL), 160, 162, 163, 164, 170, 171(TL), 178, 185, 186, 192, 193, 195, 202, 206, 207, 208, 211, 217, 219, 226, 227(TL), 228, 229, 231, 232, 236, 240, 268, 274, 278, 285, 299, 314, 315, 320, 324, 328; Michal Heron Photography 29(BR), 70(CL); Ingenix, Inc. 304, 305; Library of Congress 21; Matt Meadows/Science Photo Library/Photo Researchers, Inc. 194; Michael Newman/PhotoEdit, Inc. 269; Nova Biomedical 197; Omni-Photo Communications, Inc. 227(BR); Photo Researchers, Inc. 18; Southern Illinois University/Photo Researchers, Inc. 28(BL); Paul Steel/Corbis/Stock Market 42, 43; Tom Stewart/Corbis/Stock Market 28(TL); Stockbyte 3(BR), 65(BR); William Taufic/Corbis/Stock Market 196, 248; The Stock Photo Shop, Inc. 30(TL); US Health-Care 273; Brian Warling/American Association for Medical Assistants 9; Brian Warling/International Museum of Surgical Science 14, 15(TL), 16, 19, 22, 30(BL), 56; Brian Warling/Japan Airlines 218; Brian Warling/Pearson Education/Prentice Hall College 302

Illustrations Credits

All illustration created by Imagineering Inc. for Prentice Hall.

Additional Acknowledgments

Employment Forms Courtesy of Bibbero Systems, Inc., Petaluma, CA, (800) 242-2374, www.bibbero.com, 330
RMA Duty Pin Courtesy of the American Medical Technologists, 9

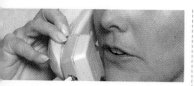

Successful Connections

Pearson's Administrative Medical Assisting

Volume One

This is the first book to connect skills in the classroom and skills on the job, by helping medical assistant students achieve success in school and in their careers.

With *Pearson's Administrative Medical Assisting*, students learn what to do and how to do it. Strong integration of tips, hints, and guidelines help students avoid common performance problems, including timeliness, presentation, and interpersonal relations.

Skills in the Classroom

- Preparing for the Certification Exam
- applied learning activities
- Open design makes using the text easy and clear to the student
- Role Delineation Chart shows student and instructor which skills and competencies will be covered in the chapter

Skills on the Job

- Case Study
- Legal and Ethical Issues
- Cultural Considerations
- Lifespan Considerations
- Professionalism
- Patient Education
- Preparing for Externship

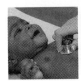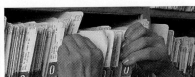

Chapter Opener Features...

Role Delineation Chart

Role Delineation Chart sets the stage and directly links the material that students need to master for passing the Certification Exam.

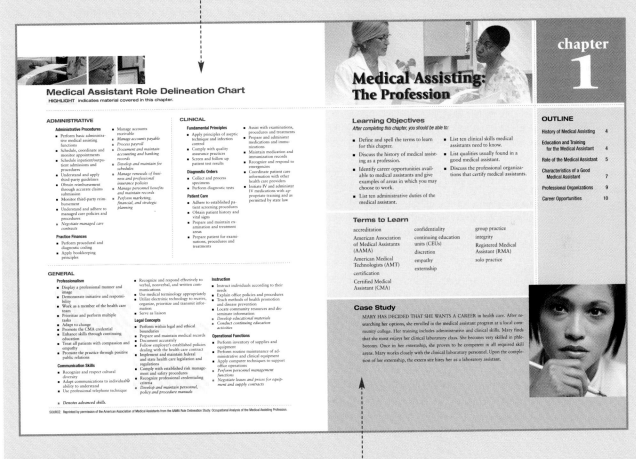

Medical Assistant Role Delineation Chart

HIGHLIGHT indicates material covered in this chapter.

ADMINISTRATIVE

Administrative Procedures
- Perform basic administrative medical assisting functions
- Schedule, coordinate and monitor appointments
- Schedule inpatient/outpatient admissions and procedures
- Understand and apply third-party guidelines
- Obtain reimbursement through accurate claims submission
- Monitor third-party reimbursement
- Understand and adhere to managed care policies and procedures
- *Negotiate managed care contracts*

Practice Finances
- Perform procedural and diagnostic coding
- Apply bookkeeping principles

- Manage accounts receivable
- *Manage accounts payable*
- *Process payroll*
- *Document and maintain accounting and banking records*
- *Develop and maintain fee schedules*
- *Manage renewals of business and professional insurance policies*
- *Manage personnel benefits and maintain records*
- *Perform marketing, financial, and strategic planning*

CLINICAL

Fundamental Principles
- Apply principles of aseptic technique and infection control
- Comply with quality assurance practices
- Screen and follow up patient test results

Diagnostic Orders
- Collect and process specimens
- Perform diagnostic tests

Patient Care
- Adhere to established patient screening procedures
- Obtain patient history and vital signs
- Prepare and maintain examination and treatment areas
- Prepare patient for examinations, procedures and treatments

- Assist with examinations, procedures and treatments
- Prepare and administer medications and immunizations
- Maintain medication and immunization records
- Recognize and respond to emergencies
- Coordinate patient care information with other health care providers
- Initiate IV and administer IV medications with appropriate training and as permitted by state law

GENERAL

Professionalism
- Display a professional manner and image
- Demonstrate initiative and responsibility
- Work as a member of the health care team
- Prioritize and perform multiple tasks
- Adapt to change
- Promote the CMA credential
- Enhance skills through continuing education
- Treat all patients with compassion and empathy
- Promote the practice through positive public relations

Communication Skills
- Recognize and respect cultural diversity
- Adapt communications to individual's ability to understand
- Use professional telephone technique

■ *Denotes advanced skills.*

- Recognize and respond effectively to verbal, nonverbal, and written communications
- Use medical terminology appropriately
- Utilize electronic technology to receive, organize, prioritize and transmit information
- Serve as liaison

Legal Concepts
- Perform within legal and ethical boundaries
- Prepare and maintain medical records
- Document accurately
- Follow employer's established policies dealing with the health care contract
- Implement and maintain federal and state health care legislation and regulations
- Comply with established risk management and safety procedures
- Recognize professional credentialing criteria
- *Develop and maintain personnel, policy and procedure manuals*

Instruction
- Instruct individuals according to their needs
- Explain office policies and procedures
- Teach methods of health promotion and disease prevention
- Locate community resources and disseminate information
- *Develop educational materials*
- *Conduct continuing education activities*

Operational Functions
- Perform inventory of supplies and equipment
- Perform routine maintenance of administrative and clinical equipment
- Apply computer techniques to support office operations
- *Perform personnel management functions*
- *Negotiate leases and prices for equipment and supply contracts*

SOURCE: Reprinted by permission of the American Association of Medical Assistants from the AAMA Role Delineation Study: Occupational Analysis of the Medical Assisting Profession.

Medical Assisting: The Profession

chapter 1

Learning Objectives

After completing this chapter, you should be able to:

- Define and spell the terms to learn for this chapter.
- Discuss the history of medical assisting as a profession.
- Identify career opportunities available to medical assistants and give examples of areas in which you may choose to work.
- List ten administrative duties of the medical assistant.
- List ten clinical skills medical assistants need to know.
- List qualities usually found in a good medical assistant.
- Discuss the professional organizations that certify medical assistants.

Terms to Learn

accreditation
American Association of Medical Assistants (AAMA)
American Medical Technologists (AMT)
certification
Certified Medical Assistant (CMA)

confidentiality
continuing education units (CEUs)
discretion
empathy
externship

group practice
integrity
Registered Medical Assistant (RMA)
solo practice

Case Study

MARY HAS DECIDED THAT SHE WANTS A CAREER in health care. After researching her options, she enrolled in the medical assistant program at a local community college. Her training includes administrative and clinical skills. Mary finds that she most enjoys her clinical laboratory class. She becomes very skilled in phlebotomy. Once in her externship, she proves to be competent in all required skill areas. Mary works closely with the clinical laboratory personnel. Upon the completion of her externship, the extern site hires her as a laboratory assistant.

OUTLINE

Case Study

Case Study provides brief vignettes that help students understand how the chapter information relates to their careers. It increases retention of chapter material because students have a context for the topics.

Additional Features...

Open design is ideal for visual learners. Material is presented in smaller chunks with relevant applications to provide context.

Legal and Ethical Issues

Licensure and continuing medical education (CME) are two areas in which you can assist the physician. The renewal of licenses is usually dependent on the completion of re-registration forms and filing these forms on time with the necessary fees. Always take care to maintain accurate records of continuing medical education units earned by the physician since CME is an important part of the licensing process. Be alert to this legal obligation and remind your employing physician in advance of such renewals.

Medical assistants dedicate themselves to the care and well-being of all patients, according to the American Association of Medical Assistants code of ethics. In addition, medical assistants should take the Oath of Hippocrates, "do no harm to the patient" as seriously as the physicians who state it at the time of their graduation from medical school. As a medical assistant, you will act as a representative of the physician and must be well versed on all legal issues that affect the physician's practice.

Legal and Ethical Issues

Legal and Ethical Issues address the complex topics in a practical and relevant manner, making it easier for students to apply.

Professionalism

Your work reflects your professionalism. If patient records are strewn about the office, or if your system precludes your being able to pull the file you need quickly, it is a reflection on your skills as a medical assistant. If your filing system is sloppy, then you are probably sloppy too. Be sure to file all records accurately, neatly, and in a timely manner.

Professionalism

Professionalism is one of the most important keys to career success. These featured highlights help students understand the importance of adopting and maintaining a professional demeanor.

Cultural Considerations

Cultural Considerations give students the skills to connect with both patients and other health professionals from diverse backgrounds.

Cultural Considerations

You will encounter an array cultural differences when fielding calls in a medical office. When dealing with a patient, it is always best to speak directly with him or her to get the best information. However, there are some cultures that may not allow direct contact with certain members of the family. Even though it is often difficult to obtain vital information by proxy (a third person), it is sometimes necessary so as to avoid cultural clashes.

You may also deal with patients with very poor English skills. Sometimes a translator is necessary. Your main goal when taking calls is to make the patient as comfortable as possible while providing the appropriate assistance.

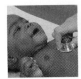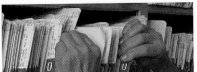

Lifespan Considerations

Care needs to be taken to keep the office child proof and kid friendly. Cover outlets with safety caps. Evaluate the placement of lamps and cords that can be pulled on or tripped over.

Lifespan Considerations

Lifespan Considerations help students develop the skills to relate to patients of all ages.

Patient Education

Most patients have difficulty understanding the details of health insurance. Practicing medical assistants often encounter patients who are convinced that, because they have paid premiums to the insurance company, they should pay nothing further to the provider of service. Tact and patience are essential in educating patients about covered and non-covered services.

Patient Education

Patient Education provides hints and important tips on how to share information with patients in a professional and complete manner.

Preparing for Externship

Preparing for Externship discusses topics and issues students may encounter during participation in an externship program.

Preparing for Externship

Appointment scheduling is an *administrative task or front office procedure. Be aware that the scheduling variation you learned in class may not be the one used at your externship site. Do not be afraid to ask questions. It is to your advantage to learn different variations. Because there is always more than one way of performing a task, you may be able to show what you learned in your office procedures class. Shared ideas sometimes lead to more effective ways of performing tasks.*

PREPARING FOR THE CERTIFICATION EXAM

1. Which of the following is a purpose of the procedure manual?
   A. standardization of procedures
   B. listing of job descriptions
   C. listing of tasks to perform within the office
   D. marketing tool
   E. listing of hospitals and clinics

2. An employee policy describing the grievance process should be contained in the
   A. general policy manual
   B. personnel policy manual
   C. employee handbook
   D. patient information booklet
   E. physician/employer file

3. What law affects the hiring of a new employee?
   A. OSHA
   B. EEOA
   C. Title VII of the Civil Rights Act
   D. EEOC
   E. AMA

4. A systems approach to office management is
   A. using outside consultants for all financial and business operations
   B. performing individual office functions in isolation
   C. integrating functio
   D. not advisable in th
   E. is the only way to

5. Arranging staff vacati
   responsibility of the
   A. physician
   B. individual who is
   C. office manager
   D. medical assistant
   E. nurse

6. The purpose of a performance evaluation is to
   A. positively encourage the continued improvement of the employee's performance
   B. negotiate a salary increase
   C. find any fault(s) in an employee's performance
   D. provide a document to compare one employee's performance with another employee's performance
   E. improve office moral

7. Employee records must be kept for all of the following EXCEPT
   A. Social Security Number
   B. net salary
   C. gross salary
   D. number of claimed exemptions (W-4 form)
   E. deductions

8. Patient instruction booklets should be used
   A. in place of individual instructions
   B. to avoid contact with difficult patients
   C. to prevent lawsuits
   D. to standardize instructions
   E. only with hearing-impaired patients

9. A new employee's probationary period is usually
   A. 30 days

Certification

Certification Exam Success end-of-the-chapter self-assessment and practice help students build exam confidence.

CRITICAL THINKING

1. Did Betsy greet Stacy appropriately?
2. What was the benefit of sending Stacy the paperwork in the mail before her visit?
3. Why did Betsy give Stacy the Notice of Privacy Practice?
4. Did Betsy handle the phone call appropriately? If not, how should she have handled it?

ON THE JOB

Dr. Morrison, a child psychiatrist, who is in solo practice, employs one medical assistant in her office. This medical assistant is multiskilled, like all medical assistants, and, essentially, handles all of the administrative and clinical tasks in the office.

It is 3:00 P.M. and a parent has just arrived for a 3:30 P.M. appointment with her 10-year old daughter. The child is a new patient of Dr. Morrison and was referred by her attending physician. She has a relatively long history of combative and destructive behavior and the referring pediatrician is seeking a psychological evaluation from Dr. Morrison. Psychotropic medication of some sort may be a viable treatment option. The medical assistant has asked the mother and daughter to please be seated and to fill out some registration forms. The child is acting out—pulling cushions off of the reception room couch, wildly ripping the pages of the magazines, whining and kicking at her mother. The behavior seems to be escalating as the mother tries to frantically control her child while, at the same time, follow the instructions of the medical assistant and fill out the registration forms.

What is your response?

1. What if anything, should the medical assistant do?
2. Would it be appropriate, for example, for the medical assistant to interrupt Dr. Morrison's current session?
3. Might this be considered a medical emergency?

INTERNET ACTIVITY

1. Find out how HIPAA has changed the way the medical office handles patient reception.
2. Look for companies that produce forms that can be used by a medical receptionist.

MediaLink   More on patient reception in the medical office environment, including interactive resources, can be found on the Student CD-ROM accompanying this textbook.

applied learning activities

Applied learning activities like "On the Job" scenarios help students increase retention and success by linking concepts to their job functions.

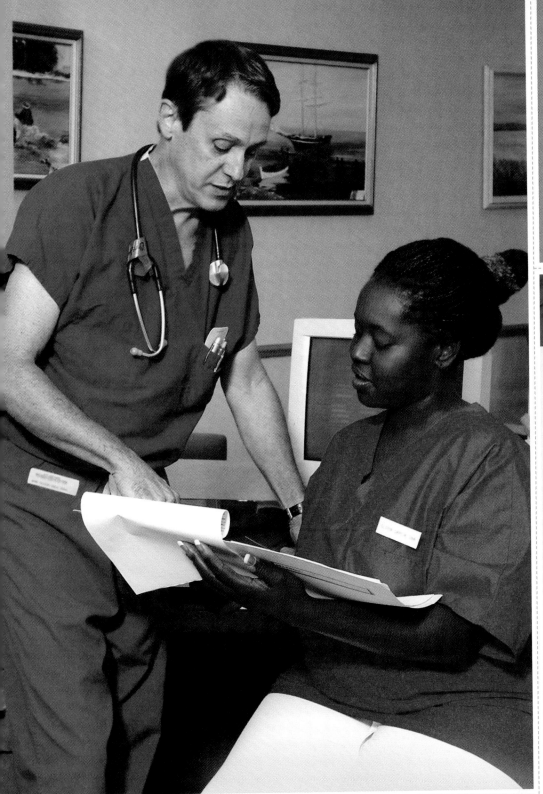

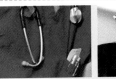

Introduction to
Health Care

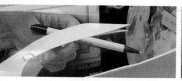

Medical Assistant Role Delineation Chart

HIGHLIGHT indicates material covered in this chapter.

ADMINISTRATIVE

Administrative Procedures

- Perform basic administrative medical assisting functions
- Schedule, coordinate and monitor appointments
- Schedule inpatient/outpatient admissions and procedures
- Understand and apply third-party guidelines
- Obtain reimbursement through accurate claims submission
- Monitor third-party reimbursement
- Understand and adhere to managed care policies and procedures
- *Negotiate managed care contracts*

Practice Finances

- Perform procedural and diagnostic coding
- Apply bookkeeping principles

- Manage accounts receivable
- *Manage accounts payable*
- *Process payroll*
- *Document and maintain accounting and banking records*
- *Develop and maintain fee schedules*
- *Manage renewals of business and professional insurance policies*
- *Manage personnel benefits and maintain records*
- *Perform marketing, financial, and strategic planning*

CLINICAL

Fundamental Principles

- Apply principles of aseptic technique and infection control
- Comply with quality assurance practices
- Screen and follow up patient test results

Diagnostic Orders

- Collect and process specimens
- Perform diagnostic tests

Patient Care

- Adhere to established patient screening procedures
- Obtain patient history and vital signs
- Prepare and maintain examination and treatment areas
- Prepare patient for examinations, procedures and treatments

- Assist with examinations, procedures and treatments
- Prepare and administer medications and immunizations
- Maintain medication and immunization records
- Recognize and respond to emergencies
- Coordinate patient care information with other health care providers
- Initiate IV and administer IV medications with appropriate training and as permitted by state law

GENERAL

Professionalism

- Display a professional manner and image
- Demonstrate initiative and responsibility
- Work as a member of the health care team
- Prioritize and perform multiple tasks
- Adapt to change
- Promote the CMA credential
- Enhance skills through continuing education
- Treat all patients with compassion and empathy
- Promote the practice through positive public relations

Communication Skills

- Recognize and respect cultural diversity
- Adapt communications to individual's ability to understand
- Use professional telephone technique

- Recognize and respond effectively to verbal, nonverbal, and written communications
- Use medical terminology appropriately
- Utilize electronic technology to receive, organize, prioritize and transmit information
- Serve as liaison

Legal Concepts

- Perform within legal and ethical boundaries
- Prepare and maintain medical records
- Document accurately
- Follow employer's established policies dealing with the health care contract
- Implement and maintain federal and state health care legislation and regulations
- Comply with established risk management and safety procedures
- Recognize professional credentialing criteria
- *Develop and maintain personnel, policy and procedure manuals*

Instruction

- Instruct individuals according to their needs
- Explain office policies and procedures
- Teach methods of health promotion and disease prevention
- Locate community resources and disseminate information
- *Develop educational materials*
- *Conduct continuing education activities*

Operational Functions

- Perform inventory of supplies and equipment
- Perform routine maintenance of administrative and clinical equipment
- Apply computer techniques to support office operations
- *Perform personnel management functions*
- *Negotiate leases and prices for equipment and supply contracts*

- *Denotes advanced skills.*

SOURCE: Reprinted by permission of the American Association of Medical Assistants from the AAMA Role Delineation Study: Occupational Analysis of the Medical Assisting Profession.

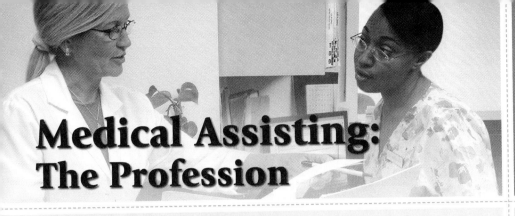

Medical Assisting: The Profession

Learning Objectives

After completing this chapter, you should be able to:

- Define and spell the terms to learn for this chapter.
- Discuss the history of medical assisting as a profession.
- Identify career opportunities available to medical assistants and give examples of areas in which you may choose to work.
- List ten administrative duties of the medical assistant.
- List ten clinical skills medical assistants need to know.
- List qualities usually found in a good medical assistant.
- Discuss the professional organizations that certify medical assistants.

Terms to Learn

accreditation

American Association of Medical Assistants (AAMA)

American Medical Technologists (AMT)

certification

Certified Medical Assistant (CMA)

confidentiality

continuing education units (CEUs)

discretion

empathy

externship

group practice

integrity

Registered Medical Assistant (RMA)

solo practice

Case Study

MARY HAS DECIDED THAT SHE WANTS A CAREER in health care. After researching her options, she enrolled in the medical assistant program at a local community college. Her training includes administrative and clinical skills. Mary finds that she most enjoys her clinical laboratory class. She becomes very skilled in phlebotomy. Once in her externship, she proves to be competent in all required skill areas. Mary works closely with the clinical laboratory personnel. Upon the completion of her externship, the extern site hires her as a laboratory assistant.

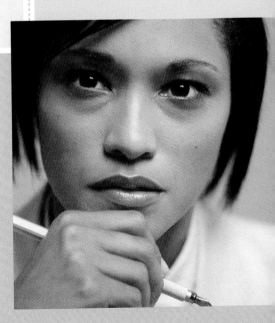

The rapidly changing health care environment has caused health care providers to rely more heavily on assistive personnel. As a result, medical assistants have become an important part the health care team. No matter the setting, these multifunctional team members provide valuable services and support. Medical assistants can be found in a variety of settings from pediatric to chiropractic offices. No matter how varied the roles or duties of the medical assistant (MA), the essential skills and personal qualities needed in all good medical assistants are quite similar.

As a well-trained, multiskilled health care professional, the medical assistant fulfills many roles in the allied health field where the challenges of everyday are balanced by opportunities for advancement, personal growth, and satisfaction. Professional organizations that oversee or regulate the education, training, and certification of medical assistants are also discussed in this chapter along with current career opportunities and the future of the medical assisting field.

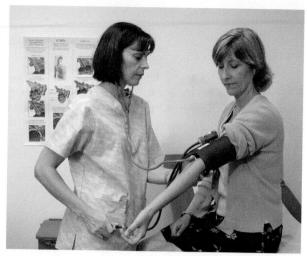

FIGURE 1-1 Medical assistants perform many functions in a physician's office or a clinic.

History of Medical Assisting

Historically, medical assistants were trained on the job by a physician. They became skilled through the day-to-day education and training provided in the medical office. Due to the increasing responsibilities, most clinics staff their offices with individuals who have received some form of formal training. Many physicians had become familiar with the clinical skills of nurses while working closely with nurses in the hospital setting, so they chose to hire registered nurses to work in their offices. When a shortage of nursing personnel occurred, physicians had to look elsewhere for professionally trained office personnel who could handle both the administrative and clinical responsibilities of a medical office practice (Figure 1-1). Patient Education addresses the need to distinguish nurses and medical assistants.

The American Association of Medical Assistants (AAMA), organized in 1956, offers the following definition of medical assisting:

Medical assisting is a multiskilled allied health profession whose practitioners work primarily in ambulatory settings such as medical offices and clinics. Medical assistants function as members of the health care delivery team and perform administrative and clinical procedures.

(From Essentials and Guidelines for an Accredited Educational Program for the Medical Assistant, adopted by the AAMA's Endowment and the American Medical Association in 1969, revised 1971, 1977, 1984, 1991, 1999, and 2003. Copyright by the American Association of Medical Assistants, Inc. Reprinted by permission.)

Education and Training for the Medical Assistant

Over the years, the education and training of medical assistants has undergone many changes and today, medical assistants are well-trained and respected practitioners in the allied health field. Students may obtain a certificate, diploma, or associate degree in the field of medical assisting.

Patient ✕ Education

Patients do not always clearly understand the distinctions among the professions of medical assistant, physician's assistant, and nurse. It is your responsibility to clarify for the patients what you are permitted to do. Do not accept being addressed as "nurse," since the nursing license carries different responsibilities and standards than does the medical assistant's certificate.

- Certificate programs: The length of the course of study varies from one institution to the next. Some programs are six weeks in length, while others may take up to a year to complete. These programs are usually offered in either vocational schools or career colleges. The focus tends to be on the development of clinical skills. Students may choose the traditional classroom setting or may opt for distance learning (online). Most certificate programs require a hands-on externship to complete the program. Depending on the accreditation, graduates of certificate programs may be eligible to sit for a national certification examination. Students who choose this training option may be supplementing prior training or may want an introduction to the health care field.

- Diploma program: These programs tend to be similar to the certificate programs. Most diploma programs are nine months to a year in length. Career and community colleges most often offer this course of study. Training focuses on developing clinical skills, as well as limited administrative skills. Completion of an externship is required and most students qualify to sit for a national certification examination. Students selecting this option may be interested in a career as a medical assistant. Others may want to use this as a stepping stone to other health care careers.

- Degree program: This course of study is approximately two years in length. It is usually offered in a traditional classroom setting at a career or community college. Along with clinical and administrative courses, courses to assist in professional development are offered as part of the curriculum. This option is usually chosen by those who know that they want a career as a medical assistant.

Accreditation

Accreditation is the process in which an institution voluntarily completes an extensive self-study after which an accrediting association visits the school to verify the self-study statements. Accreditation ensures that a school meets an established list of criteria.

Schools may also seek programmatic accreditation for their medical assisting programs. The learning outcomes for these programs are competency based. The U.S. Department of Education recognizes two agencies to accredit programs in medical assisting:

- The Commission on Accreditation of Allied Health Education Programs (CAAHEP)
- The Accrediting Bureau of Health Education Schools (ABHES)

The Joint Review Committee for Ophthalmic Medical Personnel accredits programs in ophthalmic medical assisting.

The CAAHEP Essentials state that to provide for student attainment of "*Entry-Level Competencies for the Medical Assistant,*" the curriculum—"shall include, but is not limited to the following units, modules, and/or courses of instruction:"

- Anatomy and Physiology
- Medical Terminology
- Medical Law and Ethics
- Psychology
- Communication (oral and written)
- Medical Assistant Administrative Procedures
- Medical Assisting Clinical Procedures
- Professional Components
- Externship

An externship experience is required in which students work without payment in a physician's office, clinic, or hospital setting for a specified number of hours over several weeks during the final stage of their training.

Role of the Medical Assistant

The medical assistant's main responsibility is to assist the physician in providing patient care. Central to a medical assistant's responsibilities are sound clinical skills. He or she must be able to obtain vital signs, collect specimens, administer medication, and run basic laboratory tests. It is not unusual to find medical assistants who take x-rays, conduct cardiac stress tests, and assist with minor office surgeries. Administrative duties may be part of the job description. In small clinics or physicians' offices, the medical assistant may function as the receptionist or insurance clerk.

The field of medical assisting is open to both men and women in a variety of work settings such as physicians' offices, ambulatory care clinics, government agencies, extended-care centers, hospitals, urgent care facilities, and free-standing facilities (Figure 1-2).

Responsibilities of the Medical Assistant

The list of responsibilities that medical assistants perform is extensive. For this reason, the education and training for this field is carefully designed and must involve both theory and hands-on experience. The actual duties of the medical assistant vary from office to office. However, a good medical assistant, who has received a well-rounded education, will be able to adjust to different work environments. Never perform

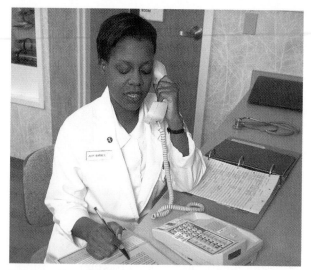

FIGURE 1-2 The medical assisting profession offers many settings in which to pursue your career. Good communication and social skills are required in each of them.

duties that are beyond your level of responsibility—education and training (Legal and Ethical Issues).

Medical assistants' responsibilities will also vary according to the size and type of setting and state laws that apply. Always familiarize yourself with federal and state regulations and guidelines governing the procedures that medical assistants are allowed to perform in whatever environment you work. Generally, the medical assistants' duties are grouped into two categories: administrative and clinical and include the following competencies.

Administrative Competencies—Business and Front Office

- Scheduling patients, including referrals to specialists
- Greeting and receiving patients
- Screening nonpatients and visitors
- Making arrangements for patient admissions to hospitals, patient tests, and procedures such as x-rays and laboratory tests
- Providing patient instruction regarding procedures and tests performed in the physician's office and hospitals
- Updating and filing patient medical records
- Coding diagnoses and procedures for insurance purposes
- Computer skills (Figure 1-3)
- Handling financial arrangements with patients
- Introduction to, or transcribing medical dictation
- Handling the telephone, reports, correspondence, and filing
- Handling mail, billing, insurance claims, credit, and collections
- Operating office equipment
- Preparing and maintaining employee records
- Handling petty cash
- Reconciling bank statements
- Maintaining records for license renewals, membership fees, and insurance premiums

Legal and Ethical Issues

It is important to fully understand what your credentials allow you to do. The medical assistant is uniquely qualified to perform the administrative and clinical procedures associated with responsibilities assigned in the particular setting by the physician. In fulfilling these responsibilities, however, you must always be aware that the potential for psychological, financial, and physical injury to the patient exists. It is your ethical responsibility to patients and your employer that you do your utmost to maintain a high level of skill performance in all that you do. The medical assistant always works as an agent of the physician.

Many of the jobs and careers discussed in this chapter require additional education, including passing a written certification examination. Be mindful that patients understand what your title—Certified Medical Assistant (CMA) or Registered Medical Assistant (RMA)—means. Never be afraid to say, "I am not qualified to do that."

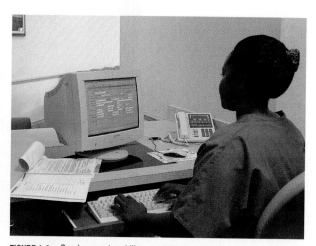

FIGURE 1-3 Good computer skills are now required to be a successful member of an office staff.

- Handling the office in the physician's absence
- Assisting the physician with articles, lectures, and manuscripts
- Utilization review of necessary procedures and referrals
- Coordinating managed-care coverage for patients and physicians
- Ensure compliance with HIPAA guidelines

Clinical Competencies—Care and Treatment of Patients

- Assisting patients in preparation for physical examinations and procedures
- Obtaining a medical history (Figure 1-4)
- Performing routine clinical and laboratory procedures under the supervision of a physician
- Collecting, preparing, and transporting laboratory specimens
- Venipuncture, where permitted
- Assisting the physician with procedures
- Instructing and educating patients on treatments and procedures
- Cleaning and sterilizing equipment
- Obtaining patient's height, weight, and vital signs
- Preparing and maintaining examination and treatment rooms
- Inventory control—ordering and storing of supplies
- Disposing of hazardous waste and other materials
- Administering medications under the supervision and orders of the physician, where permitted
- Changing bandages and dressings, and suture removal, where permitted
- Handling drug refills as directed by the physician
- Performing ECGs
- Occupational Safety and Health Administration (OSHA) guidelines compliance and employee instruction
- Performing skills relevant to a particular practice (for example: audiometry, spirometry, halter monitor)
- Disposing of contaminated supplies
- Sterilizing medical instruments
- Preparing patients for x-rays

Medical assistants who specialize will have additional duties. Some of these specialties include pediatric medical assistants, ophthalmic medical assistants, and surgical medical assistants.

Medical assistants must also meet technical standards such as bending requirements, correct bending

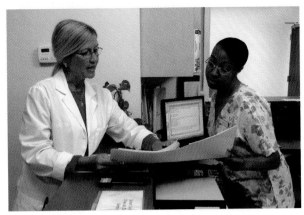

FIGURE 1-4 Helping maintain accurate patient records is a critical part of the medical assistant's work.

procedures, being able to stand for long periods of time, being able to reach overhead, and being able to lift 30 pounds.

Role Delineation

The AAMA analyzed the medical assisting field in 1979 to determine the responsibilities of the medical assistant. As a result of this survey and analysis, the AAMA used a process for developing a curriculum called DACUM (Developing A Curriculum) based on the skills performed daily by medical assistants. The DACUM philosophy is based on the belief that expert workers can describe and define their job more accurately than anyone else. In 1984 and 1990, the DACUM list was revised to reflect the major changes in medicine and the health care delivery system.

The Role Delineation Study released in 1997 and updated in 2003 by the AAMA updates and replaces DACUM. This study is the result of a composite of current competencies essential for medical assistants based upon the practice experience of an expert panel. A Role Delineation Chart, which outlines the study, identifies three major categories of competence—administrative, clinical, and general, or interdisciplinary—for entry-level medical assistants. These areas are further expanded to include competencies that should be taught in medical assisting programs. See the Role Delineation Chart included with each chapter.

Characteristics of a Good Medical Assistant

In addition to having a general medical knowledge, including medical terminology, and being able to perform administrative and clinical responsibilities, medical assistants must genuinely care about others. Cultural Considerations discusses how cultural background and personal beliefs may impact your relationship with patients.

Cultural Considerations

As a medical assistant, you will be exposed to many different cultures. It is important to first examine your culture and your beliefs. Personal beliefs are heavily influenced by cultural background and experience. Make sure that your responsibilities as a medical assistant do not conflict with your personal beliefs. Also, research the types of medical practices in which medical assistants work. For example, some women's health centers perform abortion procedures. Would working in such a facility conflict with your beliefs about abortion? Do you feel that you would treat the patient choosing an abortion the same as you would treat any other patient? Taking the time to examine your cultural background and personal beliefs can help guide you to an area of specialty with the least potential for personal conflict.

The nature of the patient and health care worker relationship demands medical assistants be able to communicate effectively and get along with others. Qualities or characteristic regularly found in good medical assistants are integrity, discretion, empathy, and the ability to safeguard the patient's right to confidentiality (Figure 1-5).

- Integrity—A medical assistant with integrity will do what is expected, when it is expected, for the simple reason that it is expected. Someone with integrity is usually honest, dependable, punctual, and dedicated to high standards.

- Empathy—The ability to work with the sick and the infirm depend on one's ability and willingness to show empathy. A medical assistant with empathy has the ability to be sensitive to or understand the feelings of another individual. An empathic person is able to stand in the shoes of another and identify with what he or she is experiencing. For example, when a medical assistant has some insight or understanding of the pain or distress a patient is feeling, he or she acts in a kindly way that expresses sensitivity to the patient's feelings.

- Discretion—A medical assistant who uses discretion is able to make decisions responsibly. Someone who uses discretion is tactful in communicating with others. It is important to be able to be fair and be familiar with policies and regulations. Discretion is important in patient interaction, as well as interaction with coworkers.

- Confidentiality—The ability to safeguard patient confidences, particularly information in the medical record regarding family history, past or current diseases or illnesses, test results, and medications is vital to the patient and health care professional relationship. No information about the patient is to be disclosed without the written permission of the patient. This is a legal and ethical issue with penalties for violating patient confidentiality. Without this trust, there can be no relationship. As the person with most frequent access to patient records and verbal confidences, the medical assistant has a serious professional responsibility to safeguard the patient's right to confidentiality.

In many cases, the medical assistant will be the first health professional with whom the patient interacts and on whom the patient bases his or her opinion of the physician (Professionalism). It is important to present a confident, professional image that helps put the patient at ease. A calm, pleasant speaking voice conveys a professional attitude. Remember, eating, drinking, or chewing gum while working are not appropriate in areas open to the public. Along with a basic understanding of human behavior and good communication skills—written, spoken, and nonverbal—the medical assistant must be able to handle tasks requiring basic mathematics, grammar, and spelling skills.

Daily habits of good personal hygiene and grooming are expected from the medical assistant. The use of strong perfumes and showy jewelry is not professional and may

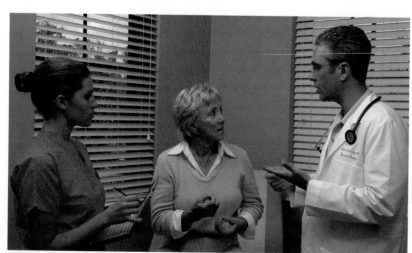

FIGURE 1-5 Medical assistants are often involved in confidential conversations between the physician and the patient.

Professionalism

As the saying goes, "First impressions are lasting impressions." This is important to remember in your daily interactions with others. This starts in the classroom. Take note of how you interact with others. You should not expect to talk to your instructors the same way you talk to your close friends.

As a medical assistant, you will be in contact with the public. How you treat the patients will be a reflection on the physician. If you treat a patient in a less than professional manner, that patient may choose to seek another physician. Health care is a service-oriented field; professional customer service skills are part of the job.

Lifespan
Considerations

Some medical clinics and physicians' offices provide care to patients within a specific age range or stage of life. Pediatric offices treat young children and adolescents. A physician who specializes in gerontology or geriatrics provides care to an elderly population of patients. Each age group is unique in its stage of physical and emotional development. Therefore, each group has different needs and considerations. You cannot expect to communicate with a five-year old patient and a 45-year old patient in the same manner. In your interactions with patients, you must consider their developmental stage and provide age appropriate care and instruction.

even be harmful. For example, strong perfume may actually trigger headaches in some individuals and loose dangling jewelry may get in the way while treating a patient. Loose, long hair and extended nails should be avoided.

Medical assistants provide the quality of care that they would wish to have given to themselves or to members of their own families. The medical assistant must have the ability to see beyond the gruff or complaining manner of the patient who is not feeling well and project a professional, pleasant, and caring attitude. Lifespan Considerations discusses patients at various life stages that medical assistants will encounter.

Professional Organizations

The American Association of Medical Assistants (AAMA), founded in 1959, is a key association in the field of medical assisting. Chicago, Illinois is national headquarters for the AAMA. This organization is responsible for the Certified Medical Assistant (CMA) certification process and offers the certification examination in January, June and in October. Certification indicates that a candidate has met the standards of the AAMA by achieving a satisfactory test result. A certificate, or legal document, is issued to such a person. The first examination given to certify medical assistants was administered in 1963.

The certification examination is offered to graduates of programs accredited by the Commission of Accreditation of Allied Health Education Program (CAAHEP) or by the Accrediting Bureau of Health Education Schools (ABHES). Upon successful completion of the certification examination, candidates will

receive a certificate, confirming them as certified medical assistants (Figure 1-6).

Membership in the AAMA is not necessary to take the certification examination. For the credential to remain current, it must be revalidated every five years, either by earning a designated number of continuing education units (CEUs) or through reexamination. The AAMA sponsors workshops, seminars, and county, state, and national conferences for medical assistants to remain current in their field.

The AAMA accredits medical assisting education/ training programs and has set the minimum standards for the entry-level in this profession. Since the AAMA is so closely allied with the medical assisting profession,

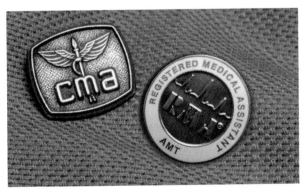

FIGURE 1-6 Becoming a Certified Medical Assistant may demonstrate your commitment to the profession and the continuing education required to maintain the CMA credential.

it is able to monitor the needs and skill education/training of the students. Education programs are periodically reevaluated by the AAMA to assure that the curriculum is adequate and maintained. Recommendations for re-accreditation are then made by the AAMA to the new accrediting agency, Commission on Accreditation of Allied Health Education Program (CAAHEP).

The American Medical Technologists (AMT) association provides oversight for the registration and testing of medical assistants, medical technologists and phlebotomists. This association, in cooperation with the AMT Institute for Education (AMTIE) has developed a continuing education (CE) program and recording system.

The AMT, a nonprofit certifying body, provides a Registered Medical Assistant (RMA) certification examination for medical assistants who meet the eligibility requirements and who can prove their competency to perform entry-level skills through written examination. The RMA is awarded to candidates who pass the AMT certification examination. The RMA certification examination is formed around the following parameters:

 I. General Medical Assisting Knowledge
  a. Anatomy and Physiology
  b. Medical Terminology
  c. Medical Law
  d. Medical Ethics
  e. Human Rights
  f. Patient Education

 II. Administrative Medical Assisting
  a. Insurance
  b. Financial Bookkeeping
  c. Medical Secretarial—Receptionist

 III. Clinical Medical Assisting
  a. Asepsis
  b. Sterilization
  c. Instruments
  d. Vital Signs
  e. Physical Examinations
  f. Clinical Pharmacology
  g. Minor Surgery
  h. Therapeutic Modalities
  i. Laboratory Procedures
  j. Electrocardiography
  k. First Aid

Career Opportunities

According to US Department of Labor Statistics (2003–2004 edition), medical assistants held about 365,000 jobs in 2002. Nearly 60 percent were employed by physicians' offices; 14 percent held positions in public and private hospitals; and almost 10 percent worked in the offices of other health care practitioners.

The medical assistant is the most frequently employed allied health professional in the physician's office and most physicians have more than one medical assistant working in their office. The US Bureau of Labor Statistics projects medical assisting to be the fastest growing occupation over the 2002–2012 period. (Bureau of Labor Statistics, US Department of Labor: Employment by Occupation and Industry, 2004, Washington, DC, US Government Printing Office.)

The anticipated need for more health professionals is based on the expected increase in the number of older adults who will require the care of a physician and the tremendous growth in the number of outpatient facilities. The wide range of health care settings presents many opportunities for the medical assistant who is trained in both clinical and administrative duties. Table 1-1 lists several inpatient and ambulatory care (outpatient) facilities or settings with descriptions of some possible job opportunities for medical assistants in each setting. Table 1-2 lists departments or specialties in which medical assistants may seek employment in either inpatient or ambulatory care settings. In some states and settings, additional education and training may be required for medical assistants to fulfill certain responsibilities. While the general category, "medical assistant," may be used in some career ads, some of the jobs title opportunities may include:

- Clinic aide
- Data processing clerk
- Billing or collection assistant
- Insurance claims coder
- Medical records clerk
- Clinical assistant
- Medical receptionist
- Multifunctional technician

With Additional Education and Credentials, You May Even Respond to Ads For:

- A medical laboratory assistant
- An electrocardiography (ECG) technician
- A phlebotomist

Experienced medical assistants may find work as office managers, medical records managers, hospital ward clerks, and teachers of medical assistants. With additional schooling, medical assistants can enter other health care occupations such as nursing, occupational therapy, physical therapy, medical and x-ray technologists.

Since your education and training includes general, administrative, and clinical skills, you can seek employment in many different types of work. Then, too, you may work for a physician who practices alone in a solo practice or one who participates in a group practice with other physicians. If you choose to work for a

TABLE 1-1   Job Opportunities for Medical Assistants in Inpatient and Ambulatory Care Settings

Inpatient Setting	Description of Job
Rehabilitation facility	Perform both clinical and administrative tasks in medical setting focused on rehabilitation and physical therapy.
Extended care center	Work with patients who require a protective environment.
Hospital	Perform both clinical and administrative tasks as a member of the health care team.
Nursing home	Perform clinical and administrative tasks working with older adult patients.
Ambulatory Care Setting	**Description of Job**
Clinic	Use clinical and administrative skills to schedule and assist with patients who require special medical attention (for example, eye clinic, orthopedic clinic, mental health clinic).
Free-standing facility	Care for patients who require immediate medical treatment.
Physician's office	Use clinical and administrative skills in the private office setting for physicians of all specialties.
Rehabilitation center	Provide care for patients recovering from illness or injury.

physician, he or she may specialize in an area of medicine such as family practice, internal medicine, pediatrics, surgery, gerontology, psychiatry, obstetrics and gynecology, sports medicine, or dermatology, just to name a few. According to the US Department of Labor Statistics (2003–2004 edition), "job prospects should be best for medical assistants with formal training or experience, particularly those with certification."

TABLE 1-2   Job Opportunities for Medical Assistants in Healthcare Departments and Specialties

Department/Specialty	Description of Job
Admissions	Handle pre-admission interviews, schedule laboratory testing, and document insurance coverage.
Billing and Insurance	Work with patients, third-party payers, insurance companies to process insurance forms, claims forms, and DRG, ICD9, CPT, and HCPC coding.
EKG/ECG Tech	Perform electrocardiogram studies on patients.
Medical Records	Use administrative skills of transcription, medical terminology, and insurance coding. Requires use of the computer.
Phlebotomy	Use clinical skills to draw blood samples for testing and blood bank use.
Surgery	Use clinical skills to sterilize surgical instruments and set up surgical trays, and assist when needed.
Treatment/Procedure/Emergency Room (ER)	Assist with minor surgeries and procedures performed in physicians' offices, hospitals, rehabilitation centers, and emergency rooms (ER).

SUMMARY

The field of medical assisting is growing in response to increasing health care needs of consumers. The profession of medical assistant offers many opportunities—roles, responsibilities, and settings for employment. Most medical assistants work in ambulatory settings such as physicians' offices where they fulfill the administrative and clinical responsibilities associated with running medical offices. The size and nature of the medical office practice will determine the number of medical assistants and the actual work they will do.

Caring individuals, who are dedicated professionals with a commitment to maintain their skills through continuing education, make the best medical assistants. The important thing to remember is the opportunities presented are many and the future of medical assisting looks attractive. A career in medical assisting is emotionally and professionally challenging.

Chapter Review

COMPETENCY REVIEW

1. Define and spell the terms to learn for this chapter.
2. List several health care facilities or specialties to work at as a medical assistant.
3. Explain the difference between administrative and clinical functions of medical assisting.
4. Name a medical assistant's professional organization.
5. What qualities are regularly found in good medical assistants?
6. Explain what the curriculum in medical assisting should include.
7. List the job titles for which a medical assistant may qualify.
8. List the educational options available to one who is interested in medical assisting.

PREPARING FOR THE CERTIFICATION EXAM

1. What is the AAMA?
   A. All American Medical Association
   B. Allied American Medical Association
   C. Administrative (division) of the American Medical Association
   D. American Association of Medical Assistants
   E. American Association of Medical Assistance

2. What are two general categories that BEST describe the responsibilities of a medical assistant?
   A. administrative and laboratory
   B. secretarial and direct patient care
   C. assisting the physician and secretarial
   D. clinical and secretarial
   E. administrative and clinical

3. Which of following is NOT a category of the AAMA Role Delineation Chart?
   A. administrative
   B. clinical
   C. professional
   D. transdisciplinary
   E. instruction

4. Which administrative tasks falls beyond the scope of practice for a medical assistant?
   A. coordinating managed care coverage
   B. handling petty cash
   C. assisting the physician with a journal article
   D. utilization review of necessary procedures
   E. posting patient information on the Internet

5. Which of the following clinical tasks falls beyond the scope of practice for a medical assistant?
   A. vital signs
   B. patient education
   C. phlebotomy
   D. handling drug refills
   E. prescribing medications

6. How many total CEUs over what period of time must a CMA obtain to remain certified?
   A. 15 CEUs over 2 years
   B. 30 CEUs over 5 years
   C. 60 CEUs over 5 years
   D. 45 CEUs over 3 years
   E. 50 CEUs over 5 years

continued on next page

7. Which of the following statements is TRUE?
   A. a MA is equivalent to a nurse
   B. a MA is equivalent to a physician assistant
   C. it is acceptable for patients to refer to a medical assistant as a "nurse"
   D. an advertisement for a medical assistant might include "medical records clerk"
   E. an advertisement for a medical assistant might include "x-ray technician"

8. As per the CAAHEP Essentials, at a minimum, the curriculum of a medical assisting school does NOT include
   A. medical assistant administrative procedures
   B. medical assistant clinical procedures
   C. medical law and ethics
   D. externship of 160 to 190 hours
   E. medical nurse training

9. Necessary characteristics of a good medical assistant should include all EXCEPT
   A. confidentiality
   B. discretion
   C. empathy
   D. integrity
   E. physical attractiveness

10. Which of the following statements is TRUE?
    A. MAs work only in physicians' offices
    B. all MA programs are diploma programs
    C. medical assistants may work as ECG technicians, with additional training
    D. MAs do not work in hospitals
    E. MAs do not need good communication skills

CRITICAL THINKING

1. Mary decides to further her health care career. What additional training will fit her interests?

2. Because Mary wants a career and not just a job as a medical assistant, what level of education might best support her goals?

3. Mary sits for the AAMA Certification Examination. What are the benefits of certification?

ON THE JOB

Darlene Smith, a CMA, has been employed six years by a Cardiology practice of three physicians. She is a graduate of a CAAHEP accredited school. Furthermore, Darlene received extensive hands-on training performing ECGs while doing her required externship.

Darlene has completed an ECG ordered by Dr. Patel for Mrs. Warner, a 76-year old patient. Dr. Patel, Darlene's boss, has telephoned her explaining that he was behind schedule doing rounds at the hospital. He asked her to do him a favor and interpret Mrs. Warner's ECG, sign his name and fax the report to Mrs. Warner's referring internist who is expecting the results.

1. Given the scope of Darlene's education, training, and years of experience as a CMA, would this "favor" fall within the AAMA guidelines of her responsibilities?

2. Would any portion of Dr. Patel's request fall within the guidelines, if so, which portion(s)? Is there ever a case for an exception to these guidelines?

3. What, if anything, should Darlene say to Dr. Patel?

INTERNET ACTIVITY

Conduct an Internet search for local medical assistant positions. How many positions require certification? What are other job titles a medical assistant would be qualified to take?

 MediaLink More on the profession of medical assisting, including interactive resources, can be found on the Student CD-ROM accompanying this textbook.

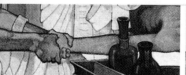

Medical Assistant Role Delineation Chart

HIGHLIGHT *indicates material covered in this chapter.*

ADMINISTRATIVE

Administrative Procedures

- Perform basic administrative medical assisting functions
- Schedule, coordinate and monitor appointments
- Schedule inpatient/outpatient admissions and procedures
- Understand and apply third-party guidelines
- Obtain reimbursement through accurate claims submission
- Monitor third-party reimbursement
- Understand and adhere to managed care policies and procedures
- *Negotiate managed care contracts*

Practice Finances

- Perform procedural and diagnostic coding
- Apply bookkeeping principles

- Manage accounts receivable
- *Manage accounts payable*
- *Process payroll*
- *Document and maintain accounting and banking records*
- *Develop and maintain fee schedules*
- *Manage renewals of business and professional insurance policies*
- *Manage personnel benefits and maintain records*
- *Perform marketing, financial, and strategic planning*

CLINICAL

Fundamental Principles

- Apply principles of aseptic technique and infection control
- Comply with quality assurance practices
- Screen and follow up patient test results

Diagnostic Orders

- Collect and process specimens
- Perform diagnostic tests

Patient Care

- Adhere to established patient screening procedures
- Obtain patient history and vital signs
- Prepare and maintain examination and treatment areas
- Prepare patient for examinations, procedures and treatments

- Assist with examinations, procedures and treatments
- Prepare and administer medications and immunizations
- Maintain medication and immunization records
- Recognize and respond to emergencies
- Coordinate patient care information with other health care providers
- Initiate IV and administer IV medications with appropriate training and as permitted by state law

GENERAL

Professionalism

- Display a professional manner and image
- Demonstrate initiative and responsibility
- Work as a member of the health care team
- Prioritize and perform multiple tasks
- Adapt to change
- Promote the CMA credential
- Enhance skills through continuing education
- Treat all patients with compassion and empathy
- Promote the practice through positive public relations

Communication Skills

- Recognize and respect cultural diversity
- Adapt communications to individual's ability to understand
- Use professional telephone technique

- Recognize and respond effectively to verbal, nonverbal, and written communications
- Use medical terminology appropriately
- Utilize electronic technology to receive, organize, prioritize and transmit information
- Serve as liaison

Legal Concepts

- Perform within legal and ethical boundaries
- Prepare and maintain medical records
- Document accurately
- Follow employer's established policies dealing with the health care contract
- Implement and maintain federal and state health care legislation and regulations
- Comply with established risk management and safety procedures
- Recognize professional credentialing criteria
- *Develop and maintain personnel, policy and procedure manuals*

Instruction

- Instruct individuals according to their needs
- Explain office policies and procedures
- Teach methods of health promotion and disease prevention
- Locate community resources and disseminate information
- *Develop educational materials*
- *Conduct continuing education activities*

Operational Functions

- Perform inventory of supplies and equipment
- Perform routine maintenance of administrative and clinical equipment
- Apply computer techniques to support office operations
- *Perform personnel management functions*
- *Negotiate leases and prices for equipment and supply contracts*

- *Denotes advanced skills.*

SOURCE: Reprinted by permission of the American Association of Medical Assistants from the AAMA Role Delineation Study: Occupational Analysis of the Medical Assisting Profession.

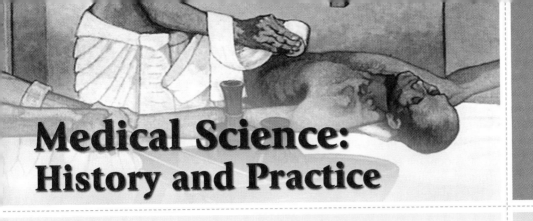

chapter 2

Medical Science: History and Practice

Learning Objectives

After completing this chapter, you should be able to:

- Define and spell the terms to learn for this chapter.

- Identify the major achievements during each of these periods: early medicine, 18th century, 19th century, 20th century, and modern medicine.

- Name three women and explain the contributions they made to medicine.

- Describe the difference between an internship and a residency in the training of physicians.

- State which type of medical practice is addressed under the medical and surgical specialties.

- Discuss ten allied health fields and the educational requirements for each of them.

- Discuss the current trends in health care that are driving changes in medical practice.

Terms to Learn

acquired immune deficiency syndrome (AIDS)

anesthesia

anthrax

bacteria

cadaver

caduceus

Diagnostic Related Groups (DRGs)

hospice

immunology

licensure

medical privilege

microbe

microorganism

morbidity rate

osteopath

pandemic

pasteurization

registration

stem cell

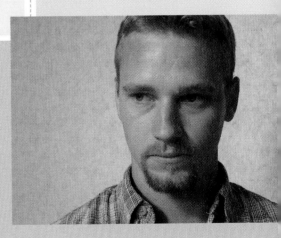

Case Study

ELIZABETH IS A MEDICAL ASSISTANT WHO HAS WORKED in a HMO in California for 6 years. One of her duties is to facilitate the provision of care as HMO subscribers transition from one type of patient care environment to another.

Elizabeth has been working with the family of a 22-year old man who is to be discharged from the hospital following acute care for depression and drug and alcohol abuse. The patient has a history of progressively worsening reactive violence and depression. He is unable to live on his own and care for himself at this time.

In addition, the family is afraid of him and do not want to assume responsibility for his care. The primary physician, medical social worker, and clinical psychologist assigned to his case recommended that he be placed in a suitable long-term care facility.

The healing art of medicine was taught and practiced before humans kept written records. This chapter describes the science and practice of medicine from the earliest evidence of healing when disease was considered to be of supernatural origin or the field of demons to the present—a time of astounding research, discovery, and healing. Contributions of many ancient peoples still influence medicine today. The discussion of present day medical codes of ethics, rules about sanitation, personal hygiene, herbal cures, acupuncture, and other medical and surgical practices highlights the specific contributions of ancient peoples and the men and women whose accomplishments catapulted the science of medicine along in leaps and bounds.

This chapter provides a picture of today's medical practitioners—issues of licensure, including evaluations, credentials, reciprocity, renewals, suspensions, and doctor's titles. In addition, current trends in health care, health care costs, types of practices, medical and surgical specialties, and roles and educational requirements of a variety of health care team members are covered.

History of Medicine

Drawings, bony remains, and some surgical tools are evidence of early human attempts to practice medicine. Folk medicine, using plants, adopted a trial-and-error method to determine which plants were poisonous and which had medicinal value. Early humans attributed supernatural origins to some ailments. In early medicine,

some diseases were considered the work of a demon, evil spirit, or an offended god who had placed some object, such as a worm, into the body of the patient. Treatment consisted of trying to remove the evil intruder.

The first doctors, "medicine men," were shaman, witch doctors, or sorcerers (Figure 2-1). In 3000 BC, Babylonian physicians practiced using the written "Code of Hammurabi." This code, named after Hammurabi, an early king of Babylon, has laws relating to the practice of medicine, which included severe penalties for errors. For example, according to the Code, a doctor who killed a patient while opening an abscess, would have his hands cut off.

Contributions of Ancient Civilizations

A study of medical practice in early Egypt offers greater insight into the basis of modern medicine. The Egyptians left behind lists of remedies, surgical treatments of wounds and injuries, and records for rules of sanitation. Personal hygiene, the sanitary preparation of food, and other matters of public health were pioneered by the practices of the Jewish religion. Other cultures contributed to moving the practice forward.

The early Greeks have records of using nonpoisonous snakes to treat the wounds of patients. The caduceus (Figure 2-2), which has become the recognized symbol for medicine, depicts a healing staff with two snakes coiled around the staff.

Herbal medical remedies from ancient India are recorded from 800 BC. The Chinese culture wrote about human blood pulses around the time of 250 BC. Early Japanese and Chinese cultures practiced acupuncture successfully.

Ancient Cures Are Today's Legacy

Early medicine, while often based on superstition, actually provided medicinal remedies that are still used today. The effect of opium produced by the poppy plant was known in ancient times and even now is used in the medication morphine to relieve severe pain. Other remedies include using:

- Nitroglycerin to treat heart patients
- Digitalis from the foxglove plant to regulate and strengthen the heartbeat
- Sulfur and cayenne pepper to stop bleeding
- Chamomile and licorice to aid digestion
- Cranberry to treat urinary tract infections

Early Medicine

Early medicine began with Hippocrates and the shift from the belief in magical sources of illness and disease to more scientific study, which looked to physical causes of disease. The medieval period from the 5th century to the 16th century was a time of little or no progress in

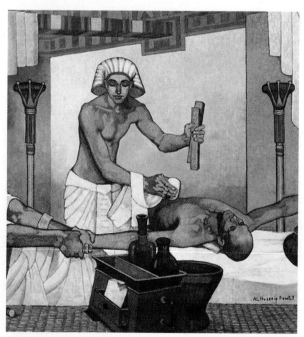

FIGURE 2-1 An early physician.

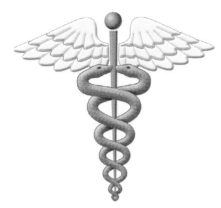

FIGURE 2-2 Caduceus, the emblem of the medical profession.

medical practices. The lack of sanitation, poor personal hygiene, and poor nutrition led to many epidemics. An epidemic is a disease, which infects a large part of a population in one region or location at the same time. The bubonic plague was a pandemic because it affected many people in different countries at the same time. It was known as the "black plague" or "black death" because the corpses appeared dark due to hemorrhage under the skin. Death was extensive in China, India, Europe, Russia, Egypt, and North Africa. The cause of bubonic plague was not discovered until 1905. It was determined then that it was bacteria which grew in the fleas of infected rats. Bacteria are microorganisms, some of which are capable of causing disease. Microorganisms are minute living organisms.

During the medieval period, medical teaching was mostly oral. Surgeons, at the time, only treated the wealthy. Other patients had to rely on the local barber to perform surgical procedures. The red and white stripe pole we are familiar with today was the sign that barbers used—a white pole wrapped with bloody bandages to solicit business. This period concludes with the introduction of the microscope and the ability to see and measure bacteria previously not observed with the naked eye.

Hippocrates (Father of Medicine)

Historically, the first scientific system of medicine is of Greek origin and is usually associated with Hippocrates (460–377 BC) who has become known as the "Father of Medicine." Hippocrates shifted medicine from the realm of mysticism and into the area of scientific practice. He stressed the body's healing nature, clinical descriptions of diseases, and the ability to discover some diseases by listening to the chest. He practiced medicine at a time in history when little was known about anatomy and physiology. Nevertheless, his writings and descriptions of symptoms remain accurate today.

The Hippocratic Oath (Box 2-1) is part of the writings of this fifth century BC physician. The oath serves as a widely used ethical guide for physicians who pledge to work for the good of the patient, to do him or her no harm, to prescribe no deadly drugs, to give no advice that could cause death, and to keep confidential medical information regarding the patient. The oath is still often administered as part of graduation ceremonies in medical schools.

Galen

Galen (130–201 AD), a Greek physician who practiced in Rome, initially followed the Hippocratic method. He stressed the value of anatomy and founded experimental physiology. He stated that arteries contained blood and not air as previously believed. Since the dissection of humans was illegal during Galen's time, he based his theories on the examination of pigs and apes. While some of his work is inaccurate due to the lack of human cadavers, or dead bodies from which to study the human anatomy, he is still known as the "Prince of Physicians."

William Harvey

In England during the 17th century, William Harvey (1578–1657) began writing on the topic of blood circulation and using the experimental method in medicine. Unfortunately for Harvey, the microscope had not yet been invented and he was never able to view capillaries.

Galileo

Galileo (1564–1642) was the first to use a telescope to study the skies. Applications of the telescope lens led to the invention of the microscope. Zacharias Janssen in Holland was an eyeglass maker who invented the microscope.

Anton van Leeuwenhoek

Anton van Leeuwenhoek (1632–1723), also in Holland, devoted his life to microscopic studies. He is known as the first person to observe and describe bacteria, which he referred to as "tiny little beasties." He is also responsible for describing spermatozoa (mature male sex cells) and protozoa. Protozoa are the simplest forms—usually one cell—of animals.

Medicine During the 18th Century

In England, formal medical training began when it was required that anyone wishing to become a doctor must first become an apprentice. Medical schools in Edinburgh and Glasgow, Scotland were developed during this era.

John Hunter

John Hunter (1728–1793) developed surgery and surgical pathology into a science. He is noted as the "Founder of Scientific Surgery." Some of his contributions to medical science include the introduction of a flexible feeding tube into the stomach. The term "surgeon" comes from the Greek word "cheir," which means hand, and "ergeon," which means work.

The Hippocratic Oath

I swear by Apollo Physician, by Asclepias, by Health, by Heal All, and by all the gods and goddesses, that according to my ability and judgment, I will keep this oath and stipulation; to reckon him who taught me this art equally dear to me as my parents, and share my substance with him and relieve his necessities if required. To regard his offspring as on the same footing with my own brothers and to teach them this art if they should wish to learn it, without fee or stipulation; and that by precept, lecture, and every other mode of instruction I will impart a knowledge of my art to my own sons and to those of my teachers and to disciples bound by a stipulation and oath according to the law of medicine, but to none others.

I will follow that method of treatment which according to my ability and judgment, I consider for the benefit of my patients, and abstain from whatever is deleterious and mischievous. I will give not deadly medicine to anyone if asked, nor suggest any counsel.

Furthermore, I will not give to a woman an instrument to produce an abortion.

With Purity and with Holiness, I will pass my life and practice my art. I will not cut a person who is suffering with a stone, but will leave this to the practitioners of this work. Into whatever houses I enter I will go into them for the benefit of the sick and will abstain from every voluntary act of mischief and corruption; and further from the seduction of females or males, bond or free.

Whatever, in connection with my professional practice, or not in connection with it, I may see or hear in the lives of men which ought not to be spoken abroad, I will not divulge, as reckoning that all such should be kept secret.

While I continue to keep this oath inviolated, may it be granted to me to enjoy life and practice the art respected by all men, at all times, but should I trespass and violate this oath, may the reverse be my lot.

Edward Jenner

Public health and hygiene began to attract attention during the 18th century. A country doctor, Edward Jenner (1749–1823), a pupil of John Hunter, observed that dairy maids who had become infected with the disease cowpox would not become infected with the deadly disease smallpox. Jenner overcame ridicule from the medical community and went on to perform the first vaccination using the smallpox vaccine.

The term vaccination comes from the Latin term "vacca" meaning cow. Cowpox was referred to as "vaccinia." Today the term vaccine means to give live or attenuated material to a person to establish resistance to disease. Vaccines come from animals other than cows today and from synthetic sources.

Rene Laennec

Another major advancement in medicine was made by Rene Laennec (1781–1826), who invented the stethoscope. His invention (Figure 2-3) was based on the use of paper wrapped into a cone shape, which was then placed over the patient's chest to listen to the heart.

Benjamin Franklin

The American statesman, Benjamin Franklin (1706–1790), was an inventor and, in addition to inventing bifocals, one of his important contributions to medical science was the discovery that colds could be passed from one person to another.

Medicine During the 19th Century

During the 19th century, the practice of medicine advanced rapidly. The documentation of accurate anatomy and physiology allowed physicians to better understand the human body. The use of sophisticated

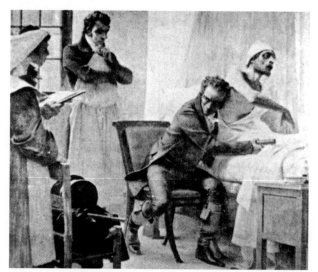

FIGURE 2-3 Rene Laennec and the stethoscope.

microscopes, injection materials, and instruments such as the ophthalmoscope all moved the practice of medicine forward.

The discovery of the cell was one of the most enlightening discoveries of this era. Many believe that the greatest achievement of the 19th century was the knowledge that certain diseases, as well as surgical wound infections, were directly caused by microorganisms. The practice of surgery changed as a result of this knowledge along with advances in the use of anesthetics.

Louis Pasteur

Louis Pasteur (1822–1895) is credited for establishing the science of bacteriology (Figure 2-4). His experiments proved that putrefaction or decay was caused by living organisms known as bacteria. His work solved many medical problems during his day including rabies, anthrax in sheep and cattle, and chicken cholera. Anthrax is a deadly infectious disease caused by *Bacillus anthracisis*. Humans can contract the disease from infected animal hair, hides, or waste. Cholera, an acute infection of the small bowel causing severe diarrhea, was determined to be a bacillus transmitted through water, milk, or food contaminated with excreta of carriers. The process of pasteurization is named after Pasteur. Pasteurization is the process during which substances, such as milk and cheese, are heated to a certain temperature to eliminate bacteria.

Joseph Lister

Joseph Lister (1827–1912) borrowed Pasteur's theories and eventually introduced the antiseptic system in surgery (Figure 2-4). Until that time, surgeons and obstetricians did not wash their hands between patients. Disease was being spread from one patient to another. Lister advised placing an antiseptic barrier between the wound and the germ-containing atmosphere. Present day aseptic techniques can be attributed to Lister's work.

Ignaz Semmelweiss

Ignaz Semmelweiss (1818–1865), an obstetrician in Vienna, advised medical students to disinfect the hands and clothing of anyone who attended a birth. During the early practice of obstetrics, a physician would wear the same "butcher's coat" for all deliveries in the hospital. Figure 2-5 shows a Cesarean section. There was a high death rate from puerperal sepsis or childbed fever. Women avoided having a baby in the hospital because of the high mortality rate or death rate. Eventually, the use of contaminated clothing and contaminated hands were traced to the spread of puerperal sepsis thanks to Dr. Semmelweiss. The term puerperal comes from the Latin word "puer" meaning child and "pario" meaning to bring forth. The term puerperium is now used to denote a period of time after a delivery.

Semmelweiss noted that the medical students would attend a mother in childbirth immediately after having

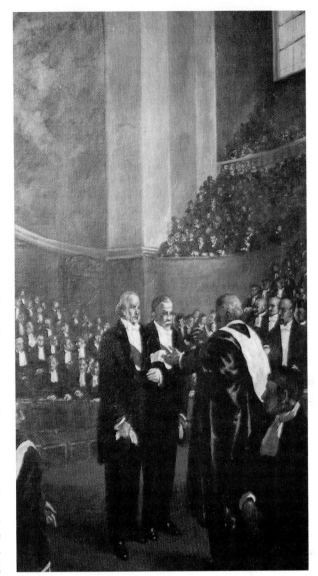

FIGURE 2-4 Louis Pasteur and Joseph Lister.

participated in an autopsy. An autopsy is an examination of the organs and tissues of a deceased body to determine the cause of death. After he advised students to disinfect their hands before attending childbirth, the incidence of disease went down dramatically. In the 1800s, the men who advocated disinfection were ridiculed and in Semmelweiss' case considered insane.

Robert Koch

Robert Koch (1843–1910) showed how bacteria could be cultivated and stained. He discovered the tubercle bacillus, the cause of tuberculosis. His investigation into the cause of cholera led to knowledge that contaminated food and water can cause disease.

Paul Ehrlich

Paul Ehrlich (1854–1915) was a pioneer in the study of microbiology. He was a pioneer in the fields of immunology, bacteriology, and the use of chemotherapy.

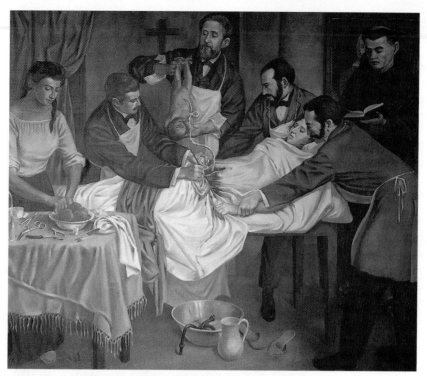

FIGURE 2-5 A cesarean section from an old medicine text book.

partial or complete sensation. An anesthetic is a substance used to produce anesthesia. These two men worked independently of each other and made possible life-saving operations that previously could not be performed without anesthetics.

WALTER REED Walter Reed (1851–1902) and others helped to conquer yellow fever, which allowed for completion of the Panama Canal by reducing the death rate for the workers. Dr. Reed gathered volunteers who allowed him to inject them with yellow fever in order to find a cure.

Medicine During the 20th Century

The first half of the 20th century resulted in major medical advances. Death rates from diseases such as tuberculosis and diphtheria dropped dramatically. The overall mortality rates decreased due to improved medical care and new emphasis was placed on morbidity rates (rates of disease and illness). Four major developments dominate this period:

- The development of chemotherapy and the specialty of oncology
- The development of immunology
- Progress in endocrinology
- Progress in nutrition

Alexander Fleming

One of the most dramatic episodes of the modern era was the discovery of antibiotics. Sir Alexander Fleming (1881–1955) accidentally discovered that a stray mold on his culture plate of staphylococci would cause the bacteria to stop growing. He called this mold Penicillium and it has became known throughout the world as penicillin. Fleming's discovery took place in 1928. He, along with two other scientists, won the Nobel Prize for their work with penicillin. The use of penicillin was one of the first examples of using chemicals to treat infections. Today, the term chemotherapy generally refers to drugs used to treat forms of cancer.

Jonas Salk and Albert Sabin

The study of immunology advanced with the discovery of vaccines against typhoid, tetanus, diphtheria, tuberculosis, yellow fever, influenza, and measles. During the 1950s, Doctors Jonas Salk (1914–1996) and

Immunology is the study of immunity, the resistance to or protection from disease. Chemotherapy is the use of chemicals including drugs to treat or control infections and disease. He developed a method for staining bacteria and cells, which eventually, led to a means for providing a differential diagnosis based on classifying organisms. He was one of the original "microbe hunters." Microbes are one-celled forms of life such as bacteria. His greatest achievement was the discovery, on his 606th attempt, of the "magic bullet" to treat syphilis. Syphilis is an infectious chronic venereal disease.

Other Major Advances During This Period

William Roentgen (1845–1923) discovered x-rays, Pierre (1859–1906) and Marie (1867–1934) Curie discovered radium, and Sigmund Freud (1856–1939) worked in the field of psychiatry.

American Medicine During This Period

Significant contributions were made to medicine through the work of William Norton, Crawford Long, and Walter Reed. The specific work of each of these individuals is highlighted here.

WILLIAM MORTON AND CRAWFORD LONG An important American contribution to the practice of medicine during this period was the discovery of anesthesia. William Morton (1819–1868), a dentist at Massachusetts General Hospital, and Crawford Long (1815–1878), a Georgia physician, are generally credited with having first demonstrated the use of ether as a general anesthetic. Anesthesia refers to the absence of

Albert Sabin (1906–1993) developed vaccines, which eradicated the crippling disease polio.

Women in Medicine

Few women were allowed to practice medicine in the early years. In part, this was due to social constraints on women appearing in public. However, many women did practice as midwives and became skilled at delivering babies. There are also some remarkable female physicians and nurses who overcame great odds to practice in their profession.

Elizabeth Blackwell

Elizabeth Blackwell (1821–1910) was the first female physician in the United States. After being turned down by several medical schools, she was finally awarded a degree in 1849 in New York. She went on to open a medical college for women and her own dispensary.

Florence Nightingale

Florence Nightingale (1820–1910) is considered the founder of modern nursing (Figure 2-6). She studied nursing in Europe and cared for wounded soldiers during the Crimean War (1850–1853). Nightingale and her fellow nurses were treated poorly by the doctors at that time.

Nightingale's attention to detail, record keeping, and compassionate nursing care changed the way nursing was practiced. She advocated the use of the nursing process and elevated nursing to an honored profession. She is referred to as "The Lady with the Lamp" due to her tireless work night and day to supervise the nursing care of wounded soldiers. She started the first school of nursing in 1860 at St. Thomas Hospital in London.

Clara Barton

Clara Barton (1821–1912) was a contemporary of Florence Nightingale, but nursed soldiers in a different war, the Civil War in the United States. She established the American Red Cross when she became aware of the need for support services for the soldiers (Figures 2-7 and 2-8). She also established the Federal Bureau of Records to help track injured and dead soldiers.

Modern Medicine and the Future

In the last 25 years, technological discoveries have permitted medical science to advance faster than in the previous one hundred years. There is the potential for greater advances in the 21st century. The average life span of ancient humans was 30 years. According to the U.S. Census Bureau (2001), a person born in 1900 had the life expectancy of 47 years and someone born in 1991 had the life expectancy of 76 years. With rapid

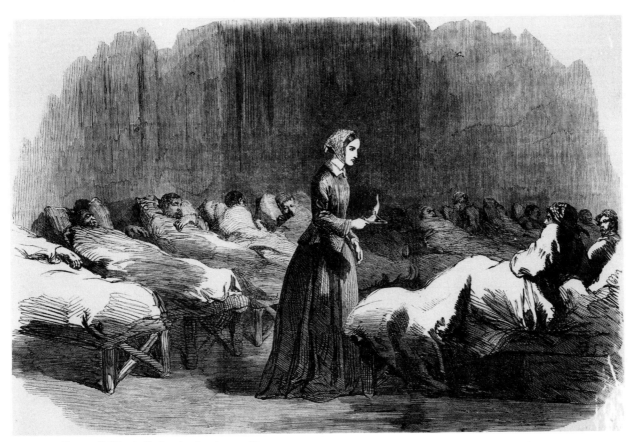

FIGURE 2-6 Florence Nightingale, the founder of modern nursing.

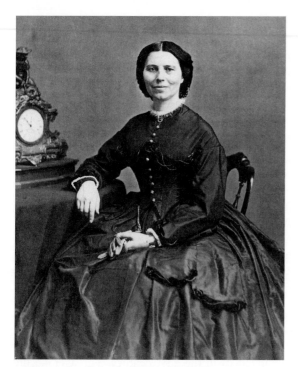

FIGURE 2-7 Clara Barton, the founder of the Red Cross.

undetectable in some people. Treatment of pregnant woman with AZT and a combination of other drugs has greatly reduced the number of HIV-positive babies. Hopefully, a cure for HIV and better treatments for AIDS will be forthcoming.

Other breakthroughs include genetic engineering during the 1980s, which permitted greater production of vaccines, the birth of the first test-tube baby in England in 1978, and the cloning of the first sheep in 1997.

Medical Frontier

The human genome project, a publicly funded international research project to sequence and identify human genes and record their positions on chromosomes, was completed in 2001. Information from the project, enables doctors to routinely screen donor eggs for many inherited diseases. Mapping human genes has

medical advancements, some estimate a life expectancy of 100 years will not be impossible.

Improved communication techniques now allow patients' results to be examined by physicians across the country. Robotics is being used in surgery. It is considered routine to successfully replace knees, hips, kidneys, and cornea. One can barely imagine the future of medical science in the 21st century.

Medical Firsts

In 1954, doctors at Brigham Hospital in Boston performed the first successful kidney transplant. In earlier attempts, patients died because physicians did not know that organs had to be compatible to have the transplant succeed. In this successful transplant, an organ was used from the patient's twin.

Dr. Michael DeBakey invented the heart pump in 1960, which made open-heart surgery possible for millions. In 1962, doctors in Boston successfully reattached the severed arm on a young boy. In 1967, Dr. Christian Barnard completed the first heart transplant. A totally implantable heart was placed in the chest of several critically ill patients in 2001.

The discovery of the human immunodeficiency virus (HIV) as the cause of AIDS in 1984 was a major breakthrough in understanding AIDS or acquired immune deficiency syndrome. AIDS is a series of illnesses that occur as a result of infection by HIV, which causes the immune system to break down. Although there is as yet no cure for AIDS, a combination of drugs has stopped HIV replication to the extent that the virus is

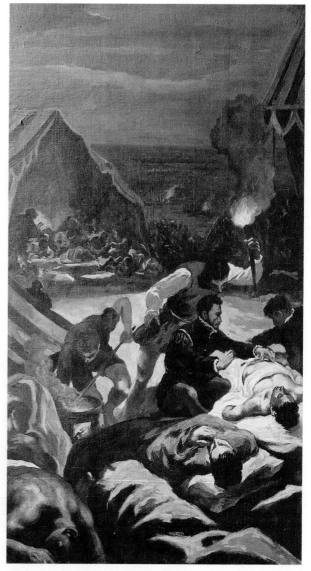

FIGURE 2-8 Healing wounded on the battlefield.

allowed for DNA testing to identify criminals, provide genetic counseling for prospective parents, and design treatments for diseases. With identification of the gene that causes Alzheimer's disease, certain types of breast cancer, and cystic fibrosis, better treatments and potential cures may be possible.

Stem cell research will play an important part in medical science in the next 20 years and beyond. A stem cell is an undifferentiated cell that can give rise to other cells of the same type or from which specialized cells can develop. Stem cell research is already being used to induce cells in the diseased pancreas of a diabetic to produce insulin.

Hopes for the future include the following:

- A cure for AIDS
- A vaccine to prevent HIV
- Cloning organs to overcome the shortage of donors
- Better treatment and outcomes for mental illness
- A cure for heart disease, cancer, and obesity
- Methods to slow aging
- Regeneration of brain and nerve cells to overcome paralysis
- Development of antibiotics that do not allow bacteria to develop a resistant strain

Medical Practitioners

The medical assistance training and skills that you receive, enable you to work for physicians who practice in a variety of specializations. You may need additional on-the-job training to work for a specialized physician, but your basic training is sufficient to apply for these positions (Preparing for Externship). As medical assistants working for physicians in a variety of specialties and different types of practices, you will encounter many allied health professionals from a wide range of fields. It is important that you understand and respect the role and educational requirements of others.

In this section, we will discuss the different types of credentials for those practicing medicine. Areas covered include fields of practice, educational requirements of medical doctors, osteopaths, and chiropractors. In addition, the Medical Practice Act and licensure issues, such as examination, reciprocity, and suspension are covered.

Title of Doctor

The title of doctor designates a person who holds a doctoral degree. Commonly doctor refers to a medical doctor or MD. The practice of medicine, which is the science of diagnosis, treatment, and prevention of disease, requires a minimum of nine to ten years of

Preparing for
Externship

As a medical assistant, you have the advantage of being multiskilled. You are preparing for a career in which you are trained in both the clinical and administrative areas. As an extern, you need to exhibit willingness to learn and behave with integrity. Showing integrity means that you hold yourself to high standards of behavior. Admitting that you have made an error is part of demonstrating integrity. Everyone makes mistakes. When you have made an error, admit it as soon as you realize what you have done. Listen to whatever comments your superior has to make about the error with a positive attitude. Take pride in your accomplishments and show initiative in the work environment.

education and training. The education and training to become a physician generally includes a four-year college degree in premedical studies, four years of medical school, and a period of internship. During the first year of residency or internship, the medical student obtains vital practical experience under the supervision of a licensed physician. At the end of residency, he or she takes a state medical board examination. If the candidate passes the state examination, he or she then becomes licensed to practice medicine in that state.

However, if the new physician wishes, he or she may seek graduate training in a specialty area or residency. This is a paid, on-the-job training position lasting anywhere from two to six years depending on the specialty chosen. Then, the resident/doctor must sit for an American Board of Medical Specialties (ABMS) examination in his or her area of study. For example, a physician who specializes in obstetrics and passes the examination would be board certified by the American Board of Obstetrics and Gynecology. At this point, the new physician chooses how and where he or she would like to practice medicine. Types of medical practices will be discussed later in this chapter.

Others with Title of Doctor

The designation doctor is also used as a proper way of addressing—verbally or in writing—someone who holds a doctoral degree of any kind. The abbreviation for doctor is "Dr." In the medical field, the title "Doctor/Dr." indicates that a person is qualified to practice medicine. In other fields, the title "Doctor/Dr." means that a person has attained the highest educational

TABLE 2-1 **Designations and Initials for Doctors**

Term	Initials
Doctor of Chiropractic	DC
Doctor Of Dental Medicine	DMD
Doctor of Dental Surgery	DDS
Doctor of Education	EdD
Doctor of Medicine	MD
Doctor of Optometry	OD
Doctor of Osteopathy	DO
Doctor of Philosophy	PhD
Doctor of Podiatric Medicine	DPM

degree in his or her field. Several designations for doctor are listed in Table 2-1 with the corresponding initials. Patient Education stresses how knowing the physician's credentials is helpful.

Doctor of Osteopathy or DO has similar educational requirements to the medical doctor. Both MDs and DOs are licensed physicians. Both categories of physicians use similar approaches to medicine, including the use of drugs, therapy, and radiation. Both groups must pass state board examinations to become licensed in their states. Doctors of Osteopathy learn the skill of manipulation therapy in schools of osteopathy. The osteopath places great emphasis on the relationship between the musculoskeletal systems and the organs of the body. In most states, the osteopath is able to perform the same procedures as a medical doctor.

A chiropractor (DC) is trained in manipulation of the spinal cord and other areas of the body. This field requires two years of premedical studies and four years of training in a licensed chiropractic school. Most states license chiropractors.

Medical Practice Acts

Each state has regulations that direct the practice of medicine in that state. While there are some slight differences from state to state, in general, these medical practice acts uphold who must be licensed to perform certain procedures. These acts also maintain the requirements for licensure (granting of a license), duties of that license, grounds on which the license can be revoked or taken away, and reports that must be made to the government. Medical practice acts also cover the penalties for practicing without a valid license.

If a physician moves to another state, he or she must obtain a license to practice in that state. It may mean taking and passing another state medical examination. See the section on reciprocity later in this chapter.

Generally, physicians in different states may consult with each other without being licensed in each other's states. Physicians who practice in governmental institutions, such as Veteran's Administration hospitals or in military service, may practice medicine without the local licensure.

Licensure

The Board of Medical Examiners in each state grants a license to practice medicine. Licensure may be granted through one of three ways: examination, endorsement, or through reciprocity.

Examination

Each state will offer its examination for licensure. This examination is usually taken before the end of medical school. Within the United States, the official medical licensing examination is called the Federation Licensing

Patient Education

Some patients require information about the physician's specialty and credentials. A patient often has questions regarding the skill level of the physician or the amount of the bill. The medical assistant can discuss these concerns with the patient. Explaining the physician's credentials, including the years of education and training required to become a doctor, particularly if the doctor specializes, often increases the patient's level of confidence in the physician.

A patient welcomes an explanation of reasons for being referred to a specialist by his or her physician. In many cases, you will provide the patient with a list of referral specialists approved by your employer. You may be required to schedule an appointment for the patient and to follow up with the patient to see that he or she visited the specialist.

Examination (FLEX). The license is then issued after an internship is completed. Successful performance on this examination entitles one to set up private practice as a general practitioner. The United States Medical Licensing Examination (USMLE), which began in 1992, provides a single licensing examination for graduates from accredited medical schools.

Endorsement

Endorsement, meaning an approval or sanction, is granted to applicants who have successfully passed the National Board Medical Examination (NBME). In fact, most physicians in the United States are licensed by endorsement. Any medical school graduate who is not licensed by endorsement is required to pass the state board examination (FLEX). Graduates of foreign medical schools must pass the same requirements as American graduates.

Reciprocity

In some cases, the state to which the physician is applying for a license will accept the state license, which the physician already holds so that the physician will not have to take another examination. This practice is known as reciprocity.

Registration

It is necessary for physicians to maintain their license by periodic re-registration either annually or bi-annually. The physician is notified by mail when to re-register and must submit the re-registration fee within a designated time period. In addition to payment of a fee to re-register, 75 hours in a three-year period of continuing medical education (CME) units are required to assure that the physician is remaining current in the field of practice. Legal and Ethical Issues discusses how a medical assistant can oversee re-registrations and renewals for the physician.

Suspension or Revoking a Medical License

A physician's license may be revoked in cases of severe misconduct, which include unprofessional conduct, commission of a crime, or personal incapacity to perform one's duties. Unprofessional conduct relates to behavior that fails to meet the ethical standards of the profession, such as inappropriate use of drugs or alcohol. Crimes include rape, murder, larceny, and narcotics convictions. Personal incapacity relates to the physician's inability to perform due to physical or mental incapacities.

Health Care Costs and Payments

Before discussing medical specialties, types of medical practices, health care facilities, and the role and education of allied health professions, it is important to look

Legal and Ethical Issues

Licensure and continuing medical education (CME) are two areas in which you can assist the physician. The renewal of licenses is usually dependent on the completion of re-registration forms and filing these forms on time with the necessary fees. Always take care to maintain accurate records of continuing medical education units earned by the physician since CME is an important part of the licensing process. Be alert to this legal obligation and remind your employing physician in advance of such renewals.

Medical assistants dedicate themselves to the care and well-being of all patients, according to the American Association of Medical Assistants code of ethics. In addition, medical assistants should take the Oath of Hippocrates, "do no harm to the patient" as seriously as the physicians who state it at the time of their graduation from medical school. As a medical assistant, you will act as a representative of the physician and must be well versed on all legal issues that affect the physician's practice.

at some health care costs and trends. Comprehending these trends and their impact on health care make you a more informed professional and will lead to a better understanding of problems that patients may have obtaining and paying for health care.

Health care has changed dramatically in the past 25 years. It has become the largest industry in the nation providing 12.9 million jobs according to the Bureau of Labor Statistics. The costs of health care are increasing faster than the cost of living. It is estimated that more than 14% of our gross national product (GNP) is spent on health care totaling about $1.5 trillion dollars per year. According to CNN Money, in 2003, 15.6% of the population or over 45 million Americans were uninsured. The costs of employer-sponsored health care increased by 13.9% between 2002 and 2003 according to Kaiser Family Foundation. The number of working Americans without health care is increasing because they cannot afford the premiums. According to Kaiser, the annual premium for a family would be more than $9,000 a year for health care coverage. The United States is the only industrialized nation that does not provide some sort of basic health care for all citizens.

What are some of the factors that are driving the skyrocketing costs of health care delivery today?

- Technological advances are expensive
- Knowledge growth and technology has led to physician specialization
- Specialization has damaged the long term doctor-patient relationship; patients do not feel close to the specialists and are more inclined to sue these doctors
- Drug costs are skyrocketing
- The population is aging and the older segment of the population uses the most health care services
- Longer life expectancy means greater need for care for a longer time
- Patients are not passive; they are active, informed consumers who demand more tests and options
- The uninsured rely on emergency room visits for primary care and do not seek medical care until absolutely necessary
- The uninsured have less or no access to preventive care and often require treatment for more advanced illness or ailments
- Social conditions, such as homelessness, substance abuse, poverty, child abuse, break up of the family unit, and increased number of people living alone, impact individual health, health care delivery systems, and health care costs

These trends need to be considered as we continue with our discussion of the types of practices, governmental regulations, and steps utilized to control the costs of health care. Insurance companies, managed care plans, such as health maintenance organizations (HMOs), Diagnostic Related Groups (DRGs), and government legislation have attempted to control costs and have had significant impact on the way health care services are delivered.

In 1983, Medicare instituted a hospital payment system called DRGS, which classifies each Medicare patient according to his or her illness. There are 467 illness categories. Under this system, hospitals receive a preset sum for treatment, regardless of the actual number of "bed days" of care used by a patient. This method of payment provides further incentive to keep costs down. However, it has also led to early discharge of patients, increased number of re-admissions, and discouraged treatment of severely ill patients. Cultural Considerations explains that community resources can be helpful to a diverse client population.

Types of Medical Practices

In the early part of the 20th century, the main form of medical practice was the solo practice. In this type of practice, a family practitioner set up a medical practice within a designated town and geographic area. Over the years, the practice of medicine and the legal environment have changed. Other forms of medical practice have become popular to meet patients' needs for around-the-clock medical coverage. Alternative forms of practice also provide the opportunity for a group of physicians to share insurance premium costs, staff, and facilities investments.

Solo Practice

In a solo practice, a physician practices alone. This is a common type of practice for dentists. However, physicians generally enter into agreements with other

Cultural Considerations

The diversity of the client population will present many challenges to you as a medical assistant. Non-English speaking patients will need brochures and handouts in their own languages if possible. Many brochures are available in Spanish for example. Often these patients are unaware of the community resources available to help them in emergency situations. In some cultures, it is considered unthinkable to ask strangers for help. Understanding how some ethnic groups dread not being self-reliant will help you treat them with more tolerance.

Names, addresses, and telephone numbers of service agencies, such as the American Red Cross, abuse hotlines, homeless shelters, soup kitchens, and poison control centers, all are available from a number of sources such as the phone book, local library, Chamber of Commerce, and the Internet. As a medical assistant, having a typed list of all facilities and information at your fingertips will enable you to be prepared for any contingency. After completing this chapter, you will have a greater understanding of the difficulties that patients face obtaining and paying for medical care. You must be ready to help them regardless of their income levels, cultural origin, race, or attitude.

physicians to provide coverage for each other's patients and to share office expenses.

Sole Proprietorship

In a sole proprietorship, one physician is still responsible for making all the administrative decisions. However, this physician may employ other physicians and pay them a salary. The physician-owner will pay all expenses and retain all assets. In the sole proprietorship form of practice, the owner is responsible and liable for the actions of all the employees.

Partnership

A partnership is a legal agreement to share in the business operation of a medical practice. A partnership is between two or more physicians. In this legal arrangement, each of the partners becomes responsible for the actions of all the partners. This refers to debts and all legal actions, unless otherwise stipulated in the legal partnership agreement.

Associate Practice

The associate practice is a legal arrangement in which physicians agree to share a facility and staff. They do not, as a general rule, share responsibility for the legal actions of each other as in the partnership. The legal contract of agreement stipulates the responsibilities of each party. The physicians act as if their practice is a sole proprietorship.

The legal arrangement must be carefully described and discussed with patients. In some cases, patients have mistakenly believed that there was a shared responsibility by all the physicians in the practice.

Group Practice

A group practice consists of three or more physicians who share the same facility (office or clinic) and practice medicine together. This is a legal form of practice in which the physicians share all expenses, income, personnel, equipment, and records. Some areas of medicine frequently found in group practice are anesthesiology, rehabilitative or obstetrical services, radiology, and pathology.

A group practice can also be designated as a health maintenance organization (HMO) or as an independent practice association (IPA). Group practices have grown rapidly during the last decade. Large groups with over 100 doctors are not uncommon. A large group practice will often form a legal corporation.

Professional Corporation

During the 1960s, state legislatures passed laws (statutes) allowing professionals, for example physicians, lawyers, and accountants, to incorporate. A corporation is managed by a board of directors and there are legal and financial benefits from incorporating.

Professional corporation members are known as shareholders. Therefore, the physician-members become the shareholders in the corporation. Some of the benefits that can be offered to employees of a corporation include medical expense reimbursement, profit sharing, pension plans, and disability insurance. These fringe benefits would not be taxable to the employee and are generally tax deductible to the employer. While a corporation can be sued, the individual assets of the members cannot be touched as in a solo practice. A corporation will remain after a member leaves or dies. Other forms of practice, such as the sole proprietorship, may die with the death of the owner.

Medical and Surgical Specialties

Due to the dramatic advances in medicine over the past two decades, there continues to be an interest in specialization among physicians. Transplant surgery, including the liver, kidneys, lungs, and pancreas, has expanded the need for medical and surgical specialties.

Medical Specialties

A description of some more common medical specialties follows.

Allergy and Immunology

An allergist treats abnormal responses or acquired hypersensitivity to substances with medical methods including testing and desensitization. Pediatricians and internists may sit for the board examination in allergy and immunology after taking several years of additional training.

Anesthesiology

An anesthesiologist is trained to administer both local and general drugs to induce a complete or partial loss of feeling (anesthesia) during a surgical procedure (Figure 2-9). This physician also provides respiratory and cardiovascular support during surgery. The anesthesiologist meets with the patient before the surgical procedure to explain the type of anesthetic that will be used. Certified registered nurse anesthesiologists (CRNA) also may administer anesthetics.

Cardiology

A cardiologist is trained to treat cardiovascular disease. This physician has received special training in the diseases and disorders of the heart and blood vessels. A cardiologist specializing in the treatment of children's heart disease would receive special training as a pediatric cardiologist.

Dermatology

A dermatologist treats injuries, growths, and infections relating to the skin, hair, and nails. This physician may treat patients either medically or surgically.

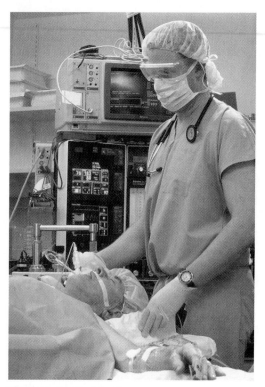

FIGURE 2-9 Anesthesiologist.

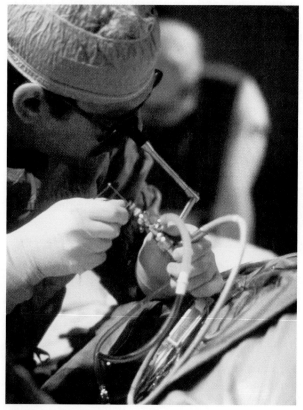

FIGURE 2-10 Nephrologist.

A dermatologist may remove growths such as warts, moles, benign cysts, birthmarks, and skin cancers.

Emergency Medicine
The physician who specializes in emergency medicine has received additional training as an emergency medical resident. Emergency medicine specialists typically work in hospital emergency rooms and freestanding, walk-in emergency centers. They acquire the ability and skills to quickly recognize and prioritize (triage) acute injuries, trauma, and illnesses. They also supervise paramedic pre-hospital care.

Family Practice (Primary Care Medicine)
The family practitioner physician will treat the entire family regardless of age and sex. In some cases, they will refer patients with specific medical conditions to specialists, such as nephrologists for the treatment of renal (kidney) diseases.

Geriatric Medicine
The practice of geriatrics is focused on the care of diseases and disorders of the elderly. Gerontology is a relatively new field of medicine and is the direct result of the larger aging population.

Hematology
Hematology is the study of blood and blood-forming tissues.

Oncology
Oncology is the study of cancer and cancer-related tumors.

Internal Medicine (Primary Medicine)
The internist is a physician who treats adult patients. This physician is skilled in diagnosis and treatment of non-surgical problems. There are subspecialties within the area of internal medicine including: cardiology, endocrinology, gastroenterology, hematology, immunology, nephrology, oncology, and pulmonary medicine.

Neurology
The neurologist treats the non-surgical patient who has a disorder or disease of the nervous system.

Nephrology
A nephrologist specializes in pathology of the kidney including disorders and diseases. A nephrologist is skilled in both medical and surgical treatments including kidney dialysis (Figure 2-10).

Nuclear Medicine
The physician specializing in this field uses radioactive substances for the diagnosis and treatment of diseases such as cancer.

Obstetrics and Gynecology

An obstetrician treats the female as she begins prenatal care and continues through labor, delivery, and the postpartum period (Figure 2-11). A gynecologist provides both medical and surgical treatment of diseases and disorders of the female reproductive system. This is a sub-specialty, which also deals with infertility, the study of a diminished capacity or inability to produce offspring.

Ophthalmology

An ophthalmologist treats disorders of the eye. The study of ophthalmology includes the diagnosis and treatment of vision problems using both medical and surgical procedures.

Orthopedics

An orthopedist or orthopod specializes in the branch of medicine that deals with the prevention and correction of disorders of the musculoskeletal system (Figure 2-12). An orthopedic surgeon specializes in surgical procedures relating to this specialty.

Otorhinolaryngology

The otorhinolaryngologist (ENT) specializes in the medical and surgical treatment of ear, nose, and throat disorders. This includes the study of otology (ear), rhinology (nose), and laryngology (throat), and is also known as otorhinolaryngology.

Pathology

A pathologist specializes in diagnosing abnormal changes in tissues that are removed during a surgical operation and in postmortem examinations. A forensic pathologist is an expert in determining the identity of a person based on such evidence as body parts, dental records, and tissue samples.

Pediatrics

The pediatrician specializes in the development and care of children from birth to maturity (Figure 2-13).

Physical Medicine and Rehabilitative Medicine

Physical medicine and/or rehabilitative medicine specialists treat patients after they have suffered an injury or disability. The purpose of treatment is to return patients to their former state of physical health if possible. This rapidly growing field is closely associated with sports medicine in which the physician treats athletes using preventive and diagnostic medicine.

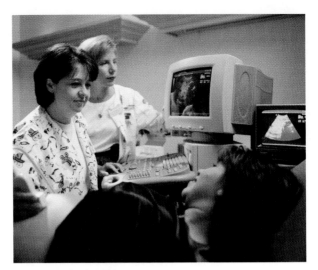

FIGURE 2-11 An obstetrician.

Psychiatry

The psychiatrist specializes in the diagnosis and treatment of patients with mental, behavioral, or emotional disorders. A psychiatrist is qualified to prescribe and administer medications. This specialist may also practice psychotherapy.

Radiology

A radiologist specializes in the study of tissue and organs that is based on x-ray visualization. This physician has been tested and approved by the American Board of Radiology.

Rheumatology

A rheumatologist treats disorders and diseases characterized by inflammation of the joints such as arthritis.

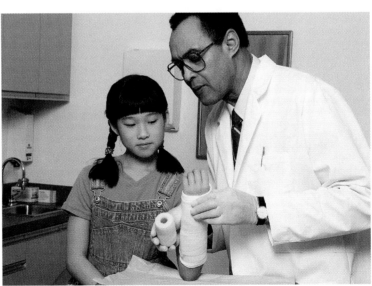

FIGURE 2-12 An orthopedist putting a cast on a young girl.

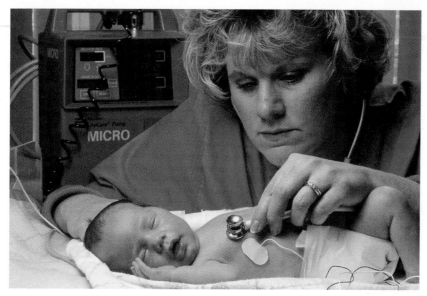

FIGURE 2-13   A pediatrician with a baby.

Surgery

A surgeon corrects illness, trauma, and deformities using an operative procedure (Figure 2-14). Surgery is any invasive procedure that requires entering the body by making an incision or passing instruments through the skin and organs.

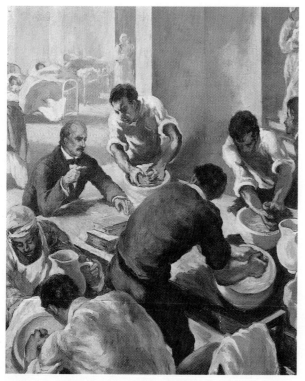

FIGURE 2-14   Surgical procedures are safer today because of hand hygiene and disinfection techniques introduced by Dr. Semmelweiss.

Surgical Specialties

General surgery includes all areas of surgery. General surgeons may restrict their practices to abdominal surgical procedures. However, many surgeons specialize in areas such as neurosurgery, cardiovascular surgery, and orthopedic surgery. Some of the more common surgical specialties are described in Table 2-2.

Health Care Institutions

Hospitals are the largest employers in the nation. According to the Bureau of Labor Statistics, in 2004, hospitals employed 41% of health care workers. In recent years, there has been increased demand from the public, government, and insurance companies to curb hospital expenses. The length of stay in the hospital has been decreasing steadily over the past decade as a result of the DRGs system of payment and better medical and surgical procedures. The result has been an increased emphasis on outpatient rather than inpatient care, especially in the area of minor surgery. Outpatient care refers to services provided to patients on a walk-in basis where no overnight stay is required; inpatient care refers to services provided to patients who are in a facility overnight or on a long-term basis.

Same-day surgery sites, home health agencies, and physical therapy/rehabilitative and sports medicine are all growing rapidly. Also, care that can be provided to older adults in their own homes is encouraged.

Hospitals

The hospital is still considered the key resource for health care in America. While the patient's primary care is delivered in the physician's office, hospitals deliver care for acute illnesses, are sites for major surgical procedures, train and educate health care professionals, conduct research, and provide educational resources to the public. Hospital sizes vary depending on the needs within the community where the hospital was built. The size is based on the number of patient beds.

As hospitals try to curb costs but maintain a rate of bed occupancy, new models are developing. Some services will be eliminated from one hospital if they are available at other nearby hospitals. Many hospitals will merge to share expenses and services or may be purchased by large national corporations.

To ensure quality health care, many hospitals seek accreditation by an association such as Joint Commission

TABLE 2-2 Surgical Specialties and Their Descriptions

Surgical Specialty	Description
Cardiovascular	Cardiovascular surgery is the surgical treatment of the heart and blood vessels.
Colorectal	Colorectal surgery involves the surgical treatment of the lower intestinal tract (colon and rectum).
Cosmetic Surgery/Plastic	Cosmetic surgery involves the reconstruction of underlying tissues. This surgical intervention is used to correct structural defects or remove scars and signs of aging.
Hand	Hand surgery is orthopedic surgery that involves surgical treatment of defects, traumas, and disorders of the hand. Hand surgeons may employ a physical therapy staff and have x-ray equipment at their disposal.
Neurosurgery	Neurosurgery involves surgical intervention for diseases and disorders of the central nervous system.
Orthopedic	Orthopedic surgery treats musculoskeletal injuries and disorders, congenital deformities, and spinal curvatures through surgical means.
Oral (Periodontics, Orthodontics)	Oral surgery involves treatment of disorders of the jaws and teeth by means of incision and surgery as well as extraction of teeth.
Thoracic	Thoracic surgery involves treatment of disorders and diseases of the chest with surgical intervention.

on the Accreditation of Health Care Organizations (JCAHO). JCAHO is a private nonprofit organization that encourages high standards of medical care. Strict guidelines must be met by the institution seeking accreditation.

There are four categories of hospitals:

- General hospital—(Figure 2-15) provides both routine care and special care such as intensive-care units and emergency rooms. They range in size from fifty beds to several hundred beds and are usually found in most towns and communities.

- Teaching hospital—provides the same type of care as in a general hospital. Teaching hospitals are generally located near a university medical school and have medical students, interns, and residents who treat patients under the supervision of staff physicians. Teaching hospitals may have more specialists on staff in order to educate and train interns and residents.

- Research hospital—provides patient care and conducts research to combat disease. Veteran's Administration hospitals throughout the nation and Shriner's hospitals for crippled children are examples of research hospitals.

- Specialty hospital—provides specialized care for certain types of patients such as children, psychiatric patients, or burn victims.

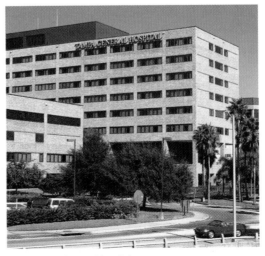

FIGURE 2-15 A general hospital.

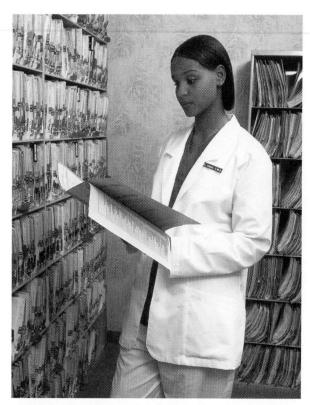

FIGURE 2-16 The medical records department.

Many larger hospitals provide all three services: general patient care, teaching, and research. The hospital organization contains many departments that interact to provide comprehensive health care for the patient. Hospital departments include emergency services, laboratory, radiology, oncology, nuclear medicine, psychiatry, pathology, immunology, respiratory, physical

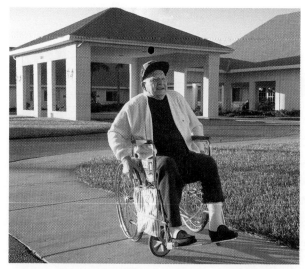

FIGURE 2-17 Skilled nursing facilities provide care for patients requiring longer stays than hospitals allow.

and occupational therapy, nursing, dietary, pharmacy, central supply, housekeeping, engineering, and health information. See Figure 2-16 for an example of a medical records department. The social services department will assist in locating medical care, treatment and/or placement for the patient after discharge from the hospital.

Physicians generally serve on the staff of more than one hospital, but seldom more than three. Physicians will then refer their patients to one of these hospitals in which they have medical privileges. Medical privileges refer to the physician's right to practice medicine in a particular hospital or other health care facility. A physician may also have "courtesy" or "visiting privileges" at a hospital where he or she may be called to see a patient on a referral basis, but in which the physician does not have admitting privileges.

Nursing Homes

Nursing homes were established in the 19th century to provide food, clothing, and shelter for the poor. Over the past century, the quality of care has improved in nursing homes and most homes care for the elderly. Many homes are owned and operated by church groups, but the majority of homes are for-profit run by nursing home corporations. There is much tighter control over the quality of care because of stricter regulations by state public health departments and Medicare. Due to the increased costs of nursing home care, some patients have to convert to Medicaid, the national health insurance for the poor, when their funds are depleted. The present day nursing home is a long-term facility that cares for elderly persons who are sick, too feeble to care for themselves, and have no other source of care. According to the U.S. Medicare Web site, approximately nine million men and women over the age of 65 needed long-term care in 2005. Seventy percent are being cared for by family and friends. The remaining thirty percent or three million needed care in long-term care facilities.

Types of Long-Term-Care Institutions

Long-term-care institutions are classified by federal regulations either as skilled nursing facilities (SNF), intermediate-care facilities (ICF), and extended-care facilities (ECF). A description of these facilities and of assisted living follows.

- Skilled nursing facility (SNF)— intended for patients who require skilled nursing care round the clock (Figure 2-17). Patients must be re-certified every 100 days to allow them to remain in a skilled-care facility.

- Intermediate-care facility (ICF)—intended for patients who are no longer able to live alone and care for themselves, but who do not require skilled nursing care on a 24-hour basis. Many ICFs also have occupational and rehabilitative therapists on their staff. Intermediate-care facilities must meet federal guidelines in order to receive federal funds for services provided to Medicare patients.

- Extended-care facility (ECF)—provides services to patients who no longer need the skilled nursing care of a hospital, but are still too ill or incapacitated to return home. Many hospitals have opened extended-care facilities for such patients (Figure 2-18). An extended-care facility provides custodial care and thus does not employ skilled personnel.

- Assisted-living facility—offers living arrangements for the older adult in which each resident or couple has a separate apartment and pays a fixed fee to have some meals and services provided. Older adults who are able to care for themselves and require a minimum of supervision are living in this relatively new environment.

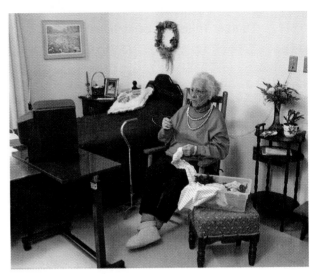

FIGURE 2-18 An extended care facility.

Hospice

Through the hospice movement, which began in medieval England, the wounded, sick, and dying were cared for by religious communities of sisters. Today's modern hospice movement emphasizes improved quality of care for the dying. Most hospice care is provided at home, but some programs also provide care in centers. This interdisciplinary program of care and supportive services facilitates the care of the patient by family members or significant others in the privacy of the patient's home or in a hospice facility.

On home visits, hospice personnel provide nursing care for the special needs of the dying patient, including pain management, but not necessarily treatment for the disease. These visits often provide great emotional support to the patient and the patient's family. Often the visiting health care worker can offer suggestions that might make the patient more comfortable. Most patients in a hospice facility are suffering from terminal illnesses, such as cancer, and Medicare currently covers part of this care in a hospice setting. Medicare (Part B) will cover a part of home care if there is a qualifying diagnosis.

Allied Health Professionals

There are many health care professions and it would be impossible to cover them all in this chapter. As a member of the health care team, it is important that you understand the role and educational require-

ments of others. Before we consider some of the specific professions, you will need an understanding of the terms certification, licensure, and registration as they relates to allied health professionals. A discussion of levels of education and degree titles will be covered as well.

Certification involves the issuing of a certificate and credentials by a professional organization to one who has met the educational/experience standards of that organization. An example would be certification as a medical assistant or CMA by the AAMA, or RMA certification by the American Medical Technologists after a candidate has passed the national examination. Registration means that a professional organization in a specific health care field administers examinations and/or maintains a list of qualified individuals. Licensure means a government agency authorizes individuals to work in a given occupation, such as registered nurses (RN), licensed practical nurses (LPN), and physical therapists (PT).

Educational requirements for health careers vary from state to state. In all cases, a high school diploma or equivalency is necessary. Post secondary education in a vocational/technical school, community college, or university may be required. Table 2-3 illustrates a career ladder in health care, educational requirements, degree designations, and some examples of professions in each category. Health care institutions may require the applicant to pass a national registration or certification examination in his or her field of study as a condition of hire. See Professionalism for continuing education requirements.

Careers in the health care field involve many types of duties or responsibilities. An extensive list of possible career choices follows and are categorized into

TABLE 2-3 Career Titles and Educational Levels

Professional	Educational Requirement	Diploma/Degree	Examples
Professional	4-year degree, advanced degree and clinical training	Bachelor (BA, BS), Master or Doctorate	Medical Doctor (MD) Patholgist
Technologist	4-year college program	Bachelor (BA, BS)	Medical Technologist (MT)
Technician	2-year community college or vocational program	Associate's degree (AS)	Medical Laboratory Technician (MLT)
Assistant	Up to 1-year classroom and clinical preparation	Diploma	Laboratory Assistant
Aide	On-the-job training	High school diploma or GED	Laboratory Aide

Professionalism

Physicians must obtain continuing education to retain their license. Medical assistants also need to keep abreast of new medical information. AAMA requires Certified Medical Assistants (CMA) to earn 60 continuing education credits (CEUs) in five years to maintain their certification. Registered Medical Assistants (RMAs) who earn certification by passing the American Medical Technologists' examination are also encouraged to earn CEUs. Being a life-long learner should be the goal of every medical assistant. The body of knowledge in health care is growing tremendously each year and you will need to be vigilant about keeping up with new information. The following are a few ideas to help you become a well-informed, life-long learner.

- Read *CMA Today*, the AAMA medical assisting journal or AMT Events, the RMA professional publications and complete the continuing education article and test in each edition if provided.

- Select an interesting condition or disease each month to research on the Internet or local library; Keep this research information in a binder for future reference.

- Subscribe to other medical publications or ask your physician if you may read some periodicals that she/he receives.

- Attend seminars provided by the local hospital, HMO, and state or local chapters of medical assisting groups.

National Heath Care Skills Standards (NHCSS) career clusters. The National Health Care Skill Standards were developed to define the body of knowledge and specific skills health care workers are expected to possess for entry-level and technical-level positions. These core standards are used by schools, colleges, and health care facilities to establish curriculum and competencies for a wide variety of fields. The health care careers discussed will be broken down according to National Health Care Skill Standards career clusters and a few examples from each category will be examined.

Therapeutic Cluster Careers

Careers in this cluster include those that involve the health care status of the patient including treatment, evaluation, collection of patient data, and evaluation of patient status.

Nurse

The term nurse refers to a diversified group of health care professionals with a range of qualifications. A description follows of a certified nursing assistant (CNA), licensed practical nurse (LPN), registered nurse (RN), and nurse practitioner (NP).

CERTIFIED NURSING ASSISTANT (CNA) A certified nursing assistant is a member of the health care team who has completed a training program and taken a state examination to qualify to assist nurses in nursing homes, hospitals, and other health care facilities. The CNA provides such patient care as bed baths, vital signs, feeding, and ambulation. Cross training of employees has led to positions such as patient care technician (PCT). The PCT may have a CNA or medical assisting background and perform more technical tasks such as drawing blood and performing EKGs. The nursing assistant may also be referred to as a nurses' aid or orderly.

LICENSED PRACTICAL NURSE (LPN) A licensed practical nurse performs some of the same, but not all, clinical nursing tasks as a registered nurse. The LPN must have graduated from a recognized one-year program and become licensed by the National Federation of Licensed Practical Nurses. In some states, the LPN is known as a licensed vocational nurse (LVN).

REGISTERED NURSE (RN) A nursing career is ideal for the person who wishes to provide hands-on patient care. Nurses work in hospitals, physicians' offices, industry, governmental agencies, ambulatory care units, emergency services, and schools. Their work ranges from managed care organizations providing direct patient care, to teaching and supervising other staff, performing research, and managing agencies. Nurses receive their education and training in either a two-year or four-year program. To become licensed as a registered nurse requires successful completion of a national licensure examination known as the National Council Licensure Examination (NCLEX). A nurse practitioner (NP) is a registered nurse who has received additional training to provide basic patient care including diagnosing and prescribing medications and treatments for common illnesses. This nurse is a masters-degree, trained individual.

Occupational Therapist (OT)

Occupational therapy provides treatment to people who are physically, mentally, developmentally, or emotionally disabled. Occupational therapists evaluate the patient's ability for self-care, work, and leisure skills. The goal of the occupational therapist is to develop programs that will help to restore the patient's ability to manage activities of daily living (ADL). Occupational therapists require a bachelor's degree from an approved program in occupational therapy. In addition, certification by the American Occupational Therapy Association (AOTA) and six months of on-the-job training are needed.

An occupational therapy assistant must complete a two-year vocational training program and be certified by AOTA. This individual works under the supervision of an OT and implements patient treatments designated by the OT.

Physical Therapist (PT)

Physical therapy is the treatment of diseases or disabilities of the joints, bones, and nerves by massage, therapeutic exercises, and heat and cold treatments. Conditions treated by means of physical therapy include: multiple sclerosis, cerebral palsy, arthritis, fractures, spinal cord injuries, and heart disease.

Practitioners work in a variety of facilities including hospitals, ambulatory care, rehabilitation centers, private practice, and schools for the physically challenged. A physical therapist is required to hold a four-year degree in physical therapy, participate in a four-month clinical internship, and successfully pass the state licensure examination. After obtaining a master's degree, some physical therapists set up private practices and provide services on a contract basis.

A physical therapy assistant may be required to have a degree from an accredited two-year college and pass a written licensure examination in some states. He or she works under the supervision of a physical therapist and implement treatments designated by the PT.

Physician's Assistant (PA)

The field of physician's assistant is relatively new, emerging since the 1970s. The goal of this profession is to assist the physician in the primary care of patients. The job description for a physician's assistant includes evaluation, monitoring, diagnostics, therapeutics, counseling, and referral skills. In nearly all states, the PA can prescribe medications. The profession has expanded to include surgeon's, pathologist's, anesthesiologist's, and radiologist's assistant, among others. The general educational program is similar to a master's level program with two years education after a bachelor's degree. In most programs, the student must have work and/or internship experience and pass an accreditation examination.

Respiratory Therapist (RT)

A respiratory therapist evaluates, treats, and cares for patients with breathing problems. A respiratory therapist tests lung capacity, administers breathing treatments, teaches self-care to patients, and provides emergency care. An RT can be employed in hospitals, cardiopulmonary laboratories, nursing homes, health maintenance organizations (HMOs), and ambulatory care facilities. To become a certified respiratory therapy technician (CRTT), the candidate must complete a one-year internship and pass a written examination given by the National Board of Respiratory Therapy.

To become a registered respiratory therapist (RRT) requires completion of a college program, an approved training program, one year's experience in the field, and the successful completion of a written examination given by the National Board of Respiratory Therapy.

Dietician

Dietitians are skilled in applying the principles of good nutrition to food selection and meal preparation. They will work closely with a patient's physician to coordinate the patient's diet with other treatments such as medications. Dietitians also provide consulting services, offer seminars, author books, counsel patients, plan food service systems, and design nutrition plans within fitness programs for athletes. A dietitian must have a bachelor's degree with a major in foods and nutrition. In addition, an internship in a dietary department is required. To become registered requires successful completion of an examination. Dietitians work in a variety of settings including hospitals, long-term-care facilities, schools, and prisons. The employment opportunities for dietitians are currently excellent.

Dental Hygienist

A dental hygienist works directly with the patient to clean teeth, take oral x-rays, teach oral health, and discusses results of dental examinations with the dentist. The dental hygienist must graduate from a two-year community college program or a four-year bachelor's program and pass both a state written and clinical examination.

Emergency Medical Technicians (EMTs)/Paramedics

Emergency medical technicians/paramedics (EMTs/paramedics) are trained in providing emergency care and transporting injured patients to a medical facility. They are skilled in recognizing emergency conditions such as cardiac arrhythmias, airway obstruction, and psychological crisis. Emergency medical technicians and paramedics always work under the direct supervision of a physician and follow a physician's orders. There are different levels of EMTs:

- Basic—the beginner EMT performs basic life support.
- Advanced—an advanced EMT has more training and advanced skills beyond the basic level.
- Paramedic—as the highest level of EMT, a paramedic is able to treat cardiac arrest, perform defibrillation, and administer certain drugs.

EMTs receive certification after completion of an approved EMT program. They must be recertified every two years and receive ongoing education and training in their field.

Diagnostic Career Cluster

The careers in this cluster are involved with procedures that create a picture of the patient's health status at a specific point in time. These careers involve measuring, evaluating, and reporting patient information.

Ultrasound Technologist (AART)

An ultrasound technologist receives training in the use of ultrasound equipment, which uses inaudible sound waves to outline shapes of tissues and organs. Ultrasound equipment produces an image of the shapes. Ultrasound images of fetal development in the uterus are commonly used to assist with fetal monitoring.

X-ray Technologist (Radiologic Technologist)

An x-ray or radiologic technologist must hold a bachelor's degree in radiologic technology, have experience in two or more radiologic disciplines such as nuclear medicine and radiation therapy, and be a registered radiologic technologist (ARRT).

Electroencephalograph Technician

Electroencephalography (EEG) is the field devoted to recording and studying the electrical activity of the brain. An EEG technician operates an electroencephalograph, which records the activity of the brain with a written tracing of the brain's electrical impulses. EEG technologists work primarily in hospitals.

Pharmacist

The field of pharmacy deals with the ordering, maintaining, preparing, and distributing prescription medications. Several pharmacy roles are described here along with the educational requirements.

A pharmacist must complete five years of education in an accredited pharmacy program. In addition, a pharmacy student must serve a one-year internship and become licensed in the state where he or she is employed. A registered pharmacist can work in a variety of institutions including hospitals, drug stores, or may open a pharmacy.

Pharmacy technicians attend a community college or private vocational program. They are able to assist the pharmacist in preparing medications. In some states, they are issued a Pharmacy Technician Certificate upon completion of an examination. A pharmacy clerk assists the pharmacist with typing prescription labels, assigning prescription numbers, and maintaining supplies and records. A high school degree is necessary for this position.

Medical Social Worker

Social work involves programs and services that are developed to meet the special needs of the ill, physically and mentally challenged, and the elderly. A medical social worker cares for the total person, including the emotional, cultural, social, and physical needs of the patient.

Medical social workers assist patients and their families in handling problems associated with a long-term illness or disability. Social workers need a thorough understanding of a community's resources for the disabled. A medical social worker requires a bachelor's degree. Many states require licensing or registration for social workers and a master's degree.

Diagnostic Imaging Technician

Diagnostic Imaging Technicians are trained in the operation of x-ray equipment such as ultrasound, computerized tomography (CT) scan, and magnetic resonance imaging (MRI). Radiology practitioners include: darkroom attendants with a minimum of education or training; radiologic technicians who are graduates of an accredited program; radiologists, who are graduates of an accredited medical school; and licensed physicians with specialized training in radiology.

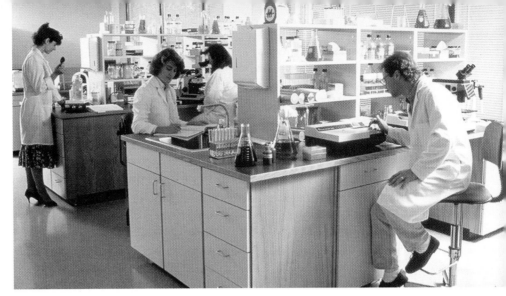

FIGURE 2-19 Hospital laboratory.

Employment opportunities are available in physicians' offices, hospitals, trauma centers, and other ambulatory care facilities.

Medical Laboratory

A medical laboratory is a facility that is equipped for testing, research, scientific experimentation, or clinical studies of materials, fluids, or tissues taken from patients. Independent laboratories provide routine analysis of patient's blood, urine, tissue, and other materials. Hospital laboratories perform tests for both inpatients and outpatients (Figure 2-19). In some instances, a physician's office (POL) will contain a small laboratory where routine tests can be conducted.

PHLEBOTOMIST OR VENIPUNCTURE TECHNICIAN A phlebotomist is skilled in drawing blood from patients. This requires the ability to maintain standard precautions, aseptic technique, excellent venipuncture technique, and good communication skills. Training in a vocational education program is required. In some cases, certification as a phlebotomist is required.

LABORATORY TECHNICIAN (MLT AND CLT) The medical laboratory technician (MLT) and the clinical laboratory technician (CLT) are laboratory technicians skilled in testing blood, urine, lymph, and body tissues. This career requires two years of training in a vocational education program and certification by the National Certification Agency for Medical Laboratory Personnel.

MEDICAL TECHNOLOGIST (MT) OR CLINICAL LABORATORY SCIENTIST (CLS). A laboratory or medical technologist must complete a four-year medical technology program in a college or university to become a certified medical technologist (CMT) or certified

laboratory scientist (CLS). This person directs the work of other laboratory staff, is responsible for maintaining quality assurance standards for all equipment, and performs laboratory analysis. The examination for this profession is prepared by the Board of Registry of the American Society of Clinical Pathologists (ASCP) or American Association of Medical Technologists.

The American Medical Technologists (AMT) certifies phlebotomists, medical laboratory technicians, and medical technologists.

Information Services Career Clusters

Careers in this cluster are involved with documenting client information, including managing, coding, analyzing, maintaining, and retrieving information.

Health Information Technology (Medical Records Technician)

Health information technology refers to the massive database known as medical records. Every person seen by a health care professional has a medical record. Medical records technicians, now more commonly referred to as health information technologists, maintain the permanent records relating to a patient's condition and treatment. The medical record is a legal document that can be used in a court of law.

A medical records technician (ART) must graduate from an accredited medical records program, have a two-year associates degree, have several years experience as a medical records clerk, and have 30 credit hours from an accredited college. Successful completion of the accredited record technical examination allows the technician to use the initials ART after his or her name.

A registered medical records administrator (RRA) requires a bachelor's degree in health information technology and the successful completion of an examination.

Medical Transcription

A medical transcriptionist types or enters into the computer dictation that is taken from a recording machine or tape. This dictation consists of medical reports from physicians and surgeons. Skills required for this profession include typing ability, good spelling understanding of medical terminology, and data processing equipment.

Office Management

The role of office manager is a choice open to some allied health professionals, including medical assistants and nurses. Office managers supervise the entire support staff. The position requires someone with a sound knowledge of the type of work performed in the office or institution, strong supervisory skills, and the ability to work closely with top management. Excellent time-management and communication skills are a must for office managers.

Unit Clerk/Communications Clerk

The unit clerk, or ward secretary, is responsible for clerical duties, reception work, and other communication duties in hospitals, long-term-care facilities, and clinics. The unit clerk in a hospital performs varied tasks, for example, taking physicians' orders from the charts and assisting the nursing staff. A knowledge of medical terminology is required.

Environmental Services Career Cluster

This career cluster includes careers involved with the patient's health care environment such as aseptic procedures, resource management, maintaining equipment, and providing sterile supplies.

Biomedical Equipment Technician

A biomedical equipment technician maintains and repairs medical testing equipment either in a health care facility or for a private company. Educational requirements vary from an associate's to a bachelor's degree.

Other health care workers in this career cluster, which do not require postsecondary education, include central supply/sterile supply workers, housekeeping staff, and food-service aides.

Centers for Disease Control (CDC)

The Centers for Disease Control (CDC), a division of Department of Health and Human Services (DHHS), was established in 1946. The CDC's main headquarters and laboratories are in Atlanta, Georgia. This is a governmental agency that employs over 8,600 people.

The purpose of the CDC is to safeguard public health by preventing and controlling disease, and act as a resource for the medical profession. The CDC seeks information about causes of disease to find cures, alerts the medical profession to potential outbreaks of diseases such as influenza, describes the group who will be at highest risk during an outbreak of disease such as the elderly, and recommends the proper treatment. In addition, the CDC conducts disease research, prevention, control, and education programs nationally and in several other countries. These programs help to train doctors, provide public health information, develop immunization services with state and local agencies, and establish standards for healthful working conditions.

SUMMARY

The medical profession contains a rich history of achievement and progress. The history of medicine can be broken into four categories: early medicine going back to 3000 BC, the 18th century, 19th century, and 20th century. Major advancements include the eradication of many deadly diseases with the advent of vaccines, the decrease of infections due to the discovery of aseptic technique and antibiotics, the harnessing of radium to treat disease, the inventions of the microscope and surgical instruments, the discovery of anesthesia, and a better understanding of anatomy and physiology.

Contemporary licensed physicians must maintain their knowledge base by completing 75 continuing medical education (CME) units over a period of three years. There are 24 medical specialty boards for the purpose of improving the quality of care by encouraging physicians to seek further education and training. The medical assistant will have the opportunity to pursue a career working for physicians in all areas of specialization.

The health care environment can be confusing and intimidating to the patient. It is important to have an understanding of the health care system and the diversity of institutions that deliver health care services. The descriptions provided in this chapter of inpatient facilities including hospitals, nursing homes, hospices, as well as ambulatory care settings and services provide a basic explanation of a rather complex structure. Patients need to know the options that are available as they seek out services and follow up on the referrals made by their primary physician for treatment, procedures, or further diagnosis. The medical assistant's understanding of the system is key to providing clear explanations to the patient. Understanding managed care plans and using the proper insurance codes (see CPT and ICD-9 in Chapter 17) for services provided to patients are necessary to assure insurance claims reimbursement.

Chapter Review

COMPETENCY REVIEW

1. Define and spell the terms to learn for this chapter.
2. State some of the major achievements in medicine during each of these periods: early medicine, 18th century, 19th century, and 20th century or modern medicine.
3. List the three methods by which a physician can become licensed.
4. Explain three circumstances that would justify the suspension or revocation of a physician's license.
5. Describe four types of medical practices.
6. Identify and explain issues in this chapter that might require patient education.
7. Find examples of four board certified physicians in your local telephone directory.
8. Describe the role of the medical assistant as it relates to patient education concerning the physician's credentials.
9. Using the local telephone directory, find examples of names and addresses of three hospitals, a hospice, an extended-care facility, and a medical laboratory.
10. Discuss the role of the medical assistant in relationship to other health care providers.

PREPARING FOR THE CERTIFICATION EXAMINATION

1. What is the symbol for healing that incorporates a staff with two coiled snakes?
   A. colliculus
   B. caisson
   C. cachination
   D. choleretic
   E. caduceus

2. The number of individual cases of a disease within a defined population is known as the
   A. morbidity rate
   B. mortality rate
   C. illness factor
   D. disease factor
   E. illness rate

3. The first written source of medical ethics for the first doctors in history is called the
   A. Code of Medical Conduct
   B. Code of Hammurabi
   C. Hippocratic Oath
   D. Code of Caduceus
   E. Oath of Medical Healing

4. One source of medicine to treat pain in early human history was
   A. the poppy plant
   B. cayenne pepper
   C. chamomile tea
   D. licorice
   E. the foxglove plant

continued on next page

5. The "father of medicine" is
   A. Caduceus
   B. Galen
   C. Hippocrates
   D. Vesalius
   E. Galileo

6. Who discovered penicillin?
   A. Sabin
   B. Salk
   C. Fleming
   D. Banting
   E. Nightingale

7. The state law which governs the licensure of physicians is the
   A. Medical Licensure Act
   B. Code of Medical Conduct and Licensure
   C. Medical Practice Act
   D. Physicians' Practice Act
   E. Physicians' Conduct Oath

8. Which physician in the late 1800s helped find a cure for yellow fever?
   A. Morton
   B. Reed
   C. Long
   D. Hahnemann
   E. Beaumont

9. Which government agency was established to safeguard public health by preventing and controlling disease through research?
   A. ICF
   B. ECF
   C. FDA
   D. HMO
   E. CDC

10. DRGs stands for
    A. Diagnostic Related Groups
    B. Diagnostic Research Groups
    C. Delivery Related Groups
    D. Drug Related Groups
    E. Drug Reactive Groups

CRITICAL THINKING

1. Is it beyond the scope of her training for Elizabeth to arrange for such care and the physical transition for this patient?

2. If yes, how could Elizabeth handle this situation with the physician and other providers that are involved in this case?

3. If no, what options could Elizabeth investigate in order to help facilitate the placement of this patient?

4. Are patient and family education merited in this particular situation or is some sort of intervention applicable?

5. Does the fact that alcohol and drug abuses are involved alter potential treatment options?

6. Because the patient has a history of violent behavior, should this fact limit the placement options?

ON THE JOB

One of the important characteristics of a medical assistant is to have a concrete foundation in the practice of medicine. This would include a complete understanding of the many medical and surgical specialties and subspecialties in which a physician can be board certified.

An important responsibility for the medical assistant is to have the ability to convey this information about the treating physician to the anxious patient and the patient's family. This is part of patient education.

Mary is employed as a medical assistant for a physician who is a pediatric cardiovascular surgeon. She is taking a history on the patient, a newborn, by interviewing the parents, Mr. and Mrs. Appleby. They are extremely anxious and upset over the condition of their newborn who was diagnosed shortly after birth with a serious, yet quite treatable, heart defect. The prognosis, should the parents agree to the corrective surgery, is quite good. However, the parents are having a difficult time understanding how the physician could help their newborn. They are not even quite sure why they were referred to this specialist and why their pediatrician could not treat the infant.

1. How could Mary comfort and reassure these parents?
2. What could she possibly say about the physician that might help the parents to understand why they were referred and how their newborn could be helped?

INTERNET ACTIVITY

Research ethical arguments for and against the use of fetal stem cells for medical treatment.

 MediaLink More on medical practices and health care environment, including interactive resources, can be found on the Student CD-ROM accompanying this textbook.

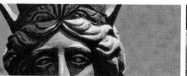

Medical Assistant Role Delineation Chart

HIGHLIGHT indicates material covered in this chapter.

ADMINISTRATIVE

Administrative Procedures

- Perform basic administrative medical assisting functions
- Schedule, coordinate and monitor appointments
- Schedule inpatient/outpatient admissions and procedures
- Understand and apply third-party guidelines
- Obtain reimbursement through accurate claims submission
- Monitor third-party reimbursement
- Understand and adhere to managed care policies and procedures
- *Negotiate managed care contracts*

Practice Finances

- Perform procedural and diagnostic coding
- Apply bookkeeping principles

- Manage accounts receivable
- *Manage accounts payable*
- *Process payroll*
- *Document and maintain accounting and banking records*
- *Develop and maintain fee schedules*
- *Manage renewals of business and professional insurance policies*
- *Manage personnel benefits and maintain records*
- *Perform marketing, financial, and strategic planning*

CLINICAL

Fundamental Principles

- Apply principles of aseptic technique and infection control
- Comply with quality assurance practices
- Screen and follow up patient test results

Diagnostic Orders

- Collect and process specimens
- Perform diagnostic tests

Patient Care

- Adhere to established patient screening procedures
- Obtain patient history and vital signs
- Prepare and maintain examination and treatment areas
- Prepare patient for examinations, procedures and treatments

- Assist with examinations, procedures and treatments
- Prepare and administer medications and immunizations
- Maintain medication and immunization records
- Recognize and respond to emergencies
- Coordinate patient care information with other health care providers
- Initiate IV and administer IV medications with appropriate training and as permitted by state law

GENERAL

Professionalism

- Display a professional manner and image
- Demonstrate initiative and responsibility
- Work as a member of the health care team
- Prioritize and perform multiple tasks
- Adapt to change
- Promote the CMA credential
- Enhance skills through continuing education
- Treat all patients with compassion and empathy
- Promote the practice through positive public relations

Communication Skills

- Recognize and respect cultural diversity
- Adapt communications to individual's ability to understand
- Use professional telephone technique

- Recognize and respond effectively to verbal, nonverbal, and written communications
- Use medical terminology appropriately
- Utilize electronic technology to receive, organize, prioritize and transmit information
- Serve as liaison

Legal Concepts

- Perform within legal and ethical boundaries
- Prepare and maintain medical records
- Document accurately
- Follow employer's established policies dealing with the health care contract
- Implement and maintain federal and state health care legislation and regulations
- Comply with established risk management and safety procedures
- Recognize professional credentialing criteria
- *Develop and maintain personnel, policy and procedure manuals*

Instruction

- Instruct individuals according to their needs
- Explain office policies and procedures
- Teach methods of health promotion and disease prevention
- Locate community resources and disseminate information
- *Develop educational materials*
- *Conduct continuing education activities*

Operational Functions

- Perform inventory of supplies and equipment
- Perform routine maintenance of administrative and clinical equipment
- Apply computer techniques to support office operations
- *Perform personnel management functions*
- *Negotiate leases and prices for equipment and supply contracts*

- *Denotes advanced skills.*

SOURCE: Reprinted by permission of the American Association of Medical Assistants from the AAMA Role Delineation Study: Occupational Analysis of the Medical Assisting Profession.

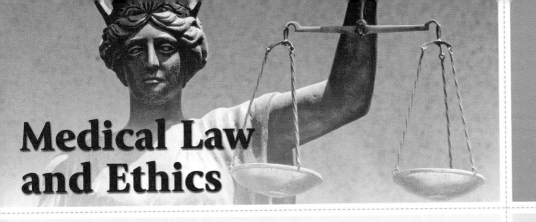

chapter 3

Medical Law and Ethics

Learning Objectives

After completing this chapter, you should be able to:

- Define and spell the terms to learn for this chapter.
- Differentiate between criminal and civil law.
- Discuss the four Ds of negligence.
- Discuss what can be done to avoid a claim of abandonment.
- Discuss informed consent.
- Discuss the role of the medical assistant relating to legal issues in the medical office.
- Explain the importance of the Hippocratic oath today.

- List the seven main points of the AMA Principles of Medical Ethics.
- List and discuss the main points of the AAMA Principles of Medical Ethics.
- Discuss what is meant by the medical assistant's standards of care.
- Describe the Patient's Bill of Rights.
- Explain the HIPAA guidelines concerning the patient's right to privacy and confidentiality in the medical office.

Terms to Learn

breach of contract
contributory negligence
defamation of character
guardian ad litem
informed consent

living will
practice of medicine
proximate cause
reasonable person standard

res ipsa loquitur
respondeat superior
standard of care
statute of limitations

Case Study

DR. BARNS IS A BOARD CERTIFIED ONCOLOGIST. Although in a solo practice, she employs a staff of five—an office manager, insurance administrator, receptionist, registered nurse, and medical assistant. They have worked in the practice together for more than three years.

Dr. Barnes has asked the medical assistant, Sue Halt, to take over the insurance administrator's duties in her absence. Since the medical assistant is multiskilled, she is the best choice on staff.

Sue was surprised to discover that insurance companies were being billed for medication that is, according to the FDA, experimental. She also was troubled by the fact that insurance companies were being billed as if the patients were being treated on an outpatient basis. In reality, many of the patients resided out of the state and had been shipped the experimental medication for self-administration.

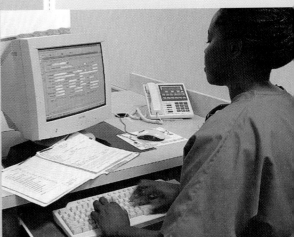

oday's health care consumer demands more of a partnership with the physician and the rest of the health care team. Patients should be part of the decision-making process regarding their care and treatment. This chapter discusses issues such as malpractice, abandonment, and litigation, as well as specific regulations and documents protecting the patient, the patient's family, physicians, and medical staff involved in care and treatment. Some examples are the Uniform Anatomical Gift Act and the Patient Self-Determination Act. Other topics presented include the public duties of the physician, documentation of medical records, regulations relating to controlled substances and the medical assistant's role in preventing liability suits.

Classification of the Law

Laws are classified into four types:

- Criminal
- Civil
- International
- Military

Only criminal and civil law are discussed here.

Criminal Law

Criminal laws are made to protect the public as a whole from the harmful acts of others.

Criminal acts fall into two categories: felony and misdemeanor. A felony carries a punishment of imprisonment in a state or federal prison or death. These crimes include murder, rape, robbery, and practicing medicine without a license. Misdemeanors are less serious offenses and carry a punishment of fines or imprisonment in jail for up to a year. They include traffic violations, disturbing the peace, and theft.

A physician's license may be revoked or taken away if he or she is convicted of a crime. Criminal cases have included revocation of a license for sexual misconduct, murder, violating narcotics laws, and practicing medicine without a license. The practice of medicine is defined as diagnosing and prescribing treatment or medication. The medical assistant must make sure that he or she always assists the physician, and does not try to treat or diagnose a patient's condition.

Civil Law

Civil law concerns relationships between individuals or between individuals and the government. Civil law includes contract law, tort law, and administrative law. Contract law includes enforceable promises and agreements between two or more persons to do or not do a particular action. Tort law covers acts that result in

TABLE 3-1 Intentional Torts

Tort	Description	Example
Assault	The threat of bodily harm to another. There does not have to be actual touching (battery) or injury for assault to take place.	Threatening to harm a patient or to perform a procedure for which he or she does not consent.
Battery	Actual bodily harm to another person without permission. This is also referred to as unlawful touching or touching without consent.	Performing surgery or a procedure without the informed consent (permission) of the patient.
False imprisonment	A violation of the personal liberty of another person through unlawful restraint.	Refusing to allow a patient to leave an office, hospital, or medical facility, when he or she requests.
Defamation of character	Damage caused to a person's reputation through spoken or written word.	Making a negative statement about another physician's ability.
Fraud	Deceitful practice.	Promising a miracle cure.
Invasion of privacy	The unauthorized publicity of information about a patient.	Allowing personal information, such as test results for HIV, to become public without the patient's permission.

harm to another. Administrative law covers regulations that are set by governmental agencies. Health care employees are most frequently involved in cases of civil law, in particular, tort and contract law.

Tort Law

A tort is a wrongful act that is committed against another person or property that results in harm. In order to meet the definition of a tort, there must be damage or injury to the patient that was caused by the physician or the physician's employee.

Intentional torts include assault, battery, false imprisonment, defamation of character, fraud, and invasion of privacy. Table 3-1 provides a description and example of these torts.

Unintentional torts, such as negligence, occur when the patient is injured as a result of the health care professional not exercising the ordinary standard of care. The health care professional must exercise the type of care that a "reasonable" person would use in a similar circumstance. This is known as the reasonable person standard.

Negligence and malpractice are the same thing. It is easier to prevent negligence than it is to defend it. Physicians can take steps to avoid negligence suits by:

- Protecting the physician-client relationship.
- Being above any reproach in the performance of their medical duties.

In order to obtain a judgment for negligence against a physician, the patient must be able to show what is referred to as the "four Ds": Duty, Dereliction or neglect of duty, Direct cause, and Damages (Box 3-1).

In legal terms, a plaintiff is a person or group of people who file a lawsuit. The defendant is the person, or group of people, who are accused of wrongdoing in a court of law.

In a case of negligence, the plaintiff must prove proximate cause. This means that the plaintiff must prove that the defendant's acts (or failure to act) directly caused the injury. For example, if a patient returns to his room after having prostate surgery and experiences severe headaches that were not present before having the surgery, the patient must prove that the physician's performance of the prostate surgery was the cause of the headaches. Contributory negligence relates to the patient's contribution to the injury, which if proven, would release the physician as the direct cause. For example, the patient did not keep an appointment causing an undetected infection to advance.

Contract Law

The branch of law known as contract law is generally concerned with a breach or neglect of an understanding between two parties.

BOX 3-1

The Four Ds of Negligence

- **Duty** refers to the physician-client relationship. The patient must prove that this relationship has been established. When the patient has made an appointment and been seen by the physician, a relationship has been established. Further office visits and treatment will establish that the physician had a duty or obligation to the patient. (Contract)
- **Dereliction or neglect of duty** refers to a physician's failure to act as any ordinary and prudent physician (a peer) within the same community would act in a similar circumstance when treating a patient. To prove dereliction or neglect of duty, a patient would have to prove that the physician's performance or treatment did not comply with the acceptable standard of care based on the norm of the ordinary and prudent physician described above. (Standard of Care)
- **Direct cause** requires the patient to prove that the physician's derelict or breach of duty was the direct cause for the injury that resulted.
- **Damages** refers to any injuries that were received by the patient. The court may award compensatory damages to pay for the patient's injuries.

A contract is a voluntary agreement that two parties enter into with the intent of mutual benefit for both parties. Something of value, which is termed *consideration*, is part of the agreement. In the medical profession, the consideration might be the performance of a hysterectomy in exchange for a specific fee. An agreement would take place between the two parties, which would include the offer ("I will perform the hysterectomy") and the acceptance of the offer ("I will allow you to perform a hysterectomy") and the consideration (performance of the hysterectomy in exchange for the fee).

In order for a contract to be legal, there are several considerations. For one thing, the concerned party (the patient) must be mentally competent at the time the contract is made. For example, the patient must not be under the influence of drugs or alcohol at the time the contract is entered.

A breach of contract occurs when either party fails to comply with the terms of the agreement. In the previous example, a breach of contract would occur if the

BOX 3-2

Premature Termination of the Physician-Patient Contract

A medical office should document any of the incidents below with a certified letter.

- Failure to pay for service.
- Missed appointments.
- Failure to follow instructions.
- The patient states (orally or in writing) that he or she is seeking the care of another physician. Reasons for seeking another physician are many. For example, the patient's insurance may have changed and the patient's physician may not be covered by the new insurance, or the patient may move.

physician removed the appendix along with the uterus during a hysterectomy without the expressed consent of the patient, or if the patient failed to pay the agreed-upon fee.

Abandonment

Once a physician has agreed to take care of a patient that contract may not be terminated improperly. The physician may be charged with abandonment of the patient if he or she does not give formal notice of withdrawal from the case. In addition, the physician must allow the patient enough time to seek the services of another physician. The best method to protect the physician from a charge of abandonment is to send a letter by certified mail.

An example of abandonment is the patient who is under treatment for a heart ailment but has not kept appointments for periodic checkups to assess his or her condition. The physician may decide that he or she can no longer accept responsibility for the medical treatment of this patient without periodic physical examinations to assess medication dosage and other factors. In this case, the physician makes a decision to no longer treat this patient. Abandonment would occur if the physician did not provide enough notice to the patient of withdrawal from the case. This notice must be sufficient for the patient to find another physician who will provide treatment. The time varies from state to state.

Termination of Contract

The termination of the contract between a physician and a patient generally occurs when the treatment has ended and the fee has been paid. However, there are serious issues that arise causing premature termination of a contract between the physician and the patient. It should be noted that both physicians and patients have the right to terminate the contractual relationship. Letters from the physician should indicate the date the physician's services will be terminated. The medical assistant needs to understand these situations and handle them correctly (Box 3-2).

Collections

Several laws have been enacted to provide protection against unscrupulous collection practices that harm individuals. The medical assistant needs to be familiar with these laws since he or she is responsible for following the administrative procedures these laws require. The laws relating to the collection process are discussed in Table 3-2.

Professional Liability

Lawsuits related to health care have greatly increased during the past decade and the average liability award granted to plaintiffs in medical malpractice cases is now over one million dollars. Professional liability is determined by the federal, state, and local laws governing the patient/physician relationship and relates to the standard of care, legal contracts, and informed consent. An important issue in the question of liability is the physician/employee relationship. Some factors impacting on this relationship are discussed here. They include respondeat superior, standard of care, malpractice, res ipsa loquitur, statute of limitations, Good Samaritan laws, and defamation of character.

Respondeat Superior

Physician/employers are especially concerned that their employees have a complete understanding of the law. The Latin term respondeat superior literally means, "Let the master answer." What this means to your employer, the physician, is that he or she is liable for the negligent actions of anyone working for him or her. In some cases and in some states, both the physician and the employee may be liable.

In effect, under respondeat superior, the physician delegates certain duties to you and if you perform them incorrectly, then the ultimate liability rests with the physician/employer. However, medical assistants and other health care workers can also be named in malpractice suits.

TABLE 3-2 Laws Governing Collection

Law	Description
Equal Credit Opportunity Act of 1975	Prohibits discrimination—unfair treatment—in the granting of credit. This law mandates that women and minorities must be issued credit if they qualify for it, based on the premise that if credit is given to one patient it should be given to all patients that request it.
Fair Debt Collection Practices Act of 1978	Provides a guide for determining what are considered the fair collections practices for creditors.
Fair Credit Reporting Act of 1971	Provides guidelines for collecting an individual's credit information. Individuals are able to learn what credit information is available about them. Consumers can correct and update this credit information.
Notice on "Use of Telephone for Debt Collection" from the Federal Communications Commission	Provides guidelines for the specific times that credit collection phone calls can be made. It prohibits using the telephone for harassment and threats. Telephone calls for the purposes of collections must be made between the hours of 8 A.M. and 9 P.M.
Truth in Lending Act of 1969	Requires a full, written disclosure concerning the payment of any fee that will be collected in more than 4 installments. Also referred to as Regulation Z of the Consumer Protection Act.

For example, if you are authorized by your employer to draw a sample of blood from a patient and you inadvertently enter a nerve causing permanent damage to the patient's arm, then you may also be liable for that patient's injury. Since the physician's medical license is in jeopardy when errors are made, it is vital that you understand the law.

Standard of Care

While a physician is under no obligation to treat everyone, once he or she does accept a patient for treatment, the physician has then entered into the physician/patient relationship and must provide a certain standard of care. This standard of care asserts that the physician must then provide the *same* knowledge, care, and skill that a similarly trained physician would provide under the same circumstances in the same locality. The law requires only reasonable, ordinary care and skill.

The physician is expected to perform the same acts that a "reasonable and prudent" physician would. This standard also states that a physician will not perform any acts that a "reasonable and prudent" physician would not. Physicians are expected to exhaust all the resources available to them when they are treating a patient. This would include:

- Taking a thorough medical history.
- Giving a complete physical examination.

- Conducting the necessary laboratory tests and x-rays.

Physicians are not expected to expose their patients to undue risk. If the physician violates this standard of care, he or she is liable for negligence.

The medical assistant must also adhere to a standard of care. This standard will depend on training, skills, experience, education, and the responsibility assigned. Employees going outside of their competency risk being sued for negligence. Preparing for Externship advises reviewing applicable laws in your state and region.

Preparing for Externship

Be sure that you have reviewed the local laws regarding the standards of care for medical assistants in your state. If you happen to move to, or work in another state, then be sure, prior to beginning working in the new state, that you are aware of applicable laws so that you can follow the regulations.

Malpractice

Professional misconduct or demonstration of an unreasonable lack of skill with the result of injury, loss, or damage to the patient is considered malpractice. It means the physician was negligent. Every mistake or error, however, is not considered malpractice. Therefore, when a treatment or diagnosis does not turn out well, the physician is not necessarily liable. The physician/employer and all staff must each act within the "standard of care" appropriate for the particular practice of medicine. All health care providers are held to this same standard.

Malpractice Insurance

In most cases, employers carry insurance to cover acts of their employees during the course of carrying out their duties. This is general liability coverage. Employees should request to see your employer's "certificate of insurance" to determine policy coverage.

Some physicians carry a rider, or addition, to their professional liability or malpractice policy to cover any negligence on the part of their clinical assistants. An example of this is the patient who slips and falls while getting off the examination table, even though you had warned the patient to sit up slowly and use the foot stool. If this type of fall were to result in a broken bone, the insurance company might settle the case even though negligence was not found.

The time taken away from the job to hire and meet with a lawyer, in order to discuss a case prior to appearing in court, as well as the court appearance itself, could become quite costly. So, if you are not covered by your employer's malpractice policy, then you must purchase your own professional liability coverage from an insurance carrier who specializes in this type of coverage.

Res Ipsa Loquitur

The doctrine of res ipsa loquitur, which means "the thing speaks for itself," applies to the law of negligence. This doctrine tells us that the breach (neglect) of duty is so obvious that it does not need further explanation or "it speaks for itself." For instance, leaving a sponge in the patient during abdominal surgery, dropping a surgical instrument causing injury to the patient, and operating on the wrong body part are all examples of res ipsa loquitur. None of these examples would have occurred without the negligence of someone involved in the procedure.

Statute of Limitations

The statute of limitations refers to the period of time during which a patient has to file a lawsuit. The court will not hear a case that is filed after the time limit has run out. This varies from state to state. In some states, the time period is one or two years.

The statute of limitations does not always start "running" when the treatment is administered. It may begin when the problem is discovered, which may be some time after the actual treatment. This is known as *the rule of discovery*. For instance, there is a case in which a physician accidentally left a surgical sponge in a patient's body during an abdominal operation. After sixteen years of abdominal discomfort, the patient required more surgery but the physician who had performed the original operation had died. So, another surgeon, who found the sponge and removed it, performed the second surgery. The patient then sued the estate of the original surgeon for malpractice and won because the statute of limitations, which was two years in that state, started running when the sponge was discovered.

The reverse of a statute "running" is a situation in which the statute is prevented from coming into play. This occurs when the injury is to a minor child. Generally, the court will appoint a guardian ad litem, an adult who will act in the court on behalf of the child. However, the child does not have to sue through a guardian ad litem as a minor, but may wait until he or she reaches adulthood. In such a case, an obstetrician and his or her assistants can be sued twenty-one years and nine months (plus the statute of limitations period in that state) after a birth injury has occurred.

Good Samaritan Laws

Good Samaritan laws are state laws that help to protect a health care professional from liability while giving emergency care to an accident victim. Such laws are in effect in all states to encourage physicians and other health care professionals to offer aid.

No one is required to provide aid in the event of an emergency, except in the state of Vermont (Figure 3-1). Someone responding in an emergency situation is only required to act within the limits of his or her skill and training. A medical assistant would not be expected, nor advised, to perform emergency treatment that is within the area practiced by physicians and nurses.

Defamation of Character

Defamation of character is a scandalous statement about someone that can injure the person's reputation. Defamation can result even when the statement is true.

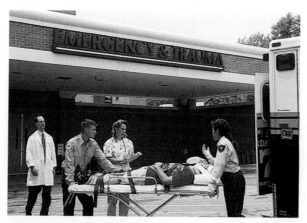

FIGURE 3-1 An accident victim gets emergency care.

Slander occurs when the defaming statement is spoken. *Libel* refers to written defamation.

As a medical assistant, you will have access to privileged information about patients that may seem harmless, but, in reality, the information could be very damaging to their reputations. For instance, a patient who has a test for an infectious disease, such as hepatitis or AIDS, may not wish an employer to know the test took place even if the test result is negative. If you call the patient's place of employment and leave a message regarding a test result of this nature, the action could be considered a breach of confidentiality and defamation.

The fact that a physician saw a patient must be kept confidential. The medical assistant should not fax information or leave messages on answering machines unless specifically instructed to do so in writing by the patient. Such instructions should be documented.

In order to protect yourself and avoid involvement in lawsuits, you must practice your skills with care, be concerned about maintaining good public relations with patients and other staff members, and understand the law.

Patient/Physician Relationship

Both physician and patient must agree to form a relationship if there is to be a contract for service and treatment. In order to receive proper treatment, the patient must confide truthfully in the physician. Failure to state all the facts may result in serious consequences for the patient. The physician is not liable if the patient has withheld critical information. Patients can expect to be treated as long as necessary.

Physician Rights

Physicians have the right to select the patients they wish to treat. They also have the right to refuse service to patients. From an ethical standpoint, most physicians do treat patients who need their skills. This is particularly true in cases of emergency.

Physicians may also state the type of services they will provide, the hours their offices will be open, and where they are located. The physician has the right to expect payment for treatment given.

Physicians have a right to take vacations and time off from their practices. Care must be taken to inform patients if their physician will be unavailable. In most cases, another physician will cover or take care of a colleague's patients while he or she is away.

Patient Rights

The patient has the right to approve or give consent or permission for all treatment. In giving consent for treatment, the patient reasonably expects that his or her physician will use the appropriate "standard of care" in providing care and treatment. That is, that the physician will use the same skill that is used by other physicians in treating patients with the same ailments. Patients also expect that all information and records about their cases will be kept confidential by the physician and staff. The patient's right to privacy prohibits the presence of unauthorized persons during physical examinations or treatments.

In addition to these rights, the patient also has certain obligations. For example, the patient is expected to follow the instructions given by the physician. And finally, the patient is expected to pay the physician for medical services.

Informed Consent

The patient can expect to receive information concerning the advantages and potential risks of all treatments. Informed consent means that the patient is informed about the possible consequences of both having and not having certain procedures and treatment. The physician must carefully explain that in some cases, the treatment may even make the patient's condition worse.

The Doctrine of Informed Consent (Figure 3-2) includes the following:

- Explanation of advantages and risks to the treatment.
- Alternatives available to the patient.
- Potential outcomes to the treatment.
- What might occur if there is no treatment.
- The use of understandable language.

Touching someone without the person's consent is referred to as battery. Since consent means to give permission or approval for something, for example, when a patient is seen for a routine examination for medical treatment, there is implied consent that the physician will touch the person during the examination. Therefore, the "touching" required for the examination would not be considered a crime of battery.

It is very difficult to "fully" inform a patient about all the things that can go wrong with a treatment. In an emergency situation in which the patient is not able to understand the explanation, nor sign a consent form, a physician is protected by law to provide care. The process of obtaining consent cannot be delegated by the physician to someone else, except in emergency situations (Figure 3-3).

Does the signed informed consent protect the physician and staff? If after the physician has carefully explained the treatment, the patient acknowledges understanding the explanation and risks involved and signs the consent form, then, generally speaking, there is some protection from lawsuits. However, patients have sued and won cases in which they were presented the risks of a procedure, signed the form, and then proceeded to sue the physician when the treatment failed.

MEMORIAL HEALTH

COMPLETE ORIGINAL IN INK FOR HOSPITAL CHART
PATIENT MUST BE AWAKE, ALERT AND ORIENTED WHEN SIGNING

DATE: _____ TIME: _____ ☐ AM ☐ PM

I AUTHORIZE THE PERFORMANCE UPON_____
OF THE FOLLOWING OPERATION (state nature and extent):_____
_____
_____
_____

TO BE PERFORMED UNDER THE DIRECTION OF DR. _____

1. I HAVE BEEN ADVISED THAT THERE IS A FAVORABLE LIKELIHOOD OF SUCCESS, BUT I UNDERSTAND THAT A COMPLETELY SUCCESSFUL OUTCOME MAY NOT BE ACHIEVABLE, AND THERE ARE NO GUARANTEES REGARDING THE OUTCOME. I ALSO UNDERSTAND THAT CERTAIN ADVERSE EVENTS COULD OCCUR AS A RESULT OF THE PERFORMANCE OF THE PROCEDURE OR TREATMENT, INCLUDING PAIN, INFECTION, LACERATION OR PUNCTURE OF INTERNAL ORGANS, BLEEDING, NERVE DAMAGE OR EVEN IN RARE CASES, DEATH. I UNDERSTAND THAT HOSPITALIZATION OR OTHER INSTITUTIONAL CARE, HOME CARE OR CARE BY HEALTH PROFESSIONALS MAY BE NEEDED FOLLOWING THE PROCEDURE OR TREATMENT, RELATED TO FULL RECOVERY, RECUPERATION OR CONVALESCENCE. I UNDERSTAND THE ALTERNATIVES TO THIS PROCEDURE, INCLUDING MY RIGHT TO REFUSE TO CONSENT TO IT, AND I NEVERTHELESS HAVE DECIDED TO CONSENT TO PERFORMANCE OF THE PROCEDURE OR TREATMENT.

2. I CONSENT TO THE PERFORMANCE OF OPERATIONS AND PROCEDURES IN ADDITION TO OR DIFFERENT FROM THOSE NOW CONTEMPLATED, WHETHER OR NOT ARISING FROM PRESENTLY UNFORESEEN CONDITIONS WHICH THE ABOVE NAMED DOCTOR OR HIS/HER ASSOCIATES OR ASSISTANTS MAY CONSIDER NECESSARY OR ADVISABLE IN THE COURSE OF THE OPERATION.

3. I CONSENT TO THE DISPOSAL BY HOSPITAL AUTHORITIES OF ANY TISSUES OR PARTS WHICH MAY BE REMOVED.

4. THE NATURE AND PURPOSE OF THE OPERATION/PROCEDURE, POSSIBLE ALTERNATIVE METHODS OF TREATMENT, THE RISK AND BENEFITS INVOLVED, AND THE COURSE OF RECUPERATION HAVE BEEN FULLY EXPLAINED TO ME. NO GUARANTEE OR ASSURANCE HAS BEEN GIVEN BY ANYONE AS TO THE RESULTS THAT MAY BE OBTAINED.

5. I UNDERSTAND AND AGREE WITH THE ABOVE INFORMATION. I HAVE NO QUESTIONS WHICH HAVE NOT BEEN ANSWERED TO MY FULL SATISFACTION. I UNDERSTAND THAT I HAVE THE RIGHT TO ASK FOR FURTHER INFORMATION BEFORE SIGNING THIS CONSENT.

I have crossed out any paragraph above which does not apply or to which I do not give consent.

PATIENT SIGNATURE: _____ WITNESS SIGNATURE: _____
(OR PARENT OR GUARDIAN IF PATIENT IS UNDER 18 YEARS OF AGE) *(OF PATIENT, PARENT OR GUARDIAN SIGNATURE)*

RELATIONSHIP: _____ WITNESS SIGNATURE: _____
☐ **TELEPHONE CONSENT** *(2ND WITNESS NEEDED FOR TELEPHONE CONSENT)*

FIGURE 3-2 Sample of an informed consent document to perform an operation, sedation, anesthetics, and other medical services.

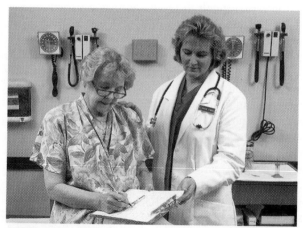

FIGURE 3-3 The patient's signature on the informed consent form indicates that the patient understands the limits and risks involved in the treatment or surgical procedure as explained by the physician.

Outpatient surgical forms or procedure forms used in clinic settings may be shorter in content. There are exceptions to the informed consent doctrine that are unique to each state. Some of the more general exceptions follow.

- A physician does not have to inform a patient about risks that are commonly known. For example, a patient could choke swallowing a pill.

- If the physician feels the disclosure of risks may be detrimental to the patient, then he or she is not responsible for disclosing them. This might occur if a patient has a severe heart condition that may be worsened by an announcement of risks.

- If the patient requests the physician not to disclose the risks, then the physician is not responsible for failing to do so.

Cultural Considerations

Medical personnel must be aware of the differences in thought and custom among different cultural groups. While the practices of groups to which one does not belong may seem unorthodox and strange, it is the medical assistant's responsibility to not make personal judgments about those practices that might interfere with the patient's health or well-being, or that might make the patient and his or her family feel uncomfortable. This includes any and all practices, such as the Christian Scientist's and Jehovah's Witness' refusal of blood transfusions, the Jewish practice of performing circumcisions by the rabbi, not the physician, and even many cultures' practice of personal hygiene. Many groups adhere to dietary regimes that are different from others. Religious practices are an area that often seems unusual if one is not a member of or an adherent to the religion. As a member of the medical community, the medical assistant should refrain from verbal or nonverbal criticisms or shows of disapproval for these differing beliefs and customs.

Patients have the right to refuse treatment. Cultural Considerations looks at accommodating different cultural groups. Some members of religious groups, such as Jehovah's Witnesses and Christian Scientists, do not wish to receive blood transfusions or certain types of medical treatment. The adults would not receive the treatment against their wishes. In the case of a minor child, the court may appoint a guardian who can then give consent for the procedure.

Rights of Minors

A minor is considered a person who has not reached the age of majority, which varies from state to state, but usually, is 18. In most states, minors are unable to give consent for treatment. Exceptions are special cases involving pregnancy, request for birth control information, abortion, testing and treatment for sexually transmitted diseases, problems with substance abuse, and a need for psychiatric care. There are two types of minors who can give consent for treatment:

- Mature minors
- Emancipated minors

A mature minor is a young person, generally under the age of 18, who possesses a maturity to understand the nature and consequences of the treatment in spite of his or her young age. Emancipated minors actually have the same legal capacity as an adult under any of the following five conditions:

- They live on their own.
- They are married.
- They are self-supporting.
- They are in the armed forces.
- Any combination of the above conditions.

Since not all states recognize the categories of mature and emancipated minors, it is wise to handle consent on a case-by-case basis. Following are some legal implications to consider when treating a minor.

- Right to confidentiality—a 16-year old who is seeking birth control information has a right to have her records remain confidential.
- Financial responsibility—the 16-year old girl seeking birth control information may not be able to pay for the office visit. Contacting her parents for payment may breach confidentiality.
- Minor's legal guardian—this is sometimes difficult to determine if the child lives with the mother but the father is financially responsible for care and treatment.

Patient Self-Determination Act

Several documents executed by the patient provide protection for the patient and physician. Such documents also provide direction for the patient's caregiver or proxy to make health-care-related decisions according to the patient's wishes at a point in time when the patient is unable to do so. These documents include the following:

Living Will

The living will allows patients to request that life-sustaining treatments and nutritional support not be used to prolong their life. This document gives patients the legal right to direct the type of care they wish to receive when their death is imminent. The document provides protection for physicians and hospitals when they follow the patient's wishes. This process is often discussed in the office with patients when they are capable of making the decision. Other family members or significant others can also be part of the discussion and decision. One copy of the living will should be kept with the patient's record.

Durable Power of Attorney

The durable power of attorney, when signed by the patient, allows an agent or representative to act on behalf of the patient. If the durable power of attorney is for health care only, then the agent may only make health-care-related decisions on behalf of the patient. The agent may be a spouse, grown child, friend, or, in some cases, an attorney.

The durable power of attorney (DPOA) is a safeguard that someone will be able to act on the patient's behalf if he or she becomes physically or mentally incapacitated. This document is in effect until the patient cancels it. A copy of the durable power of attorney should be kept with the patient's record. The person who is the patient's DPOA acts on behalf of the patient until the patient is again capable of making his or her own decisions.

Uniform Anatomical Gift Act

The Uniform Anatomical Gift Act allows persons 18 years or older and of sound mind to make a gift of any or all parts of their body for purposes of organ transplantation or medical research. One of the regulations of the act is that a physician who is not involved in the transplant will determine the time of death. No money is allowed to change hands for organ donations.

The donor will carry a card that has been signed in the presence of two witnesses. In some states, the back of the driver's license has a space to indicate the desire to be an organ donor with space for a signature.

In some cases, the family will make the decision for the donor if this was not done while the donor was alive. It is generally agreed that if a member of the family opposes the donation of organs, then the physician and hospital do not insist upon it.

Documentation

Carefully document all calls, visits, treatments, no-shows, appointment cancellations, medications, prescription refills, vital signs, and other pertinent information in the patient's chart. If an action is not recorded on the medical chart, then it is considered by most courts not to have been performed.

Use of Records in Litigation

Litigation refers to a lawsuit tried in court. For this purpose, a court of law may subpoena a medical record. When this is done, only the parts of the record that are requested should be copied and sent to the requesting attorney. Unless the original record is subpoenaed, a certified photocopy may be sent. If the original record is subpoenaed, then make a copy and return the copy to the locked file. A receipt for the subpoenaed record should then be placed in the patient's file. The patient should also be notified that his or her record has been subpoenaed. Both the subpoenaed record and the notification to the patient should be sent by certified mail.

Be especially careful when using a fax transmission for medical records. The person receiving the fax should assure you that the machine is located in a restricted area. Confidential material is not generally sent over a fax transmission. Of course, a fax is not usable when an original record is requested. A disclaimer should be placed on the fax cover sheet explaining that the records are confidential.

Should you or your employing physician receive a *subpoena duces tecum*, meaning an order to appear in court and to bring certain records or other materials to a trial or deposition, remember only the records specifically stated in the subpoena are required.

Court Testimony

Not everyone who has information relating to a case will be called into court to testify. An attorney may interrogate, or ask questions, of a witness. Another means of obtaining information from a witness to be used during a court case is to submit a deposition. In this case, a written statement is taken of oral testimony given in front of a court officer. The person who gives the oral testimony and then signs a deposition does not have to actually appear in court. An attorney submits the deposition during the court case. Arraignment occurs when a defendant is called before the court to answer a charge.

An expert witness is a person called upon to testify in court regarding what standard of care for a patient is in a similar community. An expert witness in a medical malpractice suit is generally a physician.

In the event that you are called upon to appear in court, you will want to be as comfortable as you can when giving testimony. It will be well to remember a few pointers.

- *Be professional.* You will be judged by your appearance and behavior as well as by what you say. Your attorney can advise you on this more fully.
- *Remain calm, dignified, and serious at all times.* The opposing attorney may try to make you nervous.
- *Do not answer questions you do not understand.* Simply ask the attorney to repeat the question or state, "I don't know."
- *Just present the facts surrounding the case.* Do not give any information for what is not asked. Do not insert your opinion. "The patient was shouting" is stating a fact. Stating, "He was angry," is your opinion.
- *Do not memorize your testimony ahead of time.* You will generally be allowed to take some notes with you to refresh your memory concerning dates.
- *Always tell the truth.*

Giving testimony in court is a crucial and sensitive matter. It is best to consult an attorney if you have any questions.

Public Duties of Physicians

There are responsibilities the physician has to the public. Some of these duties include reports of births, stillbirths and deaths, communicable illnesses or diseases, drug abuse, certain injuries such as rape, abuse of children, spouses, and older adults, gunshot and knife wounds, and animal bites.

Exact reporting requirements vary from state to state, so the medical assistant should be familiar with the requirements of his or her state. Office personnel, including the medical assistant, carry out many of the duties that relate to these responsibilities (Table 3-3).

Drug Regulations

The Food and Drug Administration (FDA) is the agency within the federal government that has jurisdiction over testing and approving drugs for public use. The Drug Enforcement Administration (DEA), a branch of the Justice Department, regulates the sale and use of schedule drugs.

TABLE 3-3 Public Duties of the Physician

Duty	Description
Births	Issuing of a legal certificate, which will be maintained during a person's life as proof of age. Many benefits and documents, including social security, passport, and driver's license, depend on having a valid birth certificate.
Deaths	Physicians sign a certificate indicating the cause of a natural death. Check with your state public health department to determine specific requirements. For example, in the case of a stillbirth before the 20th week of gestation, you will have to determine if both a birth and death certificate are required. A coroner or health official will have to sign a certificate in the following cases: ■ No physician present at the time of death ■ Violent death, unlawful death ■ Death as a result of criminal action ■ Death from an undetermined cause
Reportable communicable diseases	Physicians must report all diseases that can be transmitted from one person to another and are considered a general threat to the public. The list of reportable diseases differs from state to state. The report can be either by mail or phone. The following childhood vaccines and toxoids are required by law (The National Childhood Vaccine Injury Act of 1986): ■ Diphtheria, tetanus toxoids, pertussis vaccine (DTP) ■ Pertussis vaccine (whooping cough) ■ Measles, mumps, rubella (MMR) ■ Poliovirus vaccine, live ■ Poliovirus vaccine, inactivated ■ Hepatitis B vaccine ■ Tuberculosis test
Reportable injuries	Certain injuries are reportable according to state requirements. These injuries include gun or knife wounds, rape and battered persons injuries, and spousal, child, and elder abuse.
Child abuse	Questionable injuries of children, including bruises, fractured bones, and burns, must be reported. Signs of neglect, such as malnutrition, poor growth, and lack of hygiene, are reportable in some states.
Elder abuse	Physical abuse, neglect, and abandonment of older adults is reportable in most states. The reporting agency varies by state but generally includes social service agencies.
Drug abuse	Abuse of prescription drugs is reportable according to the law. Such abuse can be difficult to determine since the abuser may seek prescriptions for the same drug from several different physicians. A physician will want to see a patient before prescribing a medication.

Both the physician and the medical assistant are responsible for understanding patient education relating to legal issues. The medical assistant can assist the physician by providing good patient care and avoiding litigation by following practical recommendations. Patients must understand all papers they sign, including permission for treatment, insurance payments, and other billing materials. You may have to read and explain this material to patients if you have any doubts about their comprehension of the written materials.

The Controlled Substances Act of 1970 requires physicians to handle controlled drugs that are highly addictive in very specific ways. The physician who dispenses, purchases, administers, prescribes, or handles drugs is required to register with the Drug Enforcement Administration. The physician then receives a DEA registration number that must appear on all prescriptions for controlled substances. A DEA number is required for every location in which controlled drugs are stored. If a physician practices in two states, then two DEA numbers must be obtained. DEA registration numbers are generally printed on physician's prescription blanks. See Volume III, Chapter 48 for a sample prescription form.

Controlled drugs must be kept in a locked or even double-locked cabinet and any theft must be immediately reported to both the regional DEA office and the local police. In addition, the physician's black bag and prescription blanks should always be stored in a secure locked location.

Records must be kept to document the administering and dispensing of controlled drugs. In addition, federal regulations require a written inventory in triplicate of drug supplies, based on daily use, be made every two years and kept for two more years.

Controlled drugs are classified into five schedules, or categories that indicate levels of potential abuse. Schedule I drugs have the highest potential for addiction and abuse while Schedule V drugs have the least. In Volume III, Chapter 48, a Schedule for Controlled Substances shows the meaning of each classification and examples of drugs for each category.

The physician's medical assistant may not dispense controlled substances; however, he or she must be knowledgeable about the regulations governing the documentation and control of drugs. Only licensed personnel are permitted to dispense drugs. Be sure to report to the physician any unusual patient behavior indicating addictive drug use.

Role of the Medical Assistant

The role of the medical assistant in preventing liability suits is of paramount importance to both you and your employer. Remember that in many cases, you are the only one in the office who will hear a patient's complaint. Your ability to handle the complaint professionally and efficiently may eliminate a potential lawsuit for the physician. Patient Education discusses how providing good patient care can help to prevent litigation.

Acting under a code of ethics that compels you to safeguard any patient whose care and safety are affected by the negligent action of someone else, you must follow the chain of command, the authority structure within your office, and report to your immediate supervisor any negligent action you observe. It goes without saying that if you accidentally make an error, you will bring this to your supervisor's attention so that it can be corrected immediately (Professionalism).

You can help your employer and protect yourself, by remembering the recommendations and cautions that follow. These recommendations and cautions are clustered around major areas of responsibility you address daily in your role as a medical assistant.

Professionalism

Telling the truth is one of the most important parts of being a medical professional. Every human will make mistakes; it is part of being human. However, the most important thing any professional can do is admit that he or she made a mistake and seek to correct the mistake. However, do not offer extra information to the patient. Just state that there is a correction to be made. Be sure to speak with the supervising physician, and document clearly in the chart the mistake that was made and how it was corrected. Honesty goes a very long way in preventing litigation and providing good, quality care to all patients.

Confidentiality/Privacy

- Never make any statements about your employing physician that could be interpreted as an admission of fault. On the other hand, as a medical assistant, you cannot remain silent if you are aware that your employing physician is doing something illegal. You can be held liable for remaining silent.

- Do not participate in negative or critical discussions of the physician(s) or other practitioners in your office with your patients. Do not comment on a patient's negative criticism of a current or former physician.

- Never discuss anything about the patient outside of the office.

- Make sure that a female medical assistant is present when the physician (male or female) examines a female patient.

- Treat all patients with dignity and respect.

Office Management

- Treat all patients with the same courtesy and dignity you would expect to receive. Log and return telephone calls promptly. Explain any delays to patients who are waiting to see the physician. Offer to set up another appointment if the delay will be very long.

- Never make promises regarding what the physician can do for the patient.

- Carefully explain all fees and responsibilities for bills to the patient, relating any concerns the patient may have to the physician.

- Relay any dissatisfied patient's comments to the physician.

- If the physician will be out of town or absent from the office, post these dates. Include this announcement in the monthly billing envelopes. Also provide the name and telephone number of the physician available for patients who need care when their own physician is absent.

- If a physician is withdrawing from a case, then a certified letter must be sent to the patient declaring this. Send the letter certified mail with return receipt requested and keep a copy of the letter and receipt with the patient's record. The physician can be brought up on charges of abandonment if there is no documentation or evidence that there was a formal withdrawal.

Documentation

- Carefully sign or initial every note. Remember: medical documents are considered legal documents and may be used in a court of law.

- If the patient did not keep an appointment, be sure to document the fact as a no-show. Document canceled appointments and follow-up to determine why the patient missed the appointment.

- Document when a patient is referred to another physician and follow up to make sure the patient did see the referral physician.

- Document all patient contacts, including telephone prescription refills and tests and procedures that have been ordered. Call all patients the day after surgery to check on their progress. Document this telephone call.

- Record all care and treatment given as soon as possible after the patient's visit. This will keep patient records current and ensure appropriate follow-up treatment if it is required.

- Be sure the physician sees and initials all diagnostic reports in a timely fashion before they are filed.

- Provide all instructions to patients in writing.

Drug Regulations

- A medical assistant may administer medication only under the direct supervision of a physician. Follow the Controlled Substances Act by careful procedure and documentation. This may vary from state to state.

- Secure the supply of prescription pads from theft at all times.

- When preparing medications for administration, check the medication three times. Remember the "three befores." Check the medication **before removing it from the shelf**; check the name and dosage **again before preparing the dosage**; and check the label again **before returning the medication** to the shelf.

Certification and Licensing

- Have a thorough understanding of the limits of certification and standards of care for the medical assisting profession. Never perform any procedure for which you are not trained or qualified.

- Do not diagnose or prescribe over the telephone. This applies to all drugs even those that can be obtained over the counter. You could be charged with practicing medicine without a license.

- Do not call yourself a "nurse" or allow anyone else to refer to you as the nurse. You must be held to your own standard of care and not that of a nurse.

- Participate in continuing education and training programs to maintain your skill levels.

Informed Consent

- The physician must thoroughly explain all procedures to the patient. The medical assistant is responsible for making sure there is a signed consent form. Never have the patient sign a document that he or she does not understand.

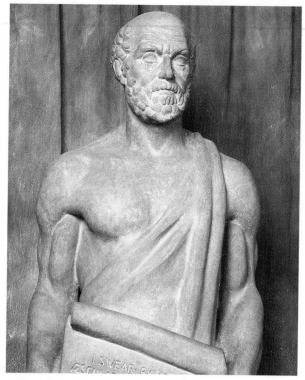

FIGURE 3-4 An artist's interpretation of Hippocrates.

- Obtain a parent or guardian's signature before any procedure is performed on a minor. The only exception is in a case of emergency, when the parent or guardian cannot be reached. File the signed consent form immediately.

Safety

- Maintain a safe environment in the office or work site for the patients and staff. Handle requests for maintenance repairs. Report any safety

hazards at once. If you knowingly overlook a hazard that a "reasonable person" would report and eliminate, you can be guilty of negligence.

- Carefully check and document medical waste disposal. Be concerned about the safety of maintenance personnel who must handle the waste containers. Always dispose of syringes and needles correctly in designated hazardous waste containers.

- Maintain and document careful quality checks on laboratory testing equipment.

Code of Ethics

Ethics is the branch of philosophy relating to morals or moral principles. It involves the examination of human character and conduct, the distinction between right and wrong, and a person's moral duty and obligations to the community. Ethics has been part of the medical profession since the early beginning of the profession.

The earliest code of ethics, or principles to govern conduct for those in medicine, dates back to around 1800 BC, to the Code of Hammurabi. In 400 BC, Hippocrates, a Greek physician referred to as the "father of medicine," wrote a statement of principles for his medical students to follow (Figure 3-4). This statement of principles is known as the Hippocratic oath, and is still important today. This oath reminds medical students of the importance of their profession, the need to teach others, and the obligation they have to act in such a way as to never knowingly harm a patient or divulge a confidence. The Hippocratic oath is still recited at medical school graduation ceremonies, and has been for centuries, as it carries an important ethical message for physicians. Modern codes of ethics have been developed as medical science has continued to advance.

Medical Ethics

Medical ethics refers to the moral conduct of people in medical professions. This moral conduct of medical professionals is governed by the high principles and standards that these professionals set for themselves and willingly choose to follow through personal dedication. Every medical profession has a "Code of Ethics" that sets moral standards that are expected to be adhered to by the members of that profession (Legal and Ethical Issues).

Ethical Standards and Behavior

Ethical standards are generally more severe than those standards that are required by law. In many cases, ethical standards are more demanding than the law. A violation of an ethical standard could mean the loss of the physician's reputation.

Legal and Ethical Issues

As an agent, or representative of the physician, the medical assistant is responsible to understand ethical standards so that he or she can respond to questions related to any office issue. It is important to remember that the medical assistant cannot diagnose or treat illnesses, although educating the patient about information the physician has given is expected. Patient confidentiality cannot be breached for any reason. Staff members should not access any chart that they do not have a specific work-related need to open.

Ethical behavior, according to the American Medical Association (AMA), refers to moral principles or practices, the customs of the medical profession, and matters of medical policy. Unethical behavior would be any actions that did not follow these ethical standards. When a physician is accused of unethical behavior or conduct in violation of these standards, he or she can be issued a warning or censure (criticism) by the AMA. The AMA Board of Examiners may recommend the expulsion or suspension of a physician from membership in the association. Expulsion, or being put out of the association, is a severe penalty for physicians since it limits the physician's ability to practice medicine. Not all physicians are members of the AMA, and the AMA does not have authority to bring legal action against nonmembers for unethical conduct. However, the State Medical Board that issued the physician his or her license may limit the physician's practice or revoke the license altogether for ethical misconduct. If it is alleged that a physician has committed a criminal act, the medical society is required to report it to the state board or governmental agency. Allege means assert or declare without proof. Violation of the law, which is followed by a conviction for the crime, may result in a fine, imprisonment, or both. The State Medical Board can then revoke the physician's license. Revocation means that the physician no longer has a license to practice medicine.

AMA Principles of Medical Ethics

In the United States, the AMA has taken a leadership role in setting standards for the ethical behavior of physicians. The AMA was organized in New York City in 1846 and the first Code of Ethics was formed shortly after that in 1847. Figure 3-5 shows a patient with a physician being assisted by a medical assistant.

The AMA Principles of Medical Ethics discusses human dignity, honesty, responsibility to society, confidentiality, the need for continued study, freedom of choice, and a responsibility of the physician to improve the community. Box 3-3 presents this statement of principles in its entirety.

Medical Assistant's Princples of Medical Ethics

Medical assistants may not be involved with the life and death ethical decisions that face the physician; however, they do face many dilemmas regarding right or wrong behavior on an almost daily basis. Examples include when a coworker violates patient confidentiality, uses foul language in front of a client, or how the team treats a patient whose body may smell of urine or alcohol. Ethical issues involve doing the right thing at the right time.

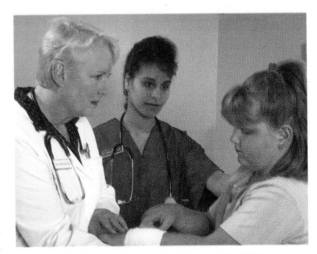

FIGURE 3-5 Medical assistant helps the physician with a patient.

Code of Ethics of the AAMA

The Code of Ethics of the American Association of Medical Assistants (AAMA) is a standard that medical assistants are expected to follow. The Code, which describes ethical and moral conduct for the medical assistant, is similar to the AMA's Principles of Medical Ethics. Box 3-4 lists the code of ethics of the AAMA. Medical assistants assume a position of trust and must try to live up to the standards of the profession as stated in the Code.

Creed of the AAMA

The Creed of the American Association of Medical Assistants can be best followed by the medical assistant who spends time reading about and discussing ethical problems, such as transplants, artificial insemination, the right to die with dignity, and abortion. To be true to this Creed, the medical assistant must know about the ethical issues the patient faces and be committed to treat the patient with respectful care regardless of the patient's religious beliefs or cultural practices.

Creed of the American Association of
Medical Assistants:

I believe in the principles and purposes of the profession of medical assisting.

I endeavor to be more effective.

I aspire to render greater service.

I protect the confidence entrusted to me.

I am dedicated to the care and well-being of all people.

I am loyal to my employer.

I am true to the ethics of my profession.

I am strengthened by compassion, courage, and faith.

BOX 3-3

AMA Principles of Medical Ethics

Preamble

The medical profession has long subscribed to a body of ethical statements developed primarily for the benefit of the patient. As a member of this profession, a physician must recognize responsibility not only to patients, but also to society, to other health professionals, and to self. The following principles adopted by the American Medical Association are not law, but standards of conduct which define the essentials of honorable behavior for the physician.

Human Dignity

I. A physician shall be dedicated to providing competent medical service with compassion and respect for human dignity.

Honesty

II. A physician shall deal honestly with patients and colleagues, and strive to expose those physicians deficient in character or competence, or who engage in fraud or deception.

Responsibility to Society

III. A physician shall respect the law and recognize a responsibility to seek changes in those requirements which are contrary to the best interests of the patient.

Confidentiality

IV. A physician shall respect the rights of patients, of colleagues, and of other health professionals, and shall safeguard patient confidence within the constraints of the law.

Continued Study

V. A physician shall continue to study, apply and advance scientific knowledge, make relevant information available to patients, colleagues, and the public, obtain consultation, and use the talents of other health professionals where needed.

Freedom of Choice

VI. A physician shall, in the provision of appropriate patient care, except in emergencies, be free to choose whom to serve, with whom to associate, and the environment in which to provide service.

Responsibility to Improved Community

VII. A physician shall recognize a responsibility to participate in activities contributing to an improved community.

Medical Assistant's Standard of Care

As a medical assistant, you must remember that your actions can have legal consequences for the physician who employs you. You are not held to the same standard of care as a physician due to differing credentials, licensure, and education. However, you will carry out your duties under the direction of a physician and, therefore, you must use the same approved methods that a physician would use. For example, you must have the same quality standard, as any physician would use when taking an electrocardiogram, drawing blood, and collecting specimens.

A medical assistant is not expected to diagnose medical conditions, interpret electrocardiograms, or prescribe medications since these are all within the area of the physician's standard of care. In fact, a med-ical assistant must continually use caution and not take on any tasks or duties for which he or she is not trained within the scope of his or her practice.

The actions of medical assistants reflect upon their physician employers. Many duties performed by medical assistants could result in harm to the patient if not done properly. There have been lawsuits in which the physician has been found guilty of negligence due to improper performance of his or her medical assistant.

The Patient's Bill of Rights

The American Hospital Association developed a statement called "The Patient's Bill of Rights," which describes the patient-physician relationship. Medical assistants also follow these guidelines when working with the physician's patients. Box 3-5 states these rights. Most offices have these rights printed for their patients.

BOX 3-4
Code of Ethics of the American Association of Medical Assistants

Preamble

The Code of Ethics of AAMA shall set forth principles of ethical and moral conduct as they relate to the medical profession and the particular practice of medical assisting.

Members of the AAMA dedicated to the conscientious pursuit of their profession, and thus desiring to merit the high regard of the entire medical profession and the respect of the general public which they serve, do hereby pledge themselves to strive always to:

Human Dignity

I. Render service with full respect for the dignity of humanity;

Confidentiality

II. Respect confidential information obtained through employment unless legally authorized or required by responsible performance of duty to divulge such information;

Honor

III. Uphold the honor and high principles of the profession and accept its disciplines;

Continued Study

IV. Seek to continually improve the knowledge and skills of medical assistants for the benefit of patients and professional colleagues;

Responsibility for Improved Community

V. Participate in additional service activities aimed toward improving the health and well-being of the community.

Copyright by the American Association of Medical Assistants, Inc. Reprinted by permission.

Confidentiality

According to the Medical Patients Rights Act, all patients have the right to have their personal privacy respected and their medical records handled with confidentiality. Any information, such as test results, patient histories, and even the fact that the patient is a patient, cannot be told to another person. No information can be given over the telephone without the patient's permission. No patient records can be given to another person or physician without the patient's written permission or unless the court has subpoenaed it. A subpoena is a court order for a person to appear in court or for documents to be presented to the court.

A further set of rules towards maintaining confidentiality is called the Health Insurance Portability and Accountability Act (HIPAA). All medical office employees must undergo HIPAA training during their orientation. HIPAA rules ensure that private patient information remains private. Without written authorization, patient information may not be shared with other entities. HIPAA extends to making sure that computers with confidential patient information cannot be seen or accessed by individuals who are not authorized to see the information. All faxes and e-mails that contain private patient information must have a note stating that the information is confidential, and if the information is accidentally transmitted to someone without clearance to read the information, they must immediately notify the office, and destroy the information.

The medical assistant's treatment and concern for the patient reflects the physician's high standards of care. The human dignity of each patient must be preserved regardless of the patient's socioeconomic background, race, age, nationality, sexual orientation, or gender (Figure 3-6). Any promise or commitment that the medical assistant makes to a patient can be legally binding to his or her physician and employer. This means that the physician can be held responsible for something the staff has said or implied with regard to the physician improving the patient's condition. Keep all matters relating to patients in confidence. If you believe that any health professional is acting in an unethical or unprofessional manner, you should discuss this with your employer or another physician.

Any information that is given to a physician by a patient is considered confidential and it may not be given to an unauthorized person. The physician's medical

BOX 3-5
The Patient's Bill of Rights

1. The patient has the right to considerate and respectful care.

2. The patient has the right to and is encouraged to obtain from physicians and other direct caregivers relevant, current, understandable information concerning diagnosis, treatment, and prognosis.

3. The patient has the right to make decisions about the plan of care prior to and during the course of treatment and to refuse a recommended treatment or plan of care to the extent permitted by law and hospital policy and to be informed of the consequences of this action.

4. The patient has the right to have an advance directive (such as a living will, health care proxy, or durable power of attorney for health care) concerning treatment or designating a surrogate decision maker with the expectation that the hospital will honor the intent of that directive to the extent permitted by law and hospital policy.

5. The patient has the right to every consideration of privacy.

6. The patient has the right to expect that all communications and records pertaining to his or her care will be treated as confidential by the hospital, except in cases such as suspected abuse and public health hazards when reporting is permitted or required by law.

7. The patient has the right to review the records pertaining to his or her medical care and to have the information explained or interpreted as necessary, except when restricted by law.

8. The patient has the right to expect that, within its capacity and policies, a hospital will make reasonable responses to the request of a patient for appropriate and medically indicated care and service.

9. The patient has the right to ask and be informed of the existence of business relationships among the hospital, educational institutions, other health care providers, or payers that may influence the patient's treatment or care.

10. The patient has the right to consent to or decline to participate in proposed research studies or human experimentation affecting care and treatment or requiring direct patient involvement, and to have those studies fully explained prior to consent.

11. The patient has the right to expect reasonable continuity of care when appropriate and to be informed by physicians and other caregivers of available and realistic patient care options when hospital care is no longer appropriate.

12. The patient has the right to be informed of hospital policies and practices that relate to patient care, treatment, and responsibilities.

assistant is considered to be an authorized person with access to the patient's file and information. This information may not be divulged without permission of the doctor or patient. The physician must be notified of any information the patient gives the medical assistant, such as the patient is not taking prescribed medications or complying with treatment (Figure 3-7).

Ethical Issues and Personal Choice

In some cases, the medical assistant may have a personal, religious, or ethical reason for wishing not to be involved in particular procedures, such as abortions or artificial insemination. This preference should be stated to the employer prior to employment, allowing for this information to be considered when making a hiring decision. In the event that the situation arises after employment begins, all concerns should be communicated to the employer immediately. It is very important not to judge what the physician is doing since he or she is acting within ethical guidelines. An individual should request to refrain from participating in the procedures in question if he or she has ethical doubts. If the medical assistant's choice to not assist the physician in a specific procedure jeopardizes the health and safety of a patient, or interferes with the physician's ability to do the procedures, it may be necessary to seek other employment.

Scientific Discovery and Ethical Issues

There are still many areas of medical ethics for which there are no conclusive answers. For instance, when should life support be withdrawn; when does a life begin; is euthanasia ever permissible; and should the

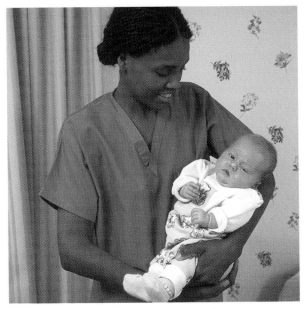

FIGURE 3-6 Patients of all socioeconomic backgrounds should be given equal care.

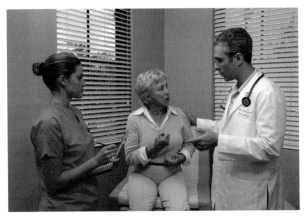

FIGURE 3-7 A medical assistant listening to the patient and physician discussing the patient's care.

unborn baby's life be sacrificed to save the mother? Scientific discoveries present new medical possibilities and choices every day. With these possibilities, there are often more complicated ethical issues to be addressed before choices can be made. The medical assistant has a responsibility to keep current on medical advances and form opinions based on sound medical ethics and practice.

SUMMARY

Medical law is based on the Hippocratic oath. Patients must be treated equally, using the best possible standards of care.

The medical and legal issues governing the medical profession and medical assistants are multifaceted. The medical assistant must be knowledgeable in many areas of the law. Laws governing medicine are different than those governing criminal behavior. Medicine is covered by civil law, often referred to as torts. It is both the physician's and the medical assistant's responsibility to be aware of these guidelines.

Chapter Review

COMPETENCY REVIEW

1. What are the elements of a contract?
2. Why is the Oath of Hippocrates still valid today?
3. Compare the principles of the AAMA or RMA with the AMA Principles of Medical Ethics.
4. What is informed consent?
5. Describe the medical assistant's responsibilities concerning medical ethics.
6. What is the difference between criminal and civil law?
7. List and describe the four Ds of negligence.
8. What are Good Samaritan laws, and how do they apply to you?
9. Why do you need thorough understanding of the law as it impacts your employer's practice?
10. State ten steps that can be taken to help protect the physician and staff from liability.

1. The earliest principles of ethical conduct, established to govern the practice of medicine, were known as
   A. Code of Hammurabi
   B. Code of Ethical Medical Practice
   C. Hippocratic oath
   D. AMA Principles of Medical Ethics
   E. Code of Medical Practice and Conduct

2. Medical ethics, by definition, refers to the
   A. regulations and standards established by the government
   B. moral conduct of medical professionals
   C. standards by which medical practice is deemed illegal
   D. ethical standards that are less severe than those required by law
   E. revocation of a physician's license to practice medicine

3. The Code of Ethics of the AAMA describes all of the following EXCEPT
   A. ethical conduct for the medical assistant
   B. moral conduct for the medical assistant
   C. a commitment to the patients to maintain their dignity and confidentiality
   D. a responsibility to improve the health and well-being of the community
   E. the legal responsibilities of the medical assistant

4. Which of the following falls INSIDE the medical assistant's standard of care?
   A. all medical assisting duties should always be under the direction of the treating physician
   B. the same standard of quality that is applicable to a physician in performing a procedure, for example, an ECG, is applicable to the medical assistant
   C. the medical assistant is allowed to, for example, prescribe over the counter medications
   D. the medical assistant is not responsible for giving physical exams
   E. the medical assistant must take a thorough medical history

5. What are the four types of written laws?
   A. misdemeanor, felony, civil, tort
   B. felony, tort, negligence, contract
   C. civil, tort, multi-national, governmental
   D. criminal, civil, tort, military
   E. civil, criminal, international, military

6. Performing surgery on a patient without the proper informed consent of the patient is an example of
   A. intentional tort
   B. abandonment
   C. breach of contract
   D. contribution negligence
   E. res ipsa loquitur

7. What might a physician be guilty of when, for example, a treatment that was below an acceptable standard of care was the direct cause of an injury?
   A. negligence
   B. malpractice
   C. abandonment
   D. A and B
   E. respondent superior

8. All actions must be carefully documented in a patient's medical chart. This would include all of the following EXCEPT
   A. calls and office visits
   B. office visits and treatments
   C. appointments and appointment cancellations
   D. personal opinions
   E. prescribed medications and their refills

9. Which, when signed by a patient, allows a representative to act on behalf of the patient in regards to medical treatment and care?
   A. durable power of attorney
   B. living will
   C. advanced directives
   D. the Uniform Anatomical Gift accord
   E. the Good Samaritan accord

10. Which statement(s) regarding patient/physician relationships is NOT true?
    A. Physicians have the right to select the patients they wish to treat.
    B. Patients expect that their physicians will use the appropriate "standard of care" in providing treatment.
    C. Consent refers to giving permission to treat.
    D. Patients can expect to receive information concerning both the advantages and potential risks of a given treatment.
    E. Patients can expect to have expensive treatment options withheld from them by their physician.

CRITICAL THINKING

1. What should Sue report to the physician?
2. Who should Sue report this to beside the physician?
3. Would Sue be legally responsible if she chooses to continue the billing practice?

ON THE JOB

Dr. Spring, a board certified obstetrician and gynecologist, has been in practice for more than ten years. He is licensed to practice medicine in both New York and Pennsylvania. Dr. Spring employs a staff that includes two medical assistants.

On Monday one of the medical assistants, Nancy Watts, took a history on a new patient that was referred to Dr. Spring by her internist. The 40-year old, married patient has had vaginal spotting for more than six weeks.

As part of the history, Nancy learned that the patient has been under the care and supervision of a fertility specialist for more than two years. In fact, although not always compliant, the patient has been on a medication treatment regime for fertility problems.

After examining the patient, Dr. Spring ordered a uterine biopsy to be performed in the office. The patient returns the following week, undergoes the biopsy and is sent home. Soon after, the patient's husband had telephoned the office, requesting to speak to Dr. Spring immediately. His wife had just been admitted to the hospital because of intense vaginal bleeding.

1. Was there anything in the patient's history that should have caused Nancy to alert the physician about performing a uterine biopsy?
2. Should Nancy have given this patient special instructions prior to the biopsy because of her history?
3. How should Nancy have handled the husband's telephone call?
4. Would it violate patient confidentiality to fax the patient's records to the emergency room physician, if requested?
5. Is this a potential case of medical negligence and malpractice? Could Nancy, as the medical assistant, have complicity in this particular case?

INTERNET ACTIVITY

Do an Internet search to explore the AAMA and AMA Web sites, especially concerning the code of ethics.

 MediaLink More on medical law and ethics, including interactive resources, can be found on the Student CD-ROM accompanying this textbook.

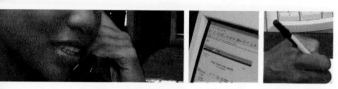

Medical Assistant Role Delineation Chart

HIGHLIGHT indicates material covered in this chapter.

ADMINISTRATIVE

Administrative Procedures

- Perform basic administrative medical assisting functions
- Schedule, coordinate and monitor appointments
- Schedule inpatient/outpatient admissions and procedures
- Understand and apply third-party guidelines
- Obtain reimbursement through accurate claims submission
- Monitor third-party reimbursement
- Understand and adhere to managed care policies and procedures
- *Negotiate managed care contracts*

Practice Finances

- Perform procedural and diagnostic coding
- Apply bookkeeping principles

- Manage accounts receivable
- *Manage accounts payable*
- *Process payroll*
- *Document and maintain accounting and banking records*
- *Develop and maintain fee schedules*
- *Manage renewals of business and professional insurance policies*
- *Manage personnel benefits and maintain records*
- *Perform marketing, financial, and strategic planning*

CLINICAL

Fundamental Principles

- Apply principles of aseptic technique and infection control
- Comply with quality assurance practices
- Screen and follow up patient test results

Diagnostic Orders

- Collect and process specimens
- Perform diagnostic tests

Patient Care

- Adhere to established patient screening procedures
- Obtain patient history and vital signs
- Prepare and maintain examination and treatment areas
- Prepare patient for examinations, procedures and treatments

- Assist with examinations, procedures and treatments
- Prepare and administer medications and immunizations
- Maintain medication and immunization records
- Recognize and respond to emergencies
- Coordinate patient care information with other health care providers
- Initiate IV and administer IV medications with appropriate training and as permitted by state law

GENERAL

Professionalism

- Display a professional manner and image
- Demonstrate initiative and responsibility
- Work as a member of the health care team
- Prioritize and perform multiple tasks
- Adapt to change
- Promote the CMA credential
- Enhance skills through continuing education
- Treat all patients with compassion and empathy
- Promote the practice through positive public relations

Communication Skills

- Recognize and respect cultural diversity
- Adapt communications to individual's ability to understand
- Use professional telephone technique

- Recognize and respond effectively to verbal, nonverbal, and written communications
- Use medical terminology appropriately
- Utilize electronic technology to receive, organize, prioritize and transmit information
- Serve as liaison

Legal Concepts

- Perform within legal and ethical boundaries
- Prepare and maintain medical records
- Document accurately
- Follow employer's established policies dealing with the health care contract
- Implement and maintain federal and state health care legislation and regulations
- Comply with established risk management and safety procedures
- Recognize professional credentialing criteria
- *Develop and maintain personnel, policy and procedure manuals*

Instruction

- Instruct individuals according to their needs
- Explain office policies and procedures
- Teach methods of health promotion and disease prevention
- Locate community resources and disseminate information
- *Develop educational materials*
- *Conduct continuing education activities*

Operational Functions

- Perform inventory of supplies and equipment
- Perform routine maintenance of administrative and clinical equipment
- Apply computer techniques to support office operations
- *Perform personnel management functions*
- *Negotiate leases and prices for equipment and supply contracts*

- *Denotes advanced skills.*

SOURCE: Reprinted by permission of the American Association of Medical Assistants from the AAMA Role Delineation Study: Occupational Analysis of the Medical Assisting Profession.

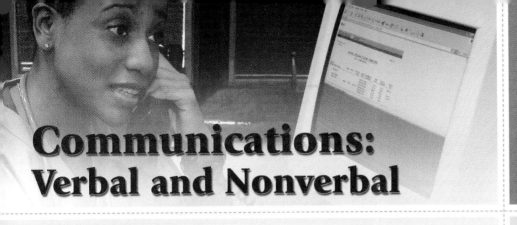

Communications: Verbal and Nonverbal

Learning Objectives

After reading this chapter, you should be able to:

- Define and spell the terms to learn for this chapter.

- Explain the importance of communication in health care today.

- Define the terms *values*, *attitudes*, and *behavior*, and explain their roles in self-awareness.

- Describe the communication process.

- Explain verbal and nonverbal communication.

- List several examples of nonverbal communication conveying impatience.

- List six guidelines for effective listening.

- Describe the difference between assertive and aggressive behavior.

- Describe two types of listening.

- List six types of defensive behavior, giving an example of each.

- Explain the importance of feedback in patient care.

Terms to Learn

active listening
aggressive
assertive
assessment
attitudes
auditory
behavior
bias
character
close-ended questions
condescending
culture

defensive behaviors
empathy
ethnicity
ethnocentric
feedback
hierarchy
Health Insurance Portability and Accountability Act (HIPAA)
holistic
kinesthetic
nonverbal communication

open-ended questions
passive listening
prejudice
rapport
risk management
stereotyping
sympathy
values
verbal communication
visual

Case Study

MARY BROWN IS A 78-YEAR-OLD NEW PATIENT in Dr. Barry's office. She is very anxious in any new situation. When she arrived a few minutes early for her appointment, she was unsure what to do. She approached the glass window, which was closed, and waited for several minutes; no one acknowledged her. Susan and the other medical assistants were all busy talking to one another and laughing at a comment someone had made.

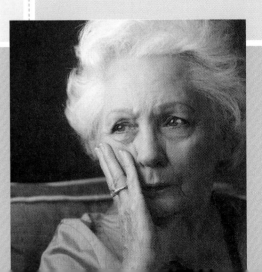

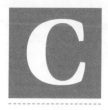Communication is a necessary requirement in any field, but is particularly essential in the health care field. As a medical assistant, you will relate to a variety of people, including sick and worried patients, your physician/employer, fellow staff members, vendors, and even some personal acquaintances of the physician. Some individuals you will interact with will be angry, frustrated, or simply ill and tired. Many patients who come into the physician's office or clinic will have physical or emotional problems that are not the main reason for their appointment. In addition, given the widely diverse population in the United States, you will be encountering people from a variety of countries and cultures. The medical assistant must be able to care for the entire patient in a holistic (viewing the overall situation) fashion and treat everyone with respect and courtesy.

It is not enough for the medical assistant to have excellent technical skills. Good interpersonal skills as well as good oral and written communication skills are needed to relate well to patients and fellow staff. In this chapter, you will learn about self-awareness and interpersonal dynamics. You will study the communication process, including directive techniques to improve effective communication, barriers to good communication, and defensive behaviors. Examining multicultural issues, communicating in special circumstances, and communicating with special needs patients will help you to be prepared for various situations you may encounter. Communication in the workplace, working as a member of a team, and understanding some conflict resolution strategies will help in your day-to-day work environment as well.

Interpersonal Dynamics

For the medical assistant to be able to provide effective communication in the delivery of health care, he or she must have a basic understanding of self. Why do you have the personality you exhibit? How do you communicate in everyday situations? Where do the impressions of others you hold originate? In other words, how did you get to be the person you are today? We will examine some concepts related to individuality and relationships with others.

Self-awareness

Understanding oneself and understanding the differences among others helps the medical assistant communicate more effectively. Personality is a sum of the traits, characteristics, and behaviors that makes us individuals. We all recognize different personalities, even among close family members.

Character is the sum of the values, attitudes, and behaviors a person exhibits. Psychologists tell us that values are a set of standards a person uses to measure the worth or importance of someone or something. Attitudes are opinions that develop from our value system. Values are acquired at home, in our family unit, and in the culture we live in and often are difficult to change. Prejudice, an opinion formed based on incorrect or irrational facts, is learned from experience and environment and colors our actions with others. An example of prejudice is viewing individuals with different skin color as inferior. Behavior, the actions others see, is based on our attitudes. To sum up, values form attitudes. Attitudes are reflected in behavior or actions that can be seen by others. Society prefers some behaviors and disapproves of others. For example, in the United States we are not permitted to have more than one spouse. In other cultures this is perfectly acceptable.

To be an effective communicator in all areas of our lives, it is important to look at our attitudes and our prejudices. How do others see us? How do we see ourselves? Examining ourselves leads to greater self-awareness and can lead to better communication skills. Patients and coworkers expect certain attitudes and professional behavior in the health care setting.

Life Stages

Understanding the stages of life through which we all pass will help the medical assistant be more sensitive to patients and their problems. Human growth and development refers not only to physical growth but also to emotional and psychological growth. Criteria, or norms, have been determined by professionals as guidelines to be used to ascertain development. The pace of development may differ widely and be irregular at times. Table 4-1 lists nine categories that make up the stages of life. Notice some corresponding characteristics listed along each stage.

Hierarchy of Needs

Along with recognizing the stages of development, it is important to understand Maslow's hierarchy, a ranked order of human needs. Psychologist Abraham Maslow established a ranking of human needs that is still widely used to help comprehend human behavior. Maslow maintained that people had needs and moved through various levels in achieving satisfaction in life. The hierarchy of needs is based on five elements or levels. These levels are:

Level I   Physiological needs such as food, water, and shelter.

Level II   Safety needs, which include physical safety as well as security—one's employment is associated with this level.

TABLE 4-1 The Nine Stages of Life

Infant (birth to 1 year)	Rapid physical growth, uncoordinated movements, may develop separation anxiety.
Toddler (1 to 2 years)	Less rapid growth, more coordination especially hands, begins walking speaking, quick mood changes.
Early childhood (3 to 5 years)	Grows taller, develops fine motor skills, becomes social, develops sense of self and body image.
Middle childhood (6 to 8 years)	Primary teeth lost, grows more slowly, begin cursive writing, begins to reason, friends are important.
Late childhood (9 to 12 years)	Muscles increase, secondary sexual signs begin, learns to communicate and compromise.
Adolescent (13 to 18 years)	Rapid physical growth, sexual maturation occurs, forms own identity, may rebel against authority.
Young adult (19 to 45 years)	Little physical growth, develops place in society, establishes family, life goals.
Middle age adult (46 to 65 years)	Aging changes occur, metabolism slows, earns most money, may question goals.
Older adult (66 years plus)	Declines in strength, slower neurological responses, hearing loss, less able to respond to stress, endures loss of family members, faces own death.

Level III Social needs, which include having a sense of belonging to a group and the need for social interaction.

Level IV Self-esteem, which includes having a sense of self-worth and pride.

Level V Self-actualization, which occurs when the individual achieves all he or she is capable of achieving and derives a sense of accomplishment.

Maslow said that he believed a person could not move to a higher level until the basic needs at a lower level were met. An understanding of Maslow's hierarchy of needs is important for the medical assistant since patients he or she will encounter daily are at different stages or levels of fulfillment of their needs.

For example, one patient may be at Level I and be concerned about how he or she will pay a medical bill. Another patient, whose Level II and Level III needs are met, may wish to see the physician about cosmetic surgery as the patient attempts to have his or her self-esteem (Level V) needs met. Patients who have life-threatening illness require that their Level II needs for future security be met. For an illustration of Maslow's hierarchy of needs, see Figure 4-1.

Health and the Mind-Body Connection

Psychologists have discovered that there is a link between stress and illness. There are predisposing factors that

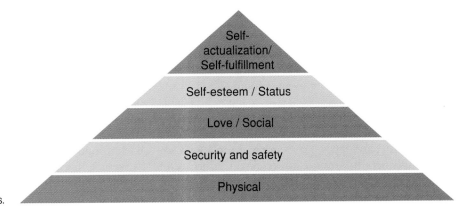

FIGURE 4-1 Maslow's hierarchy of needs.

create a tendency or susceptibility to becoming stresses. These include attitudes and feelings (emotions such as optimism or pessimism); health habits (smoking, exercise, drug use, and diet); the individual patient's methods for coping; economic and social resources; kind of job; sense of security; and the state of the patient's immune system.

The factors mentioned above also affect health care workers who have stress causing issues in their own lives and are dealing with patients who have many stress causing issues. Understanding stress factors and how to deal with them will make the medical assistant able to communicate more effectively and avoid burnout. *Burnout* is the result of experiencing prolonged periods of stress with no relief and can affect your health and career. For instance, a family member who cares for a patient with Alzheimer's disease and has no outside help may feel overwhelmed. Such a person may experience burnout and may also become ill.

Major life events, such as death of a loved one, divorce, an unexpected move away from family and friends, unemployment, or illness, can trigger stress. Some people who experience these life events may turn to unhealthy habits such as increased smoking or drinking. Others may exhibit negative behaviors such as anger outbursts, hostility, irritability, or depression. The following is a brief list of some ways to manage stress. They may be utilized by patients and caregivers alike.

- Develop a strong support system, including family and friends.
- Find a balance between striving for perfection and fear of failure.
- Eat nutritious meals.
- Avoid harmful habits such as smoking, drinking, and recreational drug use.
- Exercise regularly—walking, jogging, dancing, biking, and swimming.
- Look outward to develop social interests by understanding other people's problems and needs.
- Try to see the humor in situations.
- Limit the number of activities you engage in to a manageable few.
- Learn to budget time realistically.

Learning Styles

Examining the various styles of learning will help our self-awareness. Learning styles fall into several categories. Most of us learn by using a combination of the three styles with one style tending to be more dominant. There are three learning styles. The auditory (by hearing) learner is one who retains information better by hearing lectures, music, and tapes, for example. People who are auditory learners have difficulty retaining information presented in written format. The visual learner, as you would expect, learns better by seeing the information, by means of reading, drawings, diagrams, and films. Visual learners find it more difficult to follow lectures unless visual aids are used with the presentation. The kinesthetic (involving movement) learner learns better by hands-on activities such as experiments, games, lab exercises, and movement. Such people have difficulty grasping a procedure until they have performed it themselves. Understanding these learning styles will help prepare the medical assistant for his or her role as patient educator.

The Communication Process

The basic units of the communication process are the source, message, channel, and receiver. Think of this as the acronym S-M-C-R:

S   stands for the communication—who is sending the message?

M   represents the actual message or the actual words that are placed on paper if the message is in writing.

C   indicates the channel or channels through which the message moves from the source to the receiver. These channels include the senses: sight, smell, taste, hearing, and touch. Another set of channels consists of pathways like the telephone or interoffice mail.

R   stands for the receiver of the message.

For example, a physician (S) writes a prescription (M) that the medical assistant then reads over the telephone (C) to the pharmacist (R). If any link in this chain is broken, an incorrect message is relayed. The same holds true if you relay a message to a patient. If the medical assistant (S) explains a procedure (M) to a patient who has a hearing loss (C), then the patient (R) will not hear the message as it was intended.

The communication process, then, is a chain effect that requires a source (S) and a receiver (R). The source (S) acts upon a stimulus to encode or transmit a message (M) in a particular form. The actual message can be transmitted in a variety of ways (C), including face-to-face, over the telephone, or in written form. The receiver (R) decodes or translates the message, based on his or her emotional state, perceptions, education, socioeconomic background, and many other factors.

Add to this process, the ever-present background noises that are part of the daily functioning of a medical office, and keeping the channels of communication open is as much a daily task for the medical assistant as any other. Some examples of background noises are conversations between patients or patients and staff, background music, ringing telephones, or requests for assistance. Because of this background buzz, it is very possible that the receiver may not receive the message the sender intended.

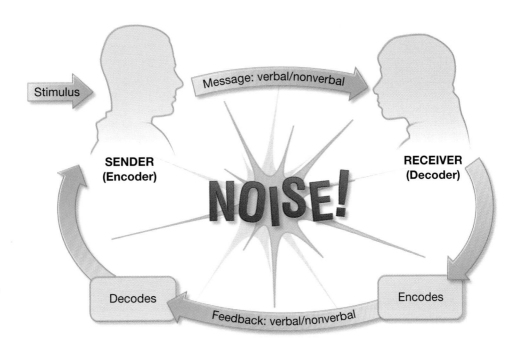

FIGURE 4-2 After face-to-face discussion, telephone conversations are probably the most frequently used channel of communication.

Channels of Communication

Channels of communication include the various means by which the spoken or written word is communicated from one person to another. Information is said to be "rich" if it conveys to the listener or reader the intent of the speaker. The greatest amount of information richness is gained from face-to-face discussion (Figure 4-2). The least amount of information is generally gained from formal numeric documents such as budget reports. When you wish to convey an important message to someone, it is better to do it face-to-face than to put the information into writing. This becomes important to remember when determining how to adequately educate patients regarding their medications. If you place all the important facts into a pamphlet, patients may never read it or might not understand your meaning. You need to consider the learning styles discussed previously and the fact that using a variety of styles better reinforces the message. However, it is important to give written instructions in addition to any verbal explanation you give the patient. Table 4-2 illustrates the varying degrees of "richness" of various information channels.

TABLE 4-2 Information Richness Channels

Information Channel	Level of Richness
Face-to-face discussion	Highest
Telephone conversations	High
Written letter/memos (individually addressed)	Moderate
Formal written documents (general bulletins or reports)	Low
Fax (facsimile)	Low
E-mail	Low
Internet	Low
Formal numeric document (printouts, budget reports)	Lowest

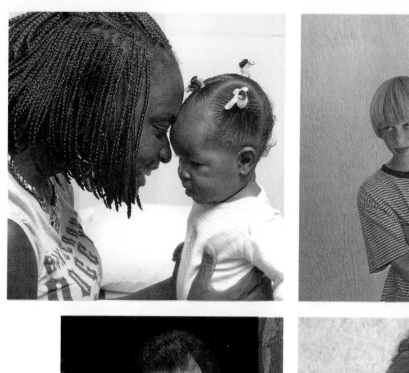
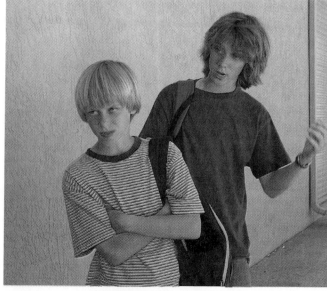
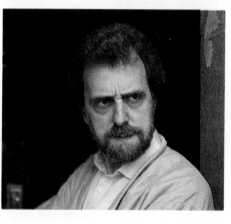
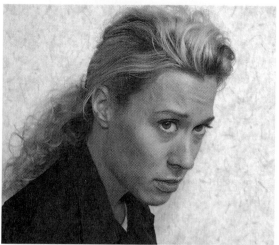

FIGURE 4-3 Nonverbal communications convey strong, powerful messages that may be negative or positive.

Verbal and Nonverbal Communication

Virtually everything a person does from birth to death is a form of communication. Smiling is a form of nonverbal communication, while talking "with a smile in your voice" is verbal communication. Nonverbal communication is the language of gesture and actions, including body language. In many cases, people are not even aware of the image they project with their bodies. The way a person holds his or her arms, makes eye contact, gestures, frowns, or turns toward or away from the speaker frequently conveys more than just words could convey (Figure 4-3). Box 4-1 offers some examples of messages that convey impatience.

Verbal Communication

Verbal communication depends on words and sounds or tone of voice. The sounds a person makes when

BOX 4-1

Communication Messages Conveying Impatience

- Interrupting people when they are speaking
- Answering telephone calls curtly
- Finishing another person's sentence
- Rushing the patient
- Eating lunch at your desk
- Looking at your watch or the clock
- Doing two things at once
- Not looking up from your work when someone approaches
- Rushing around the office

speaking cover a wide range and can convey vastly different meanings. The tone in which you speak to a patient is vitally important in making a positive impression on the patient and his or her family. Generally when someone is speaking, that person will raise his or her tone at the end of a statement when asking a question and drop the tone of voice when completing a sentence. When the speaker's tone drops it is appropriate to begin your part of the conversation. Interrupting speakers is a negative behavior that creates a barrier to good communication.

The medical assistant should speak loudly enough to be heard but not so loudly that a patient's confidentiality is compromised. Speaking clearly and properly pronouncing your words is important in conveying the message.

WORD SELECTION Choosing the right words to present a message is critical. We can all think of instances when we called a medical facility only to have been spoken to as though we were an annoyance to the person at the front desk. Other times, telephoning the medical assistant was a very pleasant experience and when the conversation was completed, we had a positive feeling. Sarcasm and ridicule have no place in the professional setting. The goal of the medical assistant is to promote an open, comfortable environment for the patient while keeping in mind that the patient is the customer. Choose your words carefully and take care not to be rude or impatient in your interpersonal relationships. See Lifespan Considerations for more on communicating with patients.

POSITIVE ATTITUDE The ability to convey a positive attitude is so important in working with people. Smiling immediately reassures the patient that he or she is welcome. When in the presence of a patient, always involve the patient in your conversation. Excluding the patient and talking "over his or her head" is disrespectful (Figure 4-4). If the conversation is of a business or confidential nature, it should be held elsewhere.

Effective medical assistants are able to demonstrate empathy but should be cautious about using sympathy for their patients. Empathy is the willingness or the ability to understand what the patient is feeling without necessarily experiencing the same thing. Sympathy, on the other hand, is feeling sorry for or pitying the patient. Patients react much better to an empathetic listener than to a sympathetic one. You can acquire the skill of empathetic listening using these simple nonverbal techniques: nodding, leaning toward the patient, or positioning yourself so you are at the patient's eye level, and indicating by your facial expression that you understand what he or she is saying (Figure 4-5).

Since we all share the same human emotions, there will be instances when you become distressed over a patient's situation. It is not possible to be a concerned health care provider and remain totally unemotional at all times. If you become upset, you can excuse yourself for a few moments. Realize that your emotions and concerns are another indication that you have chosen the correct field.

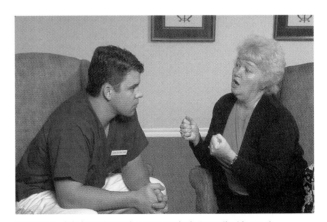

FIGURE 4-4 It is important to be concerned when a patient is upset.

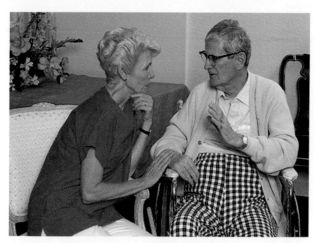

FIGURE 4-5 Empathy draws a more positive response from the patient since it is based on the willingness of the medical assistant to understand what the patient is experiencing.

Nonverbal Communication

Nonverbal communication involves facial expressions, gestures, body language, eye contact, good grooming, and mannerisms. It is important that verbal and nonverbal messages agree. Body language is learned by imitation, by being taught, and by instinct. For example, consider the hand gestures that are a normal part of communication among individuals from Italy and other Mediterranean countries. Appearance is a nonverbal form of communication. Patients expect certain types of behaviors, attitudes, and appearance in the health care setting. Unprofessional attire, visible tattoos, and overpowering perfume send a negative message. See Professionalism for more on maintaining a professional appearance.

The gesture of touch is considered a form of nonverbal communication and a form of body language. Gently touching a distraught patient's arm can reassure and comfort the patient. However, one must be cautious that the receiver does not misinterpret a

Professionalism

As a health care representative, the medical assistant should set a good example. The medical assistant sets the first impression of the office and is in many ways, the marketing representative of the practice. The medical assistant must always present a professional appearance. Good personal hygiene and grooming is a must. Nails should be kept short and unpolished, and jewelry should be kept to a minimum.

touch. In some cultures, for instance, it is considered rude to touch a child's head without permission. At times, abused children can be fearful of even innocent touching. Use caution when touching a patient unless you know him or her well.

Communication Techniques

The ability to encourage a patient to communicate effectively is critical when you wish to perform a patient assessment or evaluation to determine the patient's problems. For example, how are you to stop a patient who is talking about seemingly irrelevant issues? First of all, it is important to understand that the patient is nervous. Before we discuss specific techniques, there are several questions we need to consider as we examine the overall communication process. Each communication experience has unique qualities and must be considered carefully.

- What is the goal of your communication?
- What message do you want to give?
- What channel are you going to deliver (face-to-face, written, etc.)?
- How are you going to listen to the response (listening and observational skills)?
- How are you going to get clarification/feedback?
- Was your goal met or do you need to revise the message (assess or evaluate)?

Listening Skills

Listening involves verbal and nonverbal cues. The medical assistant must pay attention to both. Listening is either active or passive. Active listening involves paying attention to the speaker completely, concentrating on the verbal message, observing for nonverbal cues, and offering a response. It is difficult in a medical office to actively listen at times when so many things are happening at once. One skill you will gain with experience is the ability to prioritize simultaneous events. Passive listening is simply listening to someone without having to reply, such as when you are listening as a member of an audience. How we hear a message is often colored by the message being delivered. If it is criticism of your work and you disagree, you hear it one way. If it is praise for your work, you hear it another way. Sometimes we are formulating a response before the speaker is finished with his or her message. In either circumstance, the listener's mind or thoughts may wander and the message may not be delivered effectively or may be distorted. Part of effective listening is to know when it is your turn to speak and allowing enough time for the message to be completed. With

PROCEDURE

Effective Listening Skills

OBJECTIVE: Use effective listening skills to obtain chief complaint from a patient.

Equipment and Supplies
patient history form

Method
1. Identify patient.
2. Ask patient the reason for current appointment.
3. Smile and establish eye contact.
4. Seat the patient in appropriate area.
5. Focus full attention on patient.
6. Ask open-ended questions.
7. Do not interrupt patient.
8. Provide feedback by paraphrasing what the patient said.
9. Observe patient for signs of needing to give more information.
10. Restate the chief complaint before leaving patient.
11. Conclude patient interview in appropriate manner.
12. Document the chief complaint with 100% accuracy.

practice we can become good listeners. Procedure 4-1 provides steps to practice with fellow students and to employ with patients. The following are some guidelines for good listening:

- Avoid distractions.
- Face the speaker.
- Give the person your full attention.
- Maintain eye contact as suitable for culture.
- Do not be judgmental about what is said.
- Be aware of nonverbal cues.
- Note anything that seems unclear.
- Do not interrupt.
- Maintain personal space.
- Ask questions if you do not understand.

Directive Communication Techniques

The medical assistant can often assist the communication process by directing the patient's comments, using specific communication techniques so that the sharing between the patient and the medical assistant is productive.

Types of Questions

Asking questions to deliver a message and to obtain information is a directive technique. The medical assistant will be asking many questions of the patient. It is helpful to keep in mind the goal of your question before you choose the type of question to ask. Four types of questions will be discussed.

CLOSE-ENDED QUESTIONS Close-ended questions can be answered with a yes or a no. Often these types of questions are appropriate to obtain background information, such as "Is your mother still living?" However, there may be times when you ask a patient, "Do you understand what I mean," and the patient will answer, "yes" even if he or she does not comprehend what you are saying. Usually this happens because the patient does not want to be a "bother" or appear stupid. You need to consider the situation carefully when you use close-ended questions.

OPEN-ENDED QUESTIONS Open-ended questions, those that require more than yes or no responses, can be useful in gaining feedback or drawing out patient information. Using such questions or directive methods, you will be able to obtain information the physician will require to treat the patient. See Table 4-3 for a list of other directive communication techniques, including a description and an example of each technique.

PROBING QUESTIONS Probing questions are used to ask the patient for further information to more fully discuss the subject. For example, if a patient says, "My head hurts" a probing question would ask, "Where does it hurt?" or "How long have you had this pain?" In this example, other probing questions would seek information about type of pain, when it started, and when it occurs. The medical assistant is often the person the patient feels more comfortable speaking to and questioning. It is important to be empathetic and try to put the patient at ease.

TABLE 4-3   Directive Communication Techniques

Technique	Description	Example
Open-ended statement	Encourage the patient to discuss freely.	"Please describe your pain for me."
Closed-ended statement	Direct the patient to make a yes/no or simple response.	"Are you having pain?"
Reflecting	Direct the conversation back to the patient by repeating the patient's words.	Patient: "I'm afraid of what the doctor will find." MA: "You're afraid of what the doctor will find?"
Acknowledgment	Indicate understanding.	"I understand what you are saying."
Restating	State what the patient has said but in different terms.	Patient: "I can't sleep." MA: "You say you're having trouble getting to sleep at night?"
Add to an implied statement	Verbalize implied information.	Patient: "I'm usually relaxed." MA: "And today you're not relaxed?"
Seek clarification	Request more information in order to better understand.	Patient: "I don't feel good." MA: "Tell me what your symptoms are."
Silence	Remain silent or make no gesture in response to a statement.	Patient: I don't know what's wrong but something is."

LEADING QUESTIONS   Leading questions are those questions in which part of the answer is in the question. For example, when asked, "Do you have to urinate two, three, or four times a night?" the patient then has to select one answer from your choices. This may be helpful in dealing with patients who do not understand English. However, the medical assistant must be careful not to ask the specific type of leading question in order to get the exact answer he or she desires.

Feedback

Feedback, any response to a communication, is critically important when working with patients since you must determine if they really understand what they have heard. Feedback can be either verbal or nonverbal. Sometimes the verbal message and the nonverbal message that patients send do not agree. For instance, as a medical assistant you may ask, "How are you feeling?" and the patient might state, "Fine." Since the patient is walking with a painful limp, you doubt the verbal statement. Always try to ask specific questions such as, "Do you have pain?" "Tell me about your medication," or "Tell me what you need to see the doctor about." When documenting the information

that the patient provides, use the patient's words, not yours.

REFLECTING   Reflecting is a directive technique in which you mirror the patient's message back to the individual to ensure that you have understood him or her correctly. For example, you may say in response to a patient who needs an appointment, "You say you can't come in on Wednesdays?" The reflecting technique is also helpful in resolving conflicts, clearing up confusing statements, and requires more detail from the other person.

RESTATING   Restating or paraphrasing is repeating the patient's message to him or her in your own words. For example, "I heard you say that you will not be able to pay your bill this month. Is that correct?" This technique helps to confirm that both parties understand the message clearly.

CLARIFICATION   The ultimate goal in effective communication is to deliver the message so it is understood clearly. Clarification is a directive technique in which the medical assistant requests more information in order to better understand what the patient has stated. Many times patients use words such as "a lot" or "much worse" in explaining their symptoms. It is important to ask them to be more specific in order to accurately diagnose or treat them. For example, the patient says, "My right arm hurts a lot." The medical assistant should employ the directive techniques mentioned to clarify this information

The following questions are examples of follow-up questions and statements useful in this situation: "You say that your right arm hurts. Is that correct? Where on your arm do you feel the pain? What kind of pain is it? When did it start? Does it hurt all the time? Are you able to sleep? Are you taking any medications for the pain?"

Assertive versus Aggressive Behavior

Most instances of communication within the work setting involve convincing someone else to cooperate with you. Whether patient or staff communication is your goal, the methods to achieve cooperation are the same. As a medical assistant there are occasions when you will have to convince both patients and staff to listen to you. Using assertive behavior techniques can make this easier.

Being assertive means that you make a point in a positive manner by standing firm, making decisions based on your principles or values, and trusting you own ideas or instincts in the situation. Being aggressive, on the other hand, is trying to impose your point of view on others or trying to manipulate others. Aggressiveness is considered a negative behavior and indicates a type of pushiness when trying to convince others. In fact, it has been compared to making a

verbal attack against another. Many people resort to aggressive behavior in order to impose their ideas on others or when they are angry or fearful. Aggressive people are bossy and inconsiderate of the feelings of others. See Table 4-4 for a comparison of assertive and aggressive behavior.

Assertive Behavior Techniques

Acquiring the ability to use assertive behavior means that you will learn to offer new ideas or even unwanted ideas to people in such a manner that they will not feel threatened. Some assertive behaviors include being direct and honest, using positive body language, and using "I" statements such as "I feel." For instance, when calling a patient regarding nonpayment of a bill you will need to gain the patient's acceptance. The patient may become angry at the beginning of the conversation in response to an aggressive comment, such as "Are you aware that your bill is now two months overdue? When are you going to pay it?" He or she could become defensive and hang up. Since most patients know when they have not paid a bill, it is not necessary to use threatening language. A better approach would be to identify yourself and indicate that you are helping Dr. Thompson with his billings. In a calm but assertive manner, you would ask questions that would prompt a positive response from the patient. These questions might include, "How can I help you in clearing up these payments? Perhaps we can discuss your making a small payment on your account twice a month. What would be an amount that you could afford?"

Assertive Behavior Guidelines

Assertiveness is a learned skill that helps one to maintain self-confidence under stressful conditions. The basis for assertiveness is that everyone has the

---

TABLE 4-4 Comparison of Assertive and Aggressive Behavior

Assertive Behavior	Aggressive Behavior
"This medication works best when it is taken on a regular daily basis."	"You know you can't expect this medication to work when you're not taking it every day."
"Let me find someone who can answer that question for you."	"That's not my job."
"Your behavior is inappropriate."	"Why did you do that? It was stupid."
Knocking on door and then coming into an exam to say: "Excuse me, Dr. Thompson, you are needed on the telephone."	Rushing into an exam room to say: "Doctor, you've got a telephone call."

right to express opinions or beliefs in an appropriate, respectful manner without fear of being humiliated or made to feel guilty. Aggressiveness results in violation of a person's right during communication. The results of aggressive behavior are resentment and loss of respect. To practice assertive behavior use the following steps:

- Take a few deep breaths to calm yourself.
- Describe the behavior that you would like the other person to change in unemotional tones.
- Describe how you feel when the behavior occurs.
- State the positive behavior you would like to see.
- Describe the consequences that will result if the person does not change his or her behavior.
- Consequences must be appropriate, reasonable, and enforceable.
- Follow through with consequences if the behavior does not change.
- Commend the individual for the behavioral change.
- Evaluate your confrontation.

Discussing Sensitive Issues

Discussing issues involving money, such as the patient's bill and personal financial responsibility, can be very sensitive. Patients should be advised before the first visit of physician's charges for specific services or treatment. Inquiries regarding patient's medical insurance and procedure for payment of fees should also be reviewed prior to the first visit. Complying with the federal regulations regarding the patient's right to privacy of all health related information should be addressed at the first visit. The Health Insurance Portability and Accountability Act (HIPAA), is a federal act designed to improve portability and continuity of health insurance coverage; to combat waste, fraud, and abuse in health insurance and health care delivery; to promote the use of medical savings accounts; to improve access to long-term care services and coverage; to simplify the administration of health insurance and ensure the privacy of personal health information and appropriate release of that information. The medical assistant should have each patient sign a release of information form on his or her first visit.

Always consider a patient's feelings when asking questions within hearing distance of others. If questions involve personal patient health care information, HIPAA requires that the medical assistant inquire about these issues in private, where others will not overhear it. When telephoning a patient you must keep in mind that all conversation about personal health care information must be private.

The Customer-Friendly Environment

Using good interpersonal skills to set a positive environment in the health care setting generates a customer-friendly atmosphere and comfortable workplace. A warm, friendly greeting, showing respect to the patient, being sincere and sensitive, and demonstrating empathy can help set a positive tone.

Greeting Patients

A patient should be greeted within one minute of entering the office. If you are speaking on the telephone when the patient comes in, be sure to acknowledge the patient's presence with a smile and nod. Give your full attention to the patient as soon as you complete the telephone conversation.

Barriers to Communication

There are many barriers to communication. Identifying and overcoming these barriers is essential for effective communication. Some are obvious barriers, such as the distraction of loud background noise, and can be eliminated by the medical assistant. However, there are other barriers that we are not even aware of that result in either no communication or a distorted message being received. In order to understand the patient, you must overcome the barriers to effective communication (Figure 4-6).

Giving the patient false reassurance that "everything will be all right" can result in the patient's reluctance to talk to you about personal or health related fears. Such comments can also lead to liability issues for the physician if the patient believes that a promise for recovery has been made. See Legal and Ethical Issues.

The medical assistant may also put up barriers to communication without meaning to. These include not looking at the patient when he or she is speaking, interrupting the patient, abruptly changing the subject,

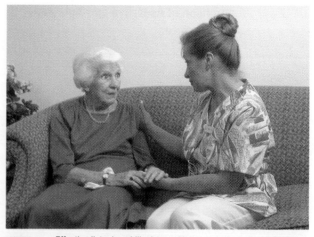

FIGURE 4-6 Effective listening skills demonstrates empathy to the patient and breaks down barriers to communication.

and using meaningless statements to soothe the patient, just to name a few. Medical assistants must remember that the patient is coming to see the physician because he or she has a problem. Patients should never be treated in a condescending manner.

Defensive Behaviors

Patients will also put up barriers to effective communication when they are under the stress of illness. These barriers are called defensive behaviors. A defensive behavior is a reaction to a perceived threat that is usually unconscious. Defensive behaviors are also referred to as coping behaviors. Not all coping behaviors are defensive or have a negative impact. For example, when trying to meet a deadline, you may have learned that using good time management skills and prioritizing tasks permits you to reach the deadline. Coping mechanisms are learned either consciously or unconsciously. As a member of the health care team, you need to be aware of your defensive behaviors in the professional setting at home. Some defensive behaviors are discussed in Table 4-5.

Use of Medical Language

You will become adept at understanding the language of medicine. The abbreviations that are used in medicine are a form of communication for people working in the health care field. However, your patients have little understanding of medical terminology. You may wish to teach patients a few simple terms so that they can better understand the physician's instructions on prescriptions. Otherwise, you must make an effort to avoid using medical terminology or abbreviations when speaking with patients. For example, abbreviations such as "NPO," meaning nothing by mouth, are not readily recognized or understood by patients. Always write out or state clear instructions regarding preparations for tests and taking medications. Patients may be reluctant to admit they do not understand. You will then assume that they have been properly instructed which is not the case. Failure to inform patients in terms they are able to understand could be construed as negligence on the part of the health care provider and increase the risk of a lawsuit.

Multicultural Issues

As a medical assistant, you will come in contact with people from many different cultures. A culture consists of the values, beliefs, attitudes, and customs shared by a group of people and passed on through the generations. Behaviors exhibited by the members of a culture are based on their beliefs and values. Health care beliefs may differ widely from those which we are accustomed. The medical assistant must be tolerant in attitude, not condescending, and treat each patient with empathy and respect. The medical assistant will encounter cultural diversity when interacting with individuals

Legal and Ethical Issues

Medical assistants must use caution when communicating with patients. Providing false hopes for recovery or implying that the physician may be able to cure a patient is not only unethical but can also result in liability for the physician and the medical assistant.

Putting incidents in writing also involves careful thought and caution. It is important to chart exactly what occurred and what the patient stated rather than the medical assistant's feelings about the situation. Recording the patient's comment, "I have an overwhelming feeling of hopelessness," is a better indication of the patient's emotional state than the comment, "I think the patient is depressed." This last comment reflects the medical assistant's judgment of the patient's appearance or what the patient said, not what the patient has said about himself or herself. As with everything that transpires in the medical environment, the HIPAA regulations must be kept in mind.

from other cultures. Cultural diversity presents its own set of barriers to effective communication. See Cultural Considerations for more on dealing with individuals from different cultures.

Language

A non-English speaking patient is at a disadvantage when trying to obtain health care. Imagine for a minute how you would feel if you were traveling in a foreign country and had an accident that required you to go to the hospital. Not only would you not understand anyone in the hospital, but also, their health care practices might be very different. The feelings of fear, frustration, and confusion you would feel would be augmented if you had no one with you to act as an interpreter.

You will encounter patients and other health care workers who speak a wide variety of languages. However, Hispanics make up the largest non-English speaking group in the United States today. It would be helpful for you to learn a few phrases and some simple words in the patient's language to help communicate with the patient and coworkers. If at all possible, you should try to get someone to interpret for the patient. Perhaps a fellow worker or family member would be able to help. If a patient has a limited ability to understand English, speak slowly and clearly, using simple

TABLE 4-5 **Defensive Behaviors**

Behavior	Description	Example
Compensation	Substitution of an attitude, feeling, or behavior with its opposite.	Mrs. Matthews believes the lump in her breast is cancer. However, she smiles and laughs whenever you talk to her about it.
Denial	Unconsciously avoiding an unwanted feeling or situation.	Mr. Morgan cancels an appointment to have a PSA (blood) test for prostate cancer in spite of having symptoms associated with prostate trouble.
Displaced anger	Expressing angry feelings toward persons or objects that are unrelated to the problem.	Mrs. Matthews is angry at being diagnosed with cancer. She takes this anger out on her family members.
Disassociation	Not connecting one event with another.	Mary Sims is a nurse who works with alcoholic patients. In her free time she drinks to excess.
Introjection	Adopting the feeling of someone else.	Mr. Morgan's friends have said that the PSA test is reliable and could relieve his anxiety about having prostate cancer. He believes them and has the test.
Projection	Placing your own feelings onto another person.	Mr. Morgan becomes irritated when the medical assistant calls to remind him of his appointment. He wrongly decides that she is irritated with him or dislikes him. In reality, he is upset with himself.
Rationalization	Justifying thoughts or behavior to avoid the truth.	Mary Sims believes that the appetite suppressant benefit of smoking offsets the risk of developing cancer.
Regression	Turning back to former behavior patterns in times of stress.	Jimmy, who is toilet trained, reverts to bedwetting during hospitalization.
Repression	Keeping unpleasant thoughts or feelings out or one's mind.	Mr. Morgan denies any urinary frequency when questioned by the physician.
Sublimation	Directing or changing unacceptable drives for security, affection or power into socially or culturally acceptable channels.	Mrs. Matthews is worried about having cancer and uses up energy cleaning her house.

words or phrases. Smiling and other positive nonverbal cues are helpful. Use pictures if they are available. It will help you be more tolerant if you put yourself in the patient's position for a moment.

Culture

People from other cultures have different views and customs relating to health care delivery. Our views and customs are not better than theirs, just different. They may have different views about the causes of illness, treatments, and the expected behavior of the health care provider. In some cultures, illness is thought to be caused by winds or forces, blood being too thick or thin, or the ill will of others.

Encouraging patients from a different culture to relate their symptoms and signs to you may be another problem. They may feel that to talk about pain is a sign of weakness or to mention psychological problems is

Cultural Considerations

Medical assistants must work with and provide care for individuals from a wide variety of racial, ethnic, cultural, religious, and socioeconomic backgrounds. In every instance, it is important to respect the individuality of everyone. Patients from other cultures may be completely unfamiliar with the Western model of medical treatment. When communicating with others who are different from ourselves we must avoid prejudging or generalizing about them. The following are just a few examples of cultural concepts or traditions you as a medical assistant may encounter: nodding the head up and down means yes to us, but it means no in some other cultures; touching someone in certain areas of the body is not permissible in some cultures; shaving body hair to prepare the patient for a procedure is not permitted in some cultures; eye contact is not acceptable in some cultures.

not permitted. One of the duties of the medical assistant is to help ensure that the patient complies with the treatment physicians prescribe whether it is in the form of medication or therapy or diagnostic examinations. It may be necessary to ask for assistance from a family member who understands the issues and can communicate more easily. See Table 4-6 for a list of some diverse cultural traditions.

Bias, Prejudice, and Stereotyping

Bias, prejudice, and stereotyping are barriers to effective communication that directly relate to cultural diversity. In order to understand these barriers, a few more definitions are in order. We defined culture as the values, attitudes, and behaviors peculiar to a group of people. Ethnicity is a classification of people based on national origin. People from the same ethnic background share similar traditions, beliefs, and language. We have all heard street names that are negative in connotation being used to describe people of specific national origin. Stereotyping results when negative generalities concerning specific characteristics of a group are applied unfairly to an entire population. Race is a classification of people based on their physical or

TABLE 4-6   **Cultural Traditions in Health Care**

Country	Sick Care Practices	Health Care Beliefs	Family Role in Care
China	Holistic and traditional includes acupuncture, herbal medicine.	Upset in body energy causes disease. Stigma attached to mental illness. Health promotion important.	Family takes care of sick even in hospital.
Former Soviet Union	Holistic, folk, and Western medical practices.	Health promotion is important. Acute sick care practiced, rehabilitation not stressed.	Family members provide care in hospital: bathing, feeding, linen change.
Philippines	Health promotion important. Mental illness a disgrace. Evil can cause illness through eyes on another.	Family may give hospital care.	Children feel obligated to care for elderly.
Vietnam	Magical and religious health care practices. Eastern, herbal medicine important. Self-care and self-medication used to treat illness.	Acute sick care only. Believe health is restoration of yin/yang and hot/cold balance.	Patient care is a family responsibility.

biological characteristics such as skin color, shape of eyes, hair, bone structure, or facial features. Race is often used to classify people unfairly and unjustly in a negative way. Bias is an unfair preference or dislike of something. A bias prevents an impartial opinion of someone or something. People who are ethnocentric believe that their cultural background is better than any other. This leads to prejudice or prejudging and stereotyping, which impact negatively on communication and acceptance of others in all relationships. To avoid these negative behaviors the medical assistant should:

- Be aware of his or her beliefs.
- Learn as much as possible about other cultures, races, and nationalities.
- Be sensitive to the feelings of others.
- Evaluate information before accepting it as a belief.
- Avoid ethnic jokes.
- Be open to differences.

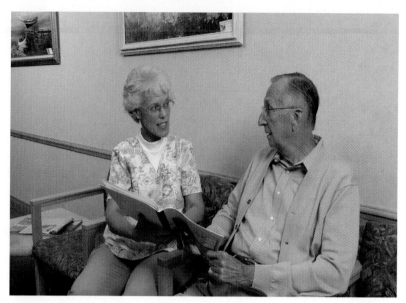

FIGURE 4-7 The medical assistant often has to reassure and comfort the patient before effective communication can take place.

Communication in Special Circumstances

The medical assistant will encounter special circumstances in the office when dealing with patients. At times, you will meet an angry patient, a patient who is terminally ill, one who is anxious, who is visually or hearing impaired, or who is mentally or emotionally impaired. Each of these types of patients must be treated with respect, empathy, and professionalism.

The Angry Patient

One of the most difficult communication problems involves the angry patient. It can be a difficult task for the medical assistant to refrain from taking the patient's comments personally. People have different styles and coping behaviors when they are frightened (Figure 4-7). Many patients who enter the physician's office are fearful of the diagnosis they may hear. Some patients become frightened of the equipment in the office or have an unwarranted fear of pain. In addition to fear, another cause of anger is loss of control. Many of us have had this feeling when we were hospitalized as a patient.

The job of the medical assistant is to remain calm and use positive communication and professional techniques to direct the patient's anger into a positive channel. Try to defuse the patient's anger. For instance, many patients will gain control over their anger when the medical assistant offers a comment such as, "I'm really sorry you feel this way. Let's see if we can solve the problem." You may have to take the patient into a private office if you cannot calm the patient immediately. Disruptive patients can upset others waiting to see the physician. While it is not necessary to give in to the unreasonable demands of a patient, realize that an upset patient is often expressing the need for you to listen carefully, without judging, and assist in solving the problem. Whenever possible, try to direct the patient's comments to the solution of the problem.

In the case of an angry caller, you must remember that no matter how angry a patient becomes, you cannot respond in anger. The role of the medical assistant is to assess or evaluate the situation. Remain calm and speak to the patient in a quiet, calm tone of voice, projecting your concern for the patient in the present situation. Often this will be enough to calm the patient down. If it does not work, however, ask your supervisor or office manager for assistance. Otherwise, ask the patient if you may return the call after you have been able to gather more information that will enable you to be of help.

In the case of a patient who becomes abusive or violent, you need to obtain assistance to protect yourself, other staff, and patients. Once the incident has been resolved, be sure to document it appropriately according to office policies.

The Anxious Patient

Many patients exhibit what is known as "white coat" syndrome. Whenever they have to encounter anyone in a white uniform, they become extremely anxious. Some signs of anxiety are trembling, flushing, perspiring, fidgeting, talking excessively, and remaining unusually quiet. Hypertensive patients who suffer from "white coat" syndrome should have their blood pressure measured at the beginning and the end of the visit to get a more representative value. To deal with anxious patients, use the communication skills you have learned in this chapter: speak calmly, reassure patients, smile, touch them respectfully on the hand, and be empathetic.

Patients with Special Needs

Meeting the needs of these patients requires some extra sensitivity, patience, and empathy on the part of the medical assistant. We will consider several types of patients individually along with some procedural guidelines.

The Hearing Impaired Patient

Hearing loss can vary from a slight loss to total deafness. Total hearing impairment is considered by many to be the most difficult of all handicaps since it keeps people isolated from communication and social interaction. If a child cannot hear, he or she will have difficulty speaking since learning speech involves imitating speech of others. Many such people communicate by means of sign language. Basic sign language is not difficult to learn. Simple phrases in sign language should be a part of every medical professional's knowledge base.

The manner in which you try to communicate will differ depending on whether the patient has a hearing aid, can lip-read, or has a family member or aid with him or her. Loss of hearing is a normal but frustrating sign of aging. The following are some guidelines to help the hearing impaired.

- Select a quiet environment to communicate with the patient.
- Reduce outside noise as much as possible.
- Never shout. Speak slowly and clearly.
- If the patient does not understand you the first time, rephrase the statement.
- Explain everything carefully before performing a procedure.
- Face the patient when speaking.
- Have a paper and pen available so that the patient can communicate in writing.

Basic hearing tests or screening tests are often performed by the medical assistant in the physician's office. An audiogram may be ordered by the physician when there is a suspicion of moderate to severe hearing loss. This test will determine the faintest sounds a patient can hear during audiometric testing. Audiometric testing, conducted by an audiologist, tests hearing ability by determining the lowest and highest intensity and frequencies that a person can distinguish. The patient may sit in a soundproof booth and receive sounds through earphones as the technician decreases the sounds or tones. Procedure 4-2 provides the steps for you to employ with the hearing impaired patient.

4-2 | **PROCEDURE**

Assisting the Hearing Impaired Patient

OBJECTIVE: Use effective communication skills to assist a hearing impaired patient prepare for a physical examination.

Equipment and Supplies
none

Method
1. Identify patient.
2. Reduce external noise as much as possible.
3. Smile and establish eye contact and face patient.
4. Speak slowly and do not shout.
5. Provide careful explanation of procedure.
6. Provide paper and pencil for patient to use if desired.
7. Use written information for the patient to reinforce message.
8. Have patient repeat your response to ensure accuracy of message, if possible.
9. Give directions using actions as well as words.
10. Be sensitive to patient's needs.
11. Employ an empathetic, professional attitude.
12. Notify physician of patient's concerns.

The Visually Impaired Patient

Blindness can be present at birth or may develop as a result of a disease such as diabetes mellitus. Patients who are blind can remain independent. The visually impaired patient cannot rely on nonverbal cues that make up much of the communication process for those with sight. The medical assistant can communicate and help the vision impaired patient by remembering to follow the guidelines suggested.

- Always speak to announce your presence when you are near a blind person.
- Offer to guide the patient into the examination room by offering your arm. Do not grab the patient without offering your arm first.
- Face the patient and speak clearly.
- Describe the patient's surroundings.
- Explain all procedures in detail before beginning.
- Try not to leave the patient alone for any length of time.
- Have available large print educational materials for patients who might benefit from them.
- Do not be condescending toward the patient.

The Terminally Ill Patient

The medical assistant will come into contact with patients who have a terminal illness. A terminal illness is one that is expected to end in death. This includes conditions and diseases such as cancer, acquired immune deficiency syndrome (AIDS), progressive heart disease, amyotrophic lateral sclerosis (Lou Gehrig's disease), cystic fibrosis, and multiple sclerosis. In such cases in which the dying process is slow for the patient, the medical assistant may encounter the patient on several office visits. While there is always hope for recovery or finding a cure through research for a disease such as AIDS, it is wise to listen to a patient express his or her fears and concerns rather than to offer false hope for a recovery. Death is a natural process that everyone must face. People have different ways of coping with death based on a variety of influences including culture, religion, personal experience, and age.

Religious, Cultural, and Personal Experience

People learn what their own culture expects of them at a very early age by observing family and friends as they handle life events such as births and deaths. In some cultures, death is considered a normal end to the life process and accepted with peace. In others, death may be feared. The terminally ill patient and family may have already established a very personal approach or method for handling death and dying. The medical assistant may also have a strong cultural attitude toward death.

Religious beliefs play an important role in the manner patients handle death and dying. Some patients will have a strong belief in an afterlife. Other patients will follow no particular religious belief. In both cases, the patient's death and dying process can be meaningful and peaceful. It is considered unacceptable for the medical assistant to attempt to convert the patient to the medical assistant's religious faith. Professionalism mandates that the medical assistant and other staff members recognize and support the patient's right to embrace his or her own religious beliefs. Table 4-7 provides a comparison of religious beliefs about birth, death, and health care practices.

The past experiences of the patient and the medical assistant will mold how they approach the topic of death. If the patient has been closely involved with the care of someone who has died a painful death, the patient may fear the same type of death for himself or herself. These patients will need to be able to discuss their fears. In the same manner, if the medical assistant has had past experiences with the death of friends or relatives, it may be easier for him or her to assist the patient.

The Stages of Grief

Dr. Elizabeth Kübler-Ross devoted much of her life to the study of the dying process and to working with dying patients. She divided the dying process into five stages that she believed all persons go through. It is helpful to understand these stages when attempting to help the dying patient. According to Kübler-Ross, all those involved with the dying process may go through five stages. This would include the patient, family members, and caregivers (such as the medical assistant).

The five stages are denial, anger, bargaining, depression, and acceptance. The stages may overlap and may not be experienced by everyone in the stated order but are all present in the dying patient according to Kübler-Ross. The five stages are discussed in Table 4-8.

As the time of death approaches, some of the earlier stages may be repeated. For example, patients may become angry when they are not able to care for themselves. The critical point to remember when assisting a patient who is dying is that the grieving period is a normal part of the dying process. At no time should the medical assistant try to tell the patient, "Don't feel that way." A patient has a right to have his or her feelings accepted unconditionally.

Hospice care, which is physical and emotional care provided to the dying person and his or her family, is a growing movement throughout the United States. The medical assistant should be acquainted with this option of care for the terminally ill.

The Mentally/Emotionally Impaired Patient

Psychology is the science of behavior and the human thought process. This behavioral science is primarily concerned with human beings acting alone or in groups.

TABLE 4-7 Religious Beliefs about Birth, Death, and Health Care

Religion	Beliefs about Birth	Beliefs about Death	Health Care Beliefs
Christian, Roman Catholic	Infant baptism is mandatory. Baptism necessary for salvation. Any Christian may perform emergency baptism.	Sacrament of anointing the sick (last rites) performed by priest. Autopsy, organ donation, and cremation permitted.	Life is sacred. Abortion and contraception prohibited. Rite of communion important.
Hinduism	No ritual at birth.	Believe in reincarnation as humans, animals, or plants. Priest ties thread around neck or wrist of deceased, pour water in mouth. Only family or friends may wash the body. Autopsy, organ donation up to individual. Cremation preferred.	Illness as punishment for sins is a belief held by some. Faith healing important to some. Will accept most medical treatments, advice.
Islam (Muslim)	No ritual at birth. Circumcision at 7 days.	Family must be present at death. Dying person must ask forgiveness of sins. Body turned toward Mecca after death. Autopsy only if required by law. Organ donation permitted. Cremation not allowed.	Illness is atonement for sins. May pray facing toward Mecca five times a day (southeastern direction in United States). Ritual washing before and after prayer. Must take medications with right hand only, left hand considered dirty.
Jehovah's Witness (Christian)	No infant baptism.	No last rites. Autopsy only when required by law and body parts must not be removed. Organ donation discouraged. Cremation permitted.	May not receive blood or blood products. Church elders pray for healing. Medications permitted if not derived from blood products.
Judaism (Orthodox)	No infant baptism, circumcision by mohel (circumcisor), child's father, or Jewish physician.	Person should never die alone. Body is ritually cleaned and dead must be buried within 24 hours. Organ donation only by permission of rabbi. Cremation forbidden.	May refuse treatments on Sabbath or holy days. Family may want to bury body parts surgically removed. Ritual hand washing on rising and before eating.

There is a distinction between normal and abnormal behavior when studying psychology. All social interactions such as those that occur during the communication process may pose a problem for some people. The medical assistant will encounter patients, family members, staff, and caregivers who exhibit a wide scope of behavior patterns. These behavior patterns may be due to diseases, mental disorders, anxiety, drug abuse, trauma, the aging process, cultural customs, or a combination of several of these causes. The medical as-

sistant must be tolerant and respectful of others in all circumstances.

When dealing with an emotionally or mentally impaired patient, it is important to determine, if possible, what level of communication the patient can understand. Often by observing the patient with a caregiver, if there is one, you will get clues on how to communicate with the patient. Speak slowly and clearly, stay calm, and keep your messages short. If you have to touch the patient for a procedure be sure to explain

TABLE 4-8 Five Stages of Grief

Stage	Description
Denial	A refusal to believe that dying is taking place. This may be a time when the patient (or family member) needs time to adjust to the reality of approaching death. This stage cannot be hurried.
Anger	At this stage, the patient may be angry at everyone and may express this intense anger at God, family, and even health care professionals. The patient may take this anger out on the closest person to him or her. Usually this is a family member. In reality the patient is angry about dying.
Bargaining	The third stage of grief involves attempting to gain time by making promises in return. Bargaining may be done between the patient and God. The patient may indicate a need to talk at this stage.
Depression	This stage is marked with a deep sadness over the loss of health, independence, and eventually life. There is an additional sadness of leaving loved ones behind. The grieving patient may become withdrawn at this time.
Acceptance	The acceptance stage is reached when there is a sense of peace and calm. The patient may make comments such as, "I have no regrets. I'm ready to die." It is better to let the patient talk and not make denial statements such as, "Don't talk like that. You're not going to die."

what you are doing first. Ask the caregiver for assistance in calming the patient, if possible.

The Non-English Speaking Patient

As mentioned in the previous discussion of cultural diversity, the non-English speaking patient is at a disadvantage in the medical environment. You should employ the communication skills discussed previously and consider the following guidelines: smile at the patient, determine if he or she has any ability to speak or understand English, speak in normal tones, use pantomime or pictures to demonstrate, and ask assistance of a family member.

Intraoffice Communication

The goal in the medical office should be to establish a sense of rapport—an environment of cooperation—with patients, coworkers, supervisors, and vendors. To create this cooperative environment, all of the communication skills we have examined in this chapter will need to be utilized.

Establishing Trust

In order to communicate effectively in the health care environment and in everyday life, we must establish trust in our relationships. Being open, honest, and firm in our convictions, presenting a professional image, and using positive body language, help create a positive environment. Some of the most difficult communication problems occur with other staff members (Figure 4-8). Good staff communication depends on positive respectful

interactions. When thoughtless or condescending comments are made, permanent damage to relationships can occur. To be condescending is to adopt a superior attitude and act as though you are better than someone else. Withdrawing from the group, feeling angry and hurt, and discussing other staff members behind their backs causes office morale to suffer. Using assertive behavior with fellow staff means that you assert your own needs without threatening theirs. For instance, if it is your turn to have a holiday off and you have been scheduled to work, it is better to state, "I'm sorry I can't work that day. Since I worked overtime on the last holiday, I have made plans for this one." An aggressive statement, such as, "It's not fair. I always have to work on holidays and the others don't," would imply that favoritism or special

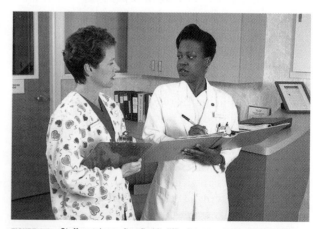

FIGURE 4-8 Staff members often find it difficult to communicate with other coworkers.

treatment has been shown to some staff members and might cause the supervisor to become defensive.

Rapport and Team Building

A positive attitude can make the difference between keeping and losing a job. A positive attitude is easier to project if you are happy in your work. The work group you are a part of is an important factor in your attitude. Work groups need to become a cohesive team. In order to do this, some degree of socializing is beneficial. Discussions about hobbies, travel, sports, family, and friends with other staff members help to establish an atmosphere of trust and understanding. However, the social aspect of staff communication should not interfere with work productivity.

Gossip is unnecessary, often negative conversation usually about someone who is not present. The medical assistant needs to learn to recognize gossip and not participate in it. Gossip can be extremely hurtful and is destructive to the atmosphere of cooperation needed in the medical facility.

Research has found that patients who have established a good relationship with their physicians and office staff are less willing to bring a lawsuit against them. It goes without saying that patients must always be provided quality medical care. However, courteous treatment of patients does pay extra dividends.

Patient as a Consumer

The patient today needs to be viewed as a consumer of health care. Patients and family members are more knowledgeable about health care options because of the Internet and other media. They no longer place the physician on a pedestal as older patients may have done when physicians made house calls. In fact, many patients can experience a certain amount of alienation from their health care providers because most physicians are specialists. Specialization can lead to viewing the patient as the sum of his or her injury or procedure—"a broken leg" or "appendectomy"—a viewpoint that is degrading. Instead, the patient should be treated holistically, and with dignity and respect. Medical assistants are the first to encounter the patient in many instances. Therefore, they are responsible for the initial impression the patient has of the practice or facility. The concept of "the customer comes first" should be a primary goal for all health care providers and needs to be considered to sustain a satisfied client base. Communication with other physicians, hospitals, and clinics is vitally important to the economic stability of practices and facilities.

Staff Arrangements

Staffing arrangements are as varied as the types of medical practices. The solo practice with its staff of one, the multi-physician practice with a variety of staff, including an office manager, the clinic with many registered nurses (RNs), and other types of allied health care workers are only a few of the types of practices in which the medical assistant may work. Regardless of the type of practice, communication is vitally important to keep conflict at a minimum, establish a positive environment, and provide quality health care.

Whatever the staffing arrangements, the physician/office manager must be clear about the chain of command and convey that information to the employees. In the solo office with one medical assistant, there is usually no problem. However, in larger practices, the health care professional with most seniority is often the unofficial office manager. This person may not be the most qualified, the most multiskilled, or an accomplished manager. Friction among coworkers is often a common problem in many of these larger practices. To avoid this problem, clearly defined areas of responsibility and authority should be established. The office policy and procedure manual can help resolve conflict about authority and responsibility.

Conflict Resolution

Inevitably there will be strife and conflict among coworkers. The procedure and policy manual is a valuable tool to begin to resolve issues. It should state clearly what standards are acceptable in all areas of the facility. Conflicts occur when there is miscommunication or misunderstanding of the message. Conflict also can occur when there are prejudices or preconceived ideas. Conflict interferes with establishing rapport and cooperation, which are essential in the workplace. To avoid conflict on a personal level, it would be helpful for you not to engage in gossip and to avoid the "downer," the negative person in the office who will try to bring you down to his or her level of pessimism. Conflict can be positive if it resolves issues of disagreement in an appropriate manner.

Critical Thinking and Problem Solving

Problem solving and critical thinking are necessary skills for health care workers. Problem solving is a way of looking at a problem and ultimately arriving at a decision. Box 4-2 lists the steps to evaluate the factors and risks involved in solving problems. Most problems have more than one solution. Weighing all the factors involved and evaluating the results will help later with other problems.

Critical thinking (Box 4-3) includes the ability to think imaginatively, solve problems, visualize situations, learn new information, and think logically. Both problem solving and critical thinking skills are important concepts to employ before trying to resolve any conflict. Box 4-4 illustrates the steps in conflict resolution.

Office Procedure and Policy Manual

A policy and procedure manual is a collection of policies and procedures for carrying out day-to-day operations in an office or facility and a vital instrument of communication in the medical office. The manual should be available to every employee, full time or part time, and must be updated on a regular basis. Every clinical procedure performed in the office should be included. For example, the procedure manual should include, but not be limited by, the following: step-by-step procedures for every test performed in the office including all reagents and calculations; quality control policies, normal values, and location and maintenance of instrumentation used. All policies related to hiring, firing, employee evaluation, personal records, job descriptions, dress code, supplies, maintenance of equipment, and rules and regulations should be included in the policy manual. The availability of policy and procedure manual to all personnel contributes to a more smoothly run office.

The Difficult Employee

A difficult or problem employee may disrupt the flow of work in an office. Negativity becomes contagious if there are no policies in place to deal with the difficult employee. Consulting the policy manual, meeting individually with the employee to obtain her side of the problem, setting goals for the employee, all may reduce the conflict. All meetings should be documented in case the positive steps recommended to the employee are not effective and termination is necessary.

Staff Meetings

Establishing a regularly scheduled staff meeting is an important step in having a smoothly functioning office. One of the most frequent complaints office managers receive is from employees who want to meet with physician/physicians and have some consistent way to address questions and concerns. The frequency of staff meetings is directly related to the type of practice, the number of staff, the office schedule, and the willingness of the practice managers/physicians.

There are many types of staff meetings. Some practices use lunch/coffee break time to gather staff. Others schedule them before or after working hours. A staff meeting may be held to offer in-service training on new equipment, updates on new procedures, to celebrate a holiday or special occasion, or any other reason office management deem appropriate. To have a successful staff meeting, you should have an agenda available ahead of time, stick to the agenda, and not let the meeting end in a gripe session. Chapter 18 will cover office management in detail.

Scope of Practice Issues

As a medical assistant, you are truly a multiskilled health care provider and are capable of functioning throughout a facility in many different areas. From the clinical

TABLE 4-9 Responses that Communicate Loyalty

Question/Comment	Sample Response
"I guess Dr. Thompson can't see me on Wednesday because he's playing golf."	"Dr. Thompson's day off is Wednesday, but he could see you on Saturday."
"I hear Dr. Thompson and his wife are divorcing?"	"I really have no information about Dr. Thompson's personal life."
"I've been waiting one hour to see Dr. Thompson. Why is he so slow?"	"I'm sorry you've had a long wait. Dr. Thompson has had many very ill patients today. May I reschedule your appointment?"

area where you have direct patient contact, to working in the front office, and including your handling of administrative procedures, you are cross-trained to effectively perform all of these duties. Other employees, like registered nurses (RNs) and licensed practical nurses (LPNs) who are working in the facility, may only be able to handle the clinical areas. Medical secretaries, coding, and billing employees usually can only perform the administrative functions. Because of your multifunctional training, you may encounter some jealousy or resentment from other staff members. It is important to work within your own scope of practice and job description. In other words, do not perform skills that are beyond your training. On the other hand, don't be afraid to promote your profession and all that it stands for.

Communicating with Superiors

In dealing with your superiors as with your coworkers, communication should be kept positive. If conflicts do arise and you need to speak with your superior, choose an appropriate time or ask for an appointment to speak with him or her. Be direct and to the point and do not promote any gossip you may have heard. If you have been given an order to do something and you need clarification on how to complete it, be sure to ask for help. Most supervisors would rather be asked a question than to have you perform a function about which you are not clear. Show initiative in your daily work. If a task needs to be done, volunteer to do it without being asked as long as it falls within your job description. Too often staff members are too busy keeping score of which employees do more or less work as compared to others.

Loyalty to Your Employer

You represent your employer or physician every time you speak to a patient or caller. You must support the physician and his or her reputation in every instance. In your position, you may become privileged to personal information about your employer. Under no circumstances, whether inside or outside of the office,

should that personal information be discussed. It is perfectly acceptable to state, "I really can't answer that," or "I'm sorry, but I don't know," in response to a patient's or other staff member's questions.

A loyal employee protects and defends an employer when other employees engage in negative conversation. See Table 4-9 for examples of loyal responses to questions or comments about your employer's personal life.

Communication and Patients' Rights

Every patient has the right to privacy and confidentiality. Any information dealing with a patient is considered privileged information. The American Hospital Association developed a statement called "The Patient's Bill of Rights," which describes the patient-physician relationship. Table 4-10 lists these rights. A copy of the "Patient's Bill of Rights" should be in every health care facility.

Confidentiality

All patients have the right to have their personal privacy respected and their medical records handled with confidentiality. Any information such as test results, patient histories, and even the fact that the patient is a patient, cannot be told to another person. No information can be given over the telephone without the patient's permission or unless a court has subpoenaed it. Your treatment and concern for the patient reflects the physician's high standards of care. The human dignity of each patient must be preserved regardless of the patient's socioeconomic background, race, age, nationality, sexual orientation, or gender.

Health Insurance Portability and Accountability Act (HIPAA)

The Health Insurance Portability and Accountability Act (HIPAA), previously mentioned, was passed in 1996 by Congress. The HIPAA Privacy Rule, which is

TABLE 4-10 Patient's Bill of Rights

1. The patient has the right to considerate and respectful care.

2. The patient has the right to and is encouraged to obtain from physicians and other direct caregivers relevant, current, understandable information concerning diagnosis, treatment, and prognosis.

3. The patient has the right to make decisions about the plan of care prior to and during the course of treatment and to refuse a recommended treatment or plan of care to the extent permitted by law and hospital policy and to be informed of the consequences of this action.

4. The patient has the right to have an advance directive (such as a living will, health care proxy, or durable power of attorney for health care) concerning treatment or designating a surrogate decision maker with the expectation that the hospital will honor the intent of that directive to the extent permitted by law and hospital policy.

5. The patient has the right to every consideration of privacy.

6. The patient has the right to expect that all communications and records pertaining to his or her care will be treated as confidential by the hospital, except in cases such as suspected abuse and public health hazards when reporting is permitted or required by law.

7. The patient has the right to review the records pertaining to his or her medical care and to have the information explained or interpreted as necessary, except when restricted by law.

8. The patient has the right to expect that, within its capacity and policies, a hospital will make reasonable response to the request of a patient for appropriate and medically indicated care and service.

9. The patient has the right to ask and be informed of the existence of business relationships among the hospital, educational institutions, other health care providers, or players that may influence the patient's treatment or care.

10. The patient has the right to consent to or decline to participate in proposed research studies or human experimentation affecting care and treatment or requiring direct patient involvement, and to have those studies fully explained prior to consent.

11. The patient has the right to expect reasonable continuity of care when appropriate and to be informed by physicians and other caregivers of available and realistic patient care options when hospital care is no longer appropriate.

12. The patient has the right to be informed of hospital policies and practices that relate to patient care, treatment, and responsibilities.

---

a part of HIPAA, provides for the federal protection of health information. This rule, while protecting patients' privacy, also allows for patients to have better access to their medical records and to have more control about how and to whom the information can be released. HIPAA designates the following information as protected health information or PHI:

- Name
- Address
- Phone numbers
- Fax numbers
- Dates (birth, death, admission, discharge, etc.)
- Social Security number
- E-mail address
- Medical record numbers

- Health plan beneficiary numbers
- Account numbers
- Certificate or license numbers
- Vehicle identifiers, serial numbers, and license plate numbers
- Device identifiers and serial numbers
- Web Universal Resource Locators (URLs)
- Internet Protocol (IP) address numbers

This means that any or all of this information cannot be given out by any means (electronic, paper, or orally) for any reason without the written authorization of the patient. The written authorization covers any information necessary for treatment, payment, and operations (TPO). If you are in doubt whether to release personal patient information, do not do it.

Check and make sure that you have obtained the appropriate authorization.

Appropriate Documentation

One way to reduce the risk of lawsuits is to document appropriately. The patient's record is a source of communication both within and outside the office necessary to provide the best quality of care. Keep in mind these steps to better documentation:

- Use the patient's own words.
- Use precise descriptions, incorporating acceptable terminology and abbreviations, and write clearly.
- Provide complete information on all forms.
- Be brief and clear when documenting and spell correctly.
- Date all entries.
- Sign all entries.
- Use ink.
- Correct and sign all charting errors appropriately.
- Maintain confidentiality.

Advising Patients

As a medical assistant, you are the physician's representative. Because you are part of the staff, wear a uniform, and assist with treatments, patients may view you as an authority figure. The physician advises the patient on a course of treatment or procedure based on his or her examination and diagnostic test results. You are not permitted to offer your opinion about the physician's diagnosis, the course of action the physician has set forth, or tell the patient what you would do in his or her position. Those opinions are beyond your scope of practice and could put you and the physician at risk of being sued. If asked by a patient, "What would you do if you were me?" you must not offer advice. Explain to the patient that the physician will be pleased to review the course of action, answer any questions, and that you will be happy to arrange for that meeting. A medical assistant giving advice to a patient could be construed as "practicing medicine without a license" and is an offense in most states.

Patient Decision Making

Patients who have received bad news from the physician or are faced with difficult choices do need help to come to a decision. Your role is to listen empathetically to the patient, ask him or her reflecting or clarifying questions, and make clear the information the physician has related to the patient to help him or her come to a decision on a course of treatment. For example, Mrs. Santos has been told by the physician that her breast biopsy was positive and mastectomy is recom-

mended as soon as possible. When the physician leaves the room, she asks you what she should do. Your response should be, "Mrs. Santos, you seem upset about having to have a mastectomy. What is concerning you about the procedure?" If she asks what you would do in her circumstances, suggest that she get a second opinion or offer to explain again in simple terms what the doctor has said. Sometimes patients are so nervous in the presence of a physician that they do not hear information correctly. It would be permissible to give her written information about the procedure, offer to bring her concerns to the physician, and encourage her to call back once she is home if she has more questions.

Risk Management

The term risk management refers to reducing the physician's risk of lawsuit in the medical setting. As a medical assistant, dealing so closely with patients, you are in a position to help reduce those risks. Communicating effectively with the patient is certainly one of primary ways to reduce the risk of being sued. On the other hand, any promise or commitment that you make to a patient can be legally binding to the physician who employs you. This means that the physician can be held responsible for something you have said or implied to the patient with regard to how the physician might improve the patient's condition. Keep all matters relating to patients' personal health information confidential. If you believe that any health professional is acting in an unethical or unprofessional manner, you should discuss this with your employer or another physician. For example, a comment such as "Did Miss Jones come in for her pregnancy test?" can result in a breach of confidentiality lawsuit against the physician if it is overheard by others.

Communication and Patient Education

The medical assistant is in a position to promote patient education. You are the staff person who interacts with the patient and spends more time with him or her than many of the other staff members. Effective communication is the goal in all interpersonal dealings. Often it falls to the medical assistant to have to explain again what the physician has already said to the patient. Many times the patient is too anxious when the physician is speaking to him or her to fully comprehend what is being said. The medical assistant should be careful not to promise outcomes. Your job is to reinforce what the physician has said, not change it. See Patient Education for additional ways to educate your patients.

Setting Goals

At times the medical assistant has to assume the role of patient educator to ensure that the patient is following through with the recommended treatments or

Patient Education

Patient education must be presented in a manner suited to the patient. In most cases, direct contact between the learner (patient) and the instructor (medical assistant) provides the best atmosphere for learning. As a medical assistant, it will be a great advantage if you are able to use the communication techniques discussed in this chapter effectively.

Life style changes can greatly affect the ability to acquire new information and some patients may use several barriers to block communication such as rationalization and denial. A patient concerned over a life-threatening diagnosis may not be in a receptive mood for education or instruction. If you sense that a patient's uncooperativeness comes from defensive or anxious behavior, you may be able to draw the person out using open-ended questions. With a mutual trust established, it is more likely that needed instruction can be given.

Brochures and pamphlets can also be helpful for explaining health care issues. Material should be clearly and simply written. The patient with a language barrier will need an interpreter when an explanation regarding treatment or medications is given. Free brochures are available to physicians through organizations, such as American Diabetes Association.

---

instructions. To this end your role may become that of "cheerleader" to encourage the compliance of the patient. Before a patient can follow through with a plan, the goals of the plan must be set. The physician sets the goal and you will reinforce it with the patient. Keep the goals simple and small. If the patient needs to lose weight to lower his or her blood pressure, it is not realistic to expect the patient to lose 5 pounds every week.

Compliance and Wellness

Health care today is frequently more wellness care than illness care. Much of the time the physician is trying to encourage healthy life styles that lead to better health overall. Often times it has been said, "if I could only give patients a pill for motivation," it would be easy. Unfortunately, this isn't possible. Positive communication—the rapport and comfort level you establish with the patient—has a direct bearing on patients' compliance with the goals that have been set. The tools already learned in this chapter can play a big role in compliance. Positive feedback—a smile, a word of praise, or a pat on the back—can help to further compliance. Be sure that you follow up on the patient's progress to encourage his or her new wellness behaviors. Written information is a powerful tool in educating the patient. However, the medical assistant should review the information with the patient to ensure that he or she understands what is written. The medical assistant should be a role model for the patient in behavior, dress, and promoting wellness.

SUMMARY

Communication is a necessary requirement for everyday living. In the health care field, the ability to communicate effectively is essential for success—for example, to call and request a prescription be renewed, to document the patient's symptoms and help the patient be diagnosed properly, to provide patient education, to arrange travel plans for the physician. The concern you have for patients will come through in your words, actions, gestures, and your tone of voice. The special needs of some patients may not be the presenting problems when they arrive in the physician's office. However, these special needs must be dealt with to accommodate the patients as much as possible. The medical assistant must remain flexible and learn to be able to handle all unusual situations professionally.

Chapter Review

COMPETENCY REVIEW

1. Define and spell the terms to learn for this chapter.
2. Explain what you would say to a patient who says that the medication Dr. Thompson gave her last week have made her sick.
3. Explain what you would say to the patient who is angry at the delay in the waiting room.
4. Explain what you would say to the patient who complains to you about Dr. Thompson.

5. What are Kübler-Ross's five stages of dying and why are they important to know?
6. Describe how to communicate to a profoundly deaf patient that or she must remove all clothing and put on a gown.
7. Describe some cultural problems that can arise when treating patients from other cultures.
8. List five impressions you believe non-Americans have of U.S. citizens.
9. Discuss several defense mechanisms that you feel you sometimes exhibit. How do they impact negatively on your relationships with others?
10. Mary Brown's neighbor calls to see if she kept her appointment because she says Mary is sometimes forgetful. What would you say?

PREPARING FOR THE CERTIFICATION EXAM

1. The basic units of the communication process are
   A. source, message, receiver, patient
   B. message, receiver
   C. channel, message, receiver, patient
   D. receiver, message, source
   E. source, message, channel, receiver

2. A nonverbal form of communication would include
   A. doing one thing at a time
   B. smiling and saying, "Hi"
   C. finishing a sentence for a patient
   D. interrupting a patient
   E. folding one's arms across one's chest

3. Consider the statement a medical assistant might make to a patient: "You say you are still in pain from your hysterectomy. On a scale of 1 to 10, with 1 being very little pain and 10 being the worst you could imagine, how would you rank your pain level at this moment?" What directive communication technique is this statement?
   A. open-ended statement
   B. closed-ended statement
   C. reflective statement
   D. acknowledgment
   E. seeking clarification

4. Which of the following statements regarding assertive versus aggressive behavior is FALSE?
   A. assertiveness is generally considered a very positive form of communication
   B. aggressiveness is generally considered a very negative form of communication
   C. assertiveness can be compared to a verbal attack against another person
   D. aggressiveness can be compared to a verbal attack against another person

E. assertiveness is trying to impose ones point of view on others

5. Placing your own feelings onto another person is an example of which of the following defensive behaviors?
   A. rationalization
   B. projection
   C. compensation
   D. displaced anger
   E. disassociation

6. When dealing with a very angry patient, which of the following statements would be BEST to defuse the situation?
   A. "I am very sorry there was an error on your billing statement. Let me see if our billing clerk can fix it while you are here."
   B. "Please come back when you are less angry. It will be easier to talk to you then."
   C. "I will not listen to you while you are expressing your anger, but I will listen soon as soon as you calm down."
   D. "I think you are feeling angry because, without a medical background like mine, you simply do not understand the situation."
   E. "I am going to refer you to my supervisor."

7. What is the best way to help a blind patient?
   A. Take the patient by the arm and lead him or her into an examination room.
   B. Speak loudly to the patient so he or she can hear you since the patient cannot read your lips.
   C. Offer your arm for the patient to take.
   D. Allow the patient to remain independent by doing as little as possible to help.
   E. Tell the patient not to go outside without assistance.

continued on next page

8. When assisting patients who have a terminal disease, the BEST method is to
   A. allow them to talk about it
   B. do not allow them to dwell on the depressing subject of death
   C. encourage them by telling them they look wonderful
   D. avoid them
   E. speak loudly and clearly

9. Defensive behavior
   A. is conscious or unconscious
   B. can alienate the patient
   C. is a natural but unacceptable response
   D. is encouraged at times
   E. is on office policy

CRITICAL THINKING

1. What should Susan do to make Mrs. Brown feel more at ease once Susan has acknowledged her presence?

2. How could the staff at Dr. Barry's office avoid making the same mistake with other patients? What would have made Mrs. Brown feel more comfortable on her first visit?

3. Have you ever experienced the same problem in a physician's office and how did it make you feel? What did you do? What would have made you feel more comfortable?

4. If you were the office manager of Dr. Barry's office, what steps would you take to correct this problem?

5. What issues discussed in this chapter are illustrated in this case study?

ON THE JOB

Amy Freeman is a new medical assistant who has recently passed the CMA examination. She has studied Dr. Kübler-Ross's five stages of dying and believes they make sense. Renee Baker, a young mother of two small children, has an appointment to see Dr. Williams for follow-up care after having been diagnosed with terminal ovarian cancer. Renee bitterly tells Amy that she is angry at the doctors for not diagnosing her condition sooner; angry at God for allowing this to happen; angry at her husband for not being more supportive; and angry at herself for not demanding better health care.

Since Renee has opened up to Amy about her feelings, Amy wants to try to help her. What should Amy do?

1. Keeping in mind Dr. Kübler-Ross's five stages of dying, what exactly should Amy say to Renee?

2. Does Amy have a responsibility to inform the physician?

INTERNET ACTIVITY

Perform a search for information on hospice care. What information can you discover that will help you communicate with Renee, the terminal ovarian cancer patient, in the above On the Job exercise?

MediaLink More on communication in the medical office environment, including interactive resources, can be found on the Student CD-ROM accompanying this textbook.

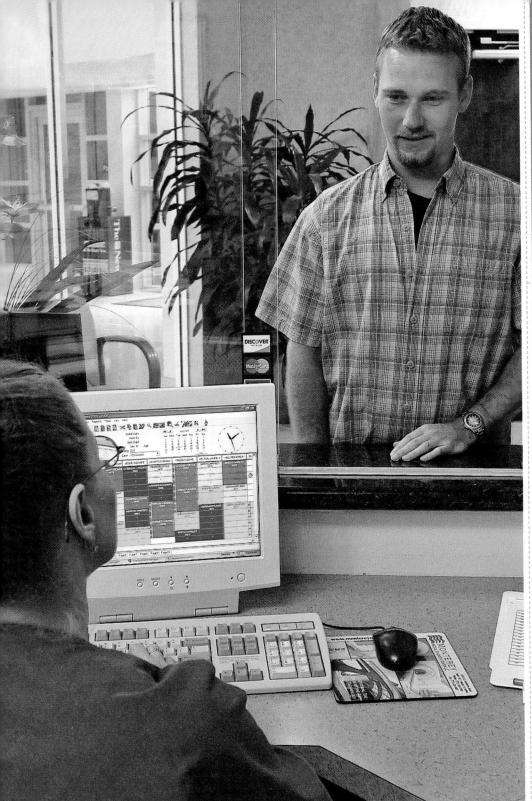

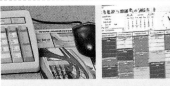

Administrative
Medical Assisting

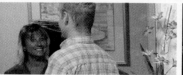

Medical Assistant Role Delineation Chart

HIGHLIGHT indicates material covered in this chapter.

ADMINISTRATIVE

Administrative Procedures

- Perform basic administrative medical assisting functions
- Schedule, coordinate and monitor appointments
- Schedule inpatient/outpatient admissions and procedures
- Understand and apply third-party guidelines
- Obtain reimbursement through accurate claims submission
- Monitor third-party reimbursement
- Understand and adhere to managed care policies and procedures
- *Negotiate managed care contracts*

Practice Finances

- Perform procedural and diagnostic coding
- Apply bookkeeping principles

- Manage accounts receivable
- *Manage accounts payable*
- *Process payroll*
- *Document and maintain accounting and banking records*
- *Develop and maintain fee schedules*
- *Manage renewals of business and professional insurance policies*
- *Manage personnel benefits and maintain records*
- *Perform marketing, financial, and strategic planning*

CLINICAL

Fundamental Principles

- Apply principles of aseptic technique and infection control
- Comply with quality assurance practices
- Screen and follow up patient test results

Diagnostic Orders

- Collect and process specimens
- Perform diagnostic tests

Patient Care

- Adhere to established patient screening procedures
- Obtain patient history and vital signs
- Prepare and maintain examination and treatment areas
- Prepare patient for examinations, procedures and treatments

- Assist with examinations, procedures and treatments
- Prepare and administer medications and immunizations
- Maintain medication and immunization records
- Recognize and respond to emergencies
- Coordinate patient care information with other health care providers
- Initiate IV and administer IV medications with appropriate training and as permitted by state law

GENERAL

Professionalism

- Display a professional manner and image
- Demonstrate initiative and responsibility
- Work as a member of the health care team
- Prioritize and perform multiple tasks
- Adapt to change
- Promote the CMA credential
- Enhance skills through continuing education
- Treat all patients with compassion and empathy
- Promote the practice through positive public relations

Communication Skills

- Recognize and respect cultural diversity
- Adapt communications to individual's ability to understand
- Use professional telephone technique

- *Denotes advanced skills.*

- Recognize and respond effectively to verbal, nonverbal, and written communications
- Use medical terminology appropriately
- Utilize electronic technology to receive, organize, prioritize and transmit information
- Serve as liaison

Legal Concepts

- Perform within legal and ethical boundaries
- Prepare and maintain medical records
- Document accurately
- Follow employer's established policies dealing with the health care contract
- Implement and maintain federal and state health care legislation and regulations
- Comply with established risk management and safety procedures
- Recognize professional credentialing criteria
- *Develop and maintain personnel, policy and procedure manuals*

Instruction

- Instruct individuals according to their needs
- Explain office policies and procedures
- Teach methods of health promotion and disease prevention
- Locate community resources and disseminate information
- *Develop educational materials*
- *Conduct continuing education activities*

Operational Functions

- Perform inventory of supplies and equipment
- Perform routine maintenance of administrative and clinical equipment
- Apply computer techniques to support office operations
- *Perform personnel management functions*
- *Negotiate leases and prices for equipment and supply contracts*

SOURCE: Reprinted by permission of the American Association of Medical Assistants from the AAMA Role Delineation Study: Occupational Analysis of the Medical Assisting Profession.

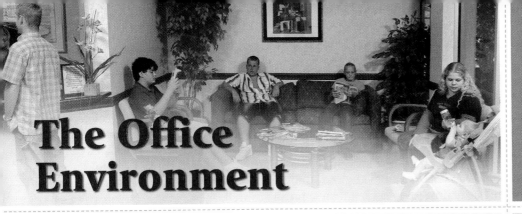

The Office Environment

chapter

5

Learning Objectives

After reading this chapter, you should be able to:

- Define and spell the terms to learn for this chapter.
- Identify six general safety measures.
- Discuss six disaster rules.
- Describe electrical, radiation, mechanical, and chemical safety hazards.
- List and describe four types of medical waste.
- Define OSHA Bloodborne Pathogens Standards.

- Describe the three points that must be included in an exposure plan.
- List and discuss five guidelines for using protective measures as indicated by OSHA.
- Discuss the importance of Universal Precautions for the medical assistant.
- List and describe six rules for proper body mechanics.

Terms to Learn

biohazard

body mechanics

ergonomics

Ground Fault Circuit Interrupter (GFCI)

incident report

Material Safety Data Sheet (MSDS)

National Committee for Quality Assurance (NCQA)

Occupational Safety and Hazard Administration (OSHA)

quality assurance (QA)

Case Study

GLORIA, A MEDICAL ASSISTANT, PREPARES A MEDICATION for Mrs. Garner that is to be given by an intramuscular injection technique. She has both safety needles and non-safety needles at hand for use in this procedure. Since she has not been told to use only the safety needles, and she feels more comfortable with the old-style, she chooses to use the non-safety needle. After giving the injection, Gloria proceeds to dispose of the needle and syringe in the sharps container. As she places the non-safety needle on the flip-lid, it begins to slide off. Gloria catches it, receiving a needle stick in the process. She continues to put the needle and syringe into the sharps container and finishes up with the patient.

After dismissing the patient, Gloria reports the needle stick to her supervisor, Linda, who then asks Gloria why she chose not to use a safety needle. Gloria explains that she didn't think she needed to and wasn't really trained to use them. Linda tells Gloria to fill out an incident report, explaining the situation in full. Then all steps are taken to provide for testing of both the patient and Gloria.

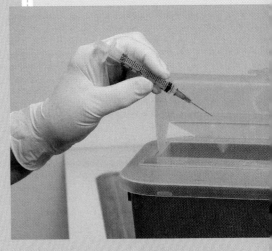

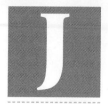ust as in any workplace, general safety measures, employee safety, housekeeping, proper body mechanics, office security, and measures to ensure a clean, pleasant environment are critical to maintaining the safety and comfort of the medical assistant and the patient in the medical office. Additional safety issues may arise in a medical workplace, including biological hazards, bloodborne pathogens, and the handling of drug samples.

General Safety Measures

The Occupational Safety and Hazard Administration (OSHA) is a governmental agency responsible for the safety of all employees of companies operating in the United States. OSHA assures the safety and health of America's workers by setting and enforcing standards; providing training, outreach, and education; establishing partnerships; and encouraging continual improvement in workplace safety and health. They have the authority to inspect a workplace without notification and to levy fines on any deficiencies they find relating to the health and safety of employees.

Many offices make the mistake of believing the only OSHA issues they need to be concerned with are the Bloodborne Pathogens Standards. While these regulations are important and will be covered later, many other safety factors fall under the regulations of OSHA.

OSHA is concerned with any workplace hazard that may impact the safety of an employee. Other governmental agencies may have standards regarding these factors as well, such as the local Fire Marshal or local law enforcement agencies. In addition, insurance companies that your office may contract might have rules and regulations above and beyond these other agencies.

A workplace hazard could be defined as any issue that could affect the health or safety of an employee—either upon immediate exposure or in the long-term. Matters surrounding workplace hazards will be discussed in the material that follows. See Guidelines 5-1 for some general safety measures to adhere to in the office.

Disaster Plan

A disaster is anything that can cause injury or damage to a group of people. Disasters in a medical office include:

5-1 GUIDELINES　　　　**General Safety Measures**

- Walk never run in a medical office. If an emergency situation occurs, move quickly without running.
- Always walk on the right-hand side of the hallway. Wheelchairs and carts bearing patients use the same hallways as do employees and visitors. Some medical facilities have a mirror on the wall or ceiling at hallway junctions so that people do not collide.
- Use handrails when using stairways.
- Never carry uncapped syringes or sharp instruments in hallways or between examination rooms.
- Keep floors clear. Immediately wipe up spills or call housekeeping to assist. Never pick up broken glass with bare hands. Use OSHA standards when cleaning up glass, spilled specimens, and liquids.
- Open doors carefully to avoid injuring someone on the other side.
- Replace burned out light bulbs immediately, especially over exit signs.
- Report all unsafe conditions immediately.
- Wear long hair pulled back and tied to prevent it from coming into contact with hazardous materials.

- Shoes should cover the entire foot. Open toe, open heel, or high heel shoes are not recommended in the medical office due to the danger of slipping and other injuries.
- Do not ever place food in the same refrigerator with laboratory specimens or refrigerated drugs.
- There should be no eating, drinking, or smoking in the medical office, except in designated areas.
- File cabinets should be mounted against the walls to avoid accidental tipping when a heavy top drawer is open.
- Floors should be clean but not so highly polished that they cause slipping. All spills must be cleaned immediately. A hazard sign should always be placed near a wet floor.
- All controlled substances (narcotics) must be stored in a locked cabinet. A record of all narcotic administration must be maintained according to the Drug Enforcement Administration (DEA) regulations. Any loss of drugs must be reported to the regional office of the DEA immediately. The local police should also be notified.

fire, flood, tornado, earthquake, or explosions. Recent events have also given rise to the need for security from terrorist attacks. Every office should have a written disaster plan in place and all employees should be familiar with the steps to be taken in any emergency. All new hires should be trained in these emergency steps within the first day of employment. This training should be documented in writing to assure compliance with OSHA regulations. If a particular medical facility has radiation equipment on site, further regulations may be required to be instituted. See Guidelines 5-2 for basic rules for handling a disaster.

Fire Safety

Floor plans showing all exits, fire extinguishers, and stairwells should be placed in conspicuous areas all around the facility. These should include arrows showing the most direct route out of the building. They should be large enough to be easily read in dim light. For each area of the facility, a person should be designated to make sure that all employees are out of that area safely.

Portable fire extinguishers should be attached to walls in areas that are no more that 75 feet away from any employee area. Appropriate types of extinguishers for medical offices are ABC types. They are capable of putting out many types of fires. Each employee should be instructed on the proper use of fire equipment.

Most medical offices are now in buildings with smoke detectors and sprinkler systems. Smoke detectors and alarms should be tested regularly. Nothing should be placed within 18 inches of a sprinkler head.

Fire drills should be held at least once a year and with all employees present. During a mandatory staff meeting would be an ideal time to hold a fire drill. The drill should reinforce the location of fire exits, how to direct people to the fire exits, and how to act in a calm manner during such an emergency.

Because of the widespread "No Smoking" policies now in place in medical facilities, cigarettes are not as much of a fire hazard as before. However, safe disposal systems should be placed in designated areas to prevent people from throwing cigarettes into wastebaskets or other trash receptacles.

The following items should be in place in the event of a fire:

- Telephone numbers of fire and police departments attached to all telephones, including extensions
- Fire extinguishers that have been properly maintained through monthly maintenance checks, the date and initials of the person responsible for testing the equipment should be legible

| 5-2 | **GUIDELINES** |

Handling a Disaster

- Remain calm. Count to 10 and assess the situation.
- Make sure that you are not in danger.
- Remove all others (patients and employees) who are in immediate danger, if it is safe for you to do so.
- Make sure that the fire department has been called in the event of a fire.
- Notify others of the emergency according to the policy of the facility.
- Use stairs, never the elevator.

- Exits and stairways that are clearly marked and free of debris, a diagram of all exits should be posted near the fire extinguishers
- Fireproof file cabinets to protect vital records

After notifying the fire department, the most important function during a fire is to see that all patients and employees are safely out of danger. All patients should be told to immediately leave the building. Any patients who need assistance should be helped. Examination rooms and bathrooms need to be inspected in the event a patient is still in the building. Use the stairs, never the elevators. See Figure 5-1 for the basic steps of a fire safety plan.

Electrical Safety

Electrical shock is a hazard in the medical office. All equipment should be grounded according to the manufacturer's instructions. Never use extension cords. They are both an electrical and a trip/fall hazard. No circuit should be overloaded. Surge protectors should be used for all electronic equipment. A power surge can short circuit or "fry" the sensitive components of electronics. You should never plug a surge protector into another surge protector to double up the number of outlets.

All electric cords to equipment should be checked regularly for any cracks, loss of insulation, or other problems. In "wet" areas, such as near sinks, a Ground Fault Circuit Interrupter (GFCI) outlet must be used. GFCIs are designed to protect people from severe or fatal electric shocks. Because a GFCI detects ground faults, it can also prevent some electrical fires and reduce the severity of others by interrupting the flow of electric current. These outlets will break the circuit if water gets into them, protecting both the user and any plugged-in equipment.

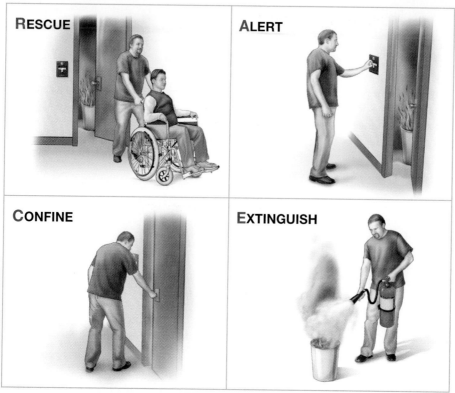

RESCUE

ALERT

CONFINE

EXTINGUISH

FIGURE 5-1   A fire safety plan like RACE saves lives.

Mechanical Safety

Many pieces of equipment in the medical office can cause harm if they are not used properly. Some of these include the centrifuge, autoclave, sterilizers, and oxygen equipment. You should always read the entire instruction manual before installing or using any type of equipment.

Chemical Hazards (OSHA Hazardous Communications)

Medical offices may contain chemicals that are hazardous to the human body. Materials may be considered harmful in several ways. Biohazards are biological substances, such as medical waste and samples of a virus or bacterium, that pose a threat to human beings and are potentially infectious. Corrosive materials cause burns, and flammable materials can burst into flame. Toxic materials can cause serious illness or death by exposure through skin contact, ingestion, or inhalation.

OSHA has very specific regulations regarding chemical hazards. These are covered under the Hazardous Communications sections. Each office should have an OSHA compliance officer who is trained and aware of all the required controls for the use and storage of such materials. All employees must have annual training for Hazardous Communications.

Each manufacturer of a product is required to provide the consumer with a Material Safety Data Sheet (MSDS), which contains written or printed material concerning a hazardous chemical. MSDSs offer basic information needed to ensure the safety and health of the user at all stages of manufacture, storage, use, and disposal of a hazardous chemical product.

MSDSs give information regarding the hazards of using the product and how to protect oneself from injury by using the appropriate Personal Protection Equipment (PPE). PPE consists of protective gloves, fluid resistant lab coats, safety glasses and a surgical mask, shield, or respirator. All MSDSs must be filed into a HAZCOM binder that is available to all employees at any time. Figure 5-2 is an example of an MSDS label that should be attached to any product that does not include a label.

Employee Safety

Safety is the responsibility of every member of the staff. While it is imperative that the practice provides a safe working environment, the staff needs to be constantly aware of their surroundings and any possible hazards. Employees must be willing to implement all safeguards to keep themselves and their patients safe.

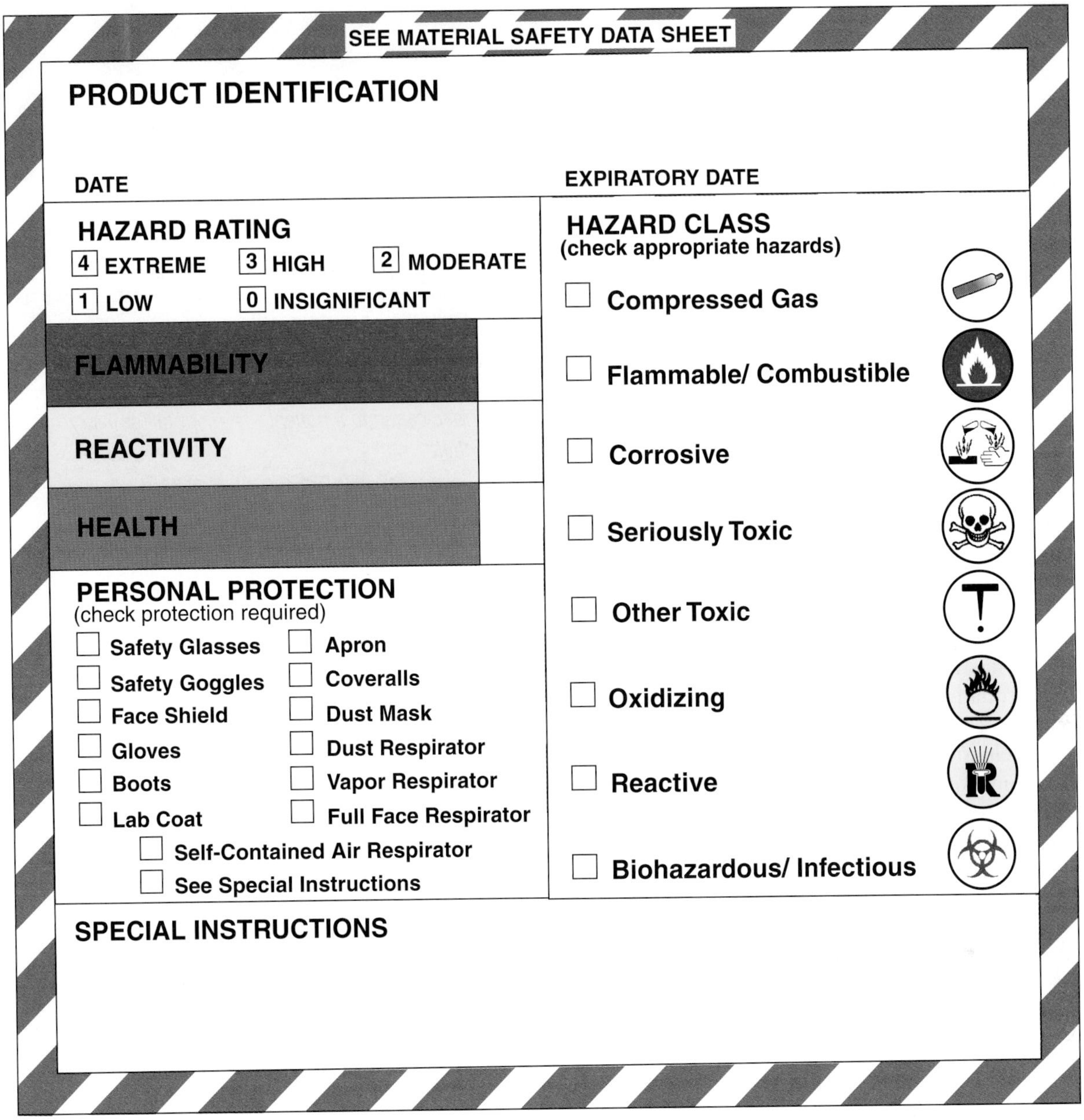

PRODUCT IDENTIFICATION

DATE | EXPIRATORY DATE

HAZARD RATING

| 4 | EXTREME | 3 | HIGH | 2 | MODERATE |
| 1 | LOW | 0 | INSIGNIFICANT |

FLAMMABILITY

REACTIVITY

HEALTH

PERSONAL PROTECTION
(check protection required)

☐ Safety Glasses ☐ Apron
☐ Safety Goggles ☐ Coveralls
☐ Face Shield ☐ Dust Mask
☐ Gloves ☐ Dust Respirator
☐ Boots ☐ Vapor Respirator
☐ Lab Coat ☐ Full Face Respirator
☐ Self-Contained Air Respirator
☐ See Special Instructions

HAZARD CLASS
(check appropriate hazards)

☐ Compressed Gas

☐ Flammable/ Combustible

☐ Corrosive

☐ Seriously Toxic

☐ Other Toxic

☐ Oxidizing

☐ Reactive

☐ Biohazardous/ Infectious

SPECIAL INSTRUCTIONS

FIGURE 5-2 An example of a Material Safety Data Sheet (MSDS).

Hazardous Medical Waste

Hospitals, dental practices, veterinary clinics, laboratories, nursing homes, medical offices, and other health care facilities generate 3.2 million tons of hazardous medical waste each year. Much of this waste is potentially infectious or radioactive. There are four major types of medical waste.

- Solid—generated in every aspect of medicine, including administration, cafeterias, patient rooms, and medical offices. It includes trash such as paper, bottles, cardboard, and cans. Solid waste is not considered hazardous but can cause pollution of the environment. Mandatory recycling can reduce the amount of solid waste produced.

- Chemical—includes substances like germicides, cleaning solvents, and pharmaceuticals. This waste can create a hazardous situation like a fire or explosion. The safe manner in which to handle and dispose of chemicals is included in the MSDS.

- Radioactive—any waste that contains or is contaminated with liquid or solid radioactive material, such as Iodine 123, Iodine 131, and Thallium 201. Radioactive waste must be clearly labeled as "radioactive" and must be removed by a licensed facility.

- Infectious—any waste material that has the potential to carry disease. It includes laboratory cultures, blood and blood products from blood banks, operating rooms, emergency rooms, doctor and dentist offices, autopsy suites, and patient rooms. Infectious waste must be separated from other solid and chemical waste at the point of origin. A licensed medical waste removal agency must dispose of these materials. This is covered in more detail under the Bloodborne Pathogens Standards section.

OSHA Bloodborne Pathogens Standards/Universal Precautions

Medical office laboratories must follow the OSHA guidelines for handling contaminated materials. These guidelines are available from the U.S. Department of Labor in Washington, DC. Most offices contract with a private company to provide assistance in meeting OSHA guidelines.

OSHA standards must be adhered to by every employee who has the possibility of occupational exposure to potentially infectious materials (Preparing for Externship). Occupational exposure is defined as a reasonable anticipation that the employee's duties will result in skin, mucous membrane, eye, or parenteral (for example, assisting with blood work) contact with infectious material. Examples of employees at risk are physicians, nurses, laboratory workers, medical assistants, dental assistants, and, in some cases, housekeeping personnel. The OSHA standards mandate that each at-risk employee must be offered the Hepatitis B vaccine series at the expense of the employer. If an employee refuses the vaccine, he or she must sign a waiver. Potential infectious materials include:

- Body fluid contaminated with blood
- Saliva in dental procedures

- Amniotic fluid
- Cerebrospinal fluid
- Human biopsy tissue or cells
- Microbiological waste (kits or inoculated culture media)
- Any unidentified body fluid
- Urine, stool, sputum, nasal secretions; vomitus and sweat are considered contaminated only if there is visible evidence of blood present

OSHA requires that each medical office have a written Exposure Control Plan to assist in minimizing employee exposure to infectious materials. This plan must be reviewed by all office staff and updated annually. An Exposure Control Plan must include:

- Exposure Determination—listing of job classifications within the office to determine at-risk employees (those with potential exposure to infectious materials).
- Method of Compliance—specific measures to reduce the risk of exposure.
- Post-Exposure—evaluation and follow-up, which specify the steps followed when an exposure incident occurs.

A record for each employee must be kept on file for 30 years after the termination of employment. This includes documentation of the employee's annual review of the Exposure Control Plan for the facility. In addition, these records must contain information regarding the administration of Hepatitis B vaccine series or waiver signed by the employee within three days of initial employment, and a copy of any exposure incident reports. These records must be confidential and kept

TABLE 5-1 **Personal Protective Equipment (PPE) and Clothing**

Clothing/Equipment	When Used
Gloves	Anticipate contact with blood, infectious material, open wounds or broken skin on hands. Examples: venipuncture, capillary stick, wound care, injections, minor surgery, cleaning contaminated equipment, such as contaminated surfaces of thermometers.
Mask	Anticipate spray with blood or infectious materials. Often used with eye shields.
Eye/Face Shield	Anticipate spray with infectious materials, droplets of blood, or other infectious matter. Example: performing blood smear.
Gowns, Lab Coats	Anticipate gross contamination of clothing during a procedure. Examples: minor surgery, laboratory procedures.

under lock and key. Legal and Ethical Issues touches on more about this issue.

Universal Precautions

The U.S. Centers for Disease Control (CDC) in Atlanta issued recommendations for protection of health care workers. These became known as the Universal Precautions. According to Universal Precautions, all blood and body fluids should be treated as if it were contaminated with any bloodborne pathogen. The most commonly noted diseases related to bloodborne exposure are HIV and HBV. Personal protective equipment (PPE) used to fulfill the recommendations includes gloves, protective eyewear, masks, and fluid resistant lab coats. Table 5-1 describes what protective clothing is appropriate, and Guidelines 5-3 lists details in the use of personal protective equipment and clothing. In addition, the MSDS will contain information regarding PPE. In 1996, the CDC issued more complete guidelines known as Standard Precautions. These guidelines are discussed more fully in Volume III, Chapter 32.

If there is a situation where infectious material has been spilled, proper procedures must be followed in the cleanup. A spill kit should be used. Commercial kits are available but a simple kit can be assembled with the following equipment:

- Plain clay kitty litter
- A small dust pan
- A biohazard bag

The kitty litter is used as a drying agent to allow sweep-up of the material without spreading it. The material is then placed in a biohazard bag to be disposed

of with other biohazardous waste. Patient Education emphasizes more about safety precautions.

Housekeeping Safety

All members of the housekeeping department must receive careful instruction regarding OSHA standards. Housekeeping personnel should not empty biohazard waste and sharps containers. They only empty office trash containers. However, since housekeeping personnel are around potentially infectious materials, they

---

5-3 **GUIDELINES**

Using Personal Protective Equipment and Clothing from OSHA

- The employer must supply the protective clothing and provide cleaning or disposal of it.
- The clothing or other equipment must be of strength to act as a barrier to infectious materials reaching the employee's street clothing, work clothing, eyes, mouth, or skin.
- Disposable gloves may not be reused.
- Protective eye equipment must have solid sides to prevent infectious material from entering the area.
- All equipment and clothing must be removed and placed in a designated container before leaving the medical office.

Safety precautions are the responsibility of all medical office personnel. The medical assistant's thorough understanding of medical office policy regarding fire safety, infectious waste, and office security results in better patient education, understanding, and protection.

Some patients are insulted when the person caring for them applies gloves before touching them. The medical assistant may need to explain to patients the rationale for wearing protective clothing by medical personnel.

must receive training. If the office contracts with an outside agency for housekeeping duties, the contract should state that all of the agency's employees should be trained in Bloodborne Pathogen Standards and Universal Precautions. The medical office is then not required to train the personnel.

If a contracted agency brings in cleaning products and does not leave them on the premises, the practice is not responsible for maintaining MSDS for those products. However, if the supplies are left in the office, MSDS must be kept in the HAZCOM (hazard communication) book and made available at all times.

Proper storage of all chemical products is essential for the safety of employees and the patients. Guidelines 5-4 presents some rules for the storage and use of cleaning products. Figures 5-3 and 5-4 show some products.

Proper Body Mechanics

Ergonomics applies scientific information and data regarding human body mechanics to the design of objects and overall environments for human use. While OSHA abandoned the ergonomic portion of the regulations, proper body mechanics—coordination of body alignment, balance, and movement—should still be a part of the medical assistant's training.

Medical assistants move, lift, and carry many things, including equipment, supplies, and even patients. Correct methods of standing and lifting objects will help prevent pain and injury. Table 5-2 describes the principles of proper body mechanics and provides a demonstration of proper lifting techniques.

Office Security

There are unique security issues in a physician's office. Medical offices make an attractive target for a thief or addict looking for drugs. Doors and windows need to have secure locks. Only a few authorized personnel should have keys for opening and closing the office. If a key is missing all locks should be changed. Many offices have electronic security systems that are activated when the last person leaves the office. In order to

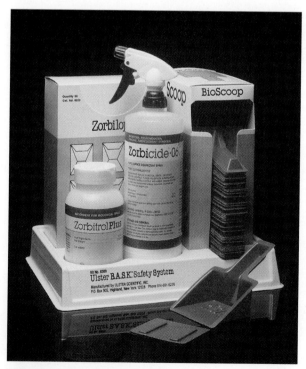

FIGURE 5-3   One type of single-use cleanup kit.

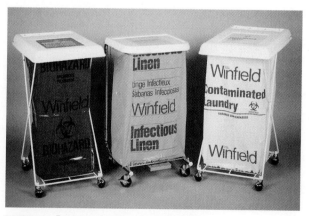

FIGURE 5-4   Examples of waste and hazard containers.

- Immediately clean and disinfect contaminated surfaces after exposure to infectious materials. Figure 5-3 shows one type of single-use cleanup kit. All surfaces must be decontaminated on a regular schedule that is posted, signed, and kept with OSHA records.
- Never pick up broken glass with hands. Use a dustpan or other mechanical device.
- Properly bag contaminated clothing and laundry in leak-proof labeled bags. Contaminated laundry should not be handled or washed at the medical office or with other noncontaminated clothing.
- Handle regulated waste (highly infectious material such as contaminated needles and surgical waste) by placing in clearly labeled biohazards waste containers (Figure 5-4). Waste must be removed by a licensed waste disposal service and incinerated or autoclaved before placing in a designated landfill area.

- Replace a damaged biohazard bag by placing a second bag around the first. Do not remove infectious material from the damaged bag.
- Use puncture-proof, sealable, biohazard sharps containers for all needles and sharps, such as razors and glass pipettes.
  - Place the container close to the work area.
  - Keep sharp container upright.
  - Never reach into the sharps container or push sharps further into the container.
  - Replace sharps container when 2/3 full.
  - Seal and label sharps containers before placing with biohazard waste for removal by disposal service.
- Perform hand hygiene both before and after using gloves.
- Personal protective equipment (PPE) may not be worn out of the laboratory areas. Failure to observe this precaution may result in an OSHA citation.

TABLE 5-2 Principles of Proper Body Mechanics

Movement	Description
Stoop	<ul><li>Do not bend from your back.</li><li>Stand close to the object you are moving.</li><li>Keep your feet 6–8 inches apart to create a base of support.</li><li>Place one foot slightly ahead of the other.</li><li>Bend at the hips and knees, keeping the back straight, and lower the body and hands down to the object (Figure 5-5).</li><li>Use the large leg muscles to assist in returning to a standing position (Figure 5-6).</li></ul> 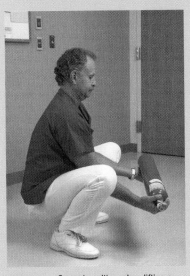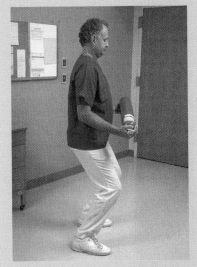 **FIGURE 5-5** Correct position when lifting a heavy object off the floor. **FIGURE 5-6** Use strong leg muscles, keeping back straight, when lifting.

(continued)

TABLE 5-2 **Principles of Proper Body Mechanics,** (*continued*)

Movement	Description
Lift firmly and smoothly	<ul><li>If you think you cannot move a heavy or awkward load, get help.</li><li>Grasp the load by using the large leg muscles.</li><li>Keep the load close to the body.</li></ul>
Use the center of gravity for carrying a load	<ul><li>Keep your back as straight as possible. (Hint: You should not be able to feel your clothing touch your back if you are standing straight.)</li><li>Keep the weight of the load close to your body and centered over the hips.</li><li>Put the load down by bending at the hips and knees.</li><li>When two or more people carry the load, have one person give the commands to lift or move the object.</li></ul>
Pull or push rather than lift or load	<ul><li>Remain close to the object you are moving.</li><li>Keep feet apart with one slightly forward.</li><li>Have a firm grasp on the object.</li><li>Crouch down with feet apart if the object is on the floor.</li><li>Bend your elbows and place hands on the load at chest level.</li><li>Keep your back straight.</li><li>Push up with your legs in order to stand up with the load.</li></ul>
Avoid reaching	<ul><li>Evaluate the distance before reaching too far for an object.</li><li>Stand close to the object.</li><li>Do not reach to the point of straining.</li><li>To change direction, point your feet in the direction you wish to go.</li><li>Keep the object close to your body as you lower it.</li></ul>
Avoid twisting	<ul><li>Do not twist your body.</li></ul>

enter the building a predetermined code has to be entered into the system. If the code is not entered within a specified number of seconds an alarm will be activated at the security system company's office. They will then alert the appropriate agency (fire, police, etc.).

Security doesn't just need to be in place when the office is closed. Procedures should take into account the need to secure patients and staff, patient medical records, computer stations, medical supplies, and, particularly, prescription pads from intruders and disorderly persons. HIPAA has raised awareness of many security issues regarding the privacy of each patient's personal medical history.

Incident Reports

Any unusual occurrence or accident is referred to as an incident in the medical setting. Following are some examples of incidents:

- A patient falls on a wet floor
- A housekeeping employee is stuck by a needle while emptying the trash
- A patient receives the wrong medication

- A patient misplaces or loses personal property, such as a hearing aid or glasses, while in the office
- Syringes or needles missing from the supply cupboard
- A medical assistant receives a needle stick from a contaminated needle
- An employee's purse is missing
- An abusive patient uses vulgar language
- A prescription pad is missing

Whenever any accident, injury, or unusual occurrence takes place, a written report must be made. This is called the incident report and can protect both the employer and the medical assistant against possible lawsuits. Some incidents should also be reported to the police or to the liability insurance carrier. For example, stolen property should be reported to the police, and a slip and fall should be reported to the insurance carrier.

Incident reports should be completed immediately in black ink. The incident should be described as simply as possible. Only objective information should be included, such as "Patient fell while getting onto exam table." Do not include subjective comment, such as "Patient was not paying attention to what he was doing." Your medical office should have its own customized form. However, most incident forms include the following information.

- Names of all persons involved
- Date and time of the incident
- Exact location of the incident (including the address of the medical facility and the location of the incident within the facility)
- Name of the person to whom the incident is reported and the time of the report
- Brief description of what happened
- Names of all witnesses
- Name and description of any equipment involved in the incident
- Action taken at the time of the incident
- Action taken to prevent a recurrence
- Signature and title of person completing the report

The incident report, like all other information relating to the patient, is subject to subpoena in litigation (lawsuits). A copy of the incident report should be placed in a master incident report file, the patient's file, and the employee's record. Figure 5-7 is an example of an incident report form. Professionalism addresses some information that can prevent incidents from occurring.

Ergonomics in the Medical Office

OSHA eliminated the ergonomics section of the regulations for medical facilities, but that doesn't mean they aren't important to the well-being and productivity of employees. If well designed, systems of work, sports and leisure, and health and safety all incorporate ergonomic principles.

In the medical setting, ergonomics applies to all aspects of the facility. The most common area for problems is the computer workstation. The keyboard should be at elbow height, the monitor at eye level, and the chair should be adjustable, with a lumbar support. The operator's feet should be able to rest on the floor comfortably, with no strain. A wrist rest and mouse wrist support should be used.

Lighting should be appropriate for the task. Overhead fluorescent lights should not reflect on the computer monitor screens, causing a glare. This can be prevented by adding an anti-glare shield to the monitor or tilting the screen so that the light does not hit it directly. Clinical areas should be well lit. Repetitive motions should be limited, and the proper tools should be available for any procedure.

Professionalism

Maintaining a professional demeanor in the medical office can prevent many incidents from occurring. Wearing the appropriate apparel, avoiding excessive jewelry, and pulling back long hair can eliminate hazards that might result in injuries.

Quality Medical Care

Quality medical care is an expectation of all patients and requires that the health care team use procedures and techniques that result in the best possible outcome for the patient. In addition, the patient must be satisfied with the care (Lifespan Considerations).

INCIDENT REPORT

Name of injured party _____ Date _____

Address _____ Telephone _____

The injured party was: ☐ Employee ☐ Patient ☐ Other _____

Date of accident/incident _____   Time of incident _____

Where did incident occur? _____

Names of witnesses (include titles):

_____

_____

What first aid/treatment was given at the time of the incident?

_____

Who administered first aid? _____

Briefly describe the incident. _____

_____

Names of employees present at time of incident/injury:

_____

What, in your opinion, caused the accident? _____

Follow-up: What steps have been taken to prevent a similar accident? _____

_____

Date _____   Employee's signature _____

Date _____   Supervisor's signature _____

FIGURE 5-7   An example of a typical incident report.

Remember that when dealing *with elderly patients, they may have balance problems or gait disabilities that make them more prone to falls. Consider this when preparing the waiting room and the examination rooms. Avoid throw rugs, extension cords, or anything that may be a trip/fall hazard.*

The major parameters or attributes of health care that are regularly examined include treatment, benefit of treatment, cost/benefit, accessibility to health care, and delivery location. The outcome factor actually requires a measurable change in the health status of the

---

BOX 5-1
The AMA's Eight Essentials of Quality Care

- Bring about the optimal in the patient's condition within the earliest time frame possible based on the patient's comfort and physical condition.
- Have an emphasis on early detection and treatment as well as health promotion and disease prevention.
- Receive treatment in a timely fashion without unnecessary delay, termination, interruption, or prolongation.
- Encourage the patient's participation in the decision process regarding his or her treatment.
- Base the treatment on skillful use of technology and the health professional's use of accepted principles of medical science.
- Demonstrate concern for the patient and patient's family, with sensitivity to the stress caused by illness.
- Achieve the treatment goal through the wise use of technology and other resources.
- Provide adequate documentation in the patient's medical record to facilitate peer evaluation and continuity of care.

patient that is a direct result of the care received. Cost/benefit refers to the expenditure or cost in terms of time, money, and effort, and the relationship of this cost to the actual benefit the patient receives. Accessibility to health care refers to the effort a patient must make to receive health care. The American Medical Association (AMA) has defined quality care by listing eight essential elements (Box 5-1).

What is Quality Assurance?

In the early 1960s, the health care industry began to feel an increasing demand from the public for accountable quality care. From that initial swell of public pressure developed a continuing effort on the part of health care providers to deliver satisfactory, achievable excellence in care. Quality assurance (QA) is gathering and evaluating information about the services provided (as well as the results achieved) and comparing this information with an accepted standard.

Quality assessment measures consist of formal, systematic evaluations of overall patterns of care. The goal of the actual programs and activities of quality assurance have a desired degree of care in a health care setting. The results of the evaluations are then compared to standard results. As deficiencies are identified, recommendations for improvement in care are made. Quality Improvement Programs (QIPs) utilize the data gathered by quality assurance/assessment to make quality improvements in health care.

Quality Assurance Program

A quality assurance program (QAP) in a hospital, ambulatory health care setting, long-term-care facility, or health maintenance organization (HMO) consists of a system for reviewing records maintained by staff. These records may consist of medical or nursing records, data regarding days of hospitalization or treatment, progress reports, and other statistics that provide a firm indication of the care received by patients. A quality assurance program must include evaluation and educational components to identify and correct problems. Quality assurance programs such as these are required in order for the facility to receive funding by the Public Health Service Act, (which defines the requirements) as well as to achieve and maintain accreditation. The basic components of a quality assurance program include the following:

- Establish a QA Committee—representatives from the entire patient care team (such as physician, nurse, and medical assistant) should be part of a QA committee (Figure 5-8).
- Review all clinical and administrative services and procedures—committee members or an

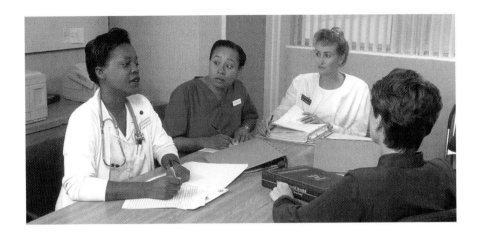

FIGURE 5-8 A quality assurance (QA) committee meeting.

assigned individual can conduct the review. All team members should have a role in the QA process, from designing the QA forms to selecting issues for review. Procedure and policy manuals are also subject to review during this process.

- Set up a structure for identifying items to review; pay particular attention to problem issues.

- Quantify all issues. For example:

    –average length of waiting time in minutes to see physician

    –number of errors in writing items on patient records

    –number of insurance claims disallowed per 100 filed

    –number of failed "needle sticks" per 50 attempts

- Limit the number of issues—set a limit to the number of issues or problems reviewed at any one session. Emphasis should be placed on taking corrective measures.

- Maintain careful records—review all records, such as incident reports and committee records, and progress or improvement with the entire medical team.

Box 5-2 lists examples of issues that a QA committee might review in a physician's office.

BOX 5-2
Issues Reviewed by a QA Committee in a Physician's Office

- Disallowed insurance claims
- Errors in dispensing medications (use incident reports)
- Errors in labeling of laboratory specimens
- Incorrect coding of diagnosis for insurance claims
- Long waiting time for patients
- Adverse reactions to treatments and/or medications (use incident reports)
- Inability to obtain venous blood on the first attempt
- Patient satisfaction (from survey/questionnaire results)
- Patients who leave the office without seeing the physician

- Patient complaints relating to confidentiality
- Appearance of office
- Handicapped parking availability
- Safety
- Provider availability
- Emergency preparations
- 16 Treatment areas
- Safety/monitoring practices for radiology and laboratory
- Medications
- Infection control
- Patient education/rights
- Medical records
- Collection procedures
- Telephone and reception behaviors

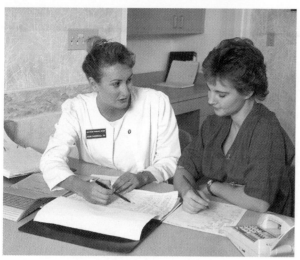

FIGURE 5-9 A medical assistant at a QA meeting.

Implementing a Quality Assurance Program (QAP)

The ultimate goal of a formal quality assurance program is to improve the quality of care so that there is no difference between what should be done and what is actually being done. Professionals in the field who are expert in a particular health care area develop these norms or standards.

To put a QAP into place, requires the development of patient-centered criteria based on acceptable stan-

---

Box 5-3
The Medical Assistant's Role in QA

- Resolve patient complaints about items such as billing questions and long waiting times in the reception room.
- Perform patient education regarding diet, laboratory and procedure instructions, and personal care.
- Perform telephone follow-up regarding a patient's condition and progress.
- Double-check laboratory tests performed in the office.
- Verify the results of laboratory tests given over the telephone. Always ask the laboratory to repeat any results that are abnormal or unclear. Request to have a written report sent by mail or fax.
- Bring patient complaints to the attention of the physician.

---

dards of care. Criteria are standards used to compare something in order to make a decision. For example, years ago some patients were discharged from a hospital without being given any formal information or education about what to do when they returned home. Now all hospitalized patients should receive instructions at discharge regarding medications, diet, activity, and follow-up appointments with the physician. This discharge plan is explained to the patient, who then signs the plan and keeps a copy. A copy of the signed plan is also put in the patient's chart, indicating this instruction took place. A quality assurance program would monitor the discharge planning process.

The Medical Assistant's Role in a QAP

The medical assistant is trained in clinical and administrative skills with the expectation for the highest level of performance. To assist the physician/employer, pay rigorous attention to the quality of care given to patients. Patient satisfaction is a key element in quality of care. The medical assistant may be the first person to respond to a patient's complaint or discomfort. Medical assistants have the opportunity to present patients' concerns or complaints at a team QA meeting so that corrective measures can be taken (Figure 5-9). Some of the areas in which to assist the physician with quality assurance are noted in Box 5-3.

Health Plan Employer Data and Information Set (HEDIS)

Under HEDIS, managed care plans that serve Medicare patients must collect data relating to eight categories of performance:

- Effectiveness of care
- Access to/availability of care
- Member satisfaction
- Informed health care choices
- Health plan descriptive information
- Cost of care
- Health plan stability
- Use of service

Medicare, HMOs, and other plans seeking accreditation from the National Committee for Quality Assurance (NCQA), must also report data. The NCQA evaluates the quality of health plans in order to help consumers and employers make more informed decisions about their health care. Eventually, most of the health plans (HMOs and PPOs) a physician contracts with will be collecting data for the medical practice.

TABLE 5-3 Clinical Laboratory Improvement Amendment (CLIA)

Category	Explanation
Simple Testing	Incorrect test results pose little risk for the patient. Laboratory is subject to random inspectors only. Some physician's laboratories fall in this category.
Intermediate-Level Testing (Level II)	Poses risk to patient if there is an incorrect test result. Must be certified by approved accrediting agency. Must be staffed by credentialed personnel. Must meet quality assurance standards.
Complex Testing (Level III)	Poses high risk to patient if there is an incorrect test result. Must be certified by approved accrediting agency. Must be staffed by credentialed personnel. Must meet quality assurance standards.

Clinical Laboratory Improvement Amendment (CLIA)

The federal government now requires that all clinical laboratories that test human specimens must be controlled. The Clinical Laboratories Improvement Amendment of 1988 (CLIA88) divides laboratories into three categories. These are described in Table 5-3. Refer to Volume III, Chapter 40 for further discussion of the Clinical Laboratory Improvement Act (CLIA), which mandates quality control of laboratory tests by categories and documentation.

SUMMARY

Safety measures including general safety, employee safety, emergency plans, such as fire, the handling of biological hazards and bloodborne pathogens, housekeeping procedures, proper body mechanics, security, and environment are essential to maintaining a safe and pleasant workplace. The efforts of a medical assistant can be critical in ensuring that all of these components are carefully regarded.

Chapter Review

COMPETENCY REVIEW

1. Define and spell the terms to learn for this chapter.
2. List six safety rules to follow in medical offices.
3. You have been asked to draft the OSHA Exposure Plan for your office. What three points must you include in this plan?

PREPARING FOR THE CERTIFICATION EXAM

1. A formal written description of an accident that has occurred in a medical setting is a/an
   A. quality assurance report
   B. incident report
   C. evaluation
   D. policy manual
   E. procedure manual

2. A material safety data sheet (MSDS) contains information about
   A. OSHA guidelines
   B. hazardous chemicals and other substances
   C. office policy
   D. vendor information
   E. medical surgical devices

continued on next page

3. OSHA guidelines are available from
   A. U.S. Department of Labor
   B. AAMA
   C. AMA
   D. FDA
   E. BNDD

4. The law regulating laboratory safety precautions is
   A. OSHA
   B. FUTA
   C. CLIA
   D. FICA
   E. A and C

5. Universal precautions mandate that
   A. all blood and bodily fluid contact is to be treated as if it contains HIV, HBV, or other bloodborne pathogens
   B. precautions must be taken only when there is visible blood present
   C. precautions are not necessary if the health care professional uses proper hand hygiene
   D. only medical assistants and nurses must follow the guidelines
   E. all employees have the Hepatitis B vaccine series

6. An OSHA citation may be issued as a result of failure to
   A. use proper telephone and reception behavior
   B. affix hazardous waste container to the wall
   C. remove street clothing before coming to and leaving from work
   D. remove PPE before leaving from work
   E. bend when lifting a heavy object

7. Medical waste consists of the following, EXCEPT
   A. radioactive waste
   B. occupational waste
   C. infectious waste
   D. chemical waste
   E. solid waste

8. Proper body mechanics involves the following muscles, EXCEPT
   A. arm
   B. back
   C. leg
   D. neck
   E. eye lid

9. OSHA reports for employee Hepatitis B vaccine records must be maintained for at least
   A. 30 years
   B. 3 years
   C. 1 year
   D. 30 months
   E. 3 months

10. The following include potential infectious materials, EXCEPT
    A. amniotic fluids
    B. body fluid with blood
    C. saliva
    D. sweat
    E. bloody vomitus

CRITICAL THINKING

1. What errors did Gloria make in preparing the injection?
2. What tests must be performed as a result of this needlestick?
3. Does Linda hold any responsibility in this situation?
4. How would this pertain to OSHA's Bloodborne Pathogens Standards?

ON THE JOB

Bonnie feels that the office is always too cold, so she keeps a heater under her desk. In order to use the heater, she needs to run an extension cord across to another electrical outlet. Several times, the safety officer in the practice asks her to discontinue using the heater. Bonnie will put the heater away for a couple of days, then bring it back out when she feels it won't be noticed. The safety officer comes by one day and confiscates the heater and extension cord. Bonnie feels that this is unfair because she is cold during the day and thinks she should be allowed to use the heater which allows her to perform her duties in comfort and more effiently.

1. What OSHA violations are of concern in this situation?
2. Did the safety officer handle the situation correctly the first few times?
3. Did the safety officer have the right to confiscate the heater and extension cord?
4. How might the situation be rectified to make Bonnie comfortable?

INTERNET ACTIVITY

Search the Internet to find private companies that are in business to provide services to prepare an office for OSHA requirements.

MediaLink More on the medical office environment, including interactive resources, can be found on the Student CD-ROM accompanying this textbook.

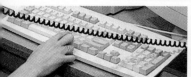

Medical Assistant Role Delineation Chart

HIGHLIGHT indicates material covered in this chapter.

ADMINISTRATIVE

Administrative Procedures

- Perform basic administrative medical assisting functions
- Schedule, coordinate and monitor appointments
- Schedule inpatient/outpatient admissions and procedures
- Understand and apply third-party guidelines
- Obtain reimbursement through accurate claims submission
- Monitor third-party reimbursement
- Understand and adhere to managed care policies and procedures
- *Negotiate managed care contracts*

Practice Finances

- Perform procedural and diagnostic coding
- Apply bookkeeping principles

- Manage accounts receivable
- *Manage accounts payable*
- *Process payroll*
- *Document and maintain accounting and banking records*
- *Develop and maintain fee schedules*
- *Manage renewals of business and professional insurance policies*
- *Manage personnel benefits and maintain records*
- *Perform marketing, financial, and strategic planning*

CLINICAL

Fundamental Principles

- Apply principles of aseptic technique and infection control
- Comply with quality assurance practices
- Screen and follow up patient test results

Diagnostic Orders

- Collect and process specimens
- Perform diagnostic tests

Patient Care

- Adhere to established patient screening procedures
- Obtain patient history and vital signs
- Prepare and maintain examination and treatment areas
- Prepare patient for examinations, procedures and treatments

- Assist with examinations, procedures and treatments
- Prepare and administer medications and immunizations
- Maintain medication and immunization records
- Recognize and respond to emergencies
- Coordinate patient care information with other health care providers
- Initiate IV and administer IV medications with appropriate training and as permitted by state law

GENERAL

Professionalism

- Display a professional manner and image
- Demonstrate initiative and responsibility
- Work as a member of the health care team
- Prioritize and perform multiple tasks
- Adapt to change
- Promote the CMA credential
- Enhance skills through continuing education
- Treat all patients with compassion and empathy
- Promote the practice through positive public relations

Communication Skills

- Recognize and respect cultural diversity
- Adapt communications to individual's ability to understand
- Use professional telephone technique

- Recognize and respond effectively to verbal, nonverbal, and written communications
- Use medical terminology appropriately
- Utilize electronic technology to receive, organize, prioritize and transmit information
- Serve as liaison

Legal Concepts

- Perform within legal and ethical boundaries
- Prepare and maintain medical records
- Document accurately
- Follow employer's established policies dealing with the health care contract
- Implement and maintain federal and state health care legislation and regulations
- Comply with established risk management and safety procedures
- Recognize professional credentialing criteria
- *Develop and maintain personnel, policy and procedure manuals*

Instruction

- Instruct individuals according to their needs
- Explain office policies and procedures
- Teach methods of health promotion and disease prevention
- Locate community resources and disseminate information
- *Develop educational materials*
- *Conduct continuing education activities*

Operational Functions

- Perform inventory of supplies and equipment
- Perform routine maintenance of administrative and clinical equipment
- Apply computer techniques to support office operations
- *Perform personnel management functions*
- *Negotiate leases and prices for equipment and supply contracts*

- *Denotes advanced skills.*

SOURCE: Reprinted by permission of the American Association of Medical Assistants from the AAMA Role Delineation Study: Occupational Analysis of the Medical Assisting Profession.

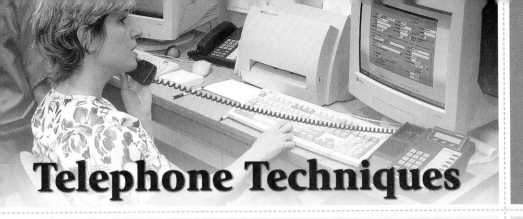

chapter 6

Telephone Techniques

Learning Objectives

After completing this chapter, you should be able to:

- Define and spell the terms to learn for this chapter.
- Take detailed and efficient telephone messages.
- Use the hold function effectively and professionally.
- Answer the telephone with a proper greeting and pleasant tone.
- Handle difficult callers.
- Understand what telephone triage is and how it is used in the medical office.
- Place long distance calls and conference calls.
- Handle emergency phone calls.

Terms to Learn

answering service

automated assistance program

caller ID

clarity

conference call

enunciation

inflection

pitch

queue

referrals

telephone triage

voice messaging system

Case Study

CINDY HAS BEEN LOOKING FOR A NEW PHYSICIAN. She has decided to try Dr. Brown since the office is near her place of work. When Cindy calls the office to set up an appointment, she is first greeted by a machine, which tells her she is calling Dr. Brown's office. She receives many options and dials "2" to schedule an appointment. Cindy then waits as the system transfers her to the appropriate person. When the transfer is done, she is greeted by Tonya, a new medical assistant in Dr. Brown's office. Tonya greets her with "Good Afternoon, this is Dr. Brown's office. This is Tonya, how may I help you?" Although Cindy is left with a cold feeling because she detects an insincere tone in Tonya's voice, she decides to ignore this and tells Tonya that she would like to make a new patient appointment. Tonya then tells Cindy to hold, and Cindy finds herself waiting and listening to rather distracting music. She has been on hold for two minutes when Tonya returns to the phone. Tonya gives no reason for the wait. At this point, Cindy is rather frustrated and informs Tonya that she will seek another physician.

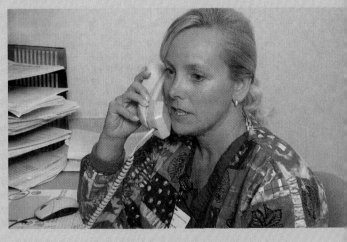

The telephone is the backbone of the medical office. It provides a key communication pathway between the physician, the staff, and the patient. As such, there are keys to using this pathway effectively. Every member of the health care team is responsible for communicating with patients and other callers and should know how to do so in the most professional way possible.

Telephone Techniques

If you work in the "front office" area, much of your day will be spent on the telephone. A fundamental rule to remember when answering your medical office's telephone is that you are not answering a home telephone. The telephone techniques used when speaking on home telephones are generally more informal and chatty than the style of conversation that is expected in a medical office. It is inappropriate to answer the office line with personal greetings, such as "Hello" or "Hi." A professional manner must always be presented to your callers.

Answering the Telephone

Your manner of answering the telephone frequently determines how the conversation will flow. It is also the first impression that callers, including potential new patients, receive of your office. Following are some important techniques that will assist you in answering your medical office's telephone in the most professional manner.

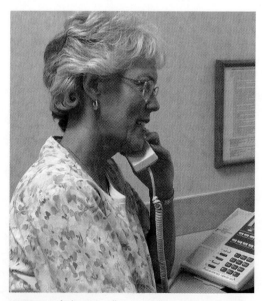

FIGURE 6-1 A pleasant smile can go a long way, even through telephone lines.

Smiling

Always answer the telephone with a smile. A human voice has so many nuances to it that most callers will be able to "hear" the warmth or indifference in your voice (Figure 6-1).

Greetings

When the medical office telephone rings, it is important that you answer the telephone quickly, usually by the third ring, and with a friendly, professional greeting. Your medical office supervisor will teach you the office's preferred method of answering the telephone. It is important that the greeting include the name of the office/physician and that all members of the staff use the same greeting. This will make the patient more comfortable in contacting your office. An example of a typical office greeting might be, "Good morning, Main Street Physicians. This is Jessica, how may I help you?"

Speech

We do not often think about how important it is to speak clearly on the telephone, but it is vital to good office management. There are four words used in reference to your speaking voice: clarity, enunciation, inflection, and pitch.

Clarity refers to the quality or state of being understandable. How clear is your voice to the caller? Are you holding the telephone receiver close to your mouth so that the best sound gets through to the caller? Many people tend to drop the receiver so that it sits just below the chin. This does not produce clear sound for the person on the other end of the telephone. You also need to make sure that there is nothing in your mouth that could garble your words. There should never be any gum, candy, or food in your mouth when addressing a caller.

Enunciation refers to the clear articulation and pronouncement of your words. Be careful not to speak too rapidly. Because you use the same greeting and phrase over and over again, it is easy to fall into the habit of speaking hurriedly. Remember to slow down, and pronounce your words slowly and properly. Avoid using regional pronunciations in the office setting. Remember that your patients come from many different cultures and may not understand your particular pronunciation. The sound of your voice ranges from high to low, depending on the context of your phrase. Have you ever noticed that when you ask a question your voice tends to rise at the end of the phrase? This is an example of the use of pitch or loudness of your voice. You will need to be aware of your voice pitch when speaking with patients. Inflection refers to the pitch and tone of your voice and the way you utter your words and phrases. Remember that speaking on the telephone is an opportunity to display excellent customer service. Try to avoid using a monotone voice (one single tone). The caller may feel you are bored and that you are not interested in helping.

Identify the Caller

Protection of a patient's information is vital in every medical office and health care facility. It is important to remember that some individuals may seek confidential information by dubious means, such as claiming to be the patient or even a specialist treating a patient. Therefore, steps must be taken to protect patient records. For example, each time a person calls in and claims to be a patient, it is a good idea to ask for some identifying information, especially his or her first and last names, social security number, and date of birth. You can check this information against the patient's computer record. You may also pull the patient's paper chart and check against that record. This will help to ensure that the person speaking is the patient.

The Business Telephone System

There are many types of business telephone systems in use today (Figure 6-2). Most medical offices will use some form of a multi-line telephone. Some may have all of the lines separate, where you must press that particular line's button to answer it, or a system that will feed calls to you from a queue or waiting line. More and more offices have systems that will answer the initial call with a recording and then feed the calls to the appropriate people.

Whether you are answering initially (without an automated system) or an automated system answers (calls are queued), remember to follow the rules of greeting callers discussed earlier.

Making Calls

Just as often as you answer calls in a medical office, you will have to make them. On most business telephones, you will be required to dial "9" to get an outside line. Some telephones may just have an outside line button that you will need to hit before you dial. Depending on the office's location, you may also need to dial the area code with all calls. Large cities have begun to make this a common practice because of the need for multiple area codes within a local calling zone. The telephone calls that you make in the office should be limited to business calls. All offices have different policies on the use of the office telephone for personal calls. Some may prohibit them all together, while others may allow them in limited number. It is important to keep in mind that the office telephone is for patients and emergencies, so you need to keep the lines open.

Using the Hold Function

One of the most sensitive issues relating to telephone courtesy is the use of the "hold" function. The hold function refers to the ability to keep more than one call on the line at a time. Holding the call is permissible when the person being called will come on the line

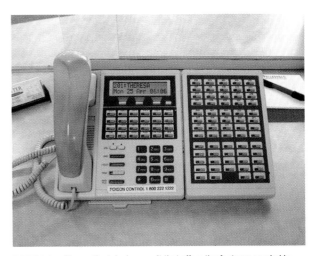

FIGURE 6-2 Choose the telephone unit that offers the features needed in your office.

within a short period of time or when you are already speaking to a caller on another line. However, the hold function is abused when callers are left "on hold" for indefinite periods of time.

If you are already speaking with a caller when a second call comes in, it is proper to ask the first caller if you may place him or her on hold for a moment in order to answer the second call. It is discourteous to handle the second caller before returning to the first call. An example of a typical conversation is as follows:

First caller: "Mrs. Brown, may I place you on hold for a moment? I have another call."

Second caller: "Good afternoon, Drs. Garcia and Jensen. Would you please hold?"

It is important to allow the second caller time to respond. If the second call is an emergency, you will need to take care of it before returning to the original call. If it is not an emergency, finish the original call before moving onto the second call. With all calls that you place on hold, try to keep the wait time to a minimum. Nobody likes to be on hold.

There are other situations where you may need to place a caller on hold. For example, you may need to pull a chart to answer a patient's question. When this happens, explain to the patient what you need to do to get the appropriate information, and then ask if you may place him or her on hold. Again, always wait for a response and then retrieve the information in the timeliest manner possible. If you have trouble getting the information and need more time, let the caller know. Do not leave callers on hold without checking back with them. To avoid forgetting that you have a caller on hold, be wary of distractions and do not do tasks that are unrelated to helping that caller.

Another situation that will require you to put a caller on hold is when a patient needs to speak with the doctor or another staff member who is not readily available. In this situation, make sure the person calling is aware that there will be a wait and offer to take a message and a number for a return call. As much as possible, it is best to keep the telephone lines open. If the caller chooses to wait, you will need to check on him or her approximately every 30 seconds. Let the caller know that the person he or she is waiting on is still unavailable. Then check to see if the caller would like to leave a name and number so as to have the call returned. See Box 6-1 for a list of things to avoid when using the hold function.

Transferring Calls

As you field calls in the medical office, you will find that it is often necessary to transfer or send them from one office telephone extension to another extension in the same office. Most business telephones will have the ability to transfer the call from your desk. There are a few steps that you should follow to make this a smooth transition for the caller.

First, once you have identified the person to whom you will be transferring the call, tell the caller the name of this person. This lets the caller know who to expect on the other end of the line as well as who to call back in case of disconnection during the transfer. If you have an extension number available, it is also helpful to provide that number to the patient before transferring him or her. When you start the transfer, make sure that the caller is aware of your actions. Do not transfer a patient without his or her prior knowledge and consent. Also, avoid transferring the call and hanging up without knowledge of whether the person was available to help the caller. Most telephones systems allow you to announce a call that you are transferring. Let the person to whom you

are transferring the call know the caller's name and the reason for the call. That person may tell you that he or she is unavailable to take the call. You may get a busy signal when you try to transfer the call. In these situations, take a message, or let the caller leave a recorded message.

Taking a Message

Medical offices are busy by nature. Medical assistants will often take messages from patients, other physicians, health care facilities, businesses, etc. Be prepared by keeping a notebook on hand to take notes while speaking with the caller. This will ensure that you have the information correct, such as the caller's name and the reason for the call. It is best not to trust your memory.

All messages should include the first and last name of the caller, a telephone number at which he or she can be reached for a callback, the reason for the call, and the name of the person he or she is trying to reach. If at any time you do not understand what a caller has stated, you will need to clarify the message with that caller. You may repeat to the caller what you believe you heard, or you may ask the caller to repeat back what was said to you. Always repeat the telephone number for a call back to the caller. The caller may interpret the lack of a return call due to an incorrect number, as lack of concern or disrespect. All telephone messages regarding a patient should be placed in the patient's chart.

It is very important to remember not to throw anything away that contains patient information. If a sheet of paper from the notepad you use to take proper messages has patient information, it must be shredded. It is a violation of the HIPAA privacy rule to throw patient information into the trash.

See Procedure 6-1 for instructions on how to take telephone messages. Legal and Ethical Issues discusses more about following office protocol.

The Voice Messaging System

In the medical office, you will deal with a voice messaging system for both incoming and outgoing calls. A voice messaging system allows for messages (voice mail) to be left or recorded when the medical assistant is unavailable to answer the telephone.

For incoming calls, your office may have a voice messaging system to record messages for you when you are away from your desk. If you are using a voice message system, remember to include your name and number in your recorded greeting. Your voice messaging system should also allow for the caller to dial "0" for immediate assistance.

When calling patients, you will find that most of them will have some form of voice messaging system, whether with a land line or cell phone. This does present a problem in the context of patient privacy. It is important to know your office's policy as to what kind of message should be left on a patient's voice messaging system.

BOX 6-1
Placing a Caller on Hold: Things to Avoid

When placing a caller on hold always avoid:
- Switching the caller to "hold" before he or she states the reason for the call
- Placing several callers on hold at the same time
- Going back to the "hold" call and asking, "Who are you waiting for?"
- Cutting off calls by careless use of the hold button
- Leaving a caller "on hold" for several minutes without checking back on the caller
- Playing loud music on the telephone line while the patient is "on hold"
- Stating rudely "Hold" or "hold please" without giving any explanation

Medical assistants must use a level of caution when speaking with patients over the telephone. Remember to never try to diagnose a patient yourself. Only the physician can diagnose. When handling calls, remember to always follow your office's protocol manual. Make sure to document every call that you have with a patient. All details— even seemingly insignificant ones—should be documented. Never throw any patient information away in a trash can. All patient information must be shredded when being disposed.

Call Forwarding

The call forwarding feature allows for a telephone user to forward calls to another telephone. For example, a physician may wish to forward his or her cell phone calls to a home telephone. You will often use this feature if your office uses an answering service. Your office calls will be forwarded to the answering services lines.

Caller ID

Caller ID is an increasingly popular telephone option. This function allows for telephone owners to know who is calling each time the telephone rings. In the office, it is unlikely that you will have caller ID, but many of your patients may have this telephone feature. It is important to understand that a medical office may need to block the office number from showing up on the patient's caller ID. This is because most offices often have multiple telephone lines, some designated for incoming calls and others for outgoing calls. Each of these lines may have a different telephone number. "Backlines"—lines meant only for incoming calls from patients—should be left open at all times. If a patient has caller ID, he or she may get the number to one of your "backlines." This can become very confusing to both the patient and the staff.

Privacy Manager

Privacy manager is a fairly recent addition to the variety of telephone options. This option allows patients to block access to their home telephones. When you call a telephone number that has privacy manager attached, you will be asked to state from where you are calling. Once you have given this information, unless you are cleared, you'll be directed to a voice mail system, where you will leave a message.

Speakerphone and Headsets

There are times when you will feel the need to free up your hands for administrative duties, while still being available to answer the telephone. There are two options that can be utilized: the speakerphone and the headset.

Most telephones have a built in speakerphone or a microphone and speaker. The speakerphone allows you

---

6-1 | **PROCEDURE**

Taking a Telephone Message

OBJECTIVE: Ensure that correct and relevant information is retrieved when taking a telephone message.

Equipment and Supplies
message form or pad with carbon or carbonless for duplicates; pen

1. Give the correct greeting.
2. Use a message form or pad with a carbon copy to keep a record of the message.
3. Print the date and time of the call.
4. Print the caller's full name and telephone number. (Always ask the caller to spell his or her name.)
5. Write the name of the person being called.
6. Write down the complete message. Avoid using abbreviations other than accepted medical abbreviations. Include symptoms such as temperature, rash, emesis, and duration of symptoms.
7. Write your initials to indicate that you took the message.

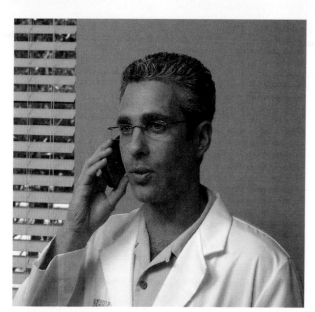

FIGURE 6-3 Many physicians use cell phones to stay in touch with their offices.

to hear and speak without having to pick up the handset of the telephone. There are a few drawbacks, however, to the speakerphone. Others nearby may overhear your conversation; also, the caller on the other end will be able to hear any background noise. Patient confidentiality should be a foremost concern when using the speakerphone.

Another hands-free feature is a headset. This is a microphone and earpiece that is worn on your head like a headband, an ergonomically safe feature. Headsets are either connected to the telephone with a cord, or they are cordless. When using a headset, you will need to remember to keep the microphone close to your mouth for the clearest delivery.

Pagers and Cell Phones

Many physicians carry pagers with them on a regular basis. It will be important for you to know if the physician(s) in your office carries a pager. This will be one of the most important methods for getting in touch with him or her in emergency situations. You will find that most pager systems are user-friendly. One simply has to call the pager number and when instructed, enter in the callback telephone number. Some offices may use a coded message system. For example, certain numbers may be designated for different types of emergencies or situations. Using a specific number will give the physician a heads up as to what the call is referencing. You will need to find out how your particular office uses the pager system.

Cell phones have become fundamental to business and social life. Most physicians and office managers now use cell phones to conduct day-to-day business

(Figure 6-3). Some have even replaced their conventional pagers with cell phones because most cell phones also have a pager function. However, cell phones do have a disadvantage in that certain parts of the hospitals do not allow them because they interfere with electronic monitors. Usually, hospital buildings are clearly marked as to where cell phones are allowed and where they are not allowed. In most of these cell-phone-free zones, pagers will still be allowed. It is important to check with the hospitals your office frequently deals with to understand their rules regarding cell phones and pagers.

Screening Telephone Calls

One of the most important ways to keep the office running smoothly and one of your key functions in the front office is to screen telephone calls effectively. When answering the telephone, you will need to determine quickly what type of call you have received and the proper way to handle it. Whenever you answer the telephone, you should ask the person the reason for the call. From there, you will either transfer the call to the appropriate person, or you will handle the call yourself. The different types of telephone calls you may receive will be discussed later in the chapter.

Making Reminder Calls and Doing Callbacks

Most offices will require medical assistants to make calls to patients to remind them of upcoming appointments. Offices might do this a week before the appointment and then again the day before the appointment.

As a medical assistant, you will also be required to make "callbacks"—return calls to patients or other callers. For instance, messages left by patients usually contain a question for the physician or deal with prescription refill requests. Your callback will relay the physician's response. Sometimes the physician may have you call a patient to check on his or her status.

When making any of these calls to a patient's house or place of business, you will need to take care in protecting the patient's privacy. Remember that this is one of the most important issues concerning a medical facility. The first thing that you should do when calling any patient is to make sure that it is the patient that you are speaking with on the telephone. Start every callback to the patient by identifying yourself, and then ask to speak to the patient. You should not indicate why you are calling until you have the patient on the telephone line. If the person who answers asks you why you are calling, explain that confidentiality laws prevent you from revealing that information.

Typical Incoming Calls

You will receive many different types of calls in the medical office. Most are from patients, but many are not. The following are some types of telephone calls you will handle on a daily basis.

Patient Calls

Most calls coming into the medical office will be from patients (Figure 6-4). We will discuss a few of the reasons why patients call.

Appointment Requests

One of the most common types of calls you receive in the office will be appointment requests. These calls will often involve patients with health problems, so you need to follow telephone triage procedures (discussed later in the chapter) to schedule them appropriately. The caller may be a current patient or a new patient. For patients who need routine appointments, give an appointment time that is convenient for both the patient and the medical office. You will learn more about scheduling appointments in Chapter 8.

Insurance and Billing Questions

It is a fact that most patients will not understand the way medical insurance works. You should anticipate receiving calls on a daily basis from patients with questions about their accounts and medical insurance. You may be able to answer some of these questions, but most will be directed to the billing department.

PROBLEMS WITH BILLS Patients will often call with the question, "Why did I receive a bill?" Many patients have the misconception that their insurance company will pay the entire bill. You may have to explain to the patient the details of what was billed. In your explanation, you will need to include what steps the insurance company has taken in regards to covering the charges. This could include discussing deductibles, co-payments, and coinsurance. You may also need to explain reasons for denial of certain charges. If you are unable to help the patient with questions concerning insurance coverage, you may refer him or her to the insurance company or to the human resources department of your employer.

ARE YOU A PARTICIPATING PROVIDER? The medical assistant should have a list of the most common insurance providers with whom the practice is affiliated. Specific questions patients have regarding provider participation should be directed to the insurance company.

Fees

Specific questions regarding fees should always be referred to the billing department. You should keep in mind that more often than not, you will be unable to give any exact figures until the patient has been seen by the physician.

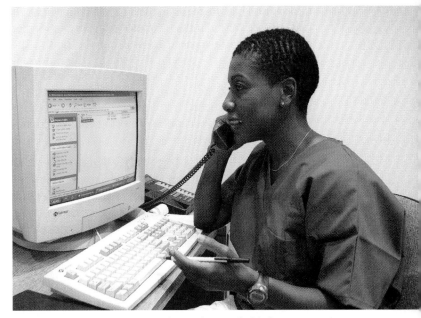

FIGURE 6-4 The medical assistant spends many hours on the telephone assisting patients.

Office Hours and Directions

Most offices now include the office hours and directions in the office's automated assistance systems. However, you may have to handle some of the calls yourself. You should have your office address and hours posted near your telephone. It is also a good idea to have directions posted near the telephone. The directions should include routes to the office from all directions—north, south, east, and west—when applicable.

Laboratory Test Results

Many patients will call the office, to get the results from recent procedures and tests. Follow your office policy regarding disseminating results to patients. Certain tests may require follow up testing or procedures. In that case, follow up is necessary to ensure that the patient performed as instructed.

Follow-Up Calls From Patients

It is common for a physician to have a patient call the office as a follow-up to certain procedures and to relate the status of certain problems. When these calls come into the office, you will need to take a message to convey this information to the physician.

Referral Requests

Many insurance companies require that patients get referrals (special paperwork) from primary care physicians when patients see a specialist. So it will often happen that a patient may call asking for the referral to be done. Referrals are done before the patient is to see the specialist and may be done over the telephone or by fax. You will need to get all of the information necessary to place the referral, including the name, address, and telephone number of the specialist's office. This information may be found in the local telephone book. It may also be found in the insurance company's provider book. You will also need to find out the reason the patient is seeing the specialist. Some of this information you may get from the patient. You may also need to check the patient's chart for the diagnosis that the referral is referencing. All referrals need to be approved by your physician before being completed and released to the patient.

Patients Who Refuse to Identify Themselves

Occasionally you will run into patients who refuse to identify themselves to you. You will need to let the caller know that you will not be of assistance without his or her name and reason for calling. Inform the caller that the physician will not return calls to patients who refuse to identify themselves.

The Persistent Talker

Every medical office has those patients who call in and draw the staff into long conversations. Unfortunately, your time is valuable and limited. You will need to end these conversations kindly, but promptly. You may simply state to the patient that you are busy helping another patient and apologize for the inconvenience.

Nonpatient Calls

Not all telephone calls to the office will be from patients. You will find that a large number of calls will come from sales people, hospitals, other physicians, and other health care facilities.

Sales Calls

Answering calls from sales representatives is part of the medical assistant's telephone responsibilities. You may have to become the wall between the sales calls and your physician and office manager. Most physicians will not take any type of sales calls while seeing patients. They may wish you to take messages or ask the sales representative to fax or email the information to them. The same will probably hold true with office managers. They will ask you to take messages from most sales calls to return the calls at a more convenient time.

Reports From Hospitals and Other Patient Care Facilities

If your physician has patients in a hospital or nursing facility, it will be common to receive calls from those facilities. The facilities will often call with status checks on patients or changes in patients' conditions. In many cases, you will need to interrupt the physician for these calls. You should knock on the examination room door and let the physician know that there is an important call.

There will also be times when you will just need to take a message for the physician. The message may just be information to relay or the physician may need to return the call. It is important that you find out whether or not the call should be returned.

BOX 6-2

Information to Request From the Patient

- Patient's name
- The caller's name, if different from the patient
- Telephone number
- Date of the call
- Time of the call
- The patient's physician, if a multi-physician practice
- Any medications that the patient is taking
- Any allergies the patient may have
- The patient's insurance
- The manner of the patient's problem

General Office Matters

Some calls received in the office deal with general office business, including telephone calls from accountants or calls regarding rented office equipment and suppliers. These calls should be handled on a case-by-case basis. It is important to screen calls from your suppliers carefully. Make sure the supplier gives you his or her name, the business' name, address, and telephone number.

Physician's Personal Calls

The physician will also receive personal calls in the office. Physicians work long hours and often encourage family members to call them at the office. Most physicians will instruct you on how they wish their personal calls to be handled. In some cases, they will want you to knock on the examination room door and simply state, "Doctor, you are wanted on the telephone." In other cases, physicians may ask you to give them telephone messages as soon as they come out of the examination room. Generally, family members do not wish to interrupt the physician during a patient examination.

Calls From Another Physician

Personal calls from other physicians are handled in a similar manner. Physicians may wish to talk to other physicians as soon as the call comes into the office. These calls may relate to a patient consultation question that needs to be answered immediately. Again, you may take a message to be delivered to the physician as he or she exits the examination room, or you may interrupt the physician with the call. You will need to follow the wishes of your employer.

Obscene or Prank Calls

It is a fact that if you have a telephone, you are at risk for receiving prank calls. You should hang up immediately if you receive obscene or prank calls. You may also report the call to the telephone operator, especially if it is an ongoing problem involving the same caller. Usually, the telephone company can trace the call.

Prescription Refill Requests

One of the most common telephone calls received in the office are requests for prescription refills. Because of the high volume of calls, many offices will have a voice mail system answer most of these calls. The medical assistant is often responsible for taking these messages off the voice mail system and responding to them. This will need to be done more than just once a day. The messages should be checked a minimum of twice a day and in larger offices, even more frequently. All of the prescription refill requests will need to be signed-off by the physician. Some physicians will request to have the patient's chart with the message before giving it an okay. It is advisable to be prepared and attach the message to the chart ahead of time. See Procedure 6-2 for important information on taking a prescription refill message.

Telephone Triage

Triage is a process used to determine the order in which patients should be treated. The patient's severity of illness or injury determines the order of treatment. Telephone triage—determining the order to take patient calls—is an issue for the telephone screening process. By asking specific questions, the medical assistant can determine how to handle a patient's problem. Each office should have a procedure manual that will outline the office's preferred method of screening telephone calls.

Most of your patients will be calling because they feel they need to see the physician. It will be one of your responsibilities to see that the patient is helped in the most appropriate manner. You will need to gather information from the patient. As with all telephone calls, the first thing you'll need to find out is

the patient's name and telephone number, in case you become disconnected. Remember to have the patient spell out his or her name to avoid mistakes. During the course of your conversation, you should ask for some basic demographic information as well as for medical information. Box 6-2 lists information that you should request from the patient. When scheduling the patient, make sure to include the information that you received from the patient. Then place the information in the patient's chart. This will help you or another medical assistant know how to prepare for the appointment. Cultural Considerations discusses more about obtaining information from patients.

The medical assistant must be careful when screening patients on the telephone. You will be assessing a patient's symptoms. This, however, is very close to going outside of the medical assistant's scope of practice. Make sure that you are closely following the established telephone protocols that were agreed upon by the physician. If ever a situation arises that is not covered in the procedure manual, the medical assistant will need to ask the physician how to handle that particular problem. Physicians will often purchase one of many triage manuals that are available on the market. Again, remember to follow only the protocols that the physician has approved. Lifespan Considerations addresses more on assessing symptoms.

If a patient refuses to tell you the reason for the call, you should explain the need for specific information so as to assist him or her. Try to make the caller comfortable in sharing the information with you.

Handling Difficult Calls

The most important thing to remember when dealing with a difficult patient is not to lose your temper. There are many types of problematic calls that you may receive. They can vary from patients who are angry and yelling, to people attempting to get confidential information. With any difficult caller, you must try and keep the situation as calm as possible. It is best to keep in mind that the patient, more often than not, is displacing anger and is probably frustrated with some other situation. It could be anything from worry over an illness, to having had a bad day, to suffering from pain.

When you have a difficult patient on the telephone line, the best approach is to be empathetic while remaining in control of the situation. Take the time to listen and find out the exact problem. Once you determine where the problem lies, then you can begin to help.

Using a Telephone Directory

When calling most insurance companies and hospitals, you will find that they have an automated telephone directory or automated assistance program—telephone systems that direct callers to the appropriate people through a series of questions.

After the call is answered, the caller is presented with options so that the telephone system can direct him or her to the proper person or department to handle the call. Be aware that many large business systems will also provide additional options. When using one of these systems, it is important to pay close attention to the options that are being offered. It can be easy to miss your cue. When you hear an option, the system will instruct you either to press the appropriate button or to state the option verbally. Keep in mind that in most systems, if you cannot find an option to fit your needs, you can dial "0" to have the operator of the system direct you manually. Patient Education highlights more uses of an automatic assistance program.

The term telephone directory can also pertain to the telephone book. These books are provided to you by your local telephone company. They come in two main forms, white pages and yellow pages. The white pages list the name, address, and telephone number of the telephone customers; the yellow pages are used to list the name, address, and telephone number of local businesses. It does cost to have your business listed. Some resources that are provided in the telephone book

---

6-2 **PROCEDURE**

Taking a Prescription Refill Message

OBJECTIVE: Ensure that correct information is acquired when refilling a patient's prescription.

Equipment and Supplies
message pad or paper; pen

1. Print the name of the patient. (This name may be different from the name of the caller.)
2. Write down the patient's telephone number.
3. Write down the name of the medication. Ask the caller to spell the medication if you are unclear about what the caller is saying.
4. Write down how long the patient has been on the medication.

5. Write down the patient's symptoms and why the prescription is still needed.
6. Take the patient's age and weight (if a child).
7. Ask for the name and telephone number of the pharmacy and the prescription number.
8. Tell the caller you will give the message to the physician.
9. Tell the caller that you will call back if the prescription cannot be refilled.
10. Pull out the patient's chart for the physician to review and attach the telephone message to it.

The telephone system can be a great way of educating patients. The system can relay information to the patient in a number of ways.

If an automated assistance program is used, it is possible to program it to provide information to the patient. Most offices will include the office's hours and directions. Any emergency numbers are also provided. Some programs include an option that lets the patient hear about new employees, such as a new physician or other practitioner.

Another opportunity to educate patients is while they are on hold. Instead of playing music during the wait time, the program can play a message explaining new techniques or procedures that the physician is offering.

---

include emergency numbers, local government numbers, national area codes, and zip codes from your region. The telephone book is also where you will find directions on making long distance calls, including international calls.

Long Distance Calls

Occasionally, you will be asked to make long distance telephone calls for office business. For a time, a long distance call would be any call outside of your area code. This is no longer true. Many of the larger cities have had to add area codes within local calling regions. It will be necessary for you to learn what is considered long distance in your area. Long distance calls can be very costly, so your office may limit how many are made.

Telephone Logs

You will find that many offices maintain a telephone log to keep track of the long distance calls being made. When the telephone bill arrives, then the log and the bill can be compared. This can help to identify any abuses of the business telephone with personal calls. Many logs will have you list the name of the person, the facility or company being called, the number being called, the name of the person placing the call, the date and time of the call, the city and state where the call is being placed, the duration of the call, and the reason for it.

Making a Long Distance Call

Direct Distance Dialing (DDD) is the most common way of making a long distance call. To place a long distance call using DDD, dial "1," then the area code followed by the number you are calling. If you need to find an area code, you will find the listing of area codes at the front of the telephone book. The telephone book will also give you instructions for making international calls, if you are required to make them.

Another way of calling long distance is to make a collect call—reversing the call charges to the person receiving the call. When collect calls are placed, the person being called is asked by the operator whether or not he or she will accept the charges. Your office should have a policy in place regarding accepting or denying collect calls.

Conference Calls

When several people from different locations wish to have a telephone discussion, you would place a conference call. This means, for example, two physicians at a distance from each other may speak with a patient at a third location at the same time. While these calls are more expensive than regular long distance calls, they can save money in the long run, since you do not have to make several long distance calls to relay the same information.

Most business telephone systems allow you to make conference calls without using the telephone operator. You will need to look into your telephone system to see if it allows you to set up a conference call. If your system is not set up to do conference calls, you may use the operator to place the calls. See Procedure 6-3 for placing a conference call.

Time Zones

You must be aware of time zones within the United States and foreign countries when placing long distance telephone calls. The continental United States and parts of Canada are divided into four time zones based on their location in the country: eastern, central, mountain, and pacific. As you move from east to west across the United States, there is a one-hour difference (earlier) in each time zone. For example, if it is 9:00 A.M. in Ohio (eastern time zone), then it will be 8:00 A.M. in Illinois (central time zone).

It is a good idea to have a time zone map posted near your office telephone (Figure 6-5). This way you can plan long distance calls based on "office hours" in each time zone. A call placed at 3:00 P.M. in California will be received in New York at 6:00 P.M., which is usually after office closing hours.

PROCEDURE

Placing a Conference Call

OBJECTIVE: Allow for a discussion via the telephone between three or more parties from various locations.

Equipment and Supplies
Telephone numbers of participating parties

1. Gather the telephone numbers of all participants before beginning the call.
2. Determine the time that everyone will be available for the conference call. You may have to call people in advance to determine a convenient time. Be aware of time zone differences when arranging conference calls.
3. Dial "0" for operator and give the operator the name and telephone number (area code first) for each person to be called.

4. The operator will then place a call to each of the parties. When all the participants are on the line, the operator will come back to the original caller (you) and the conversation can then begin. If you are placing this call for your physician, he or she will then pick up on your line.
5. If you are setting the conference call up ahead of time, tell the operator when you wish the conference call to begin.

Using an Answering Service

Many offices use an answering service for times when no one is available in the office. This service can be in effect 24-hours a day or just at designated times, for example: during the night, during lunch, or during peak hours of the day to relieve office staff.

The system works by forwarding your office calls to the service, which is at an off-site location. The answering service personnel answer the calls that come in and inform the patients that the office is closed. They will also take some non-emergency messages, which will be delivered to the staff when you return your telephone calls back to your care. When emergency calls come in, the answering service will contact the physician by pager or telephone.

This service does have a fee attached, but many offices will consider this a necessary service. You do have the option of using an answering machine or voice messaging system while the office is closed. This option is less expensive, but the patients' problems may not be addressed as quickly. If you do use an answering machine or voice messaging system, you will need to make sure that the messages are retrieved in a timely manner and that the recorded office greeting provides a number to call in case of an emergency.

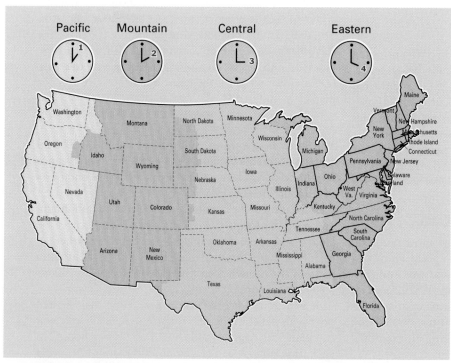

FIGURE 6-5 Having a time zone map located near the telephone will assist you with long distance calls outside your time zone.

Handling an Emergency Telephone Call

Every office should have a written protocol for handling emergency calls. Since you cannot see the telephone caller, it can be difficult to determine a true emergency by talking to someone over the telephone. It is critical to get the caller's name and telephone number immediately in case you are disconnected. You will then proceed by asking the patient specific questions. Examples of questions that you may ask, depending upon your office's procedure, are listed in Box 6-3. If an emergency is taking place during the telephone call, then alert the physician immediately.

In some cases, the patient may be hysterical or crying. Your job, in a situation such as this, is to calm the patient. If your voice remains calm and reassuring, you may be able to soothe the patient. If the caller is extremely upset, ask if there is someone else who can come to the telephone. Your role is to gain as much information from the caller as possible so that the emergency can be handled quickly. Following are some types of emergencies you may face.

- allergic reactions (anaphylactic shock)
- asthma
- broken bone
- drug overdose
- eye injury/foreign body
- gunshot/stabbing wound
- heart attack
- inability to breathe (or difficulty breathing)
- loss of consciousness
- premature labor
- profuse bleeding
- severe pain, including chest pain
- severe vomiting and/or diarrhea
- suicide attempt or suicide threats
- high temperature

BOX 6-3

Questions to Ask When Handling a Telephone Emergency

- What is your name?
- What is your telephone number?
- What is your relationship to the caller? (if a parent, spouse, friend, or passer-by is calling).
- What is the emergency?
- When did the emergency occur?
- How severe is the emergency?
- What are the patient's symptoms? (Problems breathing? Bleeding? Extreme pain? Other symptoms?)
- What has been done for the patient?
- Has anyone called an ambulance?
- Who is the patient's primary physician?
- Where is the emergency?

Note: Some specialists, such as obstetricians and cardiologists, may have additional questions they wish to have you ask the caller.

If your physician is not present, your office should have a policy in place for how to handle emergency calls. You may be required to call 911 while the patient is on the line, or you may need to instruct the patient to hang up and dial 911 directly from his or her home telephone.

Never take an emergency call lightly. Emergencies can become life-threatening if no treatment is provided. Even if you have questions as to whether the call is actually an emergency, you must always assume it is and alert the physician. Malpractice suits have been brought against medical assistants who have failed to correctly handle an emergency.

SUMMARY

A medical assistant who is working in a front desk position will find that the majority of his or her time is spent on the telephone. It is important to remember that when you are on the telephone, you are representing the medical office. Always greet the caller warmly and professionally. On a typical day, you will field many different types of calls. Take each call one at a time, and use the techniques and procedures from the chapter to work more efficiently.

COMPETENCY REVIEW

1. When it is 9:00 A.M. in New York, what time is it in Pittsburgh, PA; St. Paul, MN; Los Angeles, CA; and Denver, CO?
2. Write a telephone message for a patient who calls for a refill of *Estrace* 1 mg. daily.
3. How might you handle receiving a prank telephone call?
4. Why should you smile when answering the telephone?
5. What do you do when you are helping a patient on one line and another line begins to ring?

PREPARING FOR THE CERTIFICATION EXAM

1. When taking a prescription refill message from a patient you should include writing down the following, EXCEPT
   A. patient's name and telephone number
   B. medication and length of time the patient has been taking it
   C. patient's symptoms
   D. pharmacy's prescription number, name, and telephone number
   E. patient's social security number

2. The type of long distance call that might be used to facilitate the consultation of one physician with another is called a/an
   A. operator-assisted call
   B. DDD
   C. conference call
   D. collect call
   E. station-to-station call

3. When handling an emergency telephone call from a patient, the FIRST thing a medical assistant should do is
   A. get the caller's name and telephone number
   B. ascertain whether or not it is, in fact, an emergency
   C. gather as much information about the emergency in the shortest amount of time
   D. ask to speak with someone other than the patient/caller, who is too hysterical to communicate the details of the situation
   E. ask if an ambulance has been summoned

4. A proper initial greeting upon answering the telephone would be
   A. "Gynecology Associates."
   B. "Please hold."
   C. "Good afternoon."
   D. "This is Mary King, may I help you?"
   E. "Gynecology Associates, Ms. King speaking, may I help you?"

5. After a patient is placed on hold, it is proper to check back every
   A. 10 seconds
   B. 20 seconds
   C. 30 seconds
   D. 1 minute
   E. 2 minutes

6. When handling a request for a prescription refill, a medical assistant
   A. may call in the request, but only for a non-controlled substance
   B. should ask the patient to come into the office to obtain a written prescription
   C. may never call in a refill without the physician's direct order
   D. is certified to call in all prescription refills
   E. should call in the prescription if directed to do so by a nurse

7. A ringing telephone should be answered by the
   A. first ring
   B. second ring
   C. third ring
   D. fourth ring
   E. fifth ring

8. If a medical assistant is already speaking to a patient when another phone line rings, it is best to
   A. call to another medical assistant to answer the other line
   B. let the other line be picked up by the voice mail
   C. let the patient finish his or her question and then say, "Would you please hold?"
   D. ask the patient if you may place him or her on hold
   E. answer the second caller and handle the problem right away

continued on next page

9. A system of prioritizing patient calls according to the most ill or injured is known as
   A. classifying
   B. telephone triage
   C. insurance pre-approval
   D. mortality rate
   E. morbidity rate

10. If an emergency is taking place to the person making the telephone call, the first action the medical assistant should take is to
    A. alert the physician immediately
    B. call 911
    C. put the caller on the speaker phone
    D. record the call for liability purposes
    E. tell the person to go to the hospital immediately

CRITICAL THINKING

1. What do you think was wrong with Tonya's greeting?

2. How could Tonya improve the impressions that Cindy received so as to prevent Cindy from seeking another physician?

3. What was wrong with the way Cindy was put on hold? How could this have been improved?

4. What else in Cindy's phone call could have increased her frustration, and how could it have been helped?

ON THE JOB

For over two years, medical assistant Linda Lewis has been employed by Drs. Norek and Klein, who are gerontologists. Also on staff are two registered nurses, a medical laboratory technician, and a medical social worker. The daughter of one of the doctor's patients has just called the office. She is very distraught at the seemingly diminished capacity of her mother and insists on speaking to the doctor.

Linda explains that both of the physicians only take emergency calls during patient appointment hours, but that she will take a detailed message. The caller, however, suggests that not only should her call be considered an emergency, but that she will sue the doctor if the call is not handled accordingly.

1. What should Linda do immediately to diffuse the situation?
2. Is this clearly a case where the call should be passed on to one of the registered nurses or even the medical social worker?
3. Is this a case where, because of the threat of an impending suit, the physician should be called to the telephone?
4. How could Linda ascertain whether or not this, indeed, is an emergency? Is it even up to her as a medical assistant to make such a determination?
5. Since this is the patient's daughter, rather than the patient herself, does Linda have any reason to even enter into a conversation with the caller? Could Linda be ethically bound by confidentiality to not even admit the woman's mother is a patient?

INTERNET ACTIVITY

Use the Internet and research the ways HIPAA has affected the use of the telephone in the medical office.

MediaLink More on telephone techniques in the medical office environment, including interactive resources, can be found on the Student CD-ROM accompanying this textbook.

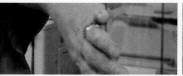

Medical Assistant Role Delineation Chart

HIGHLIGHT indicates material covered in this chapter.

ADMINISTRATIVE

Administrative Procedures

- Perform basic administrative medical assisting functions
- Schedule, coordinate and monitor appointments
- Schedule inpatient/outpatient admissions and procedures
- Understand and apply third-party guidelines
- Obtain reimbursement through accurate claims submission
- Monitor third-party reimbursement
- Understand and adhere to managed care policies and procedures
- *Negotiate managed care contracts*

Practice Finances

- Perform procedural and diagnostic coding
- Apply bookkeeping principles

- Manage accounts receivable
- *Manage accounts payable*
- *Process payroll*
- *Document and maintain accounting and banking records*
- *Develop and maintain fee schedules*
- *Manage renewals of business and professional insurance policies*
- *Manage personnel benefits and maintain records*
- *Perform marketing, financial, and strategic planning*

CLINICAL

Fundamental Principles

- Apply principles of aseptic technique and infection control
- Comply with quality assurance practices
- Screen and follow up patient test results

Diagnostic Orders

- Collect and process specimens
- Perform diagnostic tests

Patient Care

- Adhere to established patient screening procedures
- Obtain patient history and vital signs
- Prepare and maintain examination and treatment areas
- Prepare patient for examinations, procedures and treatments

- Assist with examinations, procedures and treatments
- Prepare and administer medications and immunizations
- Maintain medication and immunization records
- Recognize and respond to emergencies
- Coordinate patient care information with other health care providers
- Initiate IV and administer IV medications with appropriate training and as permitted by state law

GENERAL

Professionalism

- Display a professional manner and image
- Demonstrate initiative and responsibility
- Work as a member of the health care team
- Prioritize and perform multiple tasks
- Adapt to change
- Promote the CMA credential
- Enhance skills through continuing education
- Treat all patients with compassion and empathy
- Promote the practice through positive public relations

Communication Skills

- Recognize and respect cultural diversity
- Adapt communications to individual's ability to understand
- Use professional telephone technique

- Recognize and respond effectively to verbal, nonverbal, and written communications
- Use medical terminology appropriately
- Utilize electronic technology to receive, organize, prioritize and transmit information
- Serve as liaison

Legal Concepts

- Perform within legal and ethical boundaries
- Prepare and maintain medical records
- Document accurately
- Follow employer's established policies dealing with the health care contract
- Implement and maintain federal and state health care legislation and regulations
- Comply with established risk management and safety procedures
- Recognize professional credentialing criteria
- *Develop and maintain personnel, policy and procedure manuals*

Instruction

- Instruct individuals according to their needs
- Explain office policies and procedures
- Teach methods of health promotion and disease prevention
- Locate community resources and disseminate information
- *Develop educational materials*
- *Conduct continuing education activities*

Operational Functions

- Perform inventory of supplies and equipment
- Perform routine maintenance of administrative and clinical equipment
- Apply computer techniques to support office operations
- *Perform personnel management functions*
- *Negotiate leases and prices for equipment and supply contracts*

- *Denotes advanced skills.*

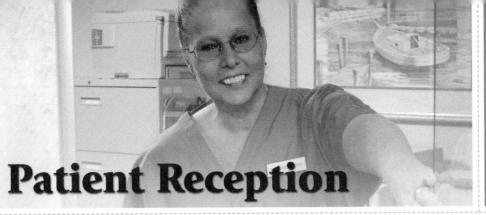

Patient Reception

Learning Objectives

After completing this chapter, you should be able to:

- Define and spell the terms to learn for this chapter.
- List the receptionist's responsibilities.
- Explain the procedure for opening the office.
- List the information to be obtained from the new patient.
- Describe how to handle the angry patient.

- Describe how to handle a waiting room emergency.
- Explain the procedure for closing the office.
- Explain the legal and ethical issues related to the duties of the receptionist.
- Describe the look of a professional medical assistant.

Terms to Learn

collating	facsimile (fax)	overbooking
co-payment	medical emergency	receptionist
demographic	no-show	

Case Study

STACY IS A NEW PATIENT COMING INTO DR. MATHIAS' OFFICE. She was sent her new patient paperwork in the mail when she made her appointment. She has the papers already completed as she goes up to the receptionist. Betsy has been the receptionist for Dr. Mathias for only three months. When Stacy comes to the window, Betsy greets her with a smile and welcomes her to the office. She then asks for Stacy's paperwork. Betsy goes through the papers to make sure that everything was signed and completed. She then asks for Stacy's insurance cards and ID to make copies. Betsy gives Stacy the HIPAA notice of privacy practice to read over and has her sign an acknowledgement of receipt. Betsy makes front and back copies of Stacy's insurance card and ID. She notes that Stacy has a $15.00 co-payment. She collects it before Stacy goes back for her appointment. During this time the phone rings, and the only person available to answer is Betsy. She answers it by the third ring, places the patient on hold, and returns to helping Stacy. Once Betsy has completed checking in Stacy, she returns to the phone call. About two minutes has elapsed and the patient on the line has hung up.

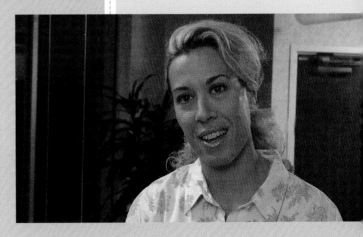

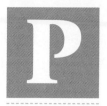

Patient reception requires a multiskilled individual whose manner, physical appearance, and tone of voice projects a professional, confident, and caring manner. A small office will have fewer employees than one with several physicians; therefore, the medical assistant in a small office will perform many of the tasks described in this chapter. In the role of receptionist, the medical assistant greets and assists incoming patients and performs many important duties, which make the office run smoothly and efficiently. Some of these duties are quiet and behind the scenes; others require constant interaction with patients. The medical assistant who functions as a receptionist must do everything possible to ensure patient safety and confidentiality at all times during the office visit.

Duties of a Receptionist

The number of patients as well as the nature of the medical practice—for example, whether it is a solo practice or a corporation of several physicians—will determine what duties or tasks the medical assistant performs in the role of receptionist (Figure 7-1).

The duties of a receptionist may include opening the office, greeting patients upon arrival, assisting a new patient with completion of the proper forms, maintaining a clean and safe environment in the reception area, managing any disturbance in the reception area, and handling a medical emergency or patient condition, which may be life threatening if left untreated. In addition, the receptionist may also handle

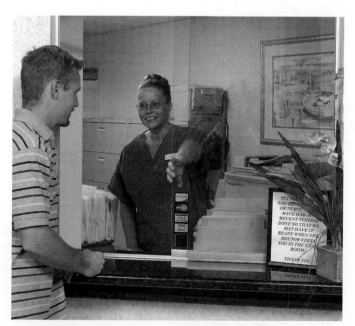

FIGURE 7-1   The medical assistant as receptionist in a medical office.

BOX 7-1
Duties of a Medical Receptionist

- Opening the office
- Pulling charts for the next day's appointments
- Collating patient records
- Checking in patients
- Greeting patients as they arrive
- Getting updated patient demographics
- Helping new patients fill out new paperwork
- Keeping the reception area clean and safe
- Managing any reception area disturbances
- Handling any reception area emergencies
- Handling some incoming calls
- Scheduling return appointments
- Possibly escorting patients to the exam rooms
- Keeping in mind the patient's time
- Documenting patient no-shows
- Closing the office

incoming telephone calls for the office, schedule returning appointments, and make reminder calls for upcoming appointments. Many of these jobs will be discussed in more detail throughout the chapter. See Box 7-1 for a list of reception duties.

The Reception Room

One of the most forgotten roles of the medical assistant will be taking care of the reception area. Many offices still refer to this area as the waiting room. However, many now call it the reception area to avoid the negative term *waiting*. This area must be kept clean and free from any hazards that may injure the patient. It is the first impression of the office that the patient gets. The receptionist will need to monitor the cleanliness of the room. If the room begins to get messy, the receptionist may need to take the time to straighten it up. Magazines, brochures, patient education documents, and toys should be arranged neatly. Any papers that may lie around need either to be thrown away or destroyed, depending upon the information they may contain. See Figure 7-2 and Professionalism for more on the reception room.

Lost and Found

It may also be the responsibility of the receptionist to take care of items left by patients in the reception area. The office may have a lost and found box in which these items may be kept. Many offices will try to contact a patient if it is known to whom the item belongs. The office may have a policy as to how long unclaimed items are kept before being thrown away or donated to a local charity.

Handling Incoming Money

The receptionist is often the person in charge of accepting office payments. They will often be responsible for collecting balances on accounts and co-payments. Co-payments are designated amounts that some medical insurance plans require patients to pay for medical services or medication, usually at the time of service. It is important to keep excellent records of all incoming money so that balancing at the end of the day is easier. See Chapter 13 for more on the handling of money in the medical office.

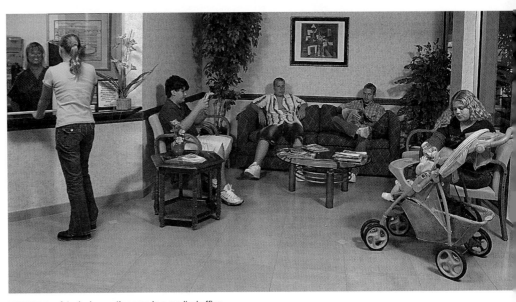

FIGURE 7-2 A typical reception area in a medical office.

Care and Maintenance of Office Equipment

The receptionist is often responsible for taking care of certain equipment such as the copiers, computers, printers, and facsimile or fax machines. It is important to learn the many functions of these machines. Knowledge of how to repair small problems, such as paper jams, is also helpful. If you are unable to fix something, it is important to know what numbers to call for service. The receptionist may also need to know how to replace certain things such as toner and ink cartridges. It is very important to make sure that these machines are filled with paper. See Chapter 11 for more information regarding the use of computers and troubleshooting.

Personal Characteristics and Physical Appearance

The receptionist is the first person a patient will see upon entering the office. Presenting a positive public image is important since your appearance reflects upon the entire staff. Careful grooming, good hygiene, and appropriate dress need to be observed. Office policy will dictate the preferred clothing. In most offices, the clinical staff wear uniforms of the same type. This can consist of scrub type pants and top with a lab coat. The advantage of this type of uniform is that it can be worn by both male and female staff and is relatively inexpensive. Colors and patterns of uniforms are usually determined by the management of the practice. Receptionists frequently wear the same style uniform as the clinical staff but without a lab coat, or they may be allowed to dress in business casual dress.

Hygiene, at a minimum, consists of daily bathing, use of a deodorant without a strong scent, good oral care, and clean, well-pressed clothing. Make-up, hairstyles, and jewelry worn by male and female medical assistants should reflect professionalism. Accessories should be conservative and minimal—generally limited to one finger ring, a watch with a second hand, name tag and a professional association pin. Long hair should be worn tied back and off the shoulders. Nails should be well trimmed and only clear polish should be used. No perfumes should be worn as patients can be allergic to certain scents. Lifespan Considerations discusses more about personal hygiene.

Name pins/tags should be visible at all times. More offices are requiring a picture ID for security reasons. These tags can serve dual purposes. With a magnetic strip, they can allow entrance into a secure area and can also be used to clock in and out the hours worked.

Professionalism

The receptionist is the first representative of the medical office that the patient is exposed to either by phone or in person. It is important that the first impression inspire confidence in the patient to the office's ability to meet his or her needs. This means that receptionists need to take great care in their appearance. Their clothes should be clean and pressed. The receptionist's hygiene influences the patient's perception of the cleanliness of the office. Receptionists need to keep their area of the office neat and organized. If patients see a messy, disorganized area, then they may wonder about the way their information will be handled.

Opening the Office

The medical assistant whose responsibility it is to open the office should arrive 15–30 minutes prior to the start of office hours. In addition to the receptionist's welcoming greeting, a well-lighted, clean, and inviting environment does much to cheer patients. The receptionist should begin checking the security alarm and disengaging it. Turn on all lights and check the general status of the reception room. It should be tidy and clean. Any area used for children's toys should be neat and safe. Magazines and books should be stacked or placed in wall racks.

Next, the medical assistant should check to see that the charts are pulled and prepared for that day's patients. Charge slips should be printed in advance for the day. The previous day's receipts should have been taken to the bank and the receptionist may have the responsibility of checking the cash box to see that the correct amount of change has been given. This will provide a way to double check the balance at the end of the day.

All office machines should be turned on and ready for use. Many copiers take several minutes to warm up in order to make copies. Be sure to add paper to the copier, fax machine, and any printers in the office. Nothing is more frustrating and time consuming than to find a fax machine with no paper and a queue of faxes waiting to be printed. Having the office machines turned on and ready can make the start of the day more efficient.

A master list of patient appointments should be printed out and copies placed on the desks of the clinical medical assistants and each of the doctors.

The final task prior to opening the office is to check the answering service and/or machine. If, additional appointments were made, pull the charts and make up a charge slip. It may be the responsibility of the opening medical assistant to make sure that all examination rooms are prepared for use. See Procedure 7-1 for more about opening the office.

Collating Records

Collating records refers to collecting all records, test results, and information pertaining to the patient, who is scheduled to be seen by the physician. Collating also refers to organizing the sub-group information (for example, laboratory and x-ray results) in records for the day's appointments as well as when filing. This should be part of pulling records, which may also be referred to as pulling charts. A record or chart refers to a medical record containing information such as laboratory and x-ray results. This is different from the patient's file. The file will refer to the financial record. It may contain billing, payment, and insurance information. The patient's file will most likely be contained on a computer, rather than on paper.

Collating records is usually done the day before patients are seen. The records of patients scheduled for a Monday are pulled and collated on the previous Friday. In some medical offices with several physicians, the number of patients seen may require collating records earlier than the day before the patient's visit. Always follow the policy of your office.

The physician's orders and notations from the previous visit must be reviewed to make sure that all necessary information has been received and is in the record. If laboratory tests or x-ray results are not present in the record, then you will have to call the laboratory or radiology department to obtain an oral report. This telephone report is written into the patient's record; however, when the originating report is received, it is placed in the patient's record also. This is quite often done by the clinical medical assistant. In some offices and laboratories, the facsimile (fax) machine can be used to send reports between facilities. A facsimile, or fax, is an electronically transmitted document containing print and/or graphic information.

In some offices, the records are to be placed in the order in which the patients will be seen. A printed appointment list is placed on top of the collated records. This list serves as a checklist to keep track of patients who have been seen by the physician. As a patient is seen, his or her name is checked off the list. A copy of this same list is placed on the physician's desk on the morning of the patient's visit. A list may also be given to the medical assistant that will be rooming patients that day, if different from the receptionist. Procedure 7-2 is provided for the process of collating records.

PROCEDURE

Opening the Office

OBJECTIVE: Prepare and set up the office to receive patients and operate efficiently.

Equipment and Supplies

checklist of opening office procedures; office keys for rooms and files; message forms or pads; master lists of scheduled patients

1. Turn on the lights in the patient reception area before the first patient arrives.
2. Check that the heating or air conditioning and computers are working properly.
3. Observe overall reception room for safety hazards such as frayed electrical cords, slippery floor, or torn carpeting. Place a warning sign near any safety hazard and report it immediately to the office manager.
4. Check magazines and recycle or discard any that are torn, damaged, or outdated.
5. Check for level of cleanliness per housekeeping services and report inadequate services.
6. Unlock file rooms or cabinets where records are kept.
7. Take calls from the answering machine or answering service. Handle any that need immediate attention.

8. Unlock any money that may be used for the day. Count and balance the money to make sure that the amount is the same as it was the day before when closing the office.
9. Unlock the outer office door.
10. Compare the master list of all patients who will be seen during the day against the patient records that were pulled during previous office hours. A patient may have been added to the schedule after the records were pulled. This patient's record must be pulled, reviewed, and added to the other records. Make phone calls to gather any laboratory test information that is missing from the record. Provide the physician(s) and nurse(s) with a copy of the list of any laboratory test information that you have called for, but has not yet been received.
11. Type and place a list of all patients who will be seen that day on the physician's desk.

PROCEDURE

Collating Records

OBJECTIVE: Prepare medical records of scheduled patients for review by the physician.

Equipment and Supplies

master list of scheduled patients; charts and records of scheduled patients

1. Print or copy the day's appointment schedule.
2. Pull all of the medical records of patients that are scheduled to be seen.
3. In each record, review the patient's last appointment and make note of any results that should have been received, including laboratory tests, x-rays results, consultation notes, and other tests.

4. If any of the results are not in the patient's chart, call the appropriate places to retrieve the results. You may take oral results, but request that the results be faxed to the office as soon as possible.
5. Make a list of all results that have been called to retrieve and any that are outstanding. Let the physician know what is still outstanding.
6. Put all information that is received onto the chart for the physician to review.

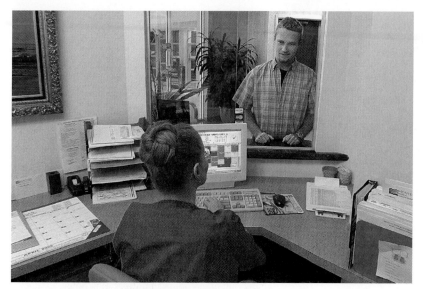
FIGURE 7-3   Each patient is greeted by the receptionist.

Greeting the Patient Upon Arrival

In the role of receptionist, the impression the medical assistant makes on the patient is often the patient's first impression of the physician and the medical office staff. The impression you make—good or bad—tends to flavor the patient's opinion of everyone related to the office. Therefore, that first impression is very, very important.

Emergency patients or those with a contagious disease should enter the office through a private office entrance (if there is one) and be escorted directly into an examination room. This is done to limit exposure to contagious germs and not to alarm the other patients.

In some offices, the receptionist sits behind a glass window, which slides open easily, allowing the receptionist to personally greet each patient entering the office (Figure 7-3). If the receptionist is on the telephone when a patient enters, then looking up and smiling is a good way to acknowledge the patient's presence. Cultural Considerations addresses more about interacting with patients.

Patients must always take precedence over other visitors to the office (for example, a medical supplier or pharmaceutical representative). Scheduling such a visit when there are few or no patients in the office might be a better solution. Nonemergency conversations with other staff persons should always be interrupted to respond to a patient.

Use caution and speak in a low voice when mentioning another patient's name over the telephone or to another staff member within hearing distance of any patients in the reception room. A violation of confidentiality can be grounds for a lawsuit. The reason for the glass enclosure is to protect the confidentiality of patients. Always close the partition when you are speaking on the telephone.

Quickly pick up ringing phones by the second ring if possible, and always take a message if you are busy with another call or a patient in the office. It is better to call the patient back if you are unable to answer a question or have to look up information rather than to leave the patient on hold. Callers should not be left on hold for longer than one minute. See Chapter 6 for more information regarding the use of the telephone. Also see Patient Education for more on patient interaction.

Signing-in

A sign-in sheet or patient register is maintained at the reception desk. The sign-in sheet, which will differ from office to office, usually has space for the patient's name, time of arrival, and the name of the physician the patient will see. The sign-in sheet allows the receptionist to maintain a continuous record of all patients who come into the office.

It is important to have every patient sign the register. The receptionist should verbally relate address and telephone information to the patient outside the hearing range of other patients, for example, "Mrs. Jones, do

Cultural Considerations

It is important to remember that different cultures have different ways of working with people. In your culture, you may feel that it is good manners to look someone in the eye when speaking with them. However, there are cultures that may be uncomfortable with looking a person in the eye because in that culture it is disrespectful. You will need to be aware of some of these cultural differences, especially if your office is located in an area in which you will deal with many people of different cultures.

you still live at 43 Home Avenue? Is your telephone number still . . . ?" The sheet should be checked for accuracy and completeness. This can be critical for billing purposes. As each patient is taken into the examination room, a check mark is placed next to the patient's name. This is only one way of patients signing in; each office develops a system that works for its flow of patients.

In some offices, the sign-in sheet is filed in a designated folder at the end of the day to provide another record of the patients seen during that day. If the office policy is to destroy the sign-in sheet to maintain confidentiality, make sure these papers are shredded. Note: Some offices are starting to move away from sign-in sheets due to confidentiality concerns. HIPAA does allow for the use of sign-in sheets, but you may not include the reason for the visit on the sign-in sheet. Only the patient's name, time of arrival, and the physicians name should be used.

Registering New Patients

New patients will need to fill out a complete patient registration form containing demographic information, which is data relating to descriptive information such as age, gender, ethnic background, education, and Social Security number (Figure 7-4). Place the registration form on a clipboard with a pen attached and have the patient complete the form while he or she is waiting to be seen by the physician. Some offices send forms to patients to be completed at home and submitted at the time of the first visit; others request new patients arrive 15–30 minutes early to complete the necessary forms. Give precise instructions. Indicate what portion of the form the patient must complete, if there are two sides to be completed, and where the patient's signature is required. Assist patients who are unable to read and write either because they are illiterate or have a physical disability. Realize that many patients who cannot read or write may be embarrassed by this. You may want to help them to fill out the form in a private area of the office.

You will need to explain to the patient your office's policies on billing and payment. Along with verbally telling him or her the policies, you may give each new patient informational brochures. Then have the patient sign an assignment of benefits form so that the insurance company may send payments directly to the physician.

Make sure that all forms are completed correctly in their entirety and that all signatures have been received. With computer-assisted registration, you can input dictation directly onto the computer terminal. Refer to Chapter 11 for more information on computer-assisted office functions.

Request to see the patient's insurance card(s). It is a good rule to ask the patient politely if any insurance information has changed. This can decrease the chances of lapsed coverage. Photocopy both sides of the card(s) and be sure that the copy is legible. Insurance billing cannot be processed without complete information. Check on the insurance card to see if there is a patient co-payment, which requires the patient pay a certain amount of the total bill. Indicate the co-payment in the appropriate place on the patient's file. The amount may be collected before or after the visit, depending upon your office's procedure.

Charge Slips

The charge slip (also referred to as encounter form or superbill) used in most medical offices is a part of the billing process. Some offices use a charge plate system or computer program that will imprint the patient's name and identification number on all forms used including the charge slip. The appropriate charge slip is attached to the medical record of each patient who is to be seen by the physician on that day. At the end of the visit, the physician indicates what treatment was given and what the charge is. The charge slip is then given to the

PATIENT REGISTRATION FORM
(Please Print)

Date: _____

Patient's
Name: _____
    First   Middle   Last

DOB: _____ / _____ / _____
    Month   Day   Year

Address: _____
    Street   City   State   Zip

Phone: _____ / _____ - _____
    (Area code)

Patient's SS#: _____-_____-_____ Driver's License #: _____ Occupation: _____

Method of payment (circle): cash check credit card insurance co-payment

Primary Insurance Co.: _____ Policy/Group #: _____

Medicare #: _____ Medicaid #: _____

Person
Responsible
For Payment: _____
    First   Middle   Last   Relationship

Address: _____
    Street   City   State   Zip

Phone: _____ / _____ - _____
    (Area code)

Employer Name: _____
    First   Middle   Last

Dept: _____

Address: _____
    Street   City   State   Zip

Phone: _____ / _____ - _____
    (Area code)

Spouse or
Nearest Relative: _____
    First   Middle   Last   Relationship

Address: _____
    Street   City   State   Zip

Phone: _____ / _____ - _____
    (Area code)

How were you referred to this office? _____

_____

Statement of Financial Responsibility: I, _____
do hereby agree to pay all medical charges incurred by the above listed patient. I further understand that these charges are my responsibility, regardless of insurance coverage.

Responsible Person's Signature: _____

FIGURE 7-4 Patient Registration Form.

receptionist or the cashier. Payment or arrangements for payment are made before the patient leaves the office.

All patients must be issued a charge slip before they leave the office. When there is no charge for the visit, as in a follow-up visit after surgery, the physician will write "no charge" or N/C on the slip. For accounting purposes there should be a charge slip number for each patient. The patient is entitled to and should receive a copy of the charges. The charge slip will contain a list of the most common current procedural terminology (CPT) and International Classification of Diseases (ICD-9). These codes identifying diagnosis-related charges used by the office.

Consideration for the Patient's Time

One of the most common complaints heard from patients is the excessive amount of time they have to spend in the reception room before being seen by a physician. Patients generally understand when they are told the physician has an emergency that has resulted in a schedule delay. However, in many cases, the physician is running behind schedule because of errors with the scheduling system, such as overbooking, when more than one patient is scheduled in the same time slot. Delays are also caused by not allowing enough time on the schedule for patient visits. This usually occurs because inaccurate information is obtained concerning the reason a patient wishes to see the doctor.

In general, a 20-minute wait is accepted by most patients. If the wait is going to be longer, then you should approach each patient and ask if the patient prefers to wait or wishes to reschedule the appointment. Patients generally respond well to a quiet explanation from the receptionist regarding how long the wait will be. Unfortunately patients after they sign in are sometimes forgotten by the receptionist. Since the patient's only contact in the office is the receptionist, it is critical that a concerned approach be used. Periodically check on your waiting patients. Know the office policy regarding which type of complaint is seen to immediately by the physician.

When a patient complains of a long delay in seeing the physician, never become angry in return or tell the patient, "It's not my fault." An empathetic medical assistant can imagine how nervous and ill the patient must feel. Make every effort to calm an angry patient so that he or she is no longer angry when going in to see the physician.

Escorting the Patient into the Examination Room

All patients should be personally escorted into the examination room (Figure 7-5). In most instances, this is done by a medical assistant assigned to patient care rather than by the receptionist. Select the correct record and clearly call the patient's name. If there is doubt that you have the correct patient, ask the patient to give you his or her name. Verify the name with the record you have requesting additional information, such as senior (Sr.) or junior (Jr.), if necessary. Make sure to also ask the patient how his or her would like to be addressed. Never call a patient by his or her first name unless the patient has asked you to do so. Walk at the patient's rate of speed and offer special assistance to patients using a wheelchair, crutches, walker, or cane. You may wish to make pleasant conversation to make the patient feel at ease.

Place the patient's record in the proper location. Do not leave the chart in the room with the patient. Often there is a slot on the outside of the examination room door for the record. Enter the room with the patient. Clearly explain exactly what articles of clothing the patient should remove. It is important to be specific because it can extend a patient's appointment time if the physician is unable to perform an examination because the patient has not been correctly prepared. Point out the gown or sheet to be used after the patient has undressed. Assist any patient who is unable to remove his or her clothing. Always protect the patient's modesty as you help the patient undress. Efforts made by medical staff to protect a patient's modesty are important to the patient.

After the examination has been completed, return to the examination room and knock before entering. Give the patient instructions about what to do next. For example, you might say to the patient, "You may dress now. The doctor will come back to talk to you shortly," or "Stop at the reception desk (or other designated area) after you have dressed, and I'll explain the test the doctor has ordered."

Make it a point to speak with each patient before he or she leaves. In some cases, the patient may need to make a payment, talk to the cashier, make another appointment, or have a specific test or procedure explained. A simple "good-bye" brings closure to each patient's office visit.

If discussion is needed, it should be done in a private area out of the hearing range and view of the other patients. Remember that HIPAA regulations prohibit discussions with patients to take place in any area where another patient may overhear.

Managing Disturbances

If a patient becomes angry or starts speaking in a loud voice, try to handle the situation immediately. It is always advisable to ask the patient to come into a quiet office where the problem can be discussed and handled.

If a private office is not available, the problem must be handled quickly and quietly in another area. Generally, people will respond to a sincere statement such as, "I'm sorry there's a problem. Let's see how we can solve it." Ask the patient to identify what he or she perceives the problem to be and then discuss the possible solutions. Frequently, the angry patient will respond well if the medical assistant uses a very quiet,

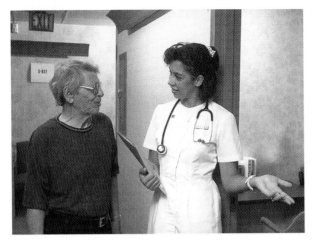

FIGURE 7-5 The medical assistant escorts the patient into the examination room.

calm manner. Keep your voice low to help calm the patient. With practice, a medical assistant can become adept at calming the angry patient. If the patient is drunk or disorderly, follow the office policy regarding when to call the police.

Children

Children pose a special challenge. Usually, children go into the examination room with the adult patient and are removed only if private areas are to be examined on the parent. If a child is left alone in the office while the parent is seen by the physician, then the medical assistant must observe that the child remains safe at all times. It is advisable to explain to the parent before he or she leaves the office that children cannot be left unattended.

On rare occasions, a physician treats a child without the parent being present. In such a case, a medical assistant or other staff person will stay with the child during the examination or procedure. Teenagers often have things to ask the doctor that they may not want their parents to hear.

Medical Emergencies in the Reception Room

There will be occasions when a medical emergency occurs in the physician's office (Figure 7-6). Ill patients may come directly to the physician's office instead of first calling the physician or 911. In this case, you must stop whatever you are doing to give assistance immediately. Ask another staff member to alert the physician. Tell available staff to give you assistance or to call 911 if emergency transport to a hospital is necessary. If all the rooms are full, you can ask the other waiting patients to step into the hall to prevent these patients becoming anxious during the emergency.

In certain emergency situations, the medical assistant may be required to start first aid procedures. It may be necessary to begin cardiopulmonary resuscitation

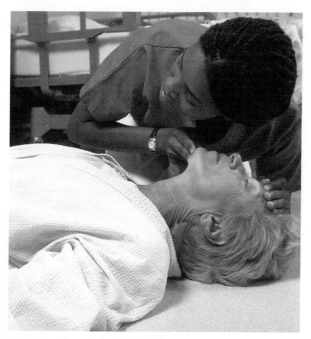

FIGURE 7-6 The medical assistant handles an emergency.

(CPR) on the patient. Your office should have guidelines set as to the proper procedure for handling this form of in-office emergency. See Legal and Ethical Issues for more about dealing with medical emergencies in the office.

If a patient's condition requires emergency treatment and equipment, which your physician is able to provide in the office setting, then immediately take the patient into an examination room. Assist the patient onto an examination table if possible. This patient should not be left unattended. Another staff member should alert the physician that the patient requires immediate attention. Many offices have an intercom system that allows communication from the reception area to all rooms in the office to quickly summon medical personnel.

If a family member who is present wishes to accompany the patient into the examination room, allow the person to do so unless prohibited by office policy. When treatment begins, a staff member should ask the family member to step out of the room.

No-Shows

No-show patients are any patients who do not keep their appointment and do not call to cancel their appointment. At the end of each day, one of the responsibilities of the receptionist is to account for these patients. Some offices have a standard practice to call the patient to determine why the appointment was not kept and to reschedule another appointment. There is sometimes a policy to charge for no-show appointments. It is important that the receptionist learn and use the procedure for "no-shows" as stated in the office's policy manual.

One person, usually the office manager, is responsible for alerting the physician to the patient "no-shows." Calling patients the day before their visits to remind them of the appointments may lower the number of no-shows.

After the patient has been rescheduled, place a notation on the patient's record about the failed appointment, the date, action taken, the result, and initials of the person performing the documentation. This documentation is important in protecting the physician should there ever be a lawsuit.

If the patient fails to keep two or more appointments, the physician should be informed. The physician may wish to send a letter declining to continue treating the patient or dismissing the patient from the practice. The letter should be sent both certified and regular mail.

Closing the Office

Closing the office at the end of the day and opening the office in the morning are two major functions of the medical assistant. These functions are key to operating a well-run office. A procedure for closing the office at the end of the day is presented in Procedure 7-3.

Closing the Office

OBJECTIVE: Secure the office properly during nonoperating hours.

Equipment and Supplies

checklist of office closing procedures; bank deposit forms and envelope/pouch; office keys for rooms and files

1. Leave at least 15 to 30 minutes at the end of the day to close the office.
2. Check all records used during the day for any orders that may have been missed. In addition, make sure that every visit is posted to be billed.
3. Records for patients who will be seen during the next day should be pulled, reviewed, and collated during the day. Place the collated records with the charge slips attached and the master list of the next day's scheduled patients together in the appropriate place. Also, make a copy of this master list of patients for each physician.
4. All money received from patient payments must either be deposited in a bank or locked in the office safe. It is wise to have the person designated to make the daily bank deposit vary the time of deposit. Many offices now use a courier for this task. For purposes of quality control, the person completing the bank deposit and the person making the deposit should not be the same. Both people should be bonded. Completing a bank deposit is discussed in Chapter 14.
5. Turn off electrical equipment and appliances. Note: Some equipment such as an incubator, fax machine, and computers, may require 24-hour operation. Check with your supervisor regarding the special requirements of your office.
6. Check all examination rooms to make sure they are clean and supplied for the next day. Note: This step may be done by the medical assistant who was in charge of rooming patients that day.
7. Straighten the reception room. Put away all magazines and pick up any toys.
8. The answering service must be activated before leaving. Know the name of the physician who is accepting emergency calls, or on call, until morning. Remind the physician who is on call.
9. Activate the security system if there is one.
10. Always double-check to make sure the door is locked.

SUMMARY

The receptionist's role can be one of the most demanding and most interesting positions in the medical office. While attending to the general running of the office, the medical assistant, as receptionist must greet all patients, assist new patients in registering while being sure to get necessary health and insurance information, answer calls, schedule patients, open and close the office, contact and document "no-shows," and more. All this requires a calm, caring, and organized individual who can keep patient information confidential and protect the safety of the patient during the office visit. The patient is most important.

Chapter Review

COMPETENCY REVIEW

1. Define and spell the terms to learn for this chapter.
2. Explain the steps you would take if you are the first person to arrive and must open the medical office.
3. Describe how a professionally groomed receptionist would appear.
4. Explain what you would do if a patient suddenly collapsed in the reception room.
5. Discuss steps a medical assistant would take to assist in preventing a claim of abandonment against a physician.
6. Describe the important characteristics of a typical waiting area.

1. At Mrs. Mendez' first appointment to see Dr. Williams, you would have the following forms for her to read and/or sign EXCEPT
   A. patient information sheet
   B. physician's emergency phone numbers
   C. authorization to pay physician form
   D. sign-in sheet
   E. bank deposit slip

2. When a patient enters the office and you are on the telephone, what is the correct procedure?
   A. continue speaking on the telephone, and after you have completed the conversation, look up and handle the walk-in patient
   B. place the telephone patient "on-hold" and tell the walk-in patient to sign in
   C. smile at the walk-in patient to indicate that you see him or her and finish talking with the patient on the telephone
   D. tell the patient on the telephone you will call back later, then handle the walk-in patient
   E. smile to answer the telephone

3. When handling the angry patient, it is best to
   A. ask the patient to have a seat
   B. calmly tell the patient you are sorry he or she is angry and take the patient to an empty examination room
   C. tell the patient that you have to cancel his appointment since you cannot have loud, angry patients in the office
   D. let the patient continue to talk until the patient's anger is gone
   E. answer the ringing telephone

4. "No-Show" appointments are documented
   A. when the staff person assigned to document "no-shows" comes in for work
   B. at the beginning of the next day
   C. at the end of the day of the failed appointment
   D. only on the sign-in sheet
   E. but do not have to be documented

5. Mr. James has walked into the office and collapsed. Dr. Williams is not there. Which of the following would a medical assistant do?
   A. alert a staff member to help Mr. James
   B. assist Mr. James and call out or ask another staff member to call 911 for help
   C. call 911 immediately and wait by the door to direct the emergency team
   D. if Mr. James is alert, advise him to go to the hospital to meet Dr. Williams, then call Dr. Williams to alert her that an emergency patient is on his way to the hospital
   E. answer the ringing telephone

6. Which of the following statements, regarding the collation of patient records is TRUE?
   A. patient records for the day's appointments are usually pulled and collated 2 days before the appointment
   B. patient records are usually pulled and collated for an appointment immediately after the reminder call
   C. only a written report of test results is entered into a patient's records not the actual laboratory report
   D. records for patients scheduled on Tuesday are pulled on Monday
   E. patient records include billing and insurance information

7. What is the name of the billing document used in most medical offices where the physician indicates a patient's treatment and charges?
   A. assignment of benefits form
   B. authorization to pay form
   C. charge slip
   D. insurance slip
   E. billing slip

8. What, in general, is the maximum acceptable amount of time for a patient to wait on the day of a scheduled appointment?
   A. 10 minutes
   B. 15 minutes
   C. 20 minutes
   D. 25 minutes
   E. 30 minutes

9. Which of the following should be considered a medical emergency in an office waiting room?
   A. a potentially contagious patient's incessant coughing
   B. a crying child with a very upset stomach
   C. a patient, whose chief complaint is nausea over the past several days, who has just vomited
   D. a disgruntled patient
   E. a patient requiring CPR

10. It is proper, when addressing patients, to
    A. call them by their surname only
    B. address them by their first name, in order to sound friendly
    C. ask them how they prefer to be addressed
    D. avoid all use of name to keep from offending the patient
    E. use a familiar nickname

CRITICAL THINKING

1. Did Betsy greet Stacy appropriately?
2. What was the benefit of sending Stacy the paperwork in the mail before her visit?
3. Why did Betsy give Stacy the Notice of Privacy Practice?
4. Did Betsy handle the phone call appropriately? If not, how should she have handled it?

ON THE JOB

Dr. Morrison, a child psychiatrist, who is in solo practice, employs one medical assistant in her office. This medical assistant is multiskilled, like all medical assistants, and, essentially, handles all of the administrative and clinical tasks in the office.

It is 3:00 P.M. and a parent has just arrived for a 3:30 P.M. appointment with her 10-year old daughter. The child is a new patient of Dr. Morrison and was referred by her attending physician. She has a relatively long history of combative and destructive behavior and the referring pediatrician is seeking a psychological evaluation from Dr. Morrison. Psychotropic medication of some sort may be a viable treatment option. The medical assistant has asked the mother and daughter to please be seated and to fill out some registration forms. The child is acting out—pulling cushions off of the reception room couch, wildly ripping the pages of the magazines, whining and kicking at her mother. The behavior seems to be escalating as the mother tries to frantically control her child while, at the same time, follow the instructions of the medical assistant and fill out the registration forms.

What is your response?

1. What if anything, should the medical assistant do?
2. Would it be appropriate, for example, for the medical assistant to interrupt Dr. Morrison's current session?
3. Might this be considered a medical emergency?

INTERNET ACTIVITY

1. Find out how HIPAA has changed the way the medical office handles patient reception.
2. Look for companies that produce forms that can be used by a medical receptionist.

 MediaLink More on patient reception in the medical office environment, including interactive resources, can be found on the Student CD-ROM accompanying this textbook.

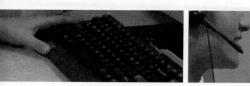

Medical Assistant Role Delineation Chart

HIGHLIGHT indicates material covered in this chapter.

ADMINISTRATIVE

Administrative Procedures

- Perform basic administrative medical assisting functions
- Schedule, coordinate and monitor appointments
- Schedule inpatient/outpatient admissions and procedures
- Understand and apply third-party guidelines
- Obtain reimbursement through accurate claims submission
- Monitor third-party reimbursement
- Understand and adhere to managed care policies and procedures
- *Negotiate managed care contracts*

- Manage accounts receivable
- *Manage accounts payable*
- *Process payroll*
- *Document and maintain accounting and banking records*
- *Develop and maintain fee schedules*
- *Manage renewals of business and professional insurance policies*
- *Manage personnel benefits and maintain records*
- *Perform marketing, financial, and strategic planning*

Practice Finances

- Perform procedural and diagnostic coding
- Apply bookkeeping principles

CLINICAL

Fundamental Principles

- Apply principles of aseptic technique and infection control
- Comply with quality assurance practices
- Screen and follow up patient test results

Diagnostic Orders

- Collect and process specimens
- Perform diagnostic tests

Patient Care

- Adhere to established patient screening procedures
- Obtain patient history and vital signs
- Prepare and maintain examination and treatment areas
- Prepare patient for examinations, procedures and treatments

- Assist with examinations, procedures and treatments
- Prepare and administer medications and immunizations
- Maintain medication and immunization records
- Recognize and respond to emergencies
- Coordinate patient care information with other health care providers
- Initiate IV and administer IV medications with appropriate training and as permitted by state law

GENERAL

Professionalism

- Display a professional manner and image
- Demonstrate initiative and responsibility
- Work as a member of the health care team
- Prioritize and perform multiple tasks
- Adapt to change
- Promote the CMA credential
- Enhance skills through continuing education
- Treat all patients with compassion and empathy
- Promote the practice through positive public relations

Communication Skills

- Recognize and respect cultural diversity
- Adapt communications to individual's ability to understand
- Use professional telephone technique

- Recognize and respond effectively to verbal, nonverbal, and written communications
- Use medical terminology appropriately
- Utilize electronic technology to receive, organize, prioritize and transmit information
- Serve as liaison

Legal Concepts

- Perform within legal and ethical boundaries
- Prepare and maintain medical records
- Document accurately
- Follow employer's established policies dealing with the health care contract
- Implement and maintain federal and state health care legislation and regulations
- Comply with established risk management and safety procedures
- Recognize professional credentialing criteria
- *Develop and maintain personnel, policy and procedure manuals*

Instruction

- Instruct individuals according to their needs
- Explain office policies and procedures
- Teach methods of health promotion and disease prevention
- Locate community resources and disseminate information
- *Develop educational materials*
- *Conduct continuing education activities*

Operational Functions

- Perform inventory of supplies and equipment
- Perform routine maintenance of administrative and clinical equipment
- Apply computer techniques to support office operations
- *Perform personnel management functions*
- *Negotiate leases and prices for equipment and supply contracts*

- *Denotes advanced skills.*

Appointment Scheduling

Learning Objectives

After completing this chapter, you should be able to:

- Define and spell the terms to learn for this chapter.
- Name and describe four scheduling systems.
- List and describe four pieces of equipment used in the scheduling process.
- Identify ten conditions that qualify as emergencies.

- Explain the importance of correct documentation when a patient does not keep an appointment.
- Describe the appointment scheduling process.
- Describe and arrange the process for scheduling a hospital admission and surgery.
- Summarize the ethical implications related to scheduling.

Terms to Learn

acute conditions
archived
cycle time
double booking
established patient

matrix
modified wave scheduling
real time
scheduling system
specific time

surgical scheduler
tickler file
time patterns
triage
wave scheduling

Case Study

MARC, CMA, IS WORKING THE FRONT DESK TODAY. He is looking ahead to tomorrow's (Friday) schedule. Fridays are Dr. Miller's short day for seeing established patients. The office usually closes from noon until 1:00 P.M. for lunch. Marc sees that Dr. Miller has the following appointments:

11:00	Laura White	2:00	Rinna Brown
	Joe Tanner		Monica Floyd
	Lucy Smith		Peter Conner
1:00	Justin Ivy		
	Ramona Pierce		
	Lucas Abrams		

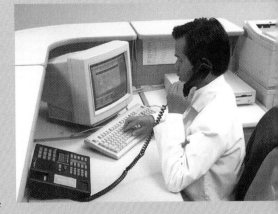

Ramona Pierce calls to cancel her appointment. Shannon Reece wants to know if she can schedule a new patient appointment for tomorrow. Marcus Fowler, a familiar drug representative, wants to know if he can drop in briefly tomorrow.

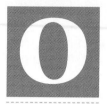

Office hours are usually determined by the physician or group of physicians in a practice. The scheduling system used in each office is dependent on a variety of factors, including the physician's preference, type and size of practice, equipment availability, staff availability, amount of flexibility required by the physician(s), insurance coverage issues, and patient needs (Figure 8-1). The two basic types of appointment scheduling systems are (1) scheduled appointments, and (2) open office hours.

There are some medical facilities, such as independent ambulatory urgent care clinics, that offer extended evening hours and may be open 24-hours a day. Independent ambulatory urgent care clinics are facilities that are prepared to handle situations requiring immediate but not life-threatening medical care. These facilities are not always attached to a hospital or other large treatment center. The patients arrive without an appointment and are generally seen in the order of arrival. A medical office or facility using such a system is said to have "open" office hours.

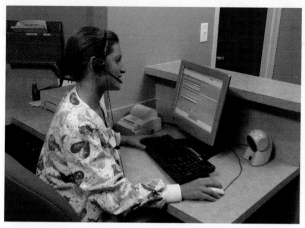

FIGURE 8-1 Scheduling patient appointments by telephone.

Appointment Schedules

Some physicians prefer to see patients according to a set schedule, depending on the specialty. As soon as a day's schedule of time slots is filled, then that day is closed to any new appointments. In this way, the physician is better able to spend an appropriate amount of time with each patient. There are several variations used for scheduling, including specified time, wave and modified wave, procedure grouping, double booking, and open hours system (Figure 8-2). All of these scheduling variations are described here along with the benefits and limitations of each type. Applying these scheduling variations in an office environment is discussed in Preparing for Externship.

Specified Time Scheduling

With specified time scheduling, each patient is given a specific time slot, which means the time allocated to each patient will depend upon the reason for the office visit or the type of examination or testing that is to be done. For example, a complete physical examination may require one and one-half hours. In an office based on 15-minute increments, or time slots, this patient would be given six time slots in a row equaling the one and one-half hours needed. This method prevents a large backlog of waiting patients or cycle time—the length of time the average patient spends in the medical office. Each staff member has a chance to maintain the office flow by reducing patient cycle time.

The drawback to specified time scheduling is that some patients may not provide enough information about their medical problems at the time the appointment is scheduled, in spite of careful questioning by the medical assistant. For instance, consider the case of a patient who is given a thirty-minute appointment but who really needs to have one or one and one-half hours for a thorough physical examination. Since not enough time was allocated for the visits, the schedule will back up. Some ways to deal with patients when the schedule backs up are discussed in Professionalism.

Some patients will discuss topics that are unrelated to the complaint that brought them into the office. This can be time consuming, frustrating for the physician, and not beneficial to the patient. It is the medical assistant's responsibility to get accurate information when scheduling patients so that the correct amount of time on the schedule is reserved for them. If the patient requires more time than was originally scheduled, the physician might have to ask the patient to make another appointment. In an attempt to prevent this from happening, many offices will build in time—known as "catch up" time—in either the morning or afternoon for emergencies.

Preparing for Externship

Appointment scheduling is an administrative task or front office procedure. Be aware that the scheduling variation you learned in class may not be the one used at your externship site. Do not be afraid to ask questions. It is to your advantage to learn different variations. Because there is always more than one way of performing a task, you may be able to show what you learned in your office procedures class. Shared ideas sometimes lead to more effective ways of performing tasks.

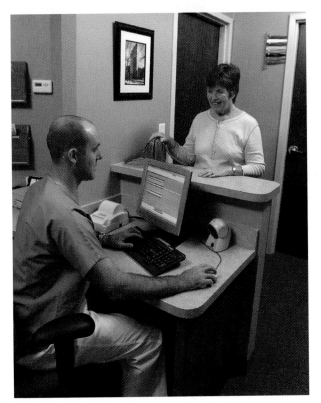

FIGURE 8-2 Scheduling appointments in a physician's office.

Wave Scheduling

Wave scheduling provides built-in flexibility to accommodate unforeseen situations, such as patients who require more time with the physician, a late arriving patient, or the patient who fails to keep an appointment (no-show). The purpose of wave scheduling is to begin and end each hour on time. Each hour is divided into equal segments of time, depending on how many patients can be seen within an hour.

For appointments averaging 20 minutes, three 20-minute appointments would be scheduled within each hour period of time, and for appointments averaging 15 minutes each, four appointments would be scheduled during the entire hour.

Using wave scheduling, all the patients are told to come in at the beginning of the hour in which they are to be seen. These patients are then seen in the order in which they arrive. Since some of the patients require more time, and others may be late, or some may not come in at all, wave scheduling allows for the actual time used by patient appointments to average out over the hour.

Modified Wave Scheduling

Wave scheduling can be modified to avoid the possibility that any patient would have to wait 40 minutes to be seen by the physician. Modified wave scheduling is also built on the hour as the base of each block of time. There are many variations of this type of scheduling.

One example would be to have three patients scheduled at intervals during the first half hour with none

scheduled for the second half hour. All three patients would be seen during the entire hour period, but the physician would not be waiting for a late arriving patient. With this system the physician can still spend 20 minutes with each patient without having to wait for any patients to arrive. Table 8-1 is a comparison chart providing examples of specified time, wave, and modified wave scheduling.

Scheduling by Grouping Procedures

Many physicians prefer to have similar procedures and examinations scheduled during a particular block of time. For example, an obstetrician may prefer to have all new patients scheduled together on two mornings a week since they will require a longer physical examination. An allergist may group all skin testing together on three afternoons a week. A pediatrician may do well-baby checkups during particular hours each day.

Double Booking Patients

Double booking, which is the practice of scheduling two patients to be seen during the same time slot without allowing for any additional time in the schedule, is considered to be an ineffective method. If each patient will need a 20-minute appointment, and both are scheduled from 1:00 P.M. to 1:20 P.M., then the entire afternoon's schedule will be late by 20 minutes, at least. Using a modified form of wave scheduling will eliminate this problem since enough time is actually allowed in the schedule for all the patients.

Open Office Hours System

An open office hours system is the least structured of all the systems. The hours in which the office is open are posted, and patients may arrive at any time during those hours. The patients are seen in the order of their arrival.

Some physicians prefer this method because the schedule is not disrupted by patients who miss appointments. The disadvantages to this method include having too many patients arrive at the same time, which frequently

Professionalism

No matter how well a scheduling system may work, there may be times when the physician gets behind schedule. It is important to communicate to patients immediately that the wait may be a little longer than anticipated. Provide updates as often as possible. Some patients may get tired of waiting and become rude and demanding. Remain courteous and assure the patient that the staff is working as quickly and safely as possible and that he or she will be seen. If the wait time is much longer, ask patients with non-urgent, less serious problems if they want to reschedule (if office policy allows).

TABLE 8-1 Comparison of Scheduling Methods

Specified Time		Wave		Modified Wave	
1:00	Ed Trombley—ear irrigation	1:00	Ed Trombley Jerry Richard Janet Orlando	1:00	Ed Trombley
1:20	Jerry Richard—well-baby checkup with vaccines			1:10	Jerry Richard
1:40	Janet Orlando—PAP smear			1:20	Janet Orlando
2:00	Lena Mezza—well-baby checkup with vaccines	2:00	Lena Mezza David Ingiolo Christina Soave	1:30	↓ ↓
2:20	David Ingiolo—BP check			1:40	↓ ↓
2:40	Christina Soave—skin rash (poss. contagious)			2:00	Lena Mezza
3:00		3:00		2:10	David Ingiolo
3:20				2:20	Christina Soave
3:40				2:30	↓ ↓
4:00		4:00		2:40	↓ ↓

results in longer patient cycle time than necessary. The physician and staff can be overworked during peak times of the day and may have no patients during other times.

Scheduling Systems

Appointment scheduling is key to the business aspects of the office process flow (Chapter 9), time management, increased efficiency, and quality patient care. A scheduling system facilitates the coordination of appropriate time segments for staff, patients, and the practice's available equipment. In order for a medical practice to coordinate time, an appointment scheduling system is applied, no matter what the practice size, specialty, and patient load. Scheduling systems establish the appropriate office process flow and coordination of time with the ability for flexibility as necessary. Appointment systems include computerized and manual. Either system can accomplish scheduling coordination of time when managed appropriately for the medical practice while adhering to HIPAA compliance guidelines.

Computerized Systems

Many medical practices of various sizes and specialties are utilizing computers to schedule appointments (Figure 8-3). Computerized systems may be purchased

based on the medical practice's specific needs. Some practices will purchase a commercial software product while others will contract a commercial appointment scheduling service. The responsibility of the medical assistant is to understand, demonstrate, and follow the computerized appointment system while adhering to HIPAA guidelines. There is no official government body or standards agency that will certify a commercial computerized product or service as a "HIPAA compliant." It is up to the health care providers to make sure

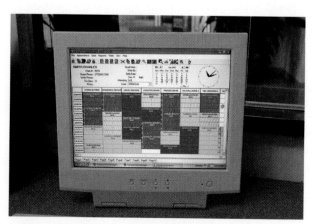

FIGURE 8-3 An example of computerized scheduling format.

the computerized product purchased for the medical practice will address the specific needs of the practice and their own HIPAA compliance issues, which will include patient safety, confidentiality, and security.

Computerized appointment systems are completed in a real time environment. Real time refers to automatically placing the appointment, patient needs, and information within the appropriate areas of the computer program versus the manual systems. The medical professional can key in the information to maximize the efficiency of the workflow. In addition, a computerized system provides the medical assistant with the ability to view times, dates, and open appointments with ease and consideration for the appointment criteria. Another advantage to computerized appointments is the ability to view and access patient appointments with a click or touch of a button. Whether a patient has a future appointment or a series of appointments, the computerized system can produce the information without the need of flipping the multiple pages in a manual schedule book.

While computerized systems maximize office process flow and patient cycle time (Chapter 9), there are some disadvantages and concerns the medical practice will need to consider. Some obvious concerns include privacy and technological factors, such as power outages, glitches within the software, and security. Computerized systems must be secured in a private space in accordance with HIPAA compliance. This can be accomplished by placing the computer in an area of the office where there is limited public walk-through traffic and visitors' ability to overhear a conversation. The computer screen should be set to a screen saver after a few short minutes to block others from viewing the screen when the medical assistant is away from the desk.

For technological concerns, in accordance with HIPAA, each medical practice should have an emergency action plan devised for such events. The medical assistant will need to back up the computerized schedule frequently to prevent loss of important information. If there were a power outage, the emergency action plan should provide information that will ensure that the medical office can operate and function for 48 to 72 hours without power. Office policies would dictate how the scheduling would be handled during the power outages, such as printing a hardcopy of the appointment schedule for the week versus one day at a time.

Another advantage of computerized appointment scheduling includes the ability to track regular

patterns within the medical practice. For example, the office could track how many no-shows, or how many patients were scheduled for the same type of appointment, i.e. flu, or even how often the physician was late within a specific period of time. These tracking features provide the medical practice with an additional tool and analytical report for audit and review of the best methods within the office. Time management could be modified as needed based on the reports.

Security concerns should be outlined in accordance with the office policies and HIPAA compliance issues. Specified security guidelines are usually dictated by the medical office functions and flow. Security includes some of the following but are not limited to them: positioning and location of the computer monitor for visibility and confidentiality, employee computer authorization and accessibility requirements, the changing of employee passwords every 30 days, proper computer firewalls for patient confidentiality, and proper computer encryption.

Manual Systems

Some medical practices have not converted to computerized systems and instead use manual appointment systems. Utilizing computers to schedule appointments often depends on the size of practices and specialties. Manual systems are comprised of a hardcopy schedule book and a pencil or pen. Appointment books are purchased from various commercial office supply companies and offer a variety of styles, sizes, and features. Each office will determine the type of book needed based on the practice needs and preferences. Refer to Figure 8-4 for a sample of an appointment book. In accordance with HIPAA compliance, the appointment book and schedule must maintain patient confidentiality at all times. The appointment book should never be left in an

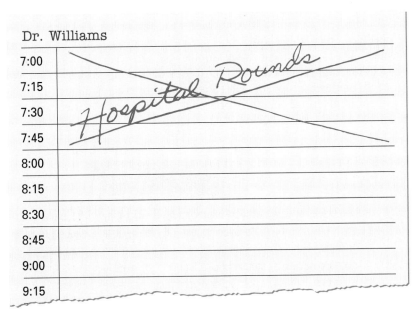

FIGURE 8-4 An example of manual appointment book.

area that is visible to visitors at the reception desk. The appointment schedule for the day should not be taped on the wall for all to view. Instead, secure a private location for required staff to reference.

The similarities and responsibilities of computerized and manual systems should be noted. The appointment book is a legal document that can be subpoenaed by the court (Legal and Ethical Issues). It is a record of the physician's day and time spent in contact with patients. Appointment books should be archived for future reference for several years in case of a court case. If there are any changes from the scheduled patients in the appointment book, such as a cancellation or no-show, these should be noted both in the appointment book and in the patient medical record. If the appointment has been rescheduled, then this should be appropriately documented. The appointment book should be archived (stored) for future reference with a hard copy or back up tape for computer scheduling. Files are archived by placing them in a storage container or facility and keeping them for several years as backup documentation.

Patient Scheduling Process

Every office will utilize its own method for appointment scheduling in accordance with the needs of the practice. However, the scheduling process remains the same for actually scheduling the appointment. The process includes either the computerized or manual system. The appointment is either entered into a manual appointment book or into the computer program.

The first step in the patient scheduling process is to be organized and efficient. Gather all required equipment, including the patient chart, computer scheduling system, pencil, manual schedule book, and office criteria requirement checklist. The medical assistant should be sure the schedule depicts all unavailable times, which is known as forming a matrix—periods of time blocked out on the daily schedule when an appointment is unavailable. Some of these blocked-out segments include times when the physician is seeing patients in the hospital, in surgery, out to lunch, on break, returning telephone calls, in meetings, and out of town. Several weeks of the schedule are blocked out or prepared at one time. It is not good practice to block out the entire schedule for the year since there may be unexpected changes in the physician's schedule. All blocking out and scheduling in the manual system is done in pencil. The medical assistant should cross out the blocks of time when the physician is unavailable, and write the reason across the line.

The next step in the process is to utilize effective communication skills. Listening to the patient's information and requests will help determine the type of appointment that is actually needed. When scheduling a patient appointment, always project a professional, caring, and willing demeanor with the patient. This can be accomplished by demonstrating effective listening and speaking skills so that the patient can understand and interpret the dialogue conveyed. Begin by asking for the patient's name, telephone contact, and purpose for the visit. Once the patient has described the purpose of his or her visit, the medical assistant should use the office criteria requirements checklist to help determine the type of and time needed for the appointment. Next, the medical assistant will need to determine the facility, equipment, and staff availability to meet the patient's needs. Based on the determination steps, the medical assistant can then discuss available dates and times with the patient. Refer to Table 8-2 for estimates of the amount of time to be allotted for specific office procedures. For more information that may need to be conveyed to patients before their appointment date, see Patient Education.

The medical assistant should offer one or two choices of dates, days and times for the patient to determine his or her availability. Be sure to always state the date, day, and time for reassurance that the patient has correctly understood when the appointment is scheduled. Once the patient and the medical assistant have mutually determined the time, either key in the information into the computer or use a pencil to enter the patient name and telephone number into the scheduled time slot in the schedule book. If the patient is making the appointment in person, write the date, day, and time on an appointment card for the patient. If the patient is on the telephone, have the patient repeat the day, date, and time. Procedure 8-1 provides information on how to schedule patients.

Missed Appointments and Delays

Appointments are cancelled for any number of reasons. Sometimes the patient experiences an unforeseen emergency, is too ill or too fatigued to get to the office, or actually forgets the appointment. Some medical practices charge patients for no-show appointments as well as rescheduled appointments. If the medical practice has a cancellation charge, the patients must be made aware of the policy prior to cancellation.

TABLE 8-2	Time Estimates for Specific Office Procedures
Procedure	**Time in Minutes**
Allergy testing	30–60
Cast check	10
Cast change	30
Complete physical with EKG	60
Blood pressure check	15
Dressing change	15
Minor surgery procedure	30–45
Office visit: Established patient	
Low complexity	5–10
Medium complexity	15–20
High complexity	20–30
Office visit: New Patient	
Low complexity	10–15
Medium complexity	15–30
Complete physical	30–45
Pelvic examination with PAP test	30
Patient education	30–45
Post-operative checkup	15–20
Prenatal examination (first visit)	30–60
Prenatal checkup	15
Prostate examination	30
School physical	15–30
Suture removal	10
Well-baby checkup	15

On the other hand, the physician may have a delay or the need to cancel appointments due to an emergency at the hospital or even a patient emergency in the office. Also, the medical office may not have all the necessary physical equipment for certain procedures, or building issues may arise as well as other unforeseen

Scheduling Patients

OBJECTIVE: Use an appointment scheduling system to schedule patients with efficiency.

Equipment and Supplies

pencil or pen (if preferred by office management); appointment schedule book

Method

1. Understand the scheduling system used in your office.
2. Use a pencil so that appointments can be erased to make changes as needed. Please note, some offices prefer the use of black or blue ink instead of pencil.
3. Set up a matrix by blocking out all time periods when the physician is not available (hospital rounds, vacation) for appointments before scheduling patients. Ideally, setting up a matrix or appointment blocking on the computer is done three months ahead of time.
4. Schedule appointments by beginning with the first empty appointment in the morning or early in the afternoon, and then fill in the day. Do not schedule appointments at the end of the day with large open gaps in between.

5. Print the patient's full first and last name next to the appropriate time on the schedule. Add Jr. for *junior* and Sr. for *senior* if there are two patients with the same name in a family.
6. Ask the patient for a current work and home telephone number, including the area code. Write these numbers next to the patient's name.
7. Write the reason for the visit on the schedule using accepted medical abbreviations.
8. Allow the correct amount of time for the appointment. If an appointment will take more than the minimum time allotted on the schedule, then use an arrow to indicate that the patient will be using 2 or 3 blocks of time. In some offices, a line is drawn across the time blocks.

NOTE: In offices where scheduling is done by computer, enter the patient information as directed by the on-screen prompts.

---

circumstances. In all cases, the medical assistant should provide patients with an explanation and reschedule appointments. Missed appointments happen with no warning, so the medical assistant has less opportunity to make satisfactory adjustments. No matter what the reason for a missed appointment, the medical assistant must contact the patient, reschedule the appointment, and document it as a missed and rescheduled appointment in the patient medical record. Careful legible documentation is necessary for HIPAA compliance as well as to legally protect the physician from a claim of patient abandonment.

Patient No-Shows

No-shows or failed appointments occur when a patient does not show up to keep an appointment. If a patient misses an appointment, write no-show (NS), or cancellation (xll) on the appointment schedule sheet and in the patient chart. Make every attempt to fill up a void in the schedule caused by a patient cancellation. One method is to call the patient who has the last appointment for

the day and ask the patient if it is possible to come in earlier. In the event that a long appointment, such as a one and one-half hour appointment for a complete physical, has been canceled, you will have to attempt to move up an entire group of patients. Many offices maintain a list of patients who wish to be called if there is an appointment open at the last minute. This approach is beneficial to maintaining good customer service as well as being an effective use of time for the office schedule.

Advance Booking

Ideally, before leaving the office, the patient will schedule his or her next appointment. This routine is known as advance booking. It is possible to book patients far in advance because most medical offices prepare the schedule books from three to six months ahead of time. Advance booking is done for regularly scheduled checkups or required follow-up appointments, such as after physical therapy treatments, or blood pressure checks. Appointment cards with the name, address, and telephone number of the physician's practice have space to write in the date and time of the next appointment and should be given to each patient at the time the next appointment is made (Figure 8-5).

Follow-up

Some offices have the patient complete a self-addressed postcard reminder to use in an appointment reminder system known as a tickler file. The tickler card is filed in a small file box (tickler file) under the date the postcard should be mailed. Such reminders are used for annual PAP tests. The tickler file is very handy for the follow-up appointments. When possible, the follow-up should be scheduled before the patient leaves the office. Follow-ups can be made in writing, by telephone, or e-mail. All follow-up methods should include the day, date, and time of the next appointment. Some offices make personal telephone calls one to two days prior to the actual appointment. Either follow-up method is considered a good approach for maintaining customer service and smart office management to decrease the no-show rate.

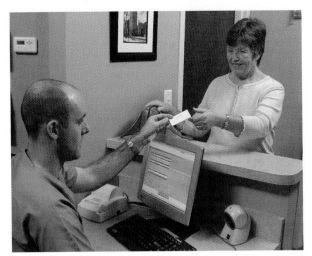

FIGURE 8-5 The medical assistant gives a patient an appointment card.

Patient Referrals

The physician will often refer patients to another facility or physician for further testing and treatment. Ideally, the appointment is scheduled as soon as possible. Whether referring a patient to another location or receiving a referral, the medical assistant must exchange pertinent information regarding the patient's name, contact number, insurance, and referral needs as well as the referral physician's name, address, and contact number. In some cases, depending on the insurance, pre-certification (approval) is necessary before scheduling the appointment.

Hospital Admission Scheduling

The medical assistant is responsible for scheduling all patient admissions to the hospital. Patients do not schedule their own hospital admissions (admits). When scheduling a direct admit to the hospital, be sure to contact the patient's insurance company for pre-admissions approval. Table 8-3 provides a description of the patient information supplied when scheduling hospital admissions.

Provide the patient with a detailed explanation of the day, date, time, and preparation needed for the admission. It is always better to place details in writing. Many offices have preprinted information to distribute to the patient. This should, however, be personalized with the patient's name. Even when preprinted materials are used, a complete, concise, verbal explanation of the important points should be given by the medical assistant.

Scheduling Surgery and Outpatient Procedures

Scheduling a surgical procedure is determined on the patient's need and diagnosis, type of surgery, insurance carrier, physician, anesthesia, and facility availability. The medical assistant will contact the surgical boarding department and arrange with the surgical boarder the necessary pre-surgical appointments (i.e. blood work, chest x-ray, etc.), the actual surgery, and postoperative appointments, if necessary. The surgical boarder may request all patient information, including legal name, telephone contacts, insurance information (prior authorization for some elective surgeries), advanced directives, or other pre-admittance information.

Sometimes the medical assistant will be asked to assist a patient in scheduling an outpatient procedure with the surgical scheduler—the person in the surgery department who schedules the procedures. Procedure 8-2 provides instructions on how to schedule inpatient surgical procedures. Procedure 8-3 reviews the steps for scheduling outpatient procedures.

Appointment Exceptions

On occasion, nonscheduled patients will contact the office with a need for an immediate appointment. These include patient emergencies and patients with acute conditions. Acute conditions are illnesses or injuries that patients suddenly experience and require treatment but may not be life threatening.

The medical assistant must listen carefully to all the patient's complaints and assess the seriousness of the patient's condition. The medical assistant will ask questions regarding where the pain is located, when it first appeared, the duration of strength or measure of the pain, and if the patient has experienced the same pain

TABLE 8-3 Patient Information Supplied when Scheduling Hospital Admissions

■ Patient's full name	Verify spelling of first and last name.
■ Address	Ask the patient to state current address.
■ Social Security number	May be taken from the patient record. (Note: This is not in compliance with HIPAA, however, medical institutions still ask for this information.)
■ Age/Date of birth	Verify birth date in patient record.
■ Telephone number	Ask patient for current number and area code.
■ Requirement	Type of room or special requirement.
■ Admitting diagnosis	Give the physician's statement from the patient record.
■ Recent prior admission	Ask the patient for last admission date in any hospital.
■ Physician's name	Give physician's name.
■ Insurance information	May fax copy of insurance card.
■ Person's name at insurance company who gave pre-approval.	Forms are also available from insurance company.

8-2   **PROCEDURE**

Scheduling Inpatient Surgical Procedures

OBJECTIVE: Perform proper procedure to schedule inpatient surgical procedures.

Equipment and Supplies
patient's chart; written instructions for patients (if required)

Method
1. Review the patient's chart for the most current information. Make sure the chart contains the physician's notes and orders regarding the surgical procedure.
2. Verify with the physician the type of procedure for which you are to schedule the patient. Then you should:
   - determine which category the surgical procedure falls under (routine, elective, urgent).
   - find out the name of the surgeon to perform the procedure.
   - obtain the surgeon's scheduling preference for this type of procedure.
   - get an estimated length of time for the procedure.
3. Gather the following information from the patient and patient's chart:
   - patient's full name, age, sex, and any other pertinent identification or information.
   - physician's current diagnosis.
   - special pre-op orders and patient instructions.
   - patient's insurance information.
4. Obtain pre-authorization from the patient's insurance company, if required.
5. Contact the surgery scheduler.
6. Follow office procedure and surgeon's request for contacting other members of the surgical team.
7. Instruct patient on special preparation and admission procedures. Provide written instructions, if available.

PROCEDURE

Scheduling an Outpatient Procedure

OBJECTIVE: To demonstrate the ability to schedule outpatient procedures in the health care setting.

Equipment and Supplies

telephone; patient's insurance card; notepad; pen

Method

1. Access the appointment system (manual or computer).
2. According to the facility policy, contact the outpatient scheduler at the local hospital or clinic and identify yourself and your office.
3. Instruct the facility about the type of procedure and amount of time the physician expects to need the operating room.
4. Determine available days at the facility.
5. Offer options to patient and have patient choose the best option.
6. Notify the facility of the date and time chosen.
7. Create patient instruction sheet to include date and time of procedure and necessary preoperative information.
8. Document conversation in the patient chart.

Charting Example

Patient has cervical conization scheduled for 12:30 p.m. on November 9, 2005. Patient was given instruction sheet and stated she understood that she would have to go for preoperative testing on November 3 and is not to eat after midnight on the night prior to surgery.

---

before. Also ask the patient for a telephone number from where he or she is calling and determine if the patient is alone. It is best for the medical assistant to use the office policy and emergency criteria list to assess the situation. The physician should always be informed immediately regarding a potential emergency.

The medical assistant will need to apply his on her triage skills. Triage is the process of sorting or grouping patients according to the seriousness of their condition. Triage becomes necessary when there is more than one seriously ill patient waiting to see the physician. In general, sudden onset of pain must be considered an emergency until otherwise determined.

If an emergency exists, such as in the case of severe chest pain, then the physician is informed of the call immediately. If a physician is not available, then the medical assistant refers the patient to the nearest emergency center. If the patient is not able to make his or her own arrangements for transportation, then the medical assistant will arrange for taxi or med-van service. Table 8-4 lists acute illnesses that will require that the patient be seen by a physician as soon a possible, while Table 8-5 lists emergency (life-threatening) conditions, which will require immediate physician assistance.

In order to eliminate the need to "squeeze in" an emergency or nonscheduled appointments and disrupt the time management office flow, the medical as-

sistant should set time patterns. Time patterns are similar to matrixing off time within the schedule for catch-up time or nonscheduled appointments. Ideally, there should be a few minutes built into the schedule between the end of one patient visit and the beginning of another patient's visit. However, most schedule systems do not allow for time between patients. Therefore, it is important to build small blocks of

TABLE 8-4 **Examples of Acute Conditions**	
Earache	Eye infection
Fever lasting more than 24 hours	Infection that is visible to patient (for example, a red, swollen area after an injury)
Pain or burning upon urination	Pain in abdomen that is not severe
Skin rash	Stabbing chest pain
Unusual discharge (for example, blood in urine)	Sore throat and/or swollen glands

TABLE 8-5 Examples of Emergency Conditions

Acute allergic reaction	Head injury
Allergic reaction with respiratory distress	Laceration
Chest pain	Loss of consciousness
Coma	Pain and/or numbness after the application of a cast for fracture
Convulsions	Poisoning
Diabetic reaction	Severe bleeding
Difficulty breathing	Severe dizziness
Drowning/near-drowning	Severe nausea, vomiting, and diarrhea lasting more than 24 hours
Drug overdose	Severe pain
Foreign object in the eye	Sudden acute illness
Fracture	Sudden paralysis of part or all of the body
Gunshot wounds	Temperature over 104° F

time into the schedule during the day when the physician can return telephone calls, catch up on charting, read mail and journals, or just rest. The best time for this is at the end of the morning's schedule and again, at the end of the day. Some physicians prefer to return all morning telephone calls when they return from lunch.

Building this free time block into the office daily schedule at the same time each day is very important. Every effort should be made not to schedule last minute appointments during this time. These "buffer" periods are excellent backup times for emergencies that may have to be seen that day.

Telephone and E-mail Scheduling

Many offices use the telephone and e-mail (electronic mail) to schedule appointments. The medical assistant will need to apply professional, legal, and effective communication skills when using these forms of technology.

Following are some professional considerations to include while communicating with the patient:

- Determine if you are speaking directly with the patient.
- Use the patient's name while addressing him or her on the telephone and in the e-mail.
- On the telephone, confirm the appointment by having the patient repeat the day, date, time, and location of the appointment.
- In an e-mail, request that the patient provide a return communication for verification of received information.
- Communicate with the patient the desire to meet his or her requested appointment time; however, an explanation may be necessary when offering an alternative time.
- Be specific and inform the patient of the office policies for cancellations and missed appointments.
- Be sure to gather all pertinent information from the patient, i.e. name, telephone contacts, e-mail address, reason for visit, insurance carrier, and whether the patient needs directions to the office.

New Patient Appointments

Scheduling a new patient's appointment requires additional time, patience, and effective organizational skills. Always project a professional and positive image with the patient. Using effective communication skills will be most beneficial from a customer service perspective, since managing this appointment will set the stage for the patient's actual in-office visit. The following steps are guidelines for scheduling a new patient:

- Assemble necessary appointment scheduling equipment.
- Obtain the patient's full legal name and correct spelling, birth date, full address, telephone contacts (home, office, cell), and e-mail address.
- Record the patient's chief complaint and symptoms.
- Request the name of the patient's insurance carrier and policy number.
- Ask how the patient was referred to the medical office (physician referral, friend, colleague, insurance company, etc.).
- Ask the patient for a preferred appointment time.
- Attempt to accommodate the new patient's request for his or her preferred appointment time.
- Confirm the day, date, and time of the appointment and have the new patient repeat the information for verification and mutual understanding.

- Provide the new patient with directions to the office.
- Inform the new patient of all materials to bring with him or her for the first visit, i.e. insurance verification, photo identification, list of current medications, past medical records (if available), current lab, x-ray, and other medical reports, as available.
- Welcome and thank the new patient by name for selecting your medical office.
- Provide all information as discussed to the new patient via mail.
- Document new patient information in a new medical record.

When scheduling pediatric and elderly patients, it is important to note that they may need specific times and may have other special needs. Lifespan Considerations discusses some ways to make the office environment more welcoming for these patients.

Lifespan Considerations

Young children often find it hard to wait patiently for extended periods of time. Try to be sensitive to this when scheduling pediatric patients. Some adult patients may have to bring their children with them. In the waiting area, have some quiet activities and magazines geared toward children. Animated and children's videos may help children wait more patiently.

Also remember that the elderly may have difficulty waiting for long periods of time. Take measures to help make them as comfortable as possible. Comfortable seating, large print reading materials, and light refreshments may be ways to make their wait easier.

Established Patient Appointments

Any patient who has been previously seen by the physician is considered an established patient. Established patients will have an existing medical record/chart that will need to be accessed each time the patient contacts the physician for an appointment. It is a good approach to verify the established patient's telephone contact, address, and insurance information prior to scheduling an appointment. Maintaining good customer service with established patients includes appointment reminders and observing patient cycle time.

Scheduling Other Types of Appointments

Medical practices may have non-patient appointments to schedule. These appointments may include, sales representatives from various companies, including office equipment, pharmaceuticals, insurance, or community service leaders. Each visitor will need an appointment to update the staff and physician on the newest product, drug(s), equipment, or community issue(s). Most offices have a policy for working with the non-patient visitors and vendor representatives.

SUMMARY

An efficiently managed medical office requires careful attention to the scheduling function. The medical assistant is responsible for carefully assessing the patient's need for an appointment. Providing the correct amount of time on the schedule for the patient visit works to ensure that the needs of patient and physician are met. However, the medical assistant must remain flexible in scheduling since patients with emergencies and acute illnesses must be seen immediately.

A professional and ethical manner is the best approach to handling a schedule that has fallen behind. Quick thinking and planning by rescheduling patients can alleviate stress for the physician who falls behind. Careful documentation and HIPAA compliance of all patients who fail to keep appointments, either through cancellation or no-show, can assist the physician in avoiding a lawsuit for abandonment of the patient.

Chapter Review

COMPETENCY REVIEW

1. Define and spell the terms to learn for this chapter.
2. Write an office policy for scheduling emergency appointments.

3. Role-play instructing a patient on admission to the hospital for a surgical procedure. Use another student as the patient.
4. Correctly document a patient appointment cancellation.
5. Use a computerized scheduling system to integrate patient information and appointment scheduling.

1. David is scheduled to have a post-operative checkup. He has been given a 15-minute appointment at 1:00 P.M. His wife, Christina, has an appointment on the same day at 1:15 P.M. What type of scheduling system is the physician using?
   A. wave scheduling
   B. specified time scheduling
   C. modified wave scheduling
   C. double booking
   E. open office hours

2. How far ahead of time should a medical office appointment schedule be "blocked out?"
   A. one year
   B. six months
   C. three months
   D. to be done when you make an appointment
   E. one week

3. What is the best method to use when a patient cancels an early afternoon one-hour appointment?
   A. move up the last appointment (15-minute exam) for the day into that slot
   B. leave the time free for the physician to get caught up with paper work
   C. do nothing since the physician is always running late
   D. call several patients who have asked to be placed on a waiting list and try to fill the entire hour
   E. try to change all of the rest of the afternoon appointments to one hour earlier

4. When the patient requires surgery, the medical assistant will
   A. give all the information to the patient so that the patient can schedule the surgery at a convenient time
   B. ask the surgeon who will be performing the surgery to schedule it
   C. call the surgery scheduler where the surgery will be performed and schedule the time
   D. place the surgery request in writing and send it to the surgical center
   E. tell the physician/employer to schedule it

5. All the following are either medical emergencies or acute conditions that require an appointment as soon as possible EXCEPT
   A. earache
   B. severe pain
   C. eye infection
   D. pain with urination
   E. fever of 99.8° F for the past two weeks

6. After a no-show and to assist the physician in avoiding a claim by a patient for abandonment, the medical assistant would
   A. tell the patient that he or she will have to find another physician for treatment
   B. screen out all patients who really do not need to be seen by the physician
   C. call the patient to attempt to re-schedule the appointment and document the telephone call
   D. nothing special needs to be done
   E. refer the patient to a specialist

7. Double booking patients
   A. is one of the most acceptable ways of patient scheduling in terms of practice time management
   B. is generally considered poor practice
   C. involves scheduling two members of the same family at the same time
   D. always forces the physician to utilize less time per patient
   E. does not cause daily scheduling problems

8. What procedure for appointment scheduling refers to crossing out periods of time when the physician is unavailable?
   A. double booking
   B. wave scheduling
   C. forming a matrix
   D. modified wave scheduling
   E. archiving

continued on next page

9. When a patient does not show up for an appointment, the medical assistant should do all of the following EXCEPT
   A. write "N/S" above the scheduled appointment
   B. record the missed appointment in the patient's record
   C. record the reason for the missed appointment in the patient's record
   D. notify the physician
   E. track down the patient

10. Which of the following is applicable to appointment cards?
   A. include the name, address and telephone number of the practice
   B. should be given to each patient whether the patient wants one or not
   C. includes all of the same information as the follow-up reminder card
   D. are generally only used for past no-shows
   E. are preprinted with the patient's name prior to the day's appointment

CRITICAL THINKING

1. What scheduling variation is in use?
2. Using a modified wave format, recreate the original schedule for Dr. Miller's Friday appointments.
3. On the new schedule, indicate Ramona Pierce's cancelled appointment.
4. The office is usually closed from 12 P.M. to 1 P.M. for lunch. New patient visits usually last about one hour. Can Shannon Reece see Dr. Miller tomorrow?
5. How should Marc handle scheduling Marcus Fowler?

ON THE JOB

A pharmaceutical representative has just arrived at the office of Dr. Joseph Henderson, a board certified orthopedic surgeon. The waiting room is literally swarming with patients waiting to see Dr. Henderson because he was delayed with an unexpectedly complicated lumbar spinal fusion and laminectomy.

The representative is very insistent, almost belligerent about seeing the physician immediately, even though she did not have an appointment to see him. In fact, the visit was totally unexpected as the representative had just been in two weeks prior to today. Last time the representative was in, she gave Dr. Henderson a variety of readily usable and dispensable medication. She has more of the same today—injectable cortisone with Novocain, muscle relaxants, NSAIDS, and even some Tylenol with codeine. Usually, Dr. Henderson is quite receptive to receiving these samples as they help ease the financial burden of his patients on whom he uses or to whom he dispenses the samples. The office is, in fact, running quite low on these particular medications because of Dr. Henderson's heavy patient load.

1. What is your response to the sales representative?
2. Should a representative ever take precedence over scheduled appointments?
3. Does the fact that Dr. Joseph is usually quite anxious to receive any and all samples for his patients enter in as a factor?
4. Does the diminished supply of these samples alter the situation?
5. Can the medical assistant ever accept delivery of any or all of these samples?

INTERNET ACTIVITY

Locate three different medical appointment scheduling software programs on the Internet. Compare and contrast the products, services, features, and costs to fit the needs of a general practitioner's medical practice. Then, locate the HIPAA compliance guidelines for appointment scheduling and develop a useful list for future reference.

 MediaLink More on scheduling appointments, including interactive resources, can be found on the Student CD-ROM accompanying this textbook.

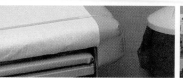

Medical Assistant Role Delineation Chart

HIGHLIGHT indicates material covered in this chapter.

ADMINISTRATIVE

Administrative Procedures

- Perform basic administrative medical assisting functions
- Schedule, coordinate and monitor appointments
- Schedule inpatient/outpatient admissions and procedures
- Understand and apply third-party guidelines
- Obtain reimbursement through accurate claims submission
- Monitor third-party reimbursement
- Understand and adhere to managed care policies and procedures
- *Negotiate managed care contracts*

Practice Finances

- Perform procedural and diagnostic coding
- Apply bookkeeping principles

- Manage accounts receivable
- *Manage accounts payable*
- *Process payroll*
- *Document and maintain accounting and banking records*
- *Develop and maintain fee schedules*
- *Manage renewals of business and professional insurance policies*
- *Manage personnel benefits and maintain records*
- *Perform marketing, financial, and strategic planning*

CLINICAL

Fundamental Principles

- Apply principles of aseptic technique and infection control
- Comply with quality assurance practices
- Screen and follow up patient test results

Diagnostic Orders

- Collect and process specimens
- Perform diagnostic tests

Patient Care

- Adhere to established patient screening procedures
- Obtain patient history and vital signs
- Prepare and maintain examination and treatment areas
- Prepare patient for examinations, procedures and treatments

- Assist with examinations, procedures and treatments
- Prepare and administer medications and immunizations
- Maintain medication and immunization records
- Recognize and respond to emergencies
- Coordinate patient care information with other health care providers
- Initiate IV and administer IV medications with appropriate training and as permitted by state law

GENERAL

Professionalism

- Display a professional manner and image
- Demonstrate initiative and responsibility
- Work as a member of the health care team
- Prioritize and perform multiple tasks
- Adapt to change
- Promote the CMA credential
- Enhance skills through continuing education
- Treat all patients with compassion and empathy
- Promote the practice through positive public relations

Communication Skills

- Recognize and respect cultural diversity
- Adapt communications to individual's ability to understand
- Use professional telephone technique

- Recognize and respond effectively to verbal, nonverbal, and written communications
- Use medical terminology appropriately
- Utilize electronic technology to receive, organize, prioritize and transmit information
- Serve as liaison

Legal Concepts

- Perform within legal and ethical boundaries
- Prepare and maintain medical records
- Document accurately
- Follow employer's established policies dealing with the health care contract
- Implement and maintain federal and state health care legislation and regulations
- Comply with established risk management and safety procedures
- Recognize professional credentialing criteria
- *Develop and maintain personnel, policy and procedure manuals*

Instruction

- Instruct individuals according to their needs
- Explain office policies and procedures
- Teach methods of health promotion and disease prevention
- Locate community resources and disseminate information
- *Develop educational materials*
- *Conduct continuing education activities*

Operational Functions

- Perform inventory of supplies and equipment
- Perform routine maintenance of administrative and clinical equipment
- Apply computer techniques to support office operations
- *Perform personnel management functions*
- *Negotiate leases and prices for equipment and supply contracts*

- *Denotes advanced skills.*

SOURCE: Reprinted by permission of the American Association of Medical Assistants from the AAMA Role Delineation Study: Occupational Analysis of the Medical Assisting Profession.

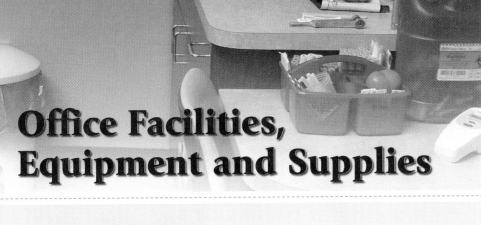

Office Facilities, Equipment and Supplies

Learning Objectives

After completing this chapter, you should be able to:

- Define and spell the terms to learn for this chapter.
- Discuss the elements of office flow.
- State the difference between capital equipment and expendable equipment.
- Discuss basic office equipment and their functions.
- Discuss HIPAA regulations as related to basic office equipment.
- State the proper procedure for handling drug samples.

Terms to Learn

American Disabilities Act (ADA)	cycle time	office flow
capital equipment	inventory	vendor
	morale	warranty

Case Study

YOU ARRIVE AT WORK TO FIND THE OFFICE CARPETS have just been cleaned and all the patient waiting room furniture is stacked in the hallway. Several patients are starting to walk in the front door. The cleaning crew cleaned the office administration area and most of the office equipment, including computers and the fax machine have been moved or unplugged. You find an entire shelf of patient records on the floor and in your work area, and you also noticed a few boxes out in the hallway that contain patient supplies.

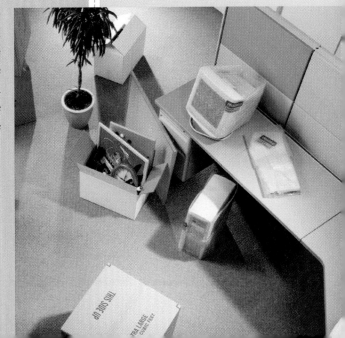

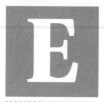

Every medical workplace should be clean to ensure employee and patient safety and health, the traffic should flow smoothly, and it should adhere to Federal, State, and local safety and health regulations. In recent years, changes have been made to many regulations that affect the medical office. As communication processes and technology become more sophisticated, it becomes necessary for the office personnel to both stay informed, and to adhere to the rules that make the medical office safe and protect everyone's right to privacy.

Medical Office Facility

The pleasant physical atmosphere created by a cheerful, clean office makes an immediate impression upon patients. It also adds to the general positive morale of the employees. Morale refers to the positive or negative state of mind of employees (regarding a feeling of well-being) with relationship to their work or work environment. Things to be considered in setting up and maintaining a medical office include the office layout and design that set the tone, attitude, climate, and culture of the office. Elements of the layout include the design of traffic flow, the color of the walls, room temperature, lighting, ventilation, furniture and placement of the furniture, equipment, supplies, and overall organization.

Facilities Planning

The medical assistant will need to view the medical office through the eyes of the patient. What does the patient see when he or she enters the doors and beyond?

One of the first considerations in planning a medical office facility is the American Disabilities Act (ADA), legislation to protect the rights of the disabled regarding access to employment, public buildings, transportation, housing, schools, and health care facilities. The American Disabilities Act allows for every public facility to be easily accessible to the handicapped, including unrestricted hallways, elevators or ramps, and handicapped restroom facilities. Furnishings should be arranged to create an easy traffic pattern for patients to follow as they enter and leave the office. There should be adequate space in the waiting room for wheelchairs to be maneuvered with ease.

All patients should walk into a medical office environment that is comfortable and bright. Some medical offices have patients walk into a reception room with a window that allows patients to look outside during their wait time. External light shines into the office making the room well lit and comfortable. Reception rooms generally should be painted with bright colors and have pleasing and tasteful art on the walls (Figure 9-1). If your office has a fish tank, it is important to regularly maintain the tank for patient safety and general cleanliness. Fish tanks are very inviting for children and adults to watch. It is important to position the tank up high enough so children cannot disturb the fish or push over the tank.

Office Layout

Medical offices are generally divided into two areas: administrative and clinical. The administrative area may contain the reception area to perform patient processing and scheduling, office equipment, file storage, payment collections, insurance, billing, and mail processing. The administrative area usually includes office equipment such as computers, printers, scanners, fax machines, postage meters, calculators, telephone system, paper shredder, dictation and transcribing equipment as well as all office supplies. The area may also include a children's play area and staff area. Child safety in the office is discussed in Lifespan Considerations.

The clinical area contains the examination rooms, physician's office and consultation room, treatment room for office surgical procedures, supply room, clean and contaminated utility areas, rest rooms, a laboratory that can house blood drawing, specimen analyzing, and electrocardiogram (ECG) equipment, and in some offices, a radiology room. Some medical facilities also have a small recovery room with a bed or cot for patients recovering from minor surgical procedures. Of course, not every

FIGURE 9-1 A reception area should be comfortable and bright.

Lifespan
Considerations

Care needs to be taken to keep the office child proof and kid friendly. Cover outlets with safety caps. Evaluate the placement of lamps and cords that can be pulled on or tripped over.

Professionalism

The professional medical assistant must be knowledgeable in many areas of the medical office. Your job may be to perform clinical duties and responsibilities on most days, performing hands-on patient care and assisting the physician. However, in the case of staff call-ins or vacations, the medical assistant must be able to cover in the front office also, assisting the office manager with the business portion of the office.

office will have all of these areas. Specialty practices may have other departments and equipment specific to the type of procedures done.

Office Flow

The medical facility generally has a flow that lends itself easily to teamwork, time management, organized and efficient office equipment usage, and patient flow. This is known as office flow. The more organized the office area, the more effective the office flow will be managed by staff and patients (Professionalism). All staff members will be involved in the office flow process from the time the patients arrive to their departure time. Each staff member has a chance to maintain the office flow by reducing patient cycle time. Cycle time is the length of time the average patient spends in the medical office. With proper office layout, the cycle time can be managed more effectively for a smoother office flow. Let's take a closer look at how these elements impact the office flow (Figure 9-2).

The first element of the office flow is the patient entrance. The first impression the patient receives begins at the medical facility door. Getting patients into the office presents the opportunity to accommodate any type of patient. The office entranceways should include handrails, elevators, ramps, wheelchair-accessible door frames, patient lifts if necessary, and well lit walkways. High steps should be marked with reflector tape and should include slip protection sheets. Doors and door handles should be marked with a push or pull indicator. Keeping doors clean and clear is vital to office aesthetics and patient safety.

Reception Area

The reception area consists of the waiting room and the reception desk. The desk should be enclosed with a glass partition that can be closed for privacy so that personal medical information cannot be overheard in the waiting room. The desk surface should be neat and not

contain confidential patient information such as records, an open appointment book, and billing information.

The medical records area should be close to the receptionist's area for quick accessibility to charts for telephone calls. The Health Insurance Portability and Accountability Act (HIPAA) states that the medical records area should not be accessible to patients and that they should not be able to read the labels of the charts. Figure 9-3 shows a typical file room.

Seating that provides good support and can be easily cleaned is most suitable for the patient reception area. Over-stuffed chairs and couches should be avoided. Housekeeping staff cannot move such furniture easily. In addition, deep chairs are difficult to get in and out of for the elderly and the infirm.

Almost every office has magazines for patients to read. All materials placed for patient reading must be screened to make sure they meet the standards of your

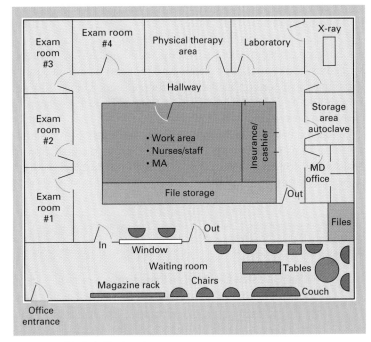

FIGURE 9-2 A typical office layout.

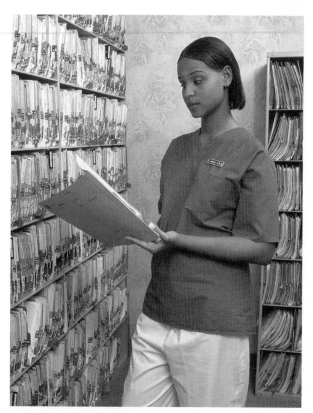

FIGURE 9-3   A typical office file room.

office and would not upset the patients. Patient Education discusses types of materials used to educate patients. It is important to organize the magazines and materials neatly in order to show that the office is clean and well maintained. Periodically, the receptionist or another staff member assigned may need to straighten up the reception area and waiting room, especially magazines and brochures.

Children's toys and books should be washable and not have small, removable parts. Large building blocks, hardcover books, and large plastic toys that can be sanitized may be placed on a small table for children. These toys should be disinfected regularly with an appropriate cleaner to prevent cross contamination.

Smoking is not allowed in medical facilities. No smoking signs should be placed at the entrance of the building. A container should be available to dispose of cigarettes before entering the building.

If a person with a communicable disease visits the office, he or she should be placed in a designated area to minimize spreading the disease. After the visit is over, the office should be disinfected immediately.

Patient orientation begins when the patient arrives in the reception area. Many medical offices prefer that a medical professional escort the patient through the office. However, this is not always possible and patients may need to get around by themselves. For patients to navigate for themselves requires clear markings that indicate the location of the registration and check-in desk, office entrance and exits, where patients should sit if there is more than one doctor in the office, and restroom locations. Hallways and walkways should be clear of any obstructions. In some offices, color-coded indicators on the floor or wall help to facilitate patient flow. It is important to have signs that show patients where they need to go.

Clearly marked areas will assist patient exits as well. When a patient is ready to leave the office, it is important to confirm the route a patient needs to take to exit the office. For example, if a patient has just been seen by a physician and you are showing the patient out, it is best to lead the way. This should prevent patients from accidentally walking into another examination room or into private areas of the office. Patients should have a direct route to the checkout desk and there should be markings on the walls to help patients to direct themselves toward the exit.

Examination Rooms

Examination rooms should only contain furnishings and equipment needed to examine a patient. Most examination rooms have only enough space for the necessities and little else. Figure 9-4 illustrates a typical patient examination room. All instruments and supplies, such as disposable gowns, towels, tissues, and sheets are kept in a sufficient number in examination room supply cabinets. Most examination tables have drawers for the convenient storage of these items. A small sink for hand hygiene, an adjustable gooseneck lamp, telephone, chair, examination table, and physician's stool are the only furnishings necessary. Examination rooms should be painted in a pleasant, comforting color. Paintings or pictures can also enhance the serenity of the room. The temperature throughout the reception

Patient   Education

Patient Education begins when the patient enters the office. Many offices now offer videotapes on various health care topics that the patients may view while waiting to be seen by the physician. Become involved in keeping all patient education pamphlets up to date and displayed on tables in the reception area or in a rack designed for literature.

area and examination rooms should be maintained at around 74° F. Patients in the examination rooms must frequently disrobe and may be chilled in just a disposable gown.

At least one examination room should be configured for a wheelchair-bound patient. It should be larger than a normal sized examination room to allow both the patient and physician to maneuver comfortably.

Examination rooms should be soundproof so that conversations cannot be heard from one room to another. The examination table should be arranged so that the patient is not exposed when the door is opened. "White noise," such as pleasant, soothing background music, can also filter sounds.

Bathrooms

Bathrooms should be kept clean and odor-free. Every bathroom should have hot and cold water, soap, paper towels or other drying system, a trashcan, and toilet tissue. Since bathrooms in the medical office are multifunctional, they should also be large enough to accommodate a wheelchair, and at least one of the bathrooms should meet ADA guidelines for a handicapped restroom facility such as handrails around the toilet. Bathrooms are used by both staff and patients. They are also used by patients who are collecting urine specimens and should have a place to set the specimen while the patient washes his or her hands after collecting the sample.

Housekeeping

Housekeeping or medical office cleaning services can be contracted to clean the front office area and the examination room every night. Regular housekeeping services are usually not responsible for handling hazardous waste containers. Instead, hazardous waste, including sharps, should be disposed of in designated containers and removed from the office or facility properly.

Office Equipment

In order for a medical office to maintain effective office flow, certain office machines and equipment are most beneficial. As mentioned above, a copier, computers, printers, scanners, fax machines (Figure 9-5), postage meters, calculators, telephone system, dictation and transcribing equipment, and paper shredder would be considered essentials for the office. This equipment and other equipment, such as examination tables, refrigerators, x-ray and EKG machines, office furnishings, and carpeting, are categorized as capital equipment.

Capital equipment refers to items that require a large dollar amount to purchase (generally over $500) and have a relatively long life. The distinguishing factor between capital equipment and general office

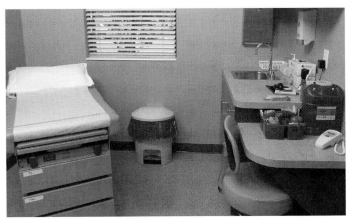

FIGURE 9-4 A patient examination room should be simple and efficiently designed.

supplies is the life expectancy (functional life period) of the product.

Capital equipment also has a financial life, which is referred to as depreciation. Depreciation is a loss in value of the product resulting from normal aging, use, or deterioration. An allowance is made for this type of loss of value for tax purposes. Therefore, the office accountant will credit capital items differently than for general office supplies. A master inventory, or list, should be detailed and maintained of all the physical assets, or capital equipment, in an office.

Determining what equipment to have begins with the office need. Obtaining the equipment requires research to gather equipment information, the actual purchase, delivery, setup, proper training, safe use, and general maintenance. Most medical offices will have the following administrative equipment.

- Calculator—used for mathematical calculation for billing and determining medication dosages.

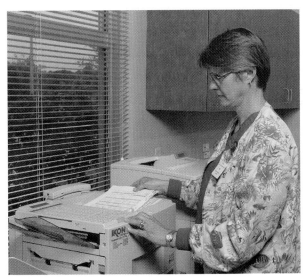

FIGURE 9-5 Fax machines are necessary in all medical offices.

- Computer—discussed in Chapter 11.
- Laser printer—used in conjunction with a computer for letter quality printing. Creates images with a laser beam and then transfers the image to paper with pressure and heat.
- Facsimile (fax) machine—used to send and receive copies to and from the office via the telephone system.
- Transcription equipment (dictation/transcription machine)—used to dictate and then transcribe information for documents and letters.
- Telephone system—discussed in Chapter 6.
- Scanners—used to "read" text and graphic files.
- Copy machine—used to copy, reduce, enlarge, and collate documents in the medical office (Figure 9-6).
- Electronic paper shredder—used to shred paper documents into thin strips so that the information on the documents cannot be retrieved.
- Postage meter—used to stamp envelopes and packages for offices with large mailings.

Transcription Equipment

The dictation equipment required for medical transcription includes transcribers, typewriters, word processing equipment, and reference materials. Newer methods of transcription include computerized voice recognition technology (VRT). Explanations of each follow.

Transcription Equipment for the Physically Challenged

There are many adaptations for persons with a physical impairment, such as lower limb paralysis, blindness, and deafness. For example, foot pedals can be replaced with hand or voice-activated equipment for a person in a wheelchair or with lower limb impairment.

The blind and visually impaired can use video magnifiers that use high-powered lenses to enlarge copy. A device called a tactile converter allows the blind person to read printed material by placing one hand inside the converter holding a printed document and "reading" the material with the index finger resting on the transmitter plate.

Blind transcriptionists are able to proofread their material through the use of a voice synthesizer. A Braille-Edit program allows blind and sighted persons to work together using a microcomputer.

The deaf or hearing-impaired are able to use a telecommunication device for the deaf (TDD) that will place sound onto paper. They can then type it into the correct format for a medical record.

Transcribers

Medical transcribers are machines that allow the transcriptionist to take oral dictation and turn this into written material and documents. These typically have an audiocassette tape (onto which the physician or other health care worker has dictated information); headphones for private listening, a speed, volume, and tone control; and a foot pedal to free the hands for typing.

The cassette mechanism of transcription equipment has the ability to play, stop, rewind, and fast-forward the tape. However, the foot pedal is used for most playing and rewinding since it is faster (Procedure 9-1).

Word Processing

Word processing has made medical transcription more efficient. The word processor has the ability to create and maneuver text without having to cut and paste a paper document. The word processor also is able to save the document. This allows the typist to work on a document, save it, retrieve it at a later time, and work on it again. Corrections during the typing process can easily be made. For example, if a dictated word or phrase is not clear on the tape, the transcriptionist can leave a blank with a question mark, speak to the dictator (physician) about the word or phrase, and add the correct word or phrase before finishing the document.

Another advantage of the word processor over the typewriter is the ability to make multiple original copies of the document.

Voice Recognition Technology (VRT)

This new technology allows the physician to speak into a microphone connected to a computer program that translates the dictation into a typed report. VRT requires the physician to provide several samples of his or her speech by reading manufacturer-provided scripts to activate the program. Since this is a time consuming process, not too many physicians have adopted this system in their offices. However, it is used in some

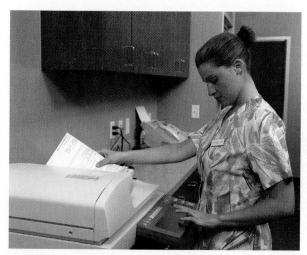

FIGURE 9-6 Copiers should meet the particular needs of the medical office.

Operating a Transcriber

OBJECTIVE: Understand basic information on how to operate a transcriber, which can produce a printed document of voice-recorded material.

Equipment and Supplies

transcriber; headset; computer; paper; printer; possibly a foot pedal

Method

1. Assure the transcriber and all ancillary equipment is turned on and is working.
2. Be sure to adjust the volume, tone, and speed controls to avoid any interruptions in the communication and transcription.
3. Listen for physician's instructions. The physician's instructions will guide the order of priority of reports and format.
4. Set all computer software formatting, such as margins, font, line spacing and indentation, and alignment.
5. Listen to the physician's recording and enter the information.
6. Complete, archive, and save all information according to the physician's procedures.

---

hospital medical records departments and as the equipment becomes more user-friendly, it will become more accessible.

Using a Postage Meter

Many offices use a postage meter that will automatically stamp large mailings. The postage can be printed directly onto an envelope with a meter. Postage can also be printed onto an adhesive backed strip that is placed directly onto a package. Metered mail does not have to be stamped when it arrives at the post office. The meter is taken into the post office for calibrating.

Purchasing Equipment

When a business determines the need for specific equipment, the purchase process begins. The medical assistant may be asked to research and compare equipment based on the manufacturer, quality, size, service, price, and other determining factors. The medical assistant can search the Internet, contact local vendors and other offices as part of the fact-gathering quest. Collecting information, printed materials, and resources will enable the physician to make the right choice when actually purchasing the equipment.

Warranties

A warranty is a guarantee in writing from the manufacturer that the product will perform correctly under normal conditions of use. The warranty provides for a replacement of defective parts at no charge within a certain period of time. An extended warranty can be purchased to cover the period of time after the warranty has expired. For example, a copier may have a one-year warranty, but an extended warranty can be purchased to cover parts replacement after that year has expired.

Some office equipment that is heavily used, such as a copy machine, has a service contract for preventive maintenance. A service contract provides maintenance and cleaning of equipment even when it is working properly to avoid a breakdown. A maintenance contract will state in detail what is actually covered by the contract. The dates and frequency of service should be noted carefully. Literature relating to warranties and preventative maintenance contracts should be kept in a designated file. Since office equipment is expensive these contracts are important.

Equipment Records

Records relating to office equipment need to be maintained. Receipts for major purchases, operating manuals, instructions, warranties, and repair and maintenance instructions need to be filed. Lists of service people with contact information should be maintained. Many offices maintain a current file of business cards representing the companies from which equipment has been purchased. Ideally, the registration and ID number of each item is maintained in a separate file from the warranty.

Remember to record any unusual occurrences of equipment in writing. Memory of what actually happened may fail over time. A written record of exactly what happened and the corrective action that was

TABLE 9-1 Equipment Inventory Record

Item	Serial #	Purchase Date	Location
Laptop	XX 12345	2/14/05	Reception
IBM Selectric II Typewriter	XC54321	2/14/05	Laboratory
IBM G40 Computer	4-190-L1001	9/19/05	Reception
Hewlett-Packard Color LaserJet Printer	JPHAC15531	9/19/05	Reception
Ricoh Copier	RC39C452	6/2/04	Billing

taken can assist in determining if something was an accident or negligence.

A list of inventory items should be kept in the procedure manual. Many inventory records are now maintained on the computer. Table 9-1 provides an example of an office inventory record.

Equipment Life and Safety

All equipment is purchased with the accompanying manufacturer's training manual to maintain the life of the machine and the safety of the user. The medical assistant should read all manuals prior to use and have the vendor provide training for the office staff. Usually, the retailer's training and manual will suggest using the equipment defaults and turning the equipment off when not in use. Training and manuals provide cleaning, maintenance and operation directions, and other important information. The suggestions usually place safety of the user first, longevity of the equipment second, and reordering or service information third. Either way, the staff should be familiar with and able to apply the general equipment features, defaults, and safety guidelines.

Legal and Ethical Issues

The medical assistant has a duty to report any incident such as equipment defects that may harm the employee. Working with inventory requires integrity. Office and medical supplies must not leave the medical office unless the physician orders them. Vendors and suppliers must be dealt with in an honest manner.

Supplies

Vendors, or suppliers, are selected based on several factors including: the quality, price, service, and availability that they provide. In general, it takes multiple vendors to provide all supplies for a medical practice. Catalog or online services can provide ease of availability, competitive pricing, and fast delivery. A wise purchaser will develop a good working relationship with vendors either in person, on the telephone, in writing, or online in preparation for negotiating a contract. Contracts or purchase agreements may include payment schedules, shipment times, product discounts, extended warranty, training sessions, and other incentives. Legal and Ethical Issues has more on equipment and supplies.

Many vendors will provide a discount on supplies when they are ordered in large quantities. This results in a unit cost savings. The drawback to this method is that many offices do not have enough storage space to handle a large inventory of supplies. Some suppliers will store excess inventory for you.

Supplies should be rotated on the shelves so that the newer supplies are in the back of the shelf and the older supplies are used first.

Expendable supplies and equipment include items that are used up in a short period of time and have a relatively inexpensive unit cost. Examples of expendable office supplies are found in Table 9-2.

Supply Inventory

Supply inventory control requires constant supervision since a medical office cannot afford to run out of supplies. Many supplies are purchased in large quantities at lower cost. It can be costly to run out and have to suddenly purchase supplies at full price with additional shipping costs for faster service.

Most offices maintain an ongoing inventory system that helps to determine when to reorder supplies. Whenever an item is removed from the supply cabinet

TABLE 9-2 Expendable Office Supplies

Paper supplies	Examination table paper, disposable gowns, drapes, paper towels, sterilization bags and tapes, stationery, photocopy paper, insurance and chart forms, laboratory order forms, appointment books, ECG paper, receipt book, appointment cards, current CPT and ICD-9 coding books.
Clinical equipment	Disposable speculums, ear and nose speculum covers, catheters, tongue blades, thermometers, cotton-tipped applicators, lubricant, needles, syringes, suture material, dressings, tape, elastic bandages, gloves, goggles.
Office Supplies	Pens, pencils, highlighters, copy paper, stapler(s), stapler removers, printer cartridge, CD-ROMs.

it is marked on the inventory sheet. A staff member is assigned the responsibility of reordering all supplies when items get to a certain level so that the supply is never totally depleted. The amount of time necessary to have the order processed and delivered should be factored in when reordering supplies. See Figure 9-7 for a sample inventory order form.

Order System

It takes experience to be able to calculate how long inventory items will last. However, records can be reviewed to determine when half the supply has been used. Then, by calculating the amount of time it takes to receive a new order, an estimate can be made when to place and how much to reorder. For example, if one printer cartridge is used in one month and there is a three-week reorder period, then a new order must be placed when half the supply has been used. Since print cartridges may be used more during a certain part of the billing periods, or when the office is busier, it would be advisable to reorder cartridges in advance to prevent running out of the supply.

Many offices use color-coded reorder reminder cards that are inserted into the stack of inventory items. As the color card comes to the top of the stack it is time to reorder. Inventory reminder cards can be maintained with a date for reorder.

Some suppliers maintain their own records and will notify the medical office when it is time to reorder. Remember to keep a list of inventory items in the procedure manual and maintain the inventory records on computer files. Some offices use an automated scanning system for inventory control and ordering system.

Drug Samples

Pharmaceutical representatives from the drug companies will often supply medical offices with samples of medications. Drug samples are small packages of a medication for distribution by the physician to the patients. An inventory list of all sample drugs should be maintained to adhere to HIPAA and in some cases, state regulations (check your local state).

Even though these drug samples are small and "free," the medical office must secure and organize the samples in a supply cupboard or drawer that is locked. It is advisable to keep all drugs together by category (for example, sedatives, antibiotics, hypertensive drugs). The expiration dates on drug samples have to be carefully monitored. All samples should be discarded in accordance with HIPAA and federal regulations when they have reached the manufactures expiration date.

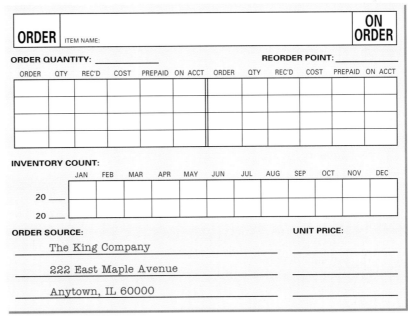

FIGURE 9-7 Sample inventory order form.

SUMMARY

The office layout contributes to the physical atmosphere, organization and impression that patients and employees will encounter. An organized office layout can affect the office flow, and decrease patient cycle time, and positively impact employee morale and patients' attitudes.

The medical assistant will maintain an inventory list for all office equipment purchased, supplies, and drug samples. All staff members should be trained on the use and operation functions of the equipment.

Chapter Review

COMPETENCY REVIEW

1. Define and spell the terms to learn for this chapter.
2. Discuss how following the manufacturer's suggestions enhances equipment longevity.
3. Discuss the importance of patient flow.
4. Discuss how inventory control methods contribute to efficient office management.
5. Discuss the handling of pharmaceutical samples in the medical office.

PREPARING FOR THE CERTIFICATION EXAM

1. Expendable medical office equipment includes the following, EXCEPT
   A. paper supplies
   B. typewriter
   C. word processor
   D. computer printer
   E. fax machine

2. Which supplies are NOT expendable clinical equipment supplies?
   A. catheters
   B. syringes
   C. gloves
   D. gloves and goggles
   E. paper towels

3. Drug samples should be kept in a locked cabinet and organized by
   A. expiration date
   B. shipment date
   C. bottle color
   D. category
   E. alphabetical order

4. A fax machine is used primarily to
   A. copy documents
   B. transcribe
   C. scan documents
   D. transmit documents
   E. store documents

5. Equipment purchase agreements may include the following, EXCEPT
   A. training
   B. warranty
   C. service
   D. price
   E. office flow

6. Office flow includes
   A. furniture placement and current periodicals
   B. traffic flow and general eye appeal
   C. temperature and lighting
   D. ventilation and clearly marked hallways
   E. purchase agreements and warranties

7. At which temperature setting should a medical office be kept?
   A. 80° F
   B. 72° F
   C. 75° F
   D. 73° F
   E. 74° F

8. What two distinct areas are set up in a medical office facility?
   A. staff room and administration offices
   B. physicians office and clinical area
   C. clinical and administrative offices
   D. staff room and reception area
   E. office and traffic flow areas

continued on next page

9. Capital equipment includes the following, EXCEPT
   A. carpeting
   B. EKG machine
   C. refrigerator
   D. files
   E. typewriter

10. When working with vendors you should expect the following, EXCEPT
    A. unit pricing
    B. inventory count
    C. competitive pricing
    D. fast delivery
    E. quality assurance

CRITICAL THINKING

1. What is the first thing you would do to fix the situation after the office carpets were cleaned?

2. How do you function in the office? Based on your knowledge about physical hazards and office safety, what precautions should you take to resolve the problem?

3. What happens to patient flow in this situation?

ON THE JOB

Develop an inventory using an electronic spreadsheet of all equipment, machines, and supplies for the clinical and administrative areas. Include purchase date, maintenance schedule, and purchase price.

INTERNET ACTIVITY

Go to the Americans with Disabilities Act Web site (www.ada.gov) and research the standards for bathrooms in public places that accommodate wheelchairs.

MediaLink More on medical office facilities, equipment, and supplies, including interactive resources, can be found in the Student CD-ROM accompanying this textbook.

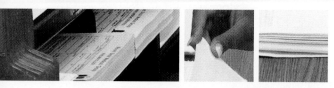

Medical Assistant Role Delineation Chart

HIGHLIGHT indicates material covered in this chapter.

ADMINISTRATIVE

Administrative Procedures

- Perform basic administrative medical assisting functions
- Schedule, coordinate and monitor appointments
- Schedule inpatient/outpatient admissions and procedures
- Understand and apply third-party guidelines
- Obtain reimbursement through accurate claims submission
- Monitor third-party reimbursement
- Understand and adhere to managed care policies and procedures
- *Negotiate managed care contracts*

Practice Finances

- Perform procedural and diagnostic coding
- Apply bookkeeping principles

- Manage accounts receivable
- *Manage accounts payable*
- *Process payroll*
- *Document and maintain accounting and banking records*
- *Develop and maintain fee schedules*
- *Manage renewals of business and professional insurance policies*
- *Manage personnel benefits and maintain records*
- *Perform marketing, financial, and strategic planning*

CLINICAL

Fundamental Principles

- Apply principles of aseptic technique and infection control
- Comply with quality assurance practices
- Screen and follow up patient test results

Diagnostic Orders

- Collect and process specimens
- Perform diagnostic tests

Patient Care

- Adhere to established patient screening procedures
- Obtain patient history and vital signs
- Prepare and maintain examination and treatment areas
- Prepare patient for examinations, procedures and treatments

- Assist with examinations, procedures and treatments
- Prepare and administer medications and immunizations
- Maintain medication and immunization records
- Recognize and respond to emergencies
- Coordinate patient care information with other health care providers
- Initiate IV and administer IV medications with appropriate training and as permitted by state law

GENERAL

Professionalism

- Display a professional manner and image
- Demonstrate initiative and responsibility
- Work as a member of the health care team
- Prioritize and perform multiple tasks
- Adapt to change
- Promote the CMA credential
- Enhance skills through continuing education
- Treat all patients with compassion and empathy
- Promote the practice through positive public relations

Communication Skills

- Recognize and respect cultural diversity
- Adapt communications to individual's ability to understand
- Use professional telephone technique

- Recognize and respond effectively to verbal, nonverbal, and written communications
- Use medical terminology appropriately
- Utilize electronic technology to receive, organize, prioritize and transmit information
- Serve as liaison

Legal Concepts

- Perform within legal and ethical boundaries
- Prepare and maintain medical records
- Document accurately
- Follow employer's established policies dealing with the health care contract
- Implement and maintain federal and state health care legislation and regulations
- Comply with established risk management and safety procedures
- Recognize professional credentialing criteria
- *Develop and maintain personnel, policy and procedure manuals*

Instruction

- Instruct individuals according to their needs
- Explain office policies and procedures
- Teach methods of health promotion and disease prevention
- Locate community resources and disseminate information
- *Develop educational materials*
- *Conduct continuing education activities*

Operational Functions

- Perform inventory of supplies and equipment
- Perform routine maintenance of administrative and clinical equipment
- Apply computer techniques to support office operations
- *Perform personnel management functions*
- *Negotiate leases and prices for equipment and supply contracts*

- *Denotes advanced skills.*

SOURCE: Reprinted by permission of the American Association of Medical Assistants from the AAMA Role Delineation Study: Occupational Analysis of the Medical Assisting Profession.

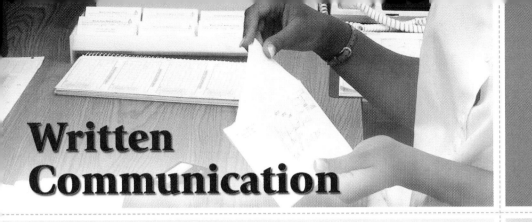

Written Communication

Learning Objectives

After completing this chapter, you should be able to:

- Define and spell the terms to learn for this chapter.
- Name and describe eight areas to consider when letter writing.
- Identify the eight parts of speech and use them correctly.
- Explain the process of proofreading and editing.
- Describe the process of drafting correspondence, using the four methods of letter styles.

- List and describe how to prepare an envelope to meet the standards of the U.S. Postal Service.
- State the four classifications of mail service.
- List and describe six special services offered by the U.S. Postal Service.
- Summarize the ethical implications related to written correspondence.
- Define an instant message and identify its purpose.

Terms to Learn

active voice	homophones	proofreading
block	modified block	redundant
gender bias	passive voice	thesaurus

Case Study

THE STUDENT IN YOUR EXTERNSHIP PROGRAM has been asked by the physician to write a letter to refer a patient to another physician for a second opinion. The student writes the letter and asks you, the medical assistant, to review it. You find many spelling and grammatical errors and address these issues with the student. Following is the letter written by the extern:

Dear Dr Johnson

I am referring a patient to your office for further evaluation. I have been seeing this patient for several years now for right metatarsal injury. It is in my opinion that this patient should seek additional information on having the right metatarsal removed. This patient has been in my office on several occasions unable to walk with much swelling.

I trust your medical opinion and would appreciate you advising the proper action to take for this patient. For your review I have enclosed past x-rays, please feel free to contact my office as soon as possible.

Sincerely,
Dr. J. Ancella

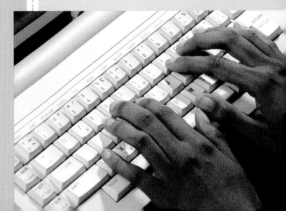

Medical assistants draft many types of correspondence to be signed by the physician/employer. These letters must reflect the professionalism of the medical practice. The physical appearance of letters depends on the quality of paper, letterhead design, and the choice of formats for the letters. However, even the most professional-looking correspondence is quickly and harshly judged when the letter is written in a negative or condescending tone, or is filled with grammatical errors. Correspondence should be positive in tone and well written.

Handling incoming mail requires efficiency in sorting, dating, and reading all correspondence. Correct handling of the mail can save money and time for the medical practice. Initiative in handling mail quickly and accurately is paramount.

Letter Writing

Letters from a medical office must be professional, courteous, business like, project a positive tone, and protect the confidentiality of the physician and the patient. This requires some diplomacy. For example, when drafting a sensitive letter requesting payment for a long overdue bill or to advise a patient to seek the services of another physician, such letters should be clear and to the point. The situation should be explained and the expected outcome presented—"Please send a check for (amount due)" or "Please call to make payment arrangements." Threats or derogatory comments are never acceptable in professional correspondence and may have legal consequences for the sender (Legal and Ethical Issues). The following letters are examples of positive and negative tones in writing.

Negative Example:

Dear Mrs. Murray:
You have repeatedly failed to take medications as prescribed and follow my recommended treatment. Since you have again failed to keep an appointment, I am forced to withdraw as your physician, and I request that you find another physician immediately.

Positive Example:

Dear Mrs. Murray:
During your last visit, we discussed the necessity of continuing medical treatment for you to recover fully from your recent medical problems. Therefore, I am concerned that you failed to keep your appointment this week and have not called the office to schedule a new appointment. Your health continues to be important to me, so I am requesting that you call me as soon as possible to discuss future treatment.

Legal and Ethical Issues

The medical assistant must carefully monitor all dated material to assure that replies are made on a timely basis. Confidential mail and correspondence including checks and payments are handled on a regular basis. This is a grave responsibility. Since the U.S. Postal Services is regulated by the federal government, any tampering or deliberate mishandling of mail is a federal offense.

A non-threatening tone of correspondence can promote the medical profession to the reader. Any attempts to threaten a patient in writing can lead to charges of harassment. Courteous language, presented in a diplomatic manner, can result in compliance and prevent a lawsuit.

An error in correspondence may not be caught by the physician before he or she signs the document. The medical assistant must carefully proofread all correspondence before it leaves the office to protect the physician from legal problems.

If we are unable to reach a mutual understanding about your medical treatment and appointment schedule, I regret that I will not be able to continue as your physician. In that event, you will receive a letter indicating that you have a month's notice in which to secure the services of another physician.

Word Choice

The use of correct words when writing office correspondence includes avoidance of the use of technical terms, gender bias (indicating either male or female by type of language used), long sentences and paragraphs, excessive use of the personal pronoun *I*, repetition, and the passive voice.

Technical Terminology

When writing a letter to medical professionals or institutions that employ medically trained staff, the use of correct medical terminology is essential. This terminology is specialized and is easily understood by medically trained professionals. Many patients are not familiar with medical terminology and, in fact, may not understand or may be intimidated by this style of writing. Table 10-1 lists selected medical terms with corresponding synonyms. The medical terms in the left-hand column are appropriate for medically trained personnel

TABLE 10-1 Medical Terms and Corresponding Synonyms

Medical Term	Synonym
Carcinoma	Cancer
Cardiac	Heart
Dermatitis	Skin irritation
Diabetes mellitus	Diabetes
Gastric	Stomach
Gynecology	Study of female diseases
Hepatic disease	Liver disease
Hyperglycemic	Excessive blood sugar
Hypertension	High blood pressure
Larynx	Voice box
Leukocytes	White blood cells
MI	Myocardial infarction
Nephroses	Kidney disease
NPO	Nothing by mouth
Otolaryngology	Study of ear and throat
Para I	First delivery
Pc	After meals
Thrombus	Blood clot

correspondence (physician to physician, physician to the medical record, medical assistant to hospital); the terms in the right-hand column are more easily understood by patients. The use and explanation of terminology in correspondence and other medical office printed matter as well as the facilitating of patient understanding with these materials is discussed in Patient Education.

Removing Gender Bias

Unfortunately it is quite common in the medical field to assume that every nurse is female and all physicians are male since this was the case many generations ago. Because this is no longer the case, gender-neutral terms are preferred. This means that any reference to a particular gender (male or female) should be eliminated. For example, a male orderly should be referred to as a medical attendant, and cleaning ladies are called housekeepers or cleaning personnel.

Written correspondence must also reflect this same neutral bias toward the genders. When writing about physicians, do not refer to them as males or nurses and medical assistants as females. For example, "The patient was referred to a hospital dietitian for diabetic diet instruction. The patient was told to ask her about a food exchange list." This wording assumes the dietitian is a female. A better statement would be, "The patient was instructed to ask the dietitian about a food exchange list." In order to write in a gender-neutral style, you may have to rewrite the sentence and choose alternate words or phrases.

Sentence and Paragraph Length

Short, concise sentences and paragraphs are preferred in medical writing. Sentence length should never exceed twenty words. Eliminate all words that are unnecessary. The paragraph should only cover one point. A good paragraph contains from two to six sentences. Your reader may stop reading if the paragraph is too long.

Patient Education

Many patient education materials used in the medical office are prepared and distributed in printed form. They include pamphlets, brochures, and letters of instructions. In many cases, the information will have to be interpreted for the patients who have language barriers, difficulty with vision, reading, or understanding medical information. This is an excellent opportunity to provide additional patient teaching. By asking the patient to repeat some of the material that has been explained, you can test the patient's understanding and comprehension.

When advising patients about correspondence, they should be cautioned about sending cash in the mail. Payments should always be made by check or money order when using the mail.

Personal Pronoun

Whenever possible, it is preferable to avoid the use of the personal pronoun *I* in professional writing. It is better to use *you* since this involves the reader. For example, a message such as, "I am asking that any overdue balance be cleared up immediately. I will have to take steps to send this account to a collection agency if it is not paid immediately," is negative. When requesting a patient to pay an overdue bill, it is better to write, "We know that you will want to clear up any overdue account. This overdue balance may have been an oversight on your part. If that is the case, would you kindly remit your payment in the enclosed envelope."

Repetition, Redundancy, and Inflated Phrases

The reader of your correspondence wants to know in concise terms what you are telling them. Avoid being redundant—repeating the same statement over again. Redundant expressions include such terms as *each and every*, *first and foremost*, and *physician's patient*. The above examples can be simplified by stating *each*, *first*, or *the patient*.

Inflated phrases can usually be eliminated without any loss of meaning. Common examples are introductory word groups such as *in my opinion*, *I think that*, *it seems that*, *one must*, and so on. Table 10-2 contains examples of inflated patterns of writing versus concise terms.

Active Versus Passive Voice

The active verbs can make writing more interesting. In the active voice, the subject of the sentence does the action; in the passive voice, the subject receives the action. Although both voices are grammatically correct, the active voice is considered more effective because it is simpler, more direct, and less wordy.

To transform a sentence from the passive to active voice, make the actor the subject of the sentence. Table 10-3 contains examples of statements in both active and passive voice.

Composing Letters

Composing letters can be a simple process when an organized approach is used. Use the guidelines presented in this chapter. The most import element in an organized letter writing approach is to get to the point quickly.

TABLE 10-2 Inflated Phrases Versus Concise Terms

Inflated	Concise
Along the lines of	Like
As a matter of fact	In fact
At all times	Always
At the present time	Now, currently
At this point in time	Now, currently
Because of the fact that	Because
By means of	By
By virtue of the fact that	Because
Due to the fact that	Because
For the purpose of	For
For the reason that	Because
Have the ability to	Be able to
In light of the fact that	Because
In the nature of	Like
In order to	To
In spite of the fact that	Although, though
In the event that	If
In the final analysis	Finally
In the neighborhood of	About
Until such time as	Until

TABLE 10-3 Active Versus Passive Voice

Active	Passive
The medical assistant took the patient's blood pressure measurement	The patient's blood pressure measurement was taken by the medical assistant.
The surgeon performed an appendectomy on the patient.	An appendectomy was performed on the patient by the surgeon.
The medical committee reached a decision.	A decision was reached by the medical committee.

TABLE 10-4 **Common Homophones**

Word	Meaning	Word	Meaning
accept	to receive	lose	to be deprived of
except	to take or leave out	pair	set of two
advice	opinion about what to do for a problem	pare	to trim
advise	to offer advice	pear	fruit
affect	to exert an influence	patience	calm endurance
effect	result; accomplishment	patients	a doctor's clients
all ready	prepared	personal	private; intimate
already	by this time	personnel	a group of employees
altar	a structure on which religious ceremonies are held	precede	to come before
alter	to change	proceed	to go forward
always	every time; forever	quiet	silent; calm
all ways	every way	quite	very
bare	naked	right	proper or just; correct
bear	to carry; to put up with	rite	a ritual
brake	something used to stop movement, to stop	write	to put words on paper
break	to split or smash	stationary	standing still
buy	to purchase	stationery	writing paper
by	near	taught	past tense of *teach*
choose	to select	taut	tight
chose	past tense of *choose*	than	besides
cite	to quote	then	at that time; next
sight	vision	their	belonging to them
site	position, place	they're	contraction of *they are*
complement	to complete	there	that place or position
compliment	praise	through	by means of; finished
conscience	sense of right and wrong	threw	past tense of *throw*
conscious	awake; aware	thorough	careful; complete
elicit	to draw or bring out	to	toward
illicit	illegal	too	also
fair	lovely; light-colored	two	one or more in number
fare	money for transportation, food or drink	waist	midsection
hear	to sense by the ear	waste	to squander
here	this place	weak	feeble
hole	hollow place	week	seven days
whole	entire; unhurt	weather	state of the atmosphere
its	of or belonging to it	whether	indicating a choice between alternatives
it's	contraction for *it is*	who's	contraction of *who is*
know	to be aware of	whose	possessive of *who*
no	opposite of yes	your	possessive of *you*
lessen	to make less	you're	contraction of *you are*
lesson	something learned		
loose	free; not secured		

Spelling

There are several words in the English language that have similar pronunciations but very different meanings and spellings. These words are called homophones. They pose problems unless the writer is careful about their usage. Table 10-4 contains some of the most common homophones.

Computer software programs cannot be depended upon to correct word use since they do not "understand" the data input or content of the correspondence. For example, use of the word *effect* or *affect* depends on the content and cannot be determined by the software program. Both spellings are correct and only the individual using the word in the sentence would be able to determine if the word is the correct choice. See Table 10-5 for examples of the most commonly misspelled medical terms. General rules for capitalization are given in Box 10-1.

Plurals

Following are some basic rules for forming plurals of words:

- Abbreviations are formed into plurals by adding an *s* (ECGs, DRGs).

TABLE 10-5 Commonly Misspelled Medical Terms

abscess	epistaxis	neuron	pneumonia
additive	eustachian	occlusion	polyp
aerosol	fissure	oscilloscope	prophylaxis
agglutination	glaucoma	osseous	prostate
albumin	gonorrhea	palliative	prosthesis
anastomosis	hemorrhage	parasite	pruritis
aneurysm	hemorrhoids	parenteral	psoriasis
anteflexion	homeostasis	parietal	pyrexia
arrhythmia	humerus	paroxysmal	respiratory
bilirubin	idiosyncrasy	pemphigus	roentgenology
bronchial	ileum	percussion	sagittal
calcaneus	ilium	perforation	sciatica
capillary	infarction	pericardium	serous
cervical	intussusception	perineum	sphincter
chromosome	ischemia	peristalsis	sphygmomanometer
cirrhosis	ischium	peritoneum	squamous
clavicle	larynx	petit mal	staphylococcus
curettage	leukemia	pharynx	suppuration
cyanosis	malaise	pituitary	trochanter
defibrillator	malleus	plantar	venous
ecchymosis	mellitus	pleura	wheal
effusion	menstruation	pleurisy	xiphoid
epididymis	metastasis		

BOX 10-1

Rules for Capitalization

First word of
- Sentences
- Expressions used as sentences
- Each item in a list or outline
- Salutation and closing of a letter

Proper name of person, place, or thing
- John F. Kennedy
- New York City
- Sears Tower

Noun that is part of a proper name
- Professor Mary King
- Dr. Beth Williams
- Michigan Avenue

- Plurals of nouns are formed by adding an *s* or an *es* (physicians, suffixes).

Basic rules for forming plurals of medical terms with specific endings are listed in Table 10-6 along with examples for each.

Numbers

In general, the numbers 1 to 10 are spelled out —one to ten— in correspondence. For numbers greater than ten, it is acceptable to use the number designation, as in

TABLE 10-6 Rules for Forming Plurals of Medical Terms (nouns)

Ending	Rule	Example
a	ae	vertebra to vertebrae
ax	aces	thorax to thoraces
ex, ix	ices	apex to apices
is	es	metastasis to metastases
on	a	ganglion to ganglia
um	a	ovum to ova
us	i	nucleus to nuclei
y	ies	biopsy to biopsies
nx	ges	phalanx to phalanges

TABLE 10-7 Use of Numbers in Correspondence

Type	Explanation of When to Use
Decimals	Write using figure without commas (23.04).
Figures	Only numbers (including 1–10) are used in tables, statistical data, dates, money, percentages, and time.
Measurements	Write out in figures (23 inches).
Percentages	Write out in figures and spell out percent (20 percent).
Tables	When typing numbers or placing them in columns align as follows: - Arabic numerals (1, 2, 3) aligned on the right. - Decimals (1.33) are aligned on the decimal. - Roman numerals (I, II, III) are aligned on the left.
Time	Do not use zeros when writing on-the-hour time. Use A.M. and P.M. with the time designation (10 A.M., not 10:00 A.M.).

128, 1020, 32. The only exception to this rule is when the number is at the beginning of a sentence. It should then be spelled out. See Table 10-7 for a further description of the use of numbers in correspondence.

Parts of Speech

Traditional grammar recognizes eight parts of speech: noun, pronoun, verb, adjective, adverb, preposition, conjunction, and interjection. Many words are able to function as more than one part of speech. For example, depending on its use in a sentence, the word *cut* can be a noun, as in "The cut is fresh," or a verb, as in "The surgeon cut into the organ." Table 10-8 provides a quick reference to parts of speech.

Error Correction in Office Correspondence

Word processing has made correspondence correction much easier. Word processing allows the writer to display the document on the computer screen, enter the

TABLE 10-8 Eight Parts of Speech

Part of Speech	Definition
Noun	Names a person, place, or thing. Example: medical assistant, office
Pronoun	Substitutes for a noun. Example: I, me, you, he, him, she, her, it, we, us, they, them
Verb	Helping verb: comes before main verb. Main verb: asserts action, being, or state of being. Example: operate, write, speak, obtain, is, are, am
Adjective	Modifies a noun or pronoun, usually answering the questions: Which one? What kind of? How many? Example: responsible medical assistant
Adverb	Modifies a verb, adjective, or adverb usually answering the questions: When? Where? Why? How? Under what conditions? To what degree? Example: gently, extremely, nicely, quietly
Preposition	Indicates the relationship between the noun and pronoun that follows it and another word in the sentence. Example: about, above, after, for, in, on, over, through
Conjunction	Connects words or word groups. Example: and, but, nor, or
Interjection	Word used to express strong feeling. Example: oh, hurrah, ouch

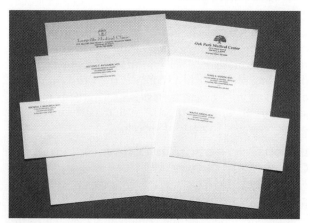

FIGURE 10-1 Different letterhead stationery and envelopes.

document, and make changes. This new document is then saved and printed.

Corrections made to letters typed on a typewriter require the use of correction ribbons, tapes, or fluids. Any corrections on correspondence should be inconspicuous. If more than a few words need correction, then the entire document needs to be retyped. It is considered unprofessional for a document to have correction fluid apparent on the document.

Standard Components of the Business Letter

All letters contain the same basic parts, starting at the top of a letter and moving down to the end. These include the heading, date, inside address, salutation, body, closing, and reference initials. In some specialized cases, such as with insurance correspondence, there may be special components added for clarification, such as the insurer's identification number.

Heading

Medical office letters are usually typed on letterhead stationery bearing the name of the physician (Beth Williams, MD) or practice (Windy City Clinic), address, telephone number, and fax number. See Figure 10-1 for an illustration of letterhead stationery. If the physician does not use letterhead stationery, the letter should be typed or printed on good quality bond paper with the return address typed above the date on the upper left side of the paper.

Date

Every correspondence must have a current date. The month must not be abbreviated, and is followed by the day and year (January 1, 2005). The date is usually placed three lines (spaces) below the letterhead or on line 15 if there is no letterhead. Four to six lines (spaces) are left after the date before the inside address.

Inside Address

The inside address contains the name, title, company name (if applicable), and address of the person who is to receive the correspondence. This is typed at the left margin and single-spaced. If there is a company name (for example, medical practice, clinic, hospital) it must be typed exactly as shown on the company's own letterhead.

All words in the inside address (such as the street name) are spelled out fully. The name of the city is followed by a comma; the two-letter state abbreviation is followed by two spaces; then the ZIP code is added. If the inside address contains a long line, it may be divided into two lines so that the inside address is in balance. The second of these two lines would be indented two spaces. See the example below.

Marvin Hammer, MD
123 Bonneymeadow
  Plaza in the Park
Chicago, IL 60610

Business courtesy recommends always including a title with the receiver's name on the inside address.

Salutation

The salutation, a courteous greeting, is typed at the left margin and spaced two lines below the inside address. The name in the salutation must agree with the name in the inside address. If the letter is going to a physician named Williams, the salutation would read, "Dear Dr. Williams:" with a colon placed after this type of salutation. If the person is well known to the writer, the first name is often used, for example "Dear Beth," followed by a comma. Guidelines 10-1 provides information on using courtesy titles in correspondence.

Body

The body contains the purpose of the letter. The body begins two spaces below the salutation and is single spaced, with a double space between each paragraph. The paragraphs of the body are either blocked or indented, depending on the style (format) of the letter. A letter may be any length, however, most letters bearing a single message are usually two to three paragraphs in length and confined to a single page.

Closing

The letter closing consists of a complimentary close containing a courtesy word(s), such as "Sincerely," "Sincerely yours," or "Yours truly." This appears two spaces below the end of the body of the letter.

The signature line is typed four spaces below the complimentary close and contains the name and title of the writer. The signature of the writer must be placed on the letter directly above the typed signature line before it is sent. If the name and title are on the same line, they are divided with a comma. The personal title of the writer (such as Mr. and Ms.) is not included in the signature line. The exception to this is when the writer may wish to indicate his or her gender to prevent the reader from being confused (for example, Ms. Leslie Lapointe or Mr. Pat Timmons).

Reference Initials

The medical professional uses reference initials to indicate who keyed the letter. Reference initials, when used, are placed at the lower left margin in lowercase, for example *bff*.

Enclosure Notation

When other documents are included along with the letter a notation is made on the letter indicating the enclosure. Examples of enclosures are x-ray films, medical records, and brochures. The abbreviation ENC. is used or the word "Enclosures" can be written out.

For example:

Enclosures (2)
x-ray lumbar spine
surgical report 12/10/20xx

| 10-1 | GUIDELINES |

Using Courtesy Titles

- *Mr.* is always an appropriate title for men.
- If there is a professional title, such as *MD* or *PhD*, this is used instead of the courtesy title.
- *Ms.* is used when the marital status of a woman is unknown.
- *Mrs.* is appropriate for a married woman if she prefers that title. However it is always safe to use *Ms.*
- *Miss* is appropriate for unmarried women who prefer that title. It is also used for young girls.
- Two people at the same address with different last names should be addressed individually. For example: Dr. Beth Williams and Mr. Allan Radde.
- A professional title, such as *owner, president, manager,* may be placed next to the name or below it depending on which is a better balance.

Allan Radde, President Dinesh Shey, PhD
Radde and Associates   Department Chair

- If there is no record of the correct spelling of a receiver's name, then call the company or office and ask for the correct spelling.

Copy Notation

A copy of all correspondence is always filed in the office. In some cases, a copy of the letter is sent to someone other than the addressee. This is noted at the bottom left of the letter by typing the initial "c:" before the recipient's name. The title of the recipient is often added.

For example:

c: Jane Paulson, Office Manager

Procedure 10-1 lists important guidelines for composing business letters.

Two-Page Letter

When the letter is too long to fit on one page, a second sheet of plain stationery is used. Letterhead stationery is used only for the top sheet. The plain, bond second sheet should be of the same quality and color as the top letterhead stationery. A margin of one inch is left at the bottom of the first page.

Form Letters

Form letters can save time for the medical assistant. A form letter is developed when the same letter is sent to several different people. Figure 10-2 illustrates an example of a form letter that can be used as a base when constructing a letter of withdrawal. The letter would be personalized with the patient's name and the signature of the physician.

PROCEDURE

Composing a Business Letter

OBJECTIVE: Compose a business letter using proper guidelines.

Equipment and Supplies
computer or typewriter; office stationery

Method

1. Gather all necessary information and supplies.
2. Determine the reason for the correspondence. Write down the main purpose of the letter.
3. Make a list of all the points you will cover in the letter. Prepare a rough draft.
4. Arrange the ideas in a logical manner. Make sure the letter has a beginning, middle, and end.
   - The beginning or introduction should be appropriate for the intended reader. Use appropriate greetings and titles.
   - The middle should contain all the supporting facts and details. Make sure the content relates to the purpose of the letter.
   - The end should be brief, pleasant, and indicate any action that is to be taken by the reader or writer.
5. Use a natural style of writing; avoid pretentious language. Avoid medical terms when writing to the layperson. Also avoid inflated phrases (refer to Table 10-2).
6. Use a positive tone—negative writing should always be avoided.
7. Pay particular attention to spelling, punctuation, and grammar.
8. Once the rough draft is satisfactory, compose the final draft of the letter. Proofread for mistakes.
9. Obtain any necessary signatures. Include any enclosures as indicated.

WINDY CITY CLINIC
Beth Williams, M.D.
123 Michigan Avenue
Chicago, IL 60610
(312) 123-1234

Date

Dear (Patient):

I find it necessary to inform you that I am withdrawing from providing you medical care for the following reason(s): _____

_____

_____

Since your condition requires medical attention, I suggest that you place yourself under the care of another physician. If you do not know of other physicians, you may wish to contact the county medical society for a referral.

I shall be available to attend to you for a reasonable time after you have received this letter, but in no event for more than 15 days.

When you have selected a new physician, I would be pleased to make available to him or her a copy of your medical chart or a summary of your treatment.

Sincerely yours,

Beth Williams, M.D.

FIGURE 10-2 A form letter is a type of letter that is sent repeatedly to many patients.

The use of a computer or a word processor with memory individualizes the form letter. The body of the letter, called the constant information, is retained in the computer's memory or on a computer disk or CD. The areas of the letter that require personalization, such as the date, inside address, and salutation, are called the *variables*. The variables can be stored on a separate CD or database and then merged into the disk or main drive of the computer, which stores the constant information. In this manner, a set of data, such as names and addresses of patients for billing purposes, can be used with a form letter enclosed with the monthly bill. Chapter 11 contains more information regarding the use of computers in the medical office.

Letter Styles

Letter styles vary depending on the purpose. Letter styles include block, modified block (standard), modified block with indented paragraphs, and a simplified letter style. Block and modified block are the most commonly used in the medical office.

The block letter style format is spaced with all lines, from the date through the signature line, flush with the left margin. There is a space separating each paragraph and between inside address, salutation, body, and close. Since there are no indentations for paragraphs, this format saves typing time.

The modified block (standard) style letter has the date, complimentary closing, and the signature line beginning at the center and moving toward the right margin. All other lines are flush with the left margin. This is often preferred since it has a professional, neat appearance. This format requires more time to type since the typist must set and use tabs. The modified block style letter with indented paragraphs is identical to the modified block except that the paragraphs are indented five spaces.

A simplified letter style format is spaced with all lines flush with the left margin. The salutation line is omitted. In its place is a subject line, which appears on the third line below the inside address. This subject line is in capital letters and draws the reader's attention to the purpose of the letter. A complimentary closing is also omitted. The signature is also typed in all capital letters on the fifth line below the body. This format is an abbreviated style of writing letters relating to patients. Figure 10-3 shows sample letter formats: block, modified block (standard), modified block with indented paragraphs, and simplified letter style.

A semi-simplified letter style format is spaced with all lines flush with the left margin except for the first line of each paragraph. The first line of each paragraph is indented five spaces. All other aspects of the simplified letter style format apply to this format.

Interoffice Memoranda

Interoffice memoranda, also called *memos*, are correspondence sent to people within the office or organization. They are used to inform personnel about meetings, general changes that affect everyone, special projects, or news items. The memo is an inexpensive means to communicate with others in the office setting. They do not require postage and are delivered through the interoffice mail route.

Memos are generally written on a short form developed for that purpose. Memos may contain a heading much like the letterhead stationery to indicate the office where they originated. They contain the word MEMORANDUM at the top of the form. Also included are the typed words DATE:, TO:, FROM:, and RE: or SUBJECT:. The memo form is meant to be used within the office setting and should never be used to send information outside of the office. Figure 10-4 illustrates an example of a memo form.

Proofreading

Proofreading or checking for errors in content and typing is critical. The professionalism of the office is judged, in part, by the appearance of correspondence

10-2 GUIDELINES

Proofreading

- Proofread and correct errors before printing the document, whenever possible.
- Use a ruler, pencil, or edge of a piece of paper to follow each line as you proofread.
- Check the content to see if it flows in a logical order.
- Check for missing and repeated words.
- Check grammar, spelling, and punctuation.
- Check where the word breaks occur.
- Verify the spelling of proper names and titles.
- Verify numbers in dates, figures, and time (hours of the day).
- Read the opening and closing carefully.
- Proofread at least twice.
- Check the general appearance of the letter for spacing and format.

and documents that come out of that office. Proofreading cannot be overemphasized. Even small omissions, such as commas, are noticed by readers. Most computer programs contain spelling and grammar check components. These should always be used before printing the document. You may have to add frequently used medical terms to the program. After printing out the document, there should be a careful reading of all correspondence to catch any content or typing errors. Pay close attention to the spelling of names and procedures. When typing figures always double-check to make sure all decimal points are placed in the correct position. Look for sound-alike terms, such as *right* and *write* or *anti-* and *ante-*. Important points to remember when proofreading letters and other documents are listed in Guidelines 10-2.

Proofreader's Marks

There are marks that are generally accepted for use when proofreading large documents. These are especially helpful when a second person is proofing the document, such as the physician. See Figure 10-5 for a list of proofreader's marks.

Editing

Editing is similar to proofreading in that you must read the final material to check for accuracy. Editing also involves reading the printed material to determine if it is clear. When editing medical reports, you cannot change the content of the report or alter the meaning in

(A)

WINDY CITY CLINIC
Beth Williams, M.D.
123 Michigan Avenue, Chicago, IL 60610
(312) 123-1234

August 1, 20xx

Thomas Moore
123 Lee Street
Louisville, KY 40223

Dear Mr. Moore:

With the season for colds and flu fast approaching, it is time once again for flu shots. Supplies have arrived and flu shots will be administered starting October 3. Please call the office to schedule a visit for your flu shot at your earliest convenience.

If you wish to wait to get your flu shot at the time of your next appointment, it is not necessary to call the office. An appointment card with the date and time of your next appointment is enclosed.

Sincerely,

Beth Williams, MD

ENC: Appointment card
c: B. Reed, Office Manager

(B)

WINDY CITY CLINIC
Beth Williams, M.D.
123 Michigan Avenue, Chicago, IL 60610
(312) 123-1234

August 1, 20xx

Thomas Moore
123 Lee Street
Louisville, KY 40223

Dear Mr. Moore:

With the season for colds and flu fast approaching, it is time once again for flu shots. Supplies have arrived and flu shots will be administered starting October 3. Please call the office to schedule a visit for your flu shot at your earliest convenience.

If you wish to wait to get your flu shot at the time of your next appointment, it is not necessary to call the office. An appointment card with the date and time of your next appointment is enclosed.

Sincerely,

Beth Williams, MD

ENC: Appointment card
c: B. Reed, Office Manager

(C)

WINDY CITY CLINIC
Beth Williams, M.D.
123 Michigan Avenue, Chicago, IL 60610
(312) 123-1234

August 1, 20xx

Thomas Moore
123 Lee Street
Louisville, KY 40223

Dear Mr. Moore:

   With the season for colds and flu fast approaching, it is time once again for flu shots. Supplies have arrived and flu shots will be administered starting October 3. Please call the office to schedule a visit for your flu shot at your earliest convenience.

   If you wish to wait to get your flu shot at the time of your next appointment, it is not necessary to call the office. An appointment card with the date and time of your next appointment is enclosed.

Sincerely,

Beth Williams, MD

ENC: Appointment card
c: B. Reed, Office Manager

(D)

WINDY CITY CLINIC
Beth Williams, M.D.
123 Michigan Avenue, Chicago, IL 60610
(312) 123-1234

August 1, 20xx

Thomas Moore
123 Lee Street
Louisville, KY 40223

RE: FLU SHOT

With the season for colds and flu fast approaching, it is time once again for flu shots. Supplies have arrived and flu shots will be administered starting October 3. Please call the office to schedule a visit for your flu shot at your earliest convenience.

If you wish to wait to get your flu shot at the time of your next appointment, it is not necessary to call the office. An appointment card with the date and time of your next appointment is enclosed.

BETH WILLIAMS, M.D.

ENC: Appointment card
c: B. Reed, Office Manager

FIGURE 10-3 Examples of four letter formats: (A) block style; (B) modified block style; (C) modified block style with indented paragraphs; and (D) simplified letter style.

```
┌─────────────────────────────────────┐
│      WINDY CITY MEDICAL CENTER      │
│             MEMORANDUM              │
│    DATE:                            │
│      TO:                            │
│    FROM:                            │
│  SUBJECT:                           │
│                                     │
│       c:                            │
└─────────────────────────────────────┘
```

FIGURE 10-4   An example of a memo form.

any way. If you believe the meaning is unclear, you must check with the writer of the report before making any editorial changes.

When editing material you have composed, such as an informational form letter to be sent to all patients, changes can be made to increase clarity.

Abbreviations

Only accepted medical abbreviations can be used in medical reports and when filing insurance documents. A list of accepted medical abbreviations is included in the appendix of this textbook.

Individual physician offices may use an abbreviation on progress notes that is related to that practice. For example, a urologist may write "L," meaning leaking urine when coughing, on his or her progress notes. While this is not an acceptable abbreviation, it can be used to conserve space and simplify documentation within that particular office. It is important that a list of those abbreviations is shared with each employee and physically posted so that all employees are clear on the meaning of each abbreviation and are using the same abbreviation for the same term.

Reference Materials

Every physician's office contains general reference books and medical dictionaries as well as textbooks related to the physician's specialization. A complete office library should include the following:

- A desk dictionary, and access to an online dictionary.
- A medical dictionary, as well as access to an online medical dictionary, assists with the correct spelling, pronunciation, acronyms, abbreviations and meaning of medical terms and diagnoses.
- A Physician's Desk Reference (PDR) to verify the correct spelling and meaning of drugs.
- Current coding books including CPT (Current Procedural Terminology), ICD-9-CM.
- A thesaurus (which provides synonyms or similar meanings for words) such as Roget's International Thesaurus and access to an online thesaurus.

Preparing Outgoing Mail

Letterhead stationery, which contains the name and address of the sender, comes in three commonly used sizes. These sizes are standard, monarch or executive, and baronial. The more common letter sizes with their matching envelope sizes are shown in Table 10-9.

The standard letterhead is used for most office correspondence. A smaller version of the standard letterhead—the monarch or executive style—is used by some physicians for their social correspondence. The baronial letterhead is a half-sheet of the standard size and is used for brief letters and memoranda. Each size of letterhead stationery has an appropriate size envelope. See Figure 10-6 for an illustration of different letter sizes.

Folding Letters and Inserting into Envelopes

Following are recommended methods for folding and inserting letters into envelopes so the contents can

TABLE 10-9   Stationery and Envelopes

Stationery	Dimensions	Envelope	Dimensions
Standard	8 1/2″ × 11″	No. 10	9 1/2″ × 4 1/8″
Monarch	7 1/4″ × 10 1/2″	No. 7	7 1/2″ × 3 7/8″
Baronial	5 1/2″ × 8 1/2	No. 6 3/4	6 1/2″ × 3 5/8″

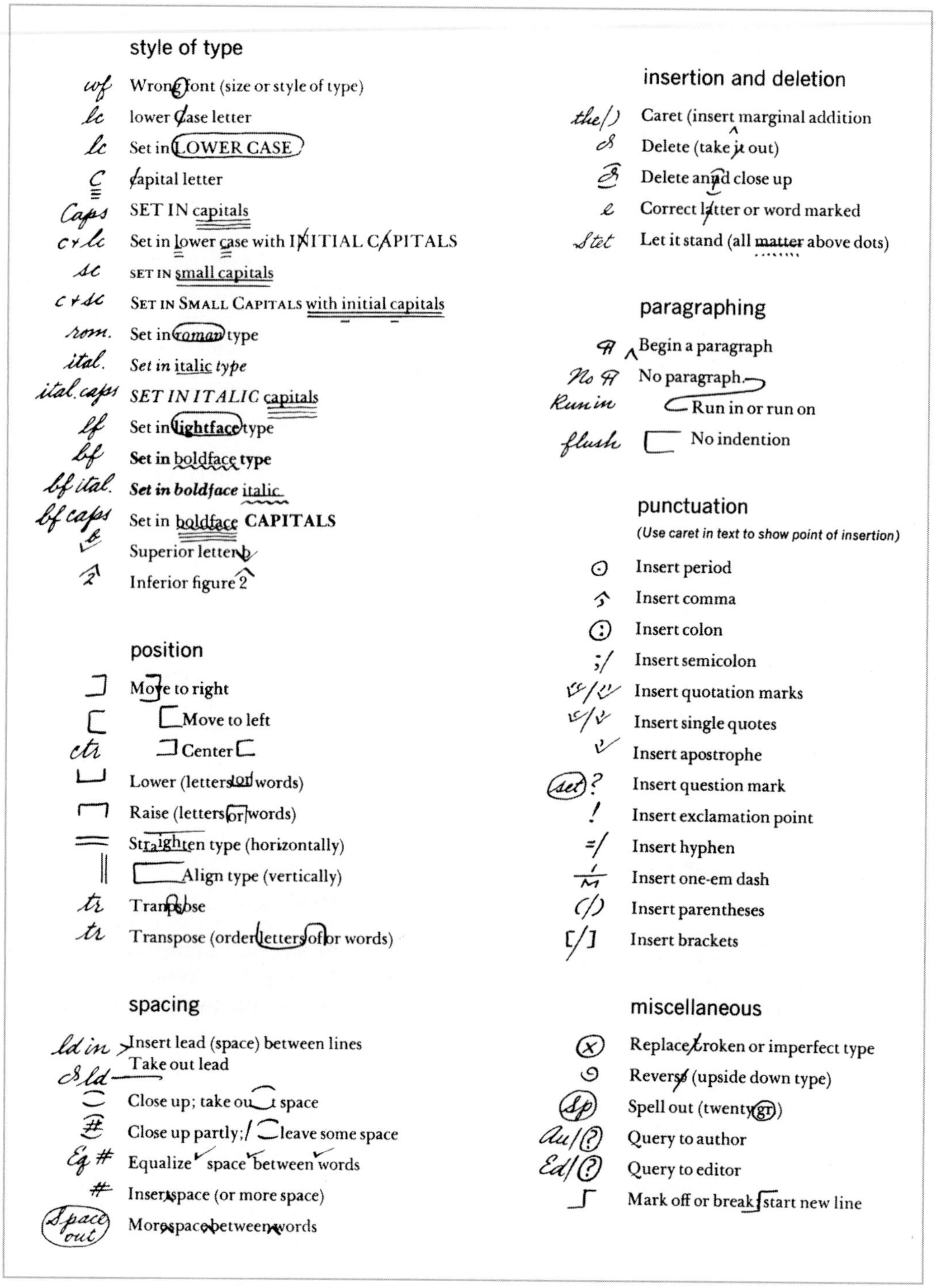

style of type

wf	Wrong font (size or style of type)
lc	lower case letter
lc	Set in LOWER CASE
C	capital letter
Caps	SET IN capitals
c + lc	Set in lower case with INITIAL CAPITALS
sc	SET IN small capitals
c + sc	SET IN SMALL CAPITALS with initial capitals
rom.	Set in roman type
ital.	Set in italic type
ital. caps	SET IN ITALIC capitals
lf	Set in lightface type
bf	Set in boldface type
bf ital.	Set in boldface italic
bf caps	Set in boldface CAPITALS
	Superior letter
	Inferior figure 2

position

⌐	Move to right
⌐	Move to left
ctr	Center
⊔	Lower (letters or words)
⊓	Raise (letters or words)
=	Straighten type (horizontally)
‖	Align type (vertically)
tr	Transpose
tr	Transpose (order letters of or words)

spacing

ld in	Insert lead (space) between lines
δ ld	Take out lead
‿	Close up; take out space
#	Close up partly; leave some space
Eq #	Equalize space between words
#	Insert space (or more space)
Space out	More space between words

insertion and deletion

the/	Caret (insert marginal addition)
δ	Delete (take it out)
δ	Delete and close up
e	Correct letter or word marked
Stet	Let it stand (all matter above dots)

paragraphing

¶	Begin a paragraph
No ¶	No paragraph.
Run in	Run in or run on
flush	No indention

punctuation

(Use caret in text to show point of insertion)

⊙	Insert period
⌃	Insert comma
⊙	Insert colon
;/	Insert semicolon
	Insert quotation marks
	Insert single quotes
ν	Insert apostrophe
set ?	Insert question mark
!	Insert exclamation point
=/	Insert hyphen
—/M	Insert one-em dash
(/)	Insert parentheses
[/]	Insert brackets

miscellaneous

(X)	Replace broken or imperfect type
ꙅ	Reverse (upside down type)
sp	Spell out (twenty gr)
Au/?	Query to author
Ed/?	Query to editor
⌐	Mark off or break start new line

FIGURE 10-5 Proofreader's marks.

remain confidential and be easily removed. See Figure 10-7 for an illustration of folding a letter.

Number 10 Envelope

1. Bring up the bottom third of the letter and fold with a crease.
2. Fold the top of the letter down to 3/8 inch from the first creased edge.
3. Make a second crease at the fold and place this edge into the envelope first.

Number 6 3/4 Envelope

1. Bring the bottom edge up to 3/8 inch from the top edge.
2. Make a crease at the fold.
3. Fold the right edge one third of the width of the paper, and press a crease at this fold.
4. Fold the left edge to 3/8 inch from the previous crease and insert this edge into the envelope first.

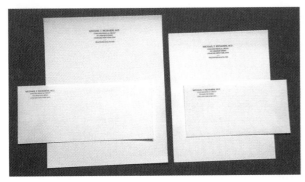

FIGURE 10-6 Letterhead stationery sizes are varied to suit the needs of the sender. Envelopes are sized to match different letter sizes.

Envelope Formats

The United States Postal Service (USPS) has recommended guidelines when typing envelopes. This is meant to improve the handling and delivery of the mail. Optical Character Recognition (OCR) equipment used by the postal service scans, reads, and sorts the envelope. For optimal efficiency of OCR scanning, the address must be typed on the envelope, using single spacing and all capital letters with no punctuation.

The last line in the address must include the city, state two-digit code, and the ZIP code. It cannot exceed 27 characters in length. See Figure 10-8 for a listing of the two digit letter abbreviations for states.

A more traditional style of typing envelopes with the initial letter in capital letters and small letters for the rest of the address is still accepted by the post office.

The bottom margin of the No. 10 envelope (business size) should be 5/8 inch with one-inch margins on the left and right sides. The No. 6 3/4 envelope should have a two-inch margin on the left side with the address 12 lines from the top of the envelope.

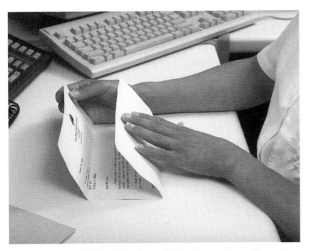

FIGURE 10-7 A well-folded letter fits easily into the envelope and is easily removed by the person who receives it.

A return address for the sender should always be placed in the upper left hand corner in the event the letter must be returned to the sender. Envelopes can be printed with the address of the sender in this position.

ZIP Codes

The five-digit ZIP code was introduced in the 1960s to increase the post office's efficiency in mail handling. ZIP codes begin on the East Coast with the number "0" eventually increasing to the number "9" on the West Coast and Hawaii. The first three numbers of the ZIP code identify the city and all five digits combine to identify the individual post office and zone within the city. Four more digits have been added to the ZIP code by the USPS. These four digits follow a hyphen behind the first five and represent the addressee's street location. The 9-digit ZIP code has eliminated many handling steps at the postal service and improved service.

Classifications of Mail

The classifications of mail vary according to weight, type, and destination. Mail is weighed in ounces and pounds. The most common types of mail are: first class, priority, second class, third class, fourth class, and express mail. Table 10-10 describes these classifications of mail.

TWO-LETTER ABBREVIATIONS

UNITED STATES and TERRITORIES

Alabama	AL	Montana	MT
Alaska	AK	Nebraska	NE
Arizona	AZ	Nevada	NV
Arkansas	AR	New Hampshire	NH
California	CA	New Jersey	NJ
Canal Zone	CZ	New Mexico	NM
Colorado	CO	New York	NY
Connecticut	CT	North Carolina	NC
Delaware	DE	North Dakota	ND
District of Columbia	DC	Ohio	OH
Florida	FL	Oklahoma	OK
Georgia	GA	Oregon	OR
Guam	GU	Pennsylvania	PA
Hawaii	HI	Puerto Rico	PR
Idaho	ID	Rhode Island	RI
Illinois	IL	South Carolina	SC
Indiana	IN	South Dakota	SD
Iowa	IA	Tennessee	TN
Kansas	KS	Texas	TX
Kentucky	KY	Utah	UT
Louisiana	LA	Vermont	VT
Maine	ME	Virgin Islands	VI
Maryland	MD	Virginia	VA
Massachusetts	MA	Washington	WA
Michigan	MI	West Virginia	WV
Minnesota	MN	Wisconsin	WI
Mississippi	MS	Wyoming	WY
Missouri	MO		

FIGURE 10-8 Every state has a two digit letter abbreviation.

TABLE 10-10 Classifications of Mail

Type	Description
First Class	Letters, postcards, business reply cards; letters weighing less than 11 ounces; sealed and unsealed, handwritten or typed material.
Priority	First class mail weighing more than 11 ounces; maximum weight of 70 pounds; postage calculated based on weight and destination.
Second Class	Newspapers and periodicals that have received second class mail authorization; copies of newspapers and periodicals mailed by the general public are not able to receive the second-class rate.
Third Class	Catalogs, books, photographs, flyers, and other printed materials (also called "bulk mail"); must be marked "Third Class;" must be sealed.
Fourth Class	Printed material, books, and merchandise not included in First and Second Class; must weigh between 16 ounces and 70 pounds; there are size limitations also.
Express Mail/Next Day Service	Available seven days a week; up to 70 pounds in weight and 108 inches around; expected delivery by noon; shipping containers are supplied; pickup service in some area.

Special Postal Services

Specialized services include certified mail, certificate of mailing, special delivery, registered mail and special handling.

Certified Mail

Mail that includes contracts, mortgages, birth certificates, deeds and checks, which are not valuable themselves but would be difficult to replace if lost, can be mailed as certified mail (Figure 10-9). They would need to be mailed at the first class rate with a special fee added for certified mail. Certified mail assists in tracking and collecting this mail. A receipt verifying delivery can be requested for a fee. Certified mail can also be sent by special delivery if the extra fee is paid. Certified mail records are maintained at the post office for two years.

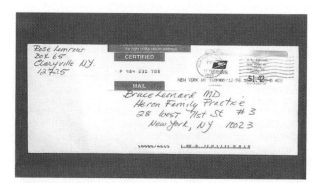

FIGURE 10-9 Items that would be difficult to replace bearing legal significance are sent by certified mail.

Certificate of Mailing

For a small fee, a certificate of mailing can be obtained at the post office. This document will demonstrate proof that mail was posted. This is useful for mailing items such as tax returns, which need to be received by a certain date.

Special Delivery

When fast delivery of an item is needed, special delivery service can be requested from the postal service. Special delivery is useful for shipping perishables, such as specimens, since the post office will deliver these items beyond the regular delivery service hours (for example, on Sundays and holidays). There is a fee for this service.

Special Handling

Special handling can be requested for third- and fourth-class items. "Special handling" is stamped across the package. The fee for this service is based on the weight of the item.

Insurance

Insurance can be purchased for third-class, fourth-class, and priority mail. The sender will then be reimbursed for the content if this mail is lost or damaged. The sender receives a receipt from the post office at the time of purchase of the insurance. This receipt along with the damaged goods must be presented when reimbursement is necessary.

Registered Mail

Registered mail is the safest way to send first-class or priority mail. A fee is paid for this service and a signed record is kept for each piece of registered mail. Registered mail is tracked as it moves throughout the mail system, which helps to reduce loss. Registered mail is insured for the value declared at the time of registration. For an additional fee the sender can request a return receipt indicating the time, place of delivery, and the receiver's signature.

Postal Money Orders

A postal money order can be purchased at the post office. The money order is replaceable if lost or stolen and can be mailed instead of the actual cash. It is available in several denominations and the fee varies according to the amount of the postal money order.

Forwarding Mail

First class is the only type of mail that can be forwarded to another address without paying an additional fee. Cross out the incorrect address and insert the new address and return to the mail carrier or post office. The post office will forward mail for up to six months.

Mail Recall

If mail has been placed into the mailbox or given to a postal carrier by mistake, it can be recalled by the sender. The sender can call the post office and request the item be held for them. When the sender goes to the post office to reclaim the mail, he or she will be asked to complete a "Sender's Application for Recall of Mail." If the mail is still at the post office, it will be returned to the sender upon completion of this form. If the mail has already left the post office, the postal clerk will call the post office where that mail has been sent and ask that the mail be returned. The sender must pay all the expenses incurred in an attempt to recall the mail, including the telephone calls placed by the postal service. If the mail has already been delivered to the addressee, the sender will be notified.

Tracing Lost Mail

All receipts for mailed goods should be retained until receipt of the mail has been acknowledged. If the mail has not arrived after a reasonable period of time, the post office will attempt to trace it for you. First class mail is not easy to trace since there is no receipt for it. The postal service requires a special form to be completed before they will trace mail.

Returned Mail

When mail has been returned and marked "undeliverable," it cannot be re-mailed until new postage is added. It is advisable to place the contents into a new envelope with the correct address, place the proper postage according to weight on the envelope, and re-mail.

Size Requirements for Mail

The USPS standardized envelope sizes in order to machine sort mail. Minimum mail sizes have been established. Domestic mail must be at least 0.0007 inch thick. A further restriction on size requires that mail 1/4 inch or less in thickness must be 3 1/2 inches in height and at least 5 inches long. All mail not meeting this requirement is considered nonstandard.

While postage is generally based on a package's weight, items that are bulky and lightweight are charged a 15-pound balloon rate surcharge. This balloon rate is applied to all Priority Mail® and Parcel Post® items that weigh less than 15 pounds and measure over 84 inches—but not more than 108 inches—in length and girth combined. Following are some general requirement guidelines for preparing mail to be metered.

- Separate all international mail from domestic mail. Separate all Canada and Mexico mail from the rest of the international mail.

- Face all letter size envelopes in the same direction. Make sure none are upside down. When mailing letter size envelopes, flaps must be sealed, tucked in, or nested (overlapped).

- Try not to overstuff letter-size envelopes. If this is not possible, you must seal the envelopes with tape.

- All envelopes larger than a No. 10 size letter envelope must be sealed before being sent.

- Keep the top right corner of each mailing piece clear of all markings. This is where the postmark will appear.

The medical assistant should always consult the USPS for specific mailing, size, weight, and pricing requirements to ensure the outgoing mail is properly prepared. This may include either a visit to the nearest postal office or browsing the USPS Web site.

Mail Handling Tips

To facilitate time management within the medical office, all mail should be handled only once. For ease and efficiency in handling large amounts of mail, follow the steps in Procedure 10-2.

Electronic Mail (E-mail)

All written materials that are transmitted electronically are referred to as electronic mail (e-mail). The documents may include letters, reports, and pictures. These e-mails may be sent over telephone lines, cables, computers, and satellites. Electronic mail allows the medical assistant to edit, correct, and transmit documents very quickly to another location. Electronic mail cannot be used if the original signature on the document

PROCEDURE

Opening the Daily Mail

OBJECTIVE: Sort and distribute the medical office's daily mail.

Equipment and Supplies

office stamps (one with date and one with name of medical office); ink pad; paper clips; pencil

Method

1. Have all supplies in one place when processing the mail.
2. Sort the mail before opening into first-class, personal/confidential, second-, third- and fourth class.
3. Discard and recycle all unwanted third-class mail.
4. Place a current date and time of arrival on each piece of mail. Purchase rubber stamp and pad from an office supply store so that the date can be changed each day.
5. Stamp the name of the medical office across all periodicals and newspapers.
6. Lay all of the envelopes flap down to reduce the motions involved in opening a large amount of mail.
7. Do not open mail marked "personal" or "confidential." Place it in the physician's box unopened unless otherwise instructed.
8. Attach all enclosures in each envelope with a paper clip. Avoid stapling since these will have to be removed later and may damage sensitive materials, such as x-rays. If an enclosure is noted within the correspondence but is not included in the envelope, write "no" next to enclosure with your initials to indicate it was not included. Clip the opened envelope to the mail until the mail is completely processed. In some cases, a return address is only on the envelope and not on the inside correspondence.
9. Open all the mail and clip together the inside contents before handling the individual correspondence.
10. Annotate the mail as soon as possible after it is opened. An annotation consists of writing a short comment in pencil to indicate the purpose of the letter, and underline the critical portions of the letter. If another document is referred to in the letter, then take initiative by pulling it from the file and attaching it to this correspondence.
11. Route the mail immediately after opening. Another department or physician may be waiting for the document.

needs to be sent. When creating e-mail, remember that e-mail is considered part of the patient's record or part of the office management, therefore all standard proofreading and confidentiality guidelines apply.

E-mail can take different forms. Just like a written letter, e-mail can take the form of a composed letter, form letter, or interoffice memorandum. Some offices use e-mail to confirm office visits. Every office has a particular format to utilize for this purpose.

Another form of e-mail is the instant message format. Instant mail can be defined as a way to communicate with another person in real-time. There are several offices that allow users to instant message each other both internally (within the office) and externally. The internal instant message format is usually connected to the office server and allows for messages to be sent quickly to each person. The external type of instant messages is generally linked to an account that is purchased from an Internet company. You would need to establish your own screen name and passwords to access and communicate with users by instant mail messages. It is important to remember that instant messages are not permanent documents and cannot be attached to a person's medical records or be used in a court of law.

If e-mail is offered to patients as a mode of communication, it is imperative to check it frequently in order to avoid liability. E-mail is not efficient to use for emergencies.

Facsimile (Fax)

Another electronic means of sending a written communication is by using a fax machine. The fax is an exact duplication of a document that is then transmitted to another location via a facsimile (fax) machine. The telephone lines are used to transmit fax documents. The original document is inserted into the fax machine, the receiver's fax phone number is dialed and when the connection is made, the document is transmitted over the telephone lines, resulting in a printed document at the receiver's fax machine. A cover sheet should be sent first, which includes information about the sender (company, name, and telephone and fax numbers) telephone number of the receiver, date, and number of pages. The cover sheet should contain verbiage to encourage the recipient to notify the sender if they have received the fax in error, and asking the recipient to destroy the document after notification.

Reflection on the Medical Practice

Medical assistants are often responsible for preparing interoffice memos and letters to patients. The letter you send is a direct reflection on the physician and the medical office as a whole. If the letter is filled with errors, incorrect diagnosis, or sent to the wrong patient, it reflects poorly on the medical office and can harm the physician's business. If your responsibilities as a medical assistant include letter writing, it is always a good idea to have someone in the office review your correspondence. To facilitate time management within the medical office, remember that you can utilize a form letter that you or the physician has created. Remember to proofread each letter and check for any inappropriate content, misspellings, grammatical or punctuation errors, and margin restrictions.

SUMMARY

The responsibilities of the medical assistant relating to office correspondence are multifaceted. These include being able to draft correspondence using correct grammar and style and efficiently handling mail. Effective mail handling includes using the most efficient and cost-saving form of mail service. These responsibilities must be handled in a professional, courteous, and diplomatic manner. Correct handling of written communication allows the medical assistant to demonstrate competence.

Chapter Review

COMPETENCY REVIEW

1. Define and spell the terms to learn for this chapter.
2. How would you track a missing piece of mail?
3. Address an envelope using the method recommended by the USPS for use with Optical Character Recognition Equipment (OCR).
4. Describe what types of material you would send by certified mail.
5. Type a short letter using both block and modified block with indented paragraph styles.
6. Why do you think companies (and medical offices) use letterhead stationery?

PREPARING FOR THE CERTIFICATION EXAM

1. Which of the following is NOT a method used for classifying mail?
   A. weight
   B. date
   C. destination
   D. type
   E. sender

2. What is the maximum weight (in pounds) for priority mail?
   A. 100
   B. 150
   C. 17
   D. 70
   E. 50

3. What is the term that means "to note the important points or items in a letter or document?"
   A. annotate
   B. announce
   C. notify
   D. proofread
   E. classify

4. Which term means "to indicate the presence of an error or correction needed on a letter or document?"
   A. annotate
   B. sort
   C. notify
   D. proofread
   E. classify

continued on next page

5. What type of mail is used to send laboratory specimens?
   A. special handling
   B. priority mail
   C. registered mail
   D. special delivery
   E. ground shipping

6. The following categories of mail can be insured EXCEPT
   A. first class
   B. second class
   C. third class
   D. fourth class
   E. first class e-mail

7. The two-letter abbreviation for Michigan is
   A. MH
   B. MN
   C. MI
   D. MG
   E. MA

8. Which of the following would NOT be used on a memorandum?
   A. writer's name
   B. subject
   C. complimentary close
   D. date
   E. receiving office

9. Which of the following is NOT found in a thesaurus?
   A. alphabetical listing
   B. index
   C. synonyms
   D. medical terminology
   E. Greek or Latin roots

10. The proofreader's mark that means "insert a space" is
    A. #
    B. //
    C. [
    D. sp
    E. tr

CRITICAL THINKING

1. According to the standard practices of written communication, what is incorrect about the student's letter?

2. What can be done to correct the problems seen in this letter?

3. In what voice is this letter written?

4. Since you have to rewrite the letter, what would you change about the letter? Why?

5. Once you have rewritten the letter, does the letter reflect the physician in a positive or negative manner? Why?

ON THE JOB

Diane Webb, a medical assistant in Dr. Williams' office, has been asked to proofread a letter that was prepared by a temporary assistant. Follow the rules for proofreading, grammar, capitalization, and spelling found in this chapter to correct the errors in this letter. Type this letter using the modified block style and prepare it for Dr. Beth Williams' signature.

Dear Docter Stacey:

I right this letter to inform you that I am pleased that you would chose me to present at your conference. Its a great complement.

Their are several cases which I can site. I would like you're recommendation since I no you will be frank with me. We must all ways be discrete and conscience of patience's rights when presenting cases relating to there conditions. We must remain mindful that patients have there legal rites.

I have the following x-ray studies which I can include: xyphoid process, greater trocanter, peretoneal abcess, left calcanus, fracture of right clavical, and a fractured ileum and ischeum. Let me know which of these rentgeneology studies you would prefer.

Please advise me on how to procede.

Sincerely yours,
Dr. Beth Williams

INTERNET ACTIVITY

Access the Internet and locate information on how to write professional medical letters and other information you may need, such as your extended ZIP code, online proofreader's marks to use as a reference tool, an online dictionary, medical dictionary, and thesaurus, and e-mail etiquette guidelines.

MediaLink More on written communication, including interactive resources, can be found on the Student CD-ROM accompanying this textbook.

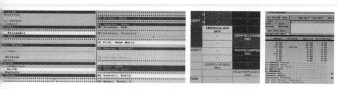

Medical Assistant Role Delineation Chart

HIGHLIGHT indicates material covered in this chapter.

ADMINISTRATIVE

Administrative Procedures

- Perform basic administrative medical assisting functions
- Schedule, coordinate and monitor appointments
- Schedule inpatient/outpatient admissions and procedures
- Understand and apply third-party guidelines
- Obtain reimbursement through accurate claims submission
- Monitor third-party reimbursement
- Understand and adhere to managed care policies and procedures
- *Negotiate managed care contracts*

Practice Finances

- Perform procedural and diagnostic coding
- Apply bookkeeping principles

- Manage accounts receivable
- *Manage accounts payable*
- *Process payroll*
- *Document and maintain accounting and banking records*
- *Develop and maintain fee schedules*
- *Manage renewals of business and professional insurance policies*
- *Manage personnel benefits and maintain records*
- *Perform marketing, financial, and strategic planning*

CLINICAL

Fundamental Principles

- Apply principles of aseptic technique and infection control
- Comply with quality assurance practices
- Screen and follow up patient test results

Diagnostic Orders

- Collect and process specimens
- Perform diagnostic tests

Patient Care

- Adhere to established patient screening procedures
- Obtain patient history and vital signs
- Prepare and maintain examination and treatment areas
- Prepare patient for examinations, procedures and treatments

- Assist with examinations, procedures and treatments
- Prepare and administer medications and immunizations
- Maintain medication and immunization records
- Recognize and respond to emergencies
- Coordinate patient care information with other health care providers
- Initiate IV and administer IV medications with appropriate training and as permitted by state law

GENERAL

Professionalism

- Display a professional manner and image
- Demonstrate initiative and responsibility
- Work as a member of the health care team
- Prioritize and perform multiple tasks
- Adapt to change
- Promote the CMA credential
- Enhance skills through continuing education
- Treat all patients with compassion and empathy
- Promote the practice through positive public relations

Communication Skills

- Recognize and respect cultural diversity
- Adapt communications to individual's ability to understand
- Use professional telephone technique

- Recognize and respond effectively to verbal, nonverbal, and written communications
- Use medical terminology appropriately
- Utilize electronic technology to receive, organize, prioritize and transmit information
- Serve as liaison

Legal Concepts

- Perform within legal and ethical boundaries
- Prepare and maintain medical records
- Document accurately
- Follow employer's established policies dealing with the health care contract
- Implement and maintain federal and state health care legislation and regulations
- Comply with established risk management and safety procedures
- Recognize professional credentialing criteria
- *Develop and maintain personnel, policy and procedure manuals*

Instruction

- Instruct individuals according to their needs
- Explain office policies and procedures
- Teach methods of health promotion and disease prevention
- Locate community resources and disseminate information
- *Develop educational materials*
- *Conduct continuing education activities*

Operational Functions

- Perform inventory of supplies and equipment
- Perform routine maintenance of administrative and clinical equipment
- Apply computer techniques to support office operations
- *Perform personnel management functions*
- *Negotiate leases and prices for equipment and supply contracts*
- *Denotes advanced skills.*

- *Denotes advanced skills.*

SOURCE: Reprinted by permission of the American Association of Medical Assistants from the AAMA Role Delineation Study: Occupational Analysis of the Medical Assisting Profession.

Computers in the Medical Office

Learning Objectives

After completing this chapter, you should be able to:

- Define and spell the terms to learn for this chapter.

- Discuss the functions and applications of the computer.

- Explain the difference between hardware and software.

- List three methods to ensure confidentiality of medical records when using a computer.

- List four methods to be ergonomically correct at your workstation.

- Describe computer maintenance and security.

- Distinguish the difference between the Internet and World Wide Web.

Terms to Learn

bandwidth

clock speed

computer

central processing unit (CPU)

floppy disk

Internet

Internet service provider (ISP)

kilobyte (K or Kb)

main memory

mass storage device

megahertz (MHz)

memory

microprocessor

monitor

mouse

printer

random-access memory (RAM)

read-only memory (ROM)

software

Telnet

universal serial bus (USB)

Usenet

World Wide Web (WWW)

Case Study

HELDA KRENZ IS A MEDICAL ASSISTANT WHO WORKS for a family practice physician. She has been asked to develop some continuing education materials for a community service project her office will conduct at the local shopping mall. She will need to locate the most current information, design and develop the materials for distribution, and include marketing materials for the event as well as her office.

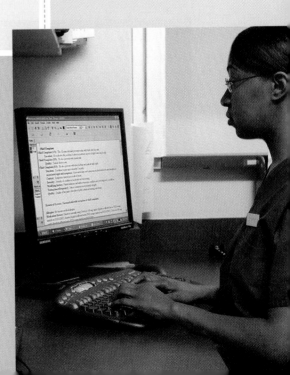

The uses of computers in medicine are many and varied. Depending on the size of the medical practice, some or all of the functions normally performed in the front office may be done with computers and specialized programs. In order to be successful in the administrative, clinical, and lab areas, the medical assistant must be familiar with computers and how they can be used.

Use of Computers in Medicine

Technology advancements have enabled medical offices to function with increased efficiency and speed using computers. Computers are considered a fundamental piece of operating equipment to perform and enhance quality patient care through data collection, eliminate duplication of work, and decrease errors. Figures 11-1 and 11-2 illustrate ways that computers have become invaluable in diagnosing, monitoring, and reporting the patient's progress. Medical assistants will be responsible for computer entries, electronic medical records, electronic bookkeeping, billing, insurance processing, appointment scheduling, inventory data, and many other functions. These responsibilities dictate the medical assistant's knowledge and application of computer literacy. Medical assistants must have competent computer skills and stay current as technology continues to advance.

Types of Computers

The types of computers used in medical offices today are microcomputers. This means that a small piece of electronic hardware, called a chip, allows the processing of information in a very small amount of space. The microchip revolutionized computers and today they

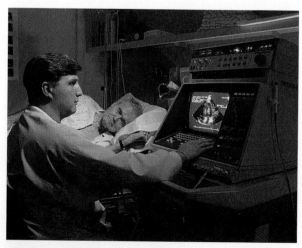

FIGURE 11-1   Echocardiography examination.

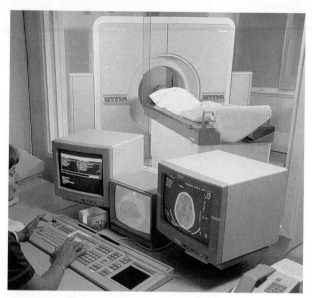

FIGURE 11-2   CT brain scanning.

can fit on a desk, in your lap, or even in a device the size of a hand-held calculator. Before the microchip was developed, computers took up a great deal of room and used a vastly different technology. In the early days, a computer that took up an entire room had the same amount of memory as what now fits on top of your desk.

As computers evolve, two characteristics have changed: size and portability. It has become more important to have computer access anywhere including in transit. Laptop computers allow users to carry their work with them (Figure 11-3). A laptop computer can fit in a case about the size of a small briefcase. Laptop computers offer the same functionality as desktop computers, only in a smaller package. Palm pilots and personal digital assistants (PDAs) are other portable devices used in the medical field. These devices store data that can be recalled as needed. Palm pilots and PDAs are so small that they can easily fit in the pocket of a lab jacket.

Basic Computer Components

A computer is a programmable machine, or system of hardware (Figure 11-4), which responds to a specific set of instructions and performs a list of instructions in programmed language called software. Table 11-1 lists the different types of hardware, software, and storage components. Generally, computers require the following components to function:

- memory makes it possible for a computer to temporarily store data and programs.
- mass storage device makes it possible for a computer to permanently retain large amounts of data. Common mass storage devices include disk drives or zip drives.

- **input** device, such as the keyboard and mouse, is a conduit through which data and instructions enter a computer.

- **output** device, such as a display screen, printer, and other devices, permits the visual capability to see what the computer has accomplished.

- central processing unit (CPU) is the brain of the computer that executes the specific set of instructions.

The CPU, or main memory of a computer, acts as a traffic controller, directing the computer's activities and sending electronic signals to the right place at the right time. The time it takes for the electronic signals to come and go is measured in megahertz (MHz). The higher the megahertz, the faster the computer can move information from one place to another. At the heart of the CPU is the microprocessor, which has a number indicating its size. Microprocessors have three differentiated characteristics: instruction set; bandwidth (the number of bits processed at one time to represent and address); and clock speed (represented in MHz for how many instructions per second the processor can execute). The higher the numbers, the more power the CPU will function.

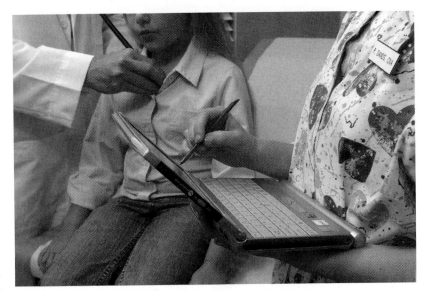

FIGURE 11-3 Medical assistant uses a laptop computer for bedside charting.

Memory

A computer's memory is measured and stored in kilobytes (Kb or K). Each kilobyte is 1,000 bytes (or characters) of information. This memory is further divided into RAM and ROM. RAM, or random-access memory, is the highest number of kilobytes a computer can hold all at once. The ROM, or read-only memory, is used to store information that is not actively being used by the computer at that moment. RAM, however, is only good as long as the computer is not turned off.

Once the computer is turned off, or powered down, all information stored in RAM is lost. The higher the number of kilobytes, the more information a particular storage media can hold.

Monitor

In order to communicate with a computer, the user needs to see what is happening. The monitor is the display screen that allows the user to observe that the computer does what it is directed to do. Monitors are categorized as monochrome, gray scale, or color. Monochrome monitors display two colors: one for the background and one for the foreground. The colors can be black and white, green and black, or amber and black. A gray scale monitor is a special type of monochrome monitor capable of displaying different shades of gray. Color or RGB (red, green, and blue) monitors display anywhere from 16 to over one million different colors (Figure 11-5). In addition to these monitor categories, monitors are available in a variety of sizes and styles similar to television screens. The screen size is measured in diagonal inches, the distance from one corner to the opposite diagonal corner.

TABLE 11-1 Hardware, Software, and Storage Components

Hardware	Software	Storage
Central processing unit (CPU)	Systems	Diskettes/floppy disks
Peripherals: monitor, printer, CD-ROM, modem, scanner, cables, and other equipment	Applications	Hard disks Magnetic tapes

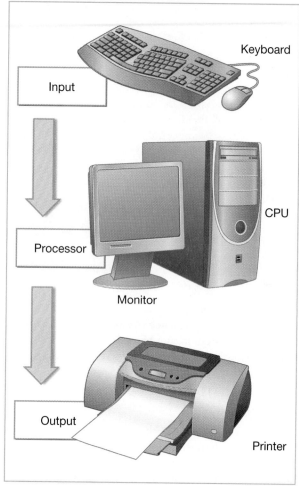

FIGURE 11-4 Components of a computer system.

Drives

Computers are based on hard-disk drive technology. By programming convention, the hard-disk drive, a magnetic storage media contained inside the computer, is usually called the "C drive." This storage area is controlled by the CPU, and information written to this magnetic media is accessed by the CPU when needed to make the computer run. Both programs and information can be stored on a hard-disk drive. The more visual the software, the larger the amount of storage space required. Disk drives can be either internal or external and there are different types of disk drives: hard-disk drive (HDD), floppy-drive (FDD), magnetic disk, and optical drive.

CD-ROM

CD-ROM stands for "Compact Disc Read-Only Memory." It is a data storage system for computers using internal or external CD-ROM players with CD-ROM. Computer programs, databases, and other large amounts of information on CD-ROM are digitally encoded and may not be changed by the user. Stored data may include simple text programs, entire encyclopedia pro-

grams, photo and sound libraries, and complex motion pictures or animations. The data is randomly accessed in the same manner as a floppy disk, which is a small flexible, magnetic disk in a rigid plastic case that stores data on and retrieves data by a computer. A CD-ROM is capable of holding or storing more information than 1,000 floppy disks.

Some computers have multimedia capabilities that allow the user to record and access a variety of sounds and music, photos, animations, and videos. Multimedia functions require the large storage capacity that a CD-ROM offers.

DVD stands for digital videodisc or digital versatile disc. DVDs use the same size disc as CD-ROMs; however they can hold much more information and can be recorded on both sides.

Removable Disk Drive

A removable disk drive uses disks mounted in cartridges. They are generally small and can fit on your key ring or in your pocket. Removable disks come in a variety of sizes ranging from 125 megabytes (MB) to 4 gigabytes (Gs). Their advantage is that multiple disks can be used to increase the amount of stored material, and that once removed, the disk can be stored away to prevent unauthorized use.

A portable universal serial bus (USB) drive, also known as jump drive, thumb drive, or flash drive, is a small portable storage device that can hold up to 4Gs of data. USB hard-disk devices can be purchased in a variety of sizes, styles, and shapes depending on the overall need.

Keyboard

Usually the keyboard is a set of keys utilized to input data. The keyboard is designed with function keys, alphanumeric keys, punctuation keys, arrow keys, and conjunction keys. Function keys serve as dual purpose

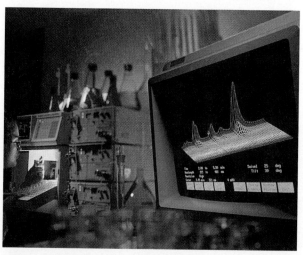

FIGURE 11-5 Color monitor for a computer system.

keys depending on the program that is running. The F1-key and the F12-key execute specific word processing operations. Conjunction keys execute directions in conjunction with the program running and at least two other keys at the same time, for example the control key+alt key+delete key = Windows task manager.

Mouse

In addition to the computer keyboard, a device that gives the user control of the computer is known as a mouse. As the mouse rolls along a hard, flat surface, it controls the movement of the cursor, or pointer on the monitor. The mouse contains at least one button, and up to three, each performing different functions depending on the program in use.

Printers

To output information from the computer monitor onto paper or hardcopy, printers are used. Popular printer options include dot matrix printers, ink-jet printers, and laser printers.

An ink-jet printer works on the dot matrix principle, so that the characters are made up of dots when the ink is blown onto the paper. Ink-jet printers are usually quieter and faster than dot matrix printers, and they can print graphics and in color if the proper ink cartridge and software have been installed. Ink-jet printers are also more costly than the dot matrix printers.

Laser printers use lasers to burn the ink onto the paper. While they are the most expensive of the three printer options, these non-impact printers are the most versatile printers available today. Laser printers are faster and quieter than either dot matrix or ink-jet printers, they can produce typewritten quality work, and they are able to add color to documents with available color print options.

Software

Software or program is the name given to the set or sets of instructions that allow the computer to perform its functions. Every computer starts with an operating system. Computer programs that work with the operating system are called "overlays." These overlay programs allow the user to choose from a menu instead of typing a command at the opening prompt. Each prompt (a symbol or message informing the user that some input is needed) directs the user what action to take. By using arrow keys, function keys, or a mouse, the user can choose the desired program from words or pictures (icons), allowing even an inexperienced user to choose a task more easily. The overlay programs that most users know are from Microsoft Windows, which lets the user choose a function from pictures or icons. Using a mouse, the user moves the cursor to the icon of the program and clicks the proper button on the mouse. The Windows program translates this command for the CPU, and the program is called to the screen.

Another layer of computer programs are called application programs. These programs can perform a special function such as spreadsheets, word processing, or data management. Spreadsheet application programs allow the user to manipulate data in table values by rows and columns. Values are input into specific cells on the spreadsheet and can be assigned a relationship between cells with formulas and labels electronically. Word processing applications provide the user the ability to create, edit, store, and print written documents such as letters, manuscripts, transmittals, and many other professional documents. Word processing programs can visually enhance the content's appearance on documents with numerous features such as bold, italics, color fonts, etc. Data management applications are similar to an electronic filing system (Figure 11-6). Data is stored in collections of information that are organized within the software application and can be sorted for quick data selection of specific desired information pieces. For example, the user would select the field for a directory of patient telephones numbers, diagnoses, or other information needed.

Advantages of medical management programs are many. After entering patient information into the program only once, the practice is able to schedule an appointment, record charges and payments, generate an insurance form, print a statement (including

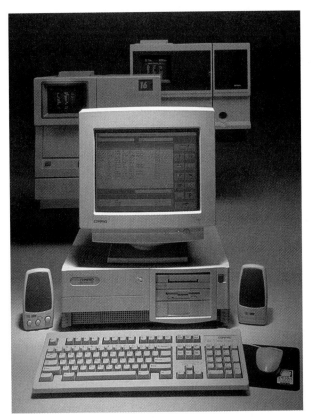

FIGURE 11-6 Patient data management system.

Most patients have now accepted computer technology as a part of conducting any business. Some patients, however, are still fearful that unauthorized persons may have access to their records. By using discretion in the handling of all medical records, the successful medical assistant conveys to the patient that confidentiality is of the utmost importance to the practice, thus reassuring the patient.

notices of delinquency accounts or aged accounts), track the number of days before payment is received from the insurance company, and write a reminder letter or postcard to the patient about an upcoming appointment.

Security for the Computer System

The same legal standards of confidentiality and the Health Insurance Portability and Accountability Act (HIPAA) compliance apply to all patient records, whether on paper or on the computer. Patient Education discusses reassuring patients about confidentiality in the medical office. It is absolutely essential for the successful medical assistant to understand that other patients should not be able to see computerized records any more easily than paper records. This may require some thought and planning when a computer system is used for record keeping in the front office.

The computer screen should be positioned so that it cannot be easily seen by patients. A privacy screen

Preparing for
Externship

Most physicians' offices have some type of computer system. As part of security, a password may be necessary to use the system. You may be issued a password so that you have access to relevant information. Remember, confidentiality still applies when using electronic devices and media. Protect your password and never allow unauthorized personnel to use your password. Once you have completed your task at the computer, remember to log off or sign off your password. This prevents others from using your password inappropriately.

around the computer workstation may be necessary, depending on the office layout. Another safeguard available is a screen saver that uses an image or texture to cover up the screen without removing any data allowing no one but the user to see it.

It is imperative that the records are accessible only to those who are authorized to use them. Keeping patient records safe may require using a password. Medical management programs often have several tiers of security, allowing one system administrator (the person in charge of the computer program) to limit access for patient records to those who need to see them. For example, the person who does appointment scheduling in a particular practice may not need to see a patient's financial records. The system administrator can "lock" the appointment scheduler out of financial records altogether, or assign limited access to the data.

Without a proper password, the user has no access to the data and must "log in" or type in his or her password, followed by an acceptance key (ENTER or RETURN) in order to use the program. It is important to guard a password carefully as discussed in Preparing for Externship. It should not be shared with coworkers or written where someone else will see it. When choosing a password, avoid using the names of children or significant others (these would be too easy for someone else to guess). Use a word or a set of numbers that has significance to you, but is also easily remembered. If you must write your password down, write it in a secure place and do not identify it as a system password. Passwords should be changed on a regular basis. Many medical offices change passwords monthly for added security and HIPAA compliance measures.

In addition to in-office security, a medical office needs to protect the computer from outside invaders (Legal and Ethical Issues). Outside invaders include hackers, crackers, viruses, or cyberbullies that access confidential information and commit identity theft. Computer security begins with regular maintenance of the computer systems such as firewalls, antivirus programs, defragmentation, deleting temporary Internet files, cookies, and the Internet history. Maintenance programs can be scheduled automatically or manually and should be run often. In addition to the internal maintenance, the external equipment should be cleaned regularly with appropriate cleaning solution to protect the user from spreading contact germs.

In order to avoid losing all data in the event of a system failure, fire, or equipment theft, it is also recommended that all data be backed up (copied onto disks or CD-ROMs) at regular intervals and that those backups be stored in a secure location outside the office. Again, confidentiality is of the utmost importance, and access to backup files should be carefully guarded.

Selecting a Computer System

Before beginning the search for a new computer system, it is important to establish the following:

- How will the computer be used?
- How many people will be using the computer system?
- How much storage space is needed now and for several years into the future?

Remember, the more visual the computer program, the more space will be required to run it. The more patients added to a particular database, the more storage space will be needed to keep pace with the size of the practice.

The second phase of the computer search should focus on the software currently being used.

- Is it meeting the needs of the practice?
- Does everyone who uses it understand how to use it?
- Will the current programs transfer to a new system?

The third critical element of a computer search is the budget and costs related to the budget, such as monthly billing and insurance claim mailings. Changing programs adds to the cost of a new computer system and must be considered carefully in any system change.

Once the hardware and software analysis has been completed, it is time to look at the products on the market.

- Are there manufacturers who have a better service record than others?
- What happens if the computer system breaks down?
- Who pays to have it fixed? Is there a warranty?

Identify a support system of computer experts who can provide ongoing technical assistance and quick on-site service for computer software and hardware problems. Purchasing a service contract to take effect when the warranty covering parts, repair,

Legal and Ethical Issues

The same standards of patient confidentiality apply to data stored on computers that apply to any and all patient records. The medical office must guard against unethical and illegal accessing and use of computer equipment for illegal purposes. Information contained within the computer must be protected, as must the computer hardware and software.

Employees of the practice must be educated and trained to understand the importance of security methods and to prevent loss or damage to valuable equipment and programs. Informed employees can follow the proper procedures to report suspicious occurrences within the workplace. The medical assistant must have an understanding of his or her own liability and the physician's liability in the processing of medical records.

and service expires is an option that you may wish to consider. Training contracts are available with firms that will provide employee training on new software and hardware.

Computer system selection is a large responsibility and while the final decision usually rests with a financial manager, the system's users can make or break the success of any given installation. Users who are unhappy with the selection are not as apt to use the system to its fullest capability, and this will, in the end, cost the practice money. Therefore, it is imperative that as many users as possible be involved in the selection process in order to make sure that the money being spent on a system is well spent. Table 11-2 lists commonly used computer terms.

The Internet

The Internet is a computer network made up of thousands of interfacing networks worldwide. Millions of computers are connected to the Internet. There are organizations that develop technical aspects of this network and set standards for creating applications on it, but no governing body is in control. Access to the Internet is through a commercial Internet service provider (ISP). Using the ISP and modem connection, you can browse the Internet for a wide variety of services: electronic mail, file transfer, vast information

TABLE 11-2 List of Frequently Used Computer Terms

Term	Definition
backup	A copy of work or software batch data stored for processing at periodic intervals.
batch	Data stored for processing at periodic intervals.
boot	To start up the computer.
catalog	List of all files stored on a storage device.
characters per second	Speed measurement for printers.
cursor	Flashing bar, arrow, or symbol that indicates where the next character will be placed.
daisy wheel printer	An impact printer that "strikes" characters onto a page, much like a typewriter; unable to produce graphic images; but does produce letter quality output.
database	Computer application that contains records or files.
data debugging	Process of eliminating errors from input data.
disk drive	A container that holds a read/write head, an access arm, and a magnetic disk for storage.
DOS	Disk operating system.
downtime	Time a computer cannot be used because of maintenance or mechanical failure.
electronic mail (e-mail)	Use of a telephone, modem, and appropriate hardware and software to allow transmission of data electronically from computer to computer.
file	A collection of related records.
file maintenance	Data entry operations including additions, deletions, and modifications.
format	Methods for setting margins, tabs, line spacing, and other layout features.
GIGO	"Garbage in, garbage out," which means if you input incorrect information you will receive incorrect output.
hard copy	A printed copy of data in a file.
hardware	The actual physical equipment that is used by a computer to process data.
input	Entering data into the computer system.
interface	Technology that allows two or more non-connected computers to exchange programs and data. Also referred to as a network.
keyboard	An input device, similar to a typewriter keyboard.
menu	A list of options available to the user.
modem	Hardware device which converts digital signals to analog signals for transfer over communication lines or links.
output	Processed data translated into final form or information to be used.
peripheral	Device required for the input, output, processing, and storage of data; Includes mouse, disk drive, keyboards, printers, and joysticks.
scrolling	Feature that allows the computer operator to control the location of the cursor within a document.
security code	A group of characters that allows an authorized computer operator access to certain programs or features. Password.
write protect	Feature of storage devices that allows the data to be seen, but not changed.

resources, interest group membership, interactive collaboration, multimedia displays, real-time broadcasting, shopping opportunities, breaking news, and much more.

With the advent of remote communications through electronic mail (e-mail) and modems, computers in one location can "talk" to computers across the street, across the state, across the country, and across the world (Professionalism).

Internet technology has allowed many medical insurance companies to offer electronic claims services or ECT (electronic claims transmission). ECT service speeds up the insurance claim process and puts the payment for services rendered into the practice's bank account in as few as three working days. Such access can be obtained through a "clearinghouse" or remote computer with transfer to multiple insurance carriers.

The World Wide Web (WWW or the Web) is a system of Internet servers. The initial purpose of the Web was to facilitate communication among its members, who were located in several countries. Rapid growth in the number of both developers and users ensued. In addition to hypertext (computer-based text), the Web began to incorporate graphics, video, and sound. The use of the Web has reached global proportions and has become a defining aspect of human culture in an amazingly short period of time.

Almost every protocol type available on the Internet is accessible on the Web. Internet protocols are sets of rules that allow for inter-machine communication on the Internet. The following is a sample of major protocols accessible on the Web:

- **E-mail** (Simple Mail Transport Protocol or SMTP)
  Distributes electronic messages and files to one or more electronic mailboxes.

- **Telnet** (Telnet Protocol)
  Facilitates login to a computer host to execute commands.

- **FTP** (File Transfer Protocol)
  Transfers text or binary files between an FTP server and client.

- **Usenet** (Network News Transfer Protocol or NNTP)
  Distributes Usenet news articles derived from topical discussions on newsgroups.

- **HTTP** (HyperText Transfer Protocol)
  Transmits hypertext over networks.

Many other protocols are available such as, the Voice over Internet Protocol (VoIP) that allows users to place a telephone call over the Web.

The World Wide Web provides almost instant access to information. The convenient and user-friendly environment of the Web makes it easy for patients to research information about a new medication, physi-

Professionalism

It is not uncommon to receive an e-mail that we wish to share with others. We may also come across Web sites of interest to others. Be careful in sharing e-mails and Web sites with others while at work. Some material may be offensive to others. It is not always appropriate to share non-work related e-mails with your coworkers while on the job. If you share an interest with a coworker and wish to exchange e-mails, ask the person for his or her personal e-mail address. E-mail him or her from your personal e-mail address while not at work.

cians to share test results with specialists assisting in diagnosing patients, or as a tool to further educate members of the health care team. Lifespan Considerations encourages you to assist older patients with making use of computers to help in their patient care. Because of the Web's ability to work with multimedia and advanced programming languages, the Web is by far the most popular component of the Internet.

Electronic Signatures

The traditional "signature" on documents is becoming a thing of the past. The traditional signature can now be converted into a mathematical process (or a set of numbers) to create an electronic signature. This set of numbers, in computing terminology a "file," will be recorded temporarily in a computer's working memory or permanently on some storage medium such as a disk. The file that constitutes the electronic document can

Lifespan
Considerations

Older patients may not be very familiar with computers and computer terminology. It may be necessary to spend more time explaining how computers are used to assist in patient care. Some may have basic knowledge of Internet use. If they wish to research a health-related topic, help them by providing a list of reputable Web sites dedicated to patient education.

be copied from place to place via telecommunication devices. An increasing proportion of both commercial and private communications takes place in purely electronic form. Some of those communications will need to be signed to achieve their intended legal effects, and even where this is not strictly necessary, the parties to a transaction are likely to wish the transaction document or communication to be signed.

HIPAA requires health care organizations to protect the privacy and security of confidential health information and calls for standard formats of electronic transactions. These standardized national requirements apply to the electronic transmission of patient history and health records such as health insurance enrollment detail and claims. The need to maintain confidentiality and privacy of medical information and rules for medical document security, including standards related to electronic signatures, is also outlined in HIPAA.

Computers and Ergonomics

If you are a long time computer user, you might have noticed the occasional discomforts that accompany spending lengthy periods of time in front of the computer. After staring at a monitor for extended amounts of time, year after year, you may start to notice the discomfort increase in frequency and severity. As use and hours on the computer continues over the years, the discomfort could become part of the daily routine when you sit down to work or game at a computer. In order to safely incorporate computer use in your daily routine and to work effectively, you should be aware of some ergonomic tips, such as appropriately positioning computer equipment (Figure 11-7).

Your Chair

When sitting in your chair, make sure that you push your hips as far back as they can go in the chair. Adjust

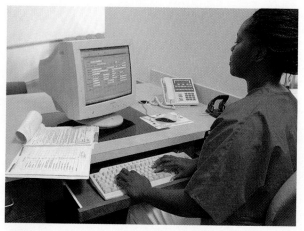

FIGURE 11-7 Ergonomically correct desk, chair and keyboard.

the seat height so your feet are flat on the floor and your knees are equal to, or slightly lower than, your hips. Adjust the back of the chair to a 100° to 110° reclined angle. Make sure your upper and lower back are supported. It may be necessary to use inflatable cushions or small pillows. If you have an active back mechanism on your chair, use it to make frequent position changes. For chairs with armrests, adjust them so that your shoulders are relaxed. If necessary, remove the armrests if they are in the way.

Your Keyboard

An articulating keyboard tray can provide optimal positioning of input devices. However, it should accommodate the mouse, enable leg clearance, and have an adjustable height and tilt mechanism. The tray should not push you too far away from other work materials such as your telephone. It is helpful if you pull up close to your keyboard and position it directly in front of your body. If possible, adjust the keyboard height so that your shoulders are relaxed, your elbows are in a slightly open position, and your wrists and hands are straight. Wrist rests can help to maintain neutral postures and pad hard surfaces. However, the wrist rest should only be used to rest the palms of the hands between keystrokes. Resting on the wrist rest while typing is not recommended.

Your Monitor

Incorrect positioning of the screen and source documents can result in awkward postures. Adjust the monitor and source documents so that your neck is in a neutral, relaxed position. Your monitor should be centered directly in front of you, above your keyboard. Position the top of the monitor approximately two to three inches above seated eye level. To reduce glare, it may be helpful to place the screen at right angles to windows and adjust curtains or blinds. Optical glass glare filters, light filters, or secondary task lights can also help reduce glare.

Your Body

Once you have correctly set up your computer workstation, use good work habits. No matter how perfect the environment, prolonged, static postures will inhibit blood circulation and take a toll on your body. Take short one to two minute stretch breaks every 20 to 30 minutes. After each hour of work, take a break or change tasks for at least five to ten minutes. Always try to get away from your computer during lunch breaks. Avoid eye fatigue by resting and refocusing your eyes periodically. Look away from the monitor and focus on something in the distance. Rest your eyes by covering them with your palms for 10 to 15 seconds. Use correct posture when working. Shift you position as much as possible.

SUMMARY

The use of computers is essential for medical offices to meet the process flow of business today. Computers enhance quality patient care through data collection, eliminate duplication of work, and decrease errors. Computers execute input, processing, output, and storage of medical data. In medical offices, computer use is especially useful in eliminating some of the more time-consuming tasks associated with appointment scheduling, charting, billing, and insurance processing.

Computers are composed of many parts including the microprocessor, CPU, monitor, keyboard, and printer. Safety on the computer includes regular maintenance, passwords, antivirus protection, HIPAA compliance, and general cleaning. The successful medical assistant is a computer literate professional who deals easily with the challenge of finding new and efficient ways to use available technology.

Chapter Review

COMPETENCY REVIEW

1. Define and spell the terms to learn for this chapter.
2. Using a microcomputer, boot up the computer. Notice what information is displayed on the screen before the computer is "ready" to work. What disk operating system is being used? Does a menu or sub-menu appear when the computer has been booted or is the computer using a version of Windows? Are any security codes required to use the programs listed? If so, what are they?
3. What type of printer is used by the computer system? Is it an impact or a non-impact printer?
4. Print a list of all the files on the hard drive.
5. Select a word processing program and type a simple letter reminding a patient that he or she is due for a blood pressure check. Use the spell-checking feature before printing the letter.
6. Enter a patient into a medical management software database. Use yourself and your own information as the data.

PREPARING FOR THE CERTIFICATION EXAM

1. Which is considered a software element of computers?
   A. hard disk
   B. central processing unit
   C. diskette
   D. kilobyte
   E. program

2. Which is NOT considered hardware?
   A. printer
   B. Windows
   C. monitor
   D. keyboard
   E. central processing unit

3. What type of printer is considered the most versatile?
   A. laser
   B. dot matrix
   C. ink jet
   D. word processor
   E. color printer

4. Which is NOT an advantage of a medical data base management program?
   A. enter patient information only once
   B. can print statements
   C. can track days before payment is received from insurer
   D. can print delinquency notices
   E. can measure storage capacity

continued on next page

5. Which is NOT recommended to establish computer security?
   A. position screen away from patients
   B. use a password that is unknown to the patient but that you can remember easily
   C. have tiers of security that limit access to patient information to authorized employees
   D. use screen savers to cover up the screen
   E. change password frequently

6. Electronic mail is
   A. entering data into the computer system
   B. a backup copy of work or software
   C. a process of eliminating errors from input data
   D. use of a telephone, modem, or hardware with software to transmit data from one computer to another
   E. physical equipment used by a computer to process data

7. A prompt is
   A. a set of instructions that tells the computer hardware what to do
   B. a reminder or hint to the user that some action must be taken
   C. processed data translated into final form
   D. methods for setting margins, tabs, and layout features
   E. a measure of storage capacity

8. The computer program that contains all records and files is known as
   A. software
   B. catalog
   C. database
   D. batch
   E. format

9. Which office function CANNOT be performed by word processing?
   A. user can input information using a typewriter-like keyboard
   B. user can see the copy that will be printed
   C. user can correct errors on the screen before printing takes place
   D. user can generate form letters
   E. user can print x-ray films

10. To protect against a loss of data and information processed by the computer, a medical assistant should
    A. change the password frequently
    B. use electronic mail
    C. use word-processing whenever possible
    D. make backup copies on a diskette
    E. handwrite a backup copy for the file

CRITICAL THINKING

1. Where should Helda begin?
2. Which software programs should she use to design and develop the educational materials and the marketing materials?
3. What should she do to become more familiar with the software features to design the materials?

ON THE JOB

Elizabeth Maxwell, a medical assistant for Dr. Casey, often works at the front desk. One of Dr. Casey's patients, Stephanie Cross, has arrived for a scheduled appointment. One her way in, Stephanie saw a neighbor leaving the office. She asks Elizabeth to look on the office system and tell her why her neighbor was in to see Dr. Casey.

Later the same day, Diana Mulderr, who sits at the desk next to Elizabeth, has forgotten her computer password. She asks to use Elizabeth's password "just for today."

1. What should Elizabeth tell Stephanie Cross?
2. Is it ever permissible to use the computer to look up information on patients for personal reasons?
3. What should Elizabeth tell Diana Mulderr?

INTERNET ACTIVITY

When researching information on the Internet, it is important that the Web sites used are reputable and provide accurate information. Perform a search using any of the search engines (a Web site that allows you to search the entire Web for related Web sites) available to you. Search for popular health-related Web sites. Make a list of ten Web sites and comment on each: ease of use, relevant information, easy to understand, etc.

MediaLink More on computers in the medical office, including interactive resources, can be found on the Student CD-ROM accompanying this textbook.

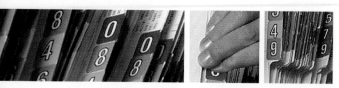

Medical Assistant Role Delineation Chart

HIGHLIGHT indicates material covered in this chapter.

ADMINISTRATIVE

Administrative Procedures

- Perform basic administrative medical assisting functions
- Schedule, coordinate and monitor appointments
- Schedule inpatient/outpatient admissions and procedures
- Understand and apply third-party guidelines
- Obtain reimbursement through accurate claims submission
- Monitor third-party reimbursement
- Understand and adhere to managed care policies and procedures
- *Negotiate managed care contracts*

- Manage accounts receivable
- *Manage accounts payable*
- *Process payroll*
- *Document and maintain accounting and banking records*
- *Develop and maintain fee schedules*
- *Manage renewals of business and professional insurance policies*
- *Manage personnel benefits and maintain records*
- *Perform marketing, financial, and strategic planning*

Practice Finances

- Perform procedural and diagnostic coding
- Apply bookkeeping principles

CLINICAL

Fundamental Principles

- Apply principles of aseptic technique and infection control
- Comply with quality assurance practices
- Screen and follow up patient test results

Diagnostic Orders

- Collect and process specimens
- Perform diagnostic tests

Patient Care

- Adhere to established patient screening procedures
- Obtain patient history and vital signs
- Prepare and maintain examination and treatment areas
- Prepare patient for examinations, procedures and treatments

- Assist with examinations, procedures and treatments
- Prepare and administer medications and immunizations
- Maintain medication and immunization records
- Recognize and respond to emergencies
- Coordinate patient care information with other health care providers
- Initiate IV and administer IV medications with appropriate training and as permitted by state law

GENERAL

Professionalism

- Display a professional manner and image
- Demonstrate initiative and responsibility
- Work as a member of the health care team
- Prioritize and perform multiple tasks
- Adapt to change
- Promote the CMA credential
- Enhance skills through continuing education
- Treat all patients with compassion and empathy
- Promote the practice through positive public relations

Communication Skills

- Recognize and respect cultural diversity
- Adapt communications to individual's ability to understand
- Use professional telephone technique

- Recognize and respond effectively to verbal, nonverbal, and written communications
- Use medical terminology appropriately
- Utilize electronic technology to receive, organize, prioritize and transmit information
- Serve as liaison

Legal Concepts

- Perform within legal and ethical boundaries
- Prepare and maintain medical records
- Document accurately
- Follow employer's established policies dealing with the health care contract
- Implement and maintain federal and state health care legislation and regulations
- Comply with established risk management and safety procedures
- Recognize professional credentialing criteria
- *Develop and maintain personnel, policy and procedure manuals*

Instruction

- Instruct individuals according to their needs
- Explain office policies and procedures
- Teach methods of health promotion and disease prevention
- Locate community resources and disseminate information
- *Develop educational materials*
- *Conduct continuing education activities*

Operational Functions

- Perform inventory of supplies and equipment
- Perform routine maintenance of administrative and clinical equipment
- Apply computer techniques to support office operations
- *Perform personnel management functions*
- *Negotiate leases and prices for equipment and supply contracts*

- *Denotes advanced skills.*

SOURCE: Reprinted by permission of the American Association of Medical Assistants from the AAMA Role Delineation Study: Occupational Analysis of the Medical Assisting Profession.

Managing Medical Records

chapter 12

Learning Objectives

After completing this chapter, you should be able to:

- Define and spell the terms to learn for this chapter.
- Describe three types of file storage units.
- State the "Rules for Filing."
- List and discuss five types of numerical filing systems.
- Describe color-coded, alphabetic, and numerical filing systems.
- State an effective system used for cross-referencing.
- Describe how to find a missing file.
- Describe a tickler file.
- Describe the process for medical transcribing and a variety of medical reports.
- Discuss quality assurance.
- Discuss ownership of the medical record.
- Discuss the medical record's statute of limitations.

Terms to Learn

active record
alphabetic filling
closed record
electronic medical record (EMR)
inactive record

medical record
microfiche
microfilm
numerical filing
problem oriented medical record (POMR)

source oriented medical record
subjective, objective, assessment, and plan (SOAP)
terminal digit filing

Case Study

YOU ARE EMPLOYED AS A MEDICAL ASSISTANT in Dr. Salpega's office. A patient, Terry Dewey, has been diagnosed with a lung cancer with metastasis to the brain. Dr. Salpega has told him that his cancer is inoperable. Mr. Dewey wants the opinion of another physician and requests that his medical records, including all test results, be released to another physician in the same city. In preparing Mr. Dewey's record, you discover that there are no x-ray results in his chart, although you know he had x-rays done. In addition, you discover that Mr. Dewey has an unpaid balance of $742.21 for services previously rendered.

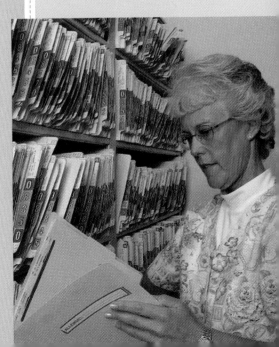

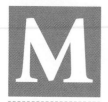edical records are the sources of all documentation relating to the patient. The medical record contains past patient history information, current diagnosis and treatment, and correspondence relating to the patient. Billing materials are often maintained in a separate accounting record. Medical records can be maintained in a variety of methods, which include paper (hard copy files), computer database files on location or off with an online separate backup system, electronic medical records (EMR), microfilm (miniaturized photographs of records) and microfiche (sheets of microfilm) and other electronic medium. Medical records management requires careful attention to accuracy, confidentiality, and proper filing and storage.

The Medical Record

The medical record contains all the written documentation that relates to the patient's health care. Each patient's medical record will contain essentially the same categories of material but information unique to each patient. Information contained in a source-oriented medical record is filed within a section with tabs. Each medical record may or may not include all standard categories based on the patient's individual health care needs. For example, not every patient will have a consultation report from another physician, or a surgical report. See Box 12-1 for a summary list of standard

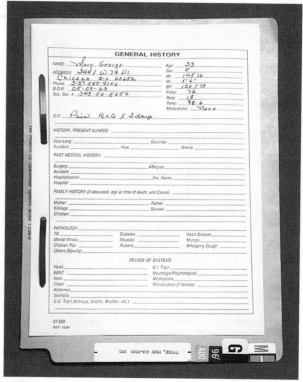

FIGURE 12-1 Handwritten documentation.

categories and reports that are covered in more detail in this chapter. Figure 12-1 is an example of handwritten documentation in a medical chart. This demonstrates just one part of what is in the standard patient's chart.

Types of Medical Records

Various medical reports are filed in the medical records with tabs that label the source, such as lab, x-ray, consultations, and special studies. These medical records are referred to as source oriented medical records.

Most medical offices and hospitals use subjective, objective, assessment, and plan (SOAP) charting and the problem oriented medical record (POMR). See Figure 12-2 for an example of SOAP charting. Volume 3, Chapter 34 contains a detailed description of the SOAP method.

For a physician to easily track the progress of a patient, the POMR system can be used. There are four sections to the POMR approach:

- Database—this section contains information about present illness, chief complaint, review of systems, laboratory reports, and physical examinations.

- Problem list—in this section each problem the patient has experienced is separately listed and numbered.

- Treatment plan—each treatment plan is numbered and corresponds to the numbered problem.

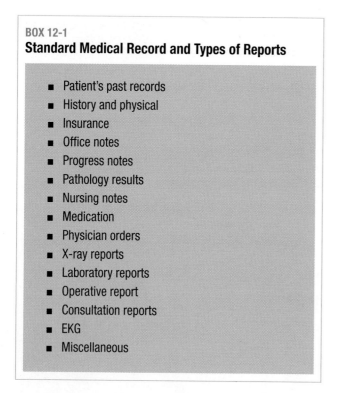

BOX 12-1
Standard Medical Record and Types of Reports

- Patient's past records
- History and physical
- Insurance
- Office notes
- Progress notes
- Pathology results
- Nursing notes
- Medication
- Physician orders
- X-ray reports
- Laboratory reports
- Operative report
- Consultation reports
- EKG
- Miscellaneous

PROGRESS NOTES

Patient's name: Jessica Lopez								Page:	1

Date	Problem Number	**S**	**O**	**A**	**P**	S = Subjective O = Objective A = Assessment P = Plan			
3/12/05	1	"I'm having dizzy spells and have not been taking my BP med."							
			BP 170/110 both arms, lying down, sitting & standing; WT. 202#						
				Hypertension					
					Rx for Norvasc 5mg daily; to monitor BP and return in 1 week				
					for BP check; placed on 1200 calorie diet to lose 20#				

FIGURE 12-2   An example of SOAP charting.

- Progress notes—every progress note entered in the chart must correspond to one of the numbered problems. Each progress note will follow the structured format of SOAP charting.

Always keep in mind that the medical record is a legal document, permanent record, and a tool used to communicate between staff members to deliver services to the patient. The patient's chart is not the place to document your opinion or internal office problems. Statements such as, "Patient not administered injection due to lack of staffing" or "Patient very angry with physician" are opinions, or subjective. All documentation should be objective, not subjective.

Everything that is done during a patient's medical visit, ordered over the telephone, or discussed with a patient over the telephone or e-mail, must be docu-

mented in the medical record. Write legibly in black ink. If you make an error, do not erase or totally obliterate the original error with commercial products like correcting fluid. If the error is made during the typing process, then it should be corrected as any other errors are corrected. However, if the error is noted later, then you must draw a line through the error, enter your initials, the date, and write in the correction. Handwritten errors on the medical chart are handled in the same manner. Procedure 12-1 lists steps the medical assistant should follow when changing or adding items to a patient's chart. Figure 12-3 is an example of a corrected chart notation.

The following items cannot be overemphasized as part of the medical assistant's responsibility to ensure an efficiently run medical office.

Date	Time	Order	Doctor	Administered by
9/9/05	3 pm	Erythromycin ~~500 mg~~ 250 mg BT 9/9	Williams	B. Tremgen RN.

FIGURE 12-3   An example of a corrected chart notation.

Adding or Changing Items on a Patient's Record

OBJECTIVE: Add an item to a patient record and correctly change an error in documentation.

Equipment and Supplies

medical record to be added to or changed; black pen; correct information or documentation to be added or changed

Method

Adding items to a record:

1. An item is added to a patient record as soon as it is discovered that the item was omitted.
2. Locate the last entry in the medical record.
3. Using a pen with black ink, on the next line of the record, immediately after the last entry, place the current date.
4. On the same line, after the date, place the statement, "Late entry."
5. Note the date on which the information to be added was gathered.
6. Enter the information that was originally omitted.

7. Sign the entry with your full name and credentials.

Changing items in a record:

1. If an entry was made in a record that was incorrect, or made in the wrong record, it must be corrected.
2. Locate the incorrect information.
3. Using a pen with black ink, draw one single line through the incorrect information, so that the incorrect information is not obscured, but can still be read.
4. NEVER erase in a medical record. NEVER use correction fluid in a medical record. NEVER mark through information so that it cannot be read.
5. Place the date of the correction, your initials, and the letters "m.e." (for mistaken entry) above the incorrect information.
6. Enter the correct information.

- Clear handwriting—the medical records that are handwritten should be easily read by anyone. Pay particular attention to numbers and spelling.

- Accurate records—keeping in mind that records are legal documents and can be used in a court of law, the physician must be able to trust the accuracy of the data. As simple as it sounds, never guessing about information and double-checking your work each time will help ensure this is the case.

- Records that are up to date and available—do not wait to update records; make it an office habit to update records either as they occur or daily. This updating should include telephone calls, lab reports, and office visits. Make sure that the files are easily accessible. If there is a patient emergency, for example, the medical history will be needed immediately.

Electronic and Computerized Medical Records

Many health care professionals remain wary of computerizing patient records because of confidentiality worries. Electronic medical records, however, are becoming more common. Here are some advantages to electronic records:

- All office workers can have immediate access to the same files; a procedure for updating files needs to be in place.

- A physician may have offsite access to records on the network.

- Records can be sent via e-mail attachments to relevant and valid heath care inquiries or to satellite offices in different cities.

- Reminders for updating files can be set for staff members when updated information is due.

Types of Forms and Reports

A standard medical record is one of the most important items in an office setting. It is imperative that you are familiar with all components of it, such as medical forms and reports, in order to maintain the integrity and accuracy of patient records.

Patient Registration

The patient registration form usually includes the patient's name, the date of the visit, as well as the patient's age, date of birth (DOB), Social Security number, driver's license number (if applicable), address, and medical insurance information. The medical assistant should also note the patient's occupation, marital status, number of children (if applicable), emergency contact information, family medical history and current medical problems, as well as the chief complaint (CC). Figure 12-4 shows an example of a chief complaint. Other information the medical assistant may wish to note is mentioned in Cultural Considerations.

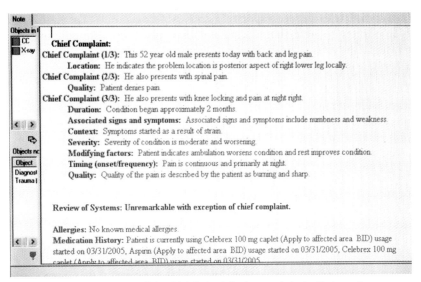

FIGURE 12-4 An example of a chief complaint chart notation in computerized patient records.

Family and Medical History

Sometimes the patient's family and medical history is listed on a separate form. This information should include the patient's past medical history of illness, surgery, allergies, current prescriptions, medications, and over-the-counter medications. It should also include herbal medications, and recreational drugs used by the patient. It should contain the patient's social and occupational history, including the amount of exercise done by the patient, whether the patient uses tobacco and the type of tobacco product, as well as alcohol use. Also, the medical assistant should note the current complaint and details of the present illness. Managed care insurances often require that the patient's current chief complaint be entered into the medical record as a history against the diagnosis. Use of the patient's own words is often requested. Relevant past family and social history is also vital, as well as the patient's medication history. Inventory of body systems is usually included as part of the patient's history.

Physical Examination Results

Not all patients receive general physical examinations. Some offices have a separate form to chart the outcome of a physical examination. The comprehensive physical examination form charts the results included in the examination, such as the patient's general appearance, nutrition, blood pressure (B/P), and head—an ear, eyes, nose, and throat examination (EENT), mouth, and scalp. Results from neck and thyroid examinations are also charted, as well as those of the thorax and breasts. Lymphadenothapy, and examinations done on the heart and lungs, the abdomen, the pelvic, genital and rectal areas, the skin, and overall impression and treatment plan also appear on the chart.

Results of All Tests

All results from tests performed on patients, such as office tests, laboratory tests, and hospital tests, should be tracked and filed in patients' records for easy accessibility should the physician need to consult them.

Records from Referred Physicians or Hospital Visits

New patients require incoming records from past offices to be placed in their records. Include a copy of the patient's written request and release for transferring records from past offices. Also, include information and relevant diagnoses from specialty physicians to whom the patient was referred for specific follow-ups.

Informed Consent Forms

A signed informed consent form documents that a patient has understood and consents to a treatment offered and has knowledge of the potential outcome and side effects of that treatment. The form must have

Cultural Considerations

Take note of the patient's cultural and ethnic background as well as that of friends or family accompanying the patient on his or her visit. It may be beneficial to make specific notes in that patient's chart regarding language spoken or other cultural considerations that the patient has mentioned in conversation.

a signature with the corresponding date. Moreover, it is important to note that the patient may withdraw consent if he or she so wishes. See Chapter 3 for more information on informed consent forms.

Diagnosis and Treatment Plan

The diagnosis and treatment plan should include the physician's diagnosis, the treatment plan, and options presented to the patient, as well as any instructions given to the patient.

Patient Correspondence and Follow-up Care

Invoices sent to the patient, procedures, follow-up visits, medical office care, and any notations involving the patient should be included in patient records. Also added to the records are documentations of telephone calls—often a separate log—as well as correspondence with or about the patient from all sources, such as laboratories, health care agencies, and referred consultations.

Consultation Report

There are many situations in which a physician will ask another physician to provide a second opinion on a patient's case. The second physician generally examines the patient, and then a report is dictated. The report is then sent to the attending physician (the requesting physician). The consultation report will include:

- Patient's name and medical record number
- Date of consultation
- Medical transcriptionist's name
- Referring physician
- Reason for the consultation
- Physical and laboratory evaluations
- Consulting physician's impression and recommendations

It is appropriate to close this report, which is supplied in letter format, with a complimentary close such as, "Thank you for allowing me to participate in the care of this patient."

Operative Note

The operative report describes a surgical procedure. The surgeon is expected to dictate this report as soon as possible, preferably immediately after the procedure is completed. The surgeon's name, date of procedure, preoperative and postoperative diagnosis, and the actual findings during the procedure are contained in this report.

This report is comprised of a description for the actual procedure, which will include location and length of the incision, the layers of skin and tissue that were incised, types of instruments used (in some cases), which organs and tissues were removed, all materials that were used in closing the wound, the estimated amount of blood loss, and a sponge count. The condition of the patient at the end of the procedure is stated, such as

"Patient tolerated procedure well," "Patient awake and responding," or "Patient taken to recovery room."

Pathology Report

The pathology report is generated by the pathologist as the result of examining tissue and organs removed during a surgical procedure (such as a biopsy) or at an autopsy. An autopsy report is generated after a patient's death to determine the cause of death. A pathology report focuses on microscopic (histology and cytology) findings as well as gross (overall) description of the tissues or organs. This report is related to disease findings and not laboratory findings, which are conducted on body fluids.

Radiology Report

A radiology report, completed by the radiologist, documents results of diagnostic procedures, such as x-rays, CT (computerized tomography) scans, MRI (magnetic resonance imaging) scans, nuclear medicine procedures (bone and thyroid scans), and other fluoroscopic examinations.

Discharge Summary

The discharge summary is completed on every hospitalized patient and summarizes the hospitalization. It explains why the patient was admitted, a summary of the patient's history, and a review of what occurred during the hospitalization. A discharge diagnosis is included in this report. The patient's condition upon leaving the hospital is noted.

Additional Reports

Other reports may be required concerning a patient, such as an emergency room report, psychiatric note, and special procedures, like a cardiac catheterization, or autopsy reports.

If information is not properly organized in the patient's medical record, errors can occur. It is very important that the medical assistant organize the patient's medical record according to facility policy. (See Procedure 12-2)

Filing

Choosing the type of file system for medical forms and reports, including the file folder coding system used in the office, is an important decision since all files must be maintained within that system. Some large offices hire an office consultant to set up a filing system. While the office staff are generally consulted when setting up a new file system, the decision is made by the physician and the office manager. There are three categories of files or records in a medical office: active, inactive, and closed.

- Active records relate to patients who have been seen in the past few years and are currently being treated. Each medical practice may have its own

PROCEDURE

Organize a Patient's Medical Record

OBJECTIVE: To update the patient's medical record verifying the right record and placing the information in the correct place in the record.

Equipment and Supplies
patient medical record; assorted documents for filing in record

Method
1. Verify that you have the right records for the patient record you have been given.

2. File documents given to you in the correct areas of the file, according to your facility policy for consistency. For example, file laboratory reports with other laboratory reports.
3. Return medical record to correct place in alphabetical order with other files.

---

policy regarding what constitutes an "active" file, but it is usually from one to five years.

- Inactive records relate to patients who have not been seen within the time period determined by office policy. These files are still maintained within the office but they are generally kept in a separate storage file cabinet. These patients have not received a formal notification that the physician has terminated caring for them. They may return when a medical problem develops.

- Closed records are those of patients who have actively terminated their contact with the physician. This occurs when they move away, ask to have their records sent to another physician, or death occurs. These files can be placed in storage boxes and are referred to as archives, since they are no longer needed but must be kept for legal reasons.

Fireproof cabinets are used to file documents, such as patient records, tax records, insurance policies, and canceled checks.

File Storage

Three types of file storage commonly used in a physician's office are vertical, lateral, and movable.

- Vertical—set up with two to four stacked pull-out drawers holding up to 100 files per drawer. This type of file storage system is heavy and space consuming.

- Lateral—set up with shelves allowing for easy access to files by pulling them off the shelves. This system often uses a color-coded method for visual recognition of files.

- Movable—set up with electrically powered or manually controlled file units that move on tracks in the floor. This type of open filing system is space saving since the file units can be moved close together when they are not needed. This system is also useful for books and journals since the floor can be reinforced when the track is installed.

File Folders

File folders are also designed to meet special needs. The top or side edge contains tabs at spaced intervals. These tabs are marked with identification labels. If files are stored with alternating tab cuts, it is easier to read the labels in the file drawer. The identification label is attached to the top tab in a vertical file cabinet or to the side edge of the file in a lateral file cabinet.

The patient's record may be placed within a separate tabbed folder that remains in the filing cabinet. The file folders may be color-coded to indicate the primary care physician. Each physician would be assigned a folder color. This helps keep files in order in large clinics. Professionalism discusses the importance of keeping files in order for any medical office, regardless of the size of the practice.

Professionalism

Your work reflects your professionalism. If patient records are strewn about the office, or if your system precludes your being able to pull the file you need quickly, it is a reflection on your skills as a medical assistant. If your filing system is sloppy, then you are probably sloppy too. Be sure to file all records accurately, neatly, and in a timely manner.

TABLE 12-1 **Rules for Alphabetic Filing**

Rules	Example
Names are filed: last name, first name, middle name (or middle initial). Each letter in the name is a separate unit.	Krause, Marvin K. is placed before Krause, Marvin L.
Initials come before a full name.	Brown, H. is placed before Brown, Henry.
Hyphenated names are treated as one unit. This applies to the names of individuals and businesses.	Amy Freeman-Smith is indexed under F for Freeman. It is considered Freemansmith for indexing purposes.
Titles (and initials) are disregarded for filing but placed in parentheses after the name.	Dr. Beth Ann Williams is indexed as Williams, Beth Ann, (Dr).
Married women are indexed using their legal name. The husband's name can be used for cross-referencing.	Mrs. Mary Jane Smith is indexed as Smith, Mary Jane (Mrs. John).
Seniority units, such as Jr. and Sr., are filed in a numerical order from first to last.	Jacob James Jurgens, Sr. comes before Jacob James Jurgens, Jr.
Numeric seniority terms are filed before alphabetic terms.	Jurgens, Jacob James III indexed before Jurgens, Jacob James, Jr.
Mac and Mc can be filed either alphabetically as they occur or grouped together depending on the preference of the office.	
Foreign language names are indexed as one unit.	Mary St. Claire is indexed as Stclaire, Mary. Carol van Damm is indexed as Vandamm, Carol.
If company names are identical, the address, by state, then city, street, may be used in the index. The ZIP code is not used to index files.	ABC Drugs, 123 Michigan Blvd., Chicago IL is indexed before ABC Drugs, 1450 N. Ash, Kalispell MT.
If individual's names are identical, use the birth date or mother's maiden name. Avoid using address since that can change.	Mark Richard Jones is indexed as Jones, Mark Richard (5/12/65) and Jones, Mark Richard (2/12/89).
Disregard apostrophes.	Megan O'Connor is indexed as OConnor, Megan.
Business organizations are indexed as they are written.	Lincoln Memorial Hospital is correct.
Disregard short terms, such as *a, and, the,* and *of.*	The Whitefish Drug Store is indexed as Whitefish Drug Store (The).
Numeric characters are indexed before alpha characters.	23rd Avenue Clinic would be indexed before the Nineteenth Street Medical Center. A separate file is set up for all numeric files.
Names with religious titles, such as Sister Mary Murphy, would be filed with the last name first, and then with the religious title.	Murphy, Sister Mary.
Compound words are filed as they are written.	South West Physician Service is filed before Southwest Physician Service.

Guides

Divider guides are used to separate files in the drawer or on the shelf. These guides are of heavy pressboard and should be placed every 1 1/2 to 2 inches to separate the file folders. The divider guide breaks the files into subsections using a letter (for example A, B, C, or A-B, Invoices) or by patient number. An out-guide is placed in the file when a file is removed to indicate where the file should be returned. The out-guide is usually a distinctive color, such as red, to indicate a file is missing.

Labels

The label on the file folder (such as the patient's name) has a main purpose of identifying what is in the file. However, the label can also include a color-coding stripe that can be used for other purposes, such as identifying the primary care physician. The label on the file drawer contains the topic and the range of files.

For example: Patient Histories

A-D

The label on the divider contains the range of files between that divider and the next.

For example: Aa-Ba

Rules for Filing

Three commonly used systems for filing are the alphabetic, numeric, and subject filing. Alphabetizing is a component of all the methods and will be explained in detail. Color-coding is used in all three systems to assist in locating files, refiling, and prevent misfiling.

Alphabetic System

Alphabetizing is the most common system for filing records in a physician's office (a hospital generally uses an ID numeric system for filing patient records). In this system, Abbott would be filed before Bacon since "A" appears before "B" in the alphabet. If the first letter is the same, then move to the second letter in the name. Abbott is filed before Acker. This does not pose problems when filing a last name since everyone understands the alphabet. However, there could be confusion when filing Jacob James Jergens, Jr. and Jacob James Jergens III, or determining how correspondence from 23rd Avenue Clinic should be filed.

The key to alphabetic filing is to divide the names and titles into units (first, second, and third). The unit is the portion of the name that is used for filing or indexing purposes. For example:

- Unit 1 Jergens
- Unit 2 Jacob
- Unit 3 James

The first letter of each unit is then used to determine where the file is to be placed. When filing a large number of files, use the first letter of the first unit and place all the files from A–Z in order. Then take each group of "A" files and use the second letter and consecutive letters to place them in order. If the entire first unit is the same, as in Smith, then move onto the second unit and third unit. For example, Smith, Loren comes before Smith, Michael, which comes before Smith, Michelle. Table 12-1 describes basic rules for alphabetic filing. Procedure 12-3 lists steps to follow when using the alphabetic filing system.

Numerical Systems

A numerical filing or patient identification system is used in hospitals and many of the larger clinics. A number is assigned to each patient's medical record. This is generally a six-digit number divided into three sections of two digits each (for example, 05-72-21). Veterans Administration hospitals use the social security number with nine digits.

There are several types of numerical filing, including straight numerical filing, filing by terminal digit, middle digit filing, unit numbering, and serial numbering.

STRAIGHT NUMERICAL FILING The simplest numerical method is the straight numerical filing system in which each record is filed sequentially based on its assigned number. The numbers used in this system begin at 01 and continue upward.

Example:	01	101	886
	02	102	887
	03	103	888
	04	104	889

In this type of system, the file space will become depleted rapidly as new files are added to one section. This requires constant re-shifting of files to make room for the new files.

TERMINAL DIGIT FILING Terminal digit filing, based on the last digits of the ID number, evenly distributes the files within the entire filing system, which eliminates the need for frequent re-shifting of files, providing enough space was designated when the filing system was set up. Filing using terminal digits requires dividing the files into 100 primary sections, starting with 00 and ending with 99. The three sections of numbers assigned to each file are designated as tertiary, secondary, and primary sections respectively. To file a record using this system, find the file section matching the patient's primary digits (21). Within that section, match up the secondary digits (72), and file the record according to the tertiary digits (05).

Example:	05	72	21
	tertiary	secondary	primary

Procedure 12-4 lists steps for using the terminal digit filing system.

PROCEDURE

Filing a Record Alphabetically

OBJECTIVE: File a patient record in the correct order, using the alphabetical method for filing.

Equipment and Supplies
patient record; alphabetical files

Method

1. Locate medical record files or medical record room.
2. Observe the name on the record to be filed.
3. Records are filed in alphabetic order by last name first, first name, then middle name or initial. Each letter in the name is a separate unit. Locate the set of records containing the same last name as the record to be filed.
4. Within the set of records containing the same last name as the record to be filed, locate the records with the same letter of the first name as the record to be filed.
5. Using the alphabet as a guide, place the record to be filed after the record that comes before it in the alphabet, but before the record that comes after it in the alphabet.
6. A name with only an initial first name is filed before a full name (Brown, H. is filed before Brown, Henry).
7. Hyphenated names are treated as one unit. (Mary Freeman-Smith is indexed as Freemansmith, Mary).
8. Disregard apostrophes (Megan O'Connor is indexed as Oconnor, Megan).
9. Titles and initials are disregarded for filing, but placed in parentheses after the name, for example, Dr. Beth Ann Williams is indexed as Williams, Beth Ann, (Dr.).
10. Married women are indexed using their legal name. The husband's name can be used for cross-referencing.
11. Seniority units, such as Jr. and Sr., are filed in numerical order from first to last.
12. Numeric seniority terms are filed before alphabetic terms.
13. After placing the file between the two records before and after it in the alphabet, check once more to be sure the file is properly placed.
14. If there is a marker or out-guide in place of the removed record, then take out the marker when replacing the file.
15. Document on the office record that the chart was filed (per office policy).

MIDDLE DIGIT FILING Using the same six-digit numbering system as with the terminal digit system, the middle digit filing system places the middle digits as the primary numbers. In this example, find the section marked 72, within that section find the 05 area, then file the record according to the tertiary digit, 21.

Example:	05	72	21
	secondary	primary	tertiary

UNIT NUMBERING This system assigns a number to patients the first time they are seen or admitted to a hospital. All other hospitalizations or hospital visits use the same number. This method requires that all the records be kept at the same location.

SERIAL NUMBERING With a serial numbering system, the patient receives a different medical record number for each hospital visit. The patient acquires multiple records that are stored at different locations. For example, a hospitalization, laboratory work, and a mammogram will all receive different numbers and be filed within their own systems.

The assigned numbers are kept in an accession record in which numbers in sequential order (1, 2, 3, 4, 5, 6 . . .) have a name placed next to them as each new name is entered. This record can also be maintained on the computer. Figure 12-5 illustrates a medical assistant filing in a medical records room.

Subject Matter

Filing by subject is used for general files, such as invoices, correspondence, resumes, and personnel records. This method is adequate as long as the files are relatively small. If these files become large, then another method, alphabetic or numerical, will have to be devised.

PROCEDURE

Filing a Record Numerically Using the Terminal Digit Filing System

OBJECTIVE: File a patient record in the correct order, using the terminal digit filing method for filing.

Equipment and supplies
patient record; numerical files

Method
1. Locate medical record files or medical record room.
2. Observe the numbers on the record to be filed.
3. Locate the set of files with the same tertiary numbers as the record to be filed (these will be the first 2 numbers on the record).
4. Within the set of records with the same tertiary numbers, locate the row of records with the same secondary numbers as the record to be filed (the secondary numbers are the second 2 numbers on the record).

5. Within the set of records with the same tertiary and secondary numbers as the record to be filed, place the record to be filed in numerical order by primary numbers (last 2 numbers on the record).
6. After placing the file in numerical order by primary numbers, check once more to be sure the file is properly placed.
7. If there is a marker or out-guide in place of the removed record, then take out the marker when replacing the file.
8. Document in the office record that the chart was filed (per office policy).

Color-Coding Systems

To decrease the number of misfiled charts and aid in file retrieval many medical record departments will use a color-coded system on their file folders. This system assigns a color for each number from 0–9. Color bars on the end of each file folder correspond to the medical record number. Usually only the three primary digits are color-coded. When files are in the correct placement, the color bands will all have the same pattern. In this manner, any misfiles are easily seen. Filing records is simplified since the correct color band can be located on the file shelf.

Color Bands

Two popular color-coding methods using a numerical system are the Ames Color File System and the Smead Manufacturing Company's method. Table 12-2 lists examples of the numerical color-coding systems used by these two systems.

There are also color-coded methods using an alphabetic system. One example is the Alpha-Z system by the Smead Manufacturing Company. This system is based on 13 colors using white letters on a colored background (for example, the white letter "A" is on a solid red background) for the first one-half of the alphabet, and the addition of a white stripe on the colored background for the second half of the alphabet

(for example, the letter "N" is a red background with a white stripe).

The Alpha-Z system uses file labels to denote the patient's name, and a color label with the letter of the alphabet to indicate the index unit. For example, Emily Jane Smith would be labeled Smith, Emily Jane with an orange color block containing a white stripe and the letter "S." Two other color blocks

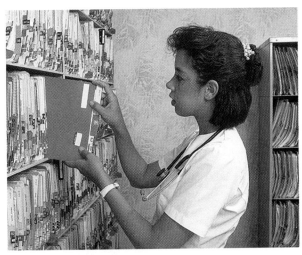

FIGURE 12-5 Medical records room.

TABLE 12-2 Numerical Color-Coding Systems

Ames Color File System	Smead Corporation System
0–red	0–yellow
1–gray	1–blue
2–blue	2–pink
3–orange	3–purple
4–purple	4–orange
5–black	5–brown
6–yellow	6–green
7–brown	7–gray
8–pink	8–red
9–green	9–black

TABLE 12-3 Alpha-Z Alphabetic Color-Coding System

Color	White Letter No Stripe	White Letter White Stripe
Red	A	N
Dark Blue	B	O
Dark Green	C	P
Light Blue	D	Q
Purple	E	R
Orange	F	S
Gray	G	T
Dark Brown	H	U
Pink	I	V
Yellow	J	W
Light Brown	K	X
Lavender	L	Y
Light Green	M	Z

would be added to the label for the secondary and tertiary letters of the index unit (in this example, "E" on a solid purple background, and "J" on a solid yellow background).

This system is ideal for the large practice with many patients having the same surnames. It can be adapted to a particular offices needs. For example, only the last name is color-coded (Joseph Evans has only one solid PURPLE color label). After the files are color-coded, they are then alphabetized within their particular "color" category.

In large practices with several physicians, each physician may have a color assigned to him or her. For example, Dr. Williams' patients might all have medical file folders with a yellow label. This color-coding system is described in Table 12-3. Figure 12-6 shows a color-coded medical record.

In some medical practices, a color-coded "year" tab is placed on folders of patients who are seen once a year. This hastens the purging of "inactive" files.

Cross-Referencing

Due to the large number of files processed in a busy office and the confusion over surnames—(for example, how are step-children's names filed for easy access?), cross-referencing of files is recommended. Cross-referencing refers to alerting the health worker that a file may be found under another name. For example, if Mrs. Henry Watts also uses her maiden name, Farideh Rahman, then a file insert into Henry Watts' file could state, "See Rahman, Farideh for Mrs. Henry Watts." Cross-referencing can be a simple, but useful tool for finding and avoiding "lost" records.

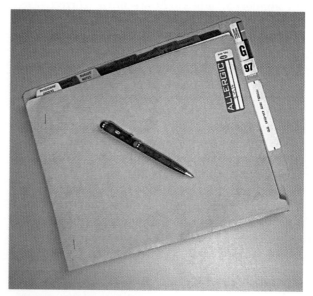

FIGURE 12-6 A color-coded record.

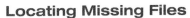

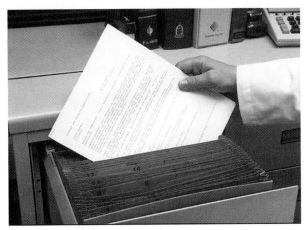

FIGURE 12-7 Tickler file using a file drawer.

Locating Missing Files

One of the most time-consuming and frustrating activities relating to medical records is locating a "missing" file. Ideally, everyone who takes a file from a cabinet should add that file name or number to a master file sheet. In addition, an out-guide should be placed in the file indicating a record was removed.

If a systematic search takes place, the file can usually be located quickly. In the case of one piece of paper that has been misfiled with other papers, it may not be located. In this case, the medical assistant will need to get another copy of the paper from the original source (for example, a laboratory or radiology report).

The best way to avoid losing a file is to file all records methodically and carefully. Guidelines 12-1 lists some ways to help you locate missing files.

Tickler Files

A tickler file is used to remind the medical assistant of an event or action that will take place at a future date. The tickler file contains patient's names and telephone numbers, dates when action or activities should occur, and actions to take. The tickler files should be reviewed on a daily basis so that actions are taken on time. For example, tickler files can be used as reminders to call patients to set appointments, to pay certain invoices, or to send fees for the physician's license renewals. Figure 12-7 is an example of a tickler file, using a file drawer. Figure 12-8 illustrates an index card tickler file.

Quality Assurance for Quality Medical Care

As discussed in Chapter 5, the primary goal of a formal quality assurance program is to improve the quality of care so that there is no difference between what should be done and what is actually being done.

Implementation of such a Quality Assurance Program (QAP) requires the development of patient-centered criteria based on acceptable standards of care. An example of this is the formalization of discharge documents from hospitals.

Incident Report

One means of documenting problem areas within the office or facility is through the incident report. In Chapter 5, an example of a typical incident report is provided. This report should be completed whenever there is an unusual occurrence, such as a fall, error in medication dispensing, needle sticks, fire, or patient complaint. The purpose is to document exactly what happened with the goal of preventing another episode.

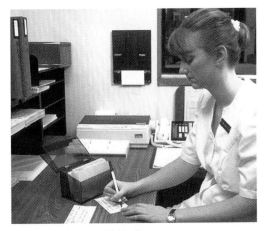

FIGURE 12-8 Index card tickler file.

Details on completing an incident report are usually included in every office's procedure manual.

Measures to Assure Quality Assurance

Quality of patient care can be assessed from within the medical profession by organized groups of physicians. It is also monitored and assessed from outside the profession through governmental or insurance provider intervention.

Joint Commission on Accreditation of Health Organizations (JCAHO)

The Joint Commission on Accreditation of Health Organizations (JCAHO), headquartered in Chicago, Illinois, is a private, nongovernmental agency that establishes guidelines for hospitals and health care agencies to follow regarding quality of care. It is supported by representatives of the American Hospital Association (AHA), American College of Surgeons, American College of Physicians, and the American Dental Association. In addition to forming guidelines for the operation of health care institutions, such as hospitals, ambulatory care facilities, and long-term care institutions, JCAHO conducts surveys and accreditation programs.

JCAHO inspectors visit a health care facility by invitation and review patient medical records, organizations of the medical staff and the general operations of the facility. Some indicators that are used during the survey and accreditation process are mortality rate, frequency of complication, nosocomial infection rate, and autopsy rate. The mortality rate refers to the number of deaths in a given population. Based on their assessment, the inspectors will issue either a full accreditation or provisional accreditation report. The Commission works with facilities to correct any deficiencies within a specified time frame.

JCAHO does not actually have authority or power to take punitive action against a physician or facility for poor treatment. However, the survey results of the JCAHO are used by other agencies, such as the Department of Health and Human Services, that do have the authority to impose a sanction or penalty.

Occupational Safety and Health Administration (OSHA)

The Occupational Safety and Health Administration (OSHA) was established by the U.S. Congress in the Occupational Safety and Health Act of 1970 "to assure so far as possible every working man and woman in the nation safe and healthful working conditions." This act covers every employer whose business affects interstate commerce.

OSHA is the federal agency that has the power to enforce regulations concerning the health and safety of employees. Every office and health care institution must be aware of OSHA recommendations and carefully monitor potential violations. For instance, the Centers for Disease Control (CDC) has issued recommendations for a set of universal precautions that all health care workers must follow when dealing with hazardous materials. The CDC has authorized OSHA to enforce these precautions.

OSHA, in cooperation with other agencies, carries out research to establish basic safety standards. OSHA inspectors carry out frequent, surprise inspections of workplaces to see that standards are maintained. OSHA safety regulations include standards for exposure to noise, asbestos, toxic chemicals, lead, pesticides and cotton dust. Violators of OSHA standards must correct the violations and pay fines if found guilty.

Since July 6, 1992, OSHA standards mandate that all health care employers must provide a means for protecting their employees from potential exposure to Hepatitis B. In fact, every health care employee must be given the choice to elect or refuse the immunization series. If refused, the employee has the right to change his or her mind and receive the immunization series at no charge. All costs associated with this immunization series must be provided by the employer.

HIPAA/Confidentiality of Records

As the demand for both access and confidentiality of medical record information grows, how does the health care provider balance the competing, often clashing, interests? The laws relating to medical recordkeeping and access have been evolving in recent years.

The privacy provisions of the federal law, the Health Insurance Portability and Accountability Act of 1996 (HIPAA), apply to health information created or maintained by health care providers who engage in certain electronic transactions, health plans, and health care clearinghouses. The Department of Health and Human Services (HHS) has issued the regulation, "Standards for Privacy of Individually Identifiable Health Information," applicable to entities covered by HIPAA. The Office for Civil Rights (OCR) is the Departmental component responsible for implementing and enforcing the privacy regulation.

The new rules require medical offices that maintain and transmit health information electronically to do the following.

- Provide reasonable and appropriate safeguards to protect the integrity and confidentiality of health care information.

- Train personnel to protect confidentiality of health care information.

- Provide policies and procedures on security and confidentiality protective measures within the medical office.

Medical information can be shared by a wide range of people, both in and out of the health care industry. Generally, access to medical records is obtained when the patient agrees to let others see them. Occasionally, patient medical information is used for health research and may be disclosed to public health agencies such as the Centers for Disease Control. Specific names are usually not given to researchers. Their use of patient information is covered by HIPAA.

Releasing Medical Records

The physician owns the medical record, but the patient has the legal right of "privileged communication" and access to his or her records. Therefore, the patient must authorize release of his or her records and state in writing that the medical records may be released. An example of a release form is seen in Figure 12-9. Since the patient has access to his or her records, the patient may also request a copy of those records. Since some records are large and require excessive duplicating time and expense, the physician may charge a fee dictated by the state to provide this service.

Health care providers have specific procedures for handling and releasing medical records because of the confidential information contained in the records and because of federal and state laws concerning HIV, mental health, and substance abuse information.

Persons Authorized to Release Records

Generally, only a patient can authorize the release of his or her own medical records. However, there are some exceptions to the rule and generally the following can sign a release:

- Parents of minor children
- Legal guardian
- Agent (someone you select to act on your behalf in a Health Care Power of Attorney)

Under some circumstances, a minor and not the parent must sign the release. If you have questions about who can authorize release of your patient records, check with your health care provider.

Specially Protected Medical Information

Federal law specially protects substance abuse treatment records. Some state laws specially protect HIV/AIDS information and mental health records. These laws are meant to encourage people with these problems to get the medical treatment they need. In order to obtain a copy of the records or have them sent somewhere, you may need to sign a form that specifically mentions this specially protected information.

Disclosure without Consent

Although medical records are confidential, there are times when they can be released without a patient's consent. In special cases, records are released to:

WINDY CITY CLINIC
Beth Williams, M.D.
123 Michigan Avenue
Chicago, IL 60610
(312) 123-1234

RECORDS RELEASE Date ______________

To ______________________________
Doctor
____
Address

I hereby authorize and request you to release

to ______________________________
Doctor
____
Address

all medical records in your possession concerning any examination, diagnosis, and/or treatment rendered to me during the period from __________ to __________

____
Signature of patient or closest relative

____
Relationship

______________________________ ______________________________
Signature of witness Address

FIGURE 12-9 A release form for medical records.

- Health care workers who have a need for the records to care for a patient.
- Qualified people or organizations that perform services, such as data processing, medical record transcription, microfilming, administrative functions, or other such related services.
- Qualified people or organizations for approved research and education functions.
- Certain government authorities, as permitted or required by law, to investigate or regulate health related issues such as child abuse, communicable diseases, and prescription drugs.
- Certain lawyers and parties in a law suit, if a patient's medical condition is an issue in the suit.

Generally, strict rules apply to those who receive medical information. For example, they are often required to have procedures to protect the patient's confidentiality and prevent release of medical information and patient identity.

Storing Medical Records

Medical records may be stored in the medical office, if there is sufficient room, or in another office or building nearby. Or, medical records storage may be outsourced to a business that specializes in managing and housing documents. Investigate the business to ensure that it is reputable and that the files will be safe and accessible. Either way, take steps to ensure that the files will be safe from fire, flood, or other damage (Legal and Ethical Issues).

Medical Transcription

Medical transcription involves translating dictated or written medical information and producing a permanent record into a typed format. The information can relate to a patient's office or hospital visit, a specific hospital report such as radiology, pathology or laboratory, or a manuscript for publication.

There is an absolute need for accuracy to ensure the correct interpretation when editing the physician's dictation. The same professional standard relating to confidentiality is necessary when handling transcription, even though the transcriptionist may never see the patient.

Medical records must be professionally prepared, following appropriate formats. They should be free of errors and correctly filed. Remember medical records are always subject to possible subpoena by a court of law.

Medical Transcriptionists

Transcriptionists are medical professionals, who have excellent typing and grammar skills, knowledge of medical terminology, and a desire for accuracy. The medical transcriptionist must understand words, where and how to apply the words, as well as have proper English grammar skills. This includes an understanding of etymology, phonetics, synonyms, acronyms, antonyms, homonyms, and eponyms.

Sound-Alike Words

Caution must be used when writing words that have the same or similar sound. When taking medical dictation off a recording device, such as a dictaphone, it can be difficult to discern the term based on the physician's pronunciation. To compound the problem, many medical terms actually sound alike when spoken, but have very different meanings.

Transcriptionists must take special precautions when transcribing tapes to make sure they have heard the correct terms. In many cases, the content of the material will determine which is the correct term. For instance, mastitis, meaning an inflammation of a mammary gland, and mastoiditis, an inflammation of the mastoid bone in the middle ear, sound alike in pronunciation. However, the mammary gland in the female breast and the mastoid bone in the ear are located in different body systems and are not generally discussed in the same context.

There are other terms, such as ureter and urethra, which are organs located in close proximity to each other in the urinary system. These two terms must never be confused. When in doubt, always ask the dictating physician to clarify the term for you. You may have to look up the exact definition of the word in a medical dictionary.

Ownership of the Medical Record

The medical assistant is frequently called upon to explain the ownership of medical records and x-ray films. Patient Education explains more about dealing with patients and medical record issues. Although the patient has paid for the film, it is the property of the medical facility that performed the x-ray. Written reports prepared by the radiologist are sent to other physicians at the request of the patient but the film generally remains in the original office. The reason being, if the film remains in one location, it can always be accessed for future examination and comparison. Once it leaves the originating facility, it can be misplaced and lost.

Physicians are able to loan their films to referring physicians for further examination. The patient has to sign a release of records form for this to take place, but the film must then be returned to the original facility. Since films are a permanent record of the patient at a particular moment, they need to be preserved carefully. It is possible, in some locations, for the patient to obtain a duplicate copy of a film. The patient would have to pay for the copy to be made.

Retention and Destruction of Medical Records

From time to time in a practice, the question will arise, "How long should we keep medical records?" While we don't have definitive answers, we can provide you with the following guidelines:

- The medical record is critical in a medical liability action, and its loss may considerably harm the physician in the defense of a claim.

- To be absolutely safe, all medical records should be retained *forever*. However, in many circumstances this is impractical. It is always a good idea to keep a patient's immunization records in case they need it in the future.

- Each state varies somewhat on the legal time limits (statute of limitations) to keep records and documents. It is usually two years and begins to run at the point of discovery of damage and the connection between that damage and the treatment. In some circumstances, this could be many years later. Special rules apply when treating a child or an incompetent patient and the time period is longer.

- Most states require all patient records be retained for two to seven years after the last treatment, or seven years after the patient reaches the age of majority (age 18 or 21 in most states), whichever comes last.

- The American Medical Association recommends keeping medical records for 10 years.

- In selected circumstances, you might consider saving the more complex records or those records with known serious patient problems for a longer period of time.

- The bottom line is there is no absolute answer and the medical assistant must be familiar with state laws.

If a physician cannot retain his or her patient records indefinitely, consideration must be given to the method of destruction. As with any office policy, a medical record destruction policy should follow a written procedure. The procedure should do the following:

- Outline the length of time records will be kept.

- Define which records will be kept on-site and which off-site.

- Designate a person to be responsible for deciding what to keep and what to purge.

- Produce a log that details which patient records have been destroyed, as well as when and how.

- Provide a method of disposal (e.g., shred, pulp, or incinerate) that destroys all information in the record. Patient confidentiality cannot be jeopardized because of an inadequate method of destruction. Many medical offices hire the services of a business that handles the destruction of medical records. That service must agree to abide by HIPAA guidelines.

SUMMARY

Handling a patient's medical record requires an efficient system, which results in few missing or misfiled records. As a medical practice grows, it may be necessary to replace an alphabetic system with a numerical or even a color-coded system. Every medical practice needs a method for alerting staff when a file has been removed from the record area. A tickler system that is used faithfully can reduce the number of omissions, such as forgetting to remind the physician to renew a medical license. Medical transcription work can be a rewarding career for a skilled typist as well.

COMPETENCY REVIEW

1. Define and spell the terms to learn for this chapter.
2. Describe where you would find Emma Holmes' file. She has not been seen by Dr. Williams for two years and there has been no communication with her. Is this an active, inactive, or closed file?
3. Set up a tickler file system for your school assignments during this semester.
4. You are missing a file for Sean Roy. Discuss what process you would use to find this file.
5. Mr. Crosby is angry and demanding that you give him his medical chart so that he can take it to another physician. How do you handle Mr. Crosby's anger and his request for his medical file?

PREPARING FOR THE CERTIFICATION EXAM

1. In filing correspondence for Janelle Louise Daniels (Mrs. Kevin Masters), 123 Valley Drive, Kalispell, MT 59999, which of the following would NOT be used as an indexing unit?
   A. Carey
   B. Daniels
   C. Jerome
   D. Masters
   E. ZIP code

2. What is the third indexing unit in the following name: Mr. Richard Allan Richards, Jr.
   A. Richards
   B. Richard
   C. Allan
   D. Jr.
   E. Mr.

3. The most commonly used filing system is based on what method?
   A. numerical
   B. color coding
   C. alphabetical
   D. unit numbering
   E. straight numbering

4. Dr. Gemma Reingold is filed as
   A. Reingold, Dr. Gemma
   B. Dr. Gemma Reingold
   C. Reingold, Gemma
   D. Reingold, Gemma (Dr.)
   E. Ms. Gemma Reingold

5. Maura Fitzpatrick has been assigned the patient ID number 239431. To search for her file, you will look under 94, then 23, then 31. What system are you using?
   A. unit numbering
   B. middle digit filing
   C. terminal digit filing
   D. straight numbering
   E. service numbering

6. Adrian Washington has been assigned a color using the Alpha-Z color-coding system. Under what color would you find his chart?
   A. lavender with white stripe
   B. light brown
   C. dark brown with white stripe
   D. yellow
   E. yellow with white stripe

7. David Jesse Montgomery III's file would be filed in what order in relation to David Jesse Montgomery, Jr.'s file?
   A. before
   B. after
   C. with David Jesse Montgomery, Jr.'s file
   D. the designations III and Jr. are ignored when filing
   E. Jr's are filed separately

8. VRT is an example of (a/an)
   A. phonetic
   B. synonym
   C. acronym
   D. antonym
   E. etymology

continued on next page

9. Transcription equipment includes all of the following EXCEPT
   A. computer
   B. typewriter
   C. transcriber
   D. word processor
   E. shredder

10. A report containing information about the tissue removed during a surgical procedure is called a/an
    A. consultation report
    B. operative note
    C. pathology report
    D. additional report
    E. history report

CRITICAL THINKING

1. How will you handle Mr. Dewey's request and unpaid balance?
2. What will you do about Mr. Dewey's missing x-ray reports?

ON THE JOB

Marissa Lopez is asked to create a patient file and records for a new patient, Jonathan Schmidt. Please walk Marissa through each step of creating a new patient file, making sure that each component of the file is complete. Use the SOAP section of this chapter as part of your solution. Show how the patient's progress will be tracked by using POMR.

INTERNET ACTIVITY

Search the Internet for the newest legislation in your home state regarding the handling of medical records. Write a summary of the article, and discuss with your class whether the legislation adds to the efficiency of dealing with medical records or creates unnecessary obstacles.

MediaLink More on managing medical records, including interactive resources, can be found on the Student CD-ROM accompanying this textbook.

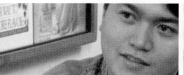

Medical Assistant Role Delineation Chart

HIGHLIGHT indicates material covered in this chapter.

ADMINISTRATIVE

Administrative Procedures

- Perform basic administrative medical assisting functions
- Schedule, coordinate and monitor appointments
- Schedule inpatient/outpatient admissions and procedures
- Understand and apply third-party guidelines
- Obtain reimbursement through accurate claims submission
- Monitor third-party reimbursement
- Understand and adhere to managed care policies and procedures
- *Negotiate managed care contracts*

Practice Finances

- Perform procedural and diagnostic coding
- Apply bookkeeping principles

- Manage accounts receivable
- *Manage accounts payable*
- *Process payroll*
- *Document and maintain accounting and banking records*
- *Develop and maintain fee schedules*
- *Manage renewals of business and professional insurance policies*
- *Manage personnel benefits and maintain records*
- *Perform marketing, financial, and strategic planning*

CLINICAL

Fundamental Principles

- Apply principles of aseptic technique and infection control
- Comply with quality assurance practices
- Screen and follow up patient test results

Diagnostic Orders

- Collect and process specimens
- Perform diagnostic tests

Patient Care

- Adhere to established patient screening procedures
- Obtain patient history and vital signs
- Prepare and maintain examination and treatment areas
- Prepare patient for examinations, procedures and treatments

- Assist with examinations, procedures and treatments
- Prepare and administer medications and immunizations
- Maintain medication and immunization records
- Recognize and respond to emergencies
- Coordinate patient care information with other health care providers
- Initiate IV and administer IV medications with appropriate training and as permitted by state law

GENERAL

Professionalism

- Display a professional manner and image
- Demonstrate initiative and responsibility
- Work as a member of the health care team
- Prioritize and perform multiple tasks
- Adapt to change
- Promote the CMA credential
- Enhance skills through continuing education
- Treat all patients with compassion and empathy
- Promote the practice through positive public relations

Communication Skills

- Recognize and respect cultural diversity
- Adapt communications to individual's ability to understand
- Use professional telephone technique

- Recognize and respond effectively to verbal, nonverbal, and written communications
- Use medical terminology appropriately
- Utilize electronic technology to receive, organize, prioritize and transmit information
- Serve as liaison

Legal Concepts

- Perform within legal and ethical boundaries
- Prepare and maintain medical records
- Document accurately
- Follow employer's established policies dealing with the health care contract
- Implement and maintain federal and state health care legislation and regulations
- Comply with established risk management and safety procedures
- Recognize professional credentialing criteria
- *Develop and maintain personnel, policy and procedure manuals*

Instruction

- Instruct individuals according to their needs
- Explain office policies and procedures
- Teach methods of health promotion and disease prevention
- Locate community resources and disseminate information
- *Develop educational materials*
- *Conduct continuing education activities*

Operational Functions

- Perform inventory of supplies and equipment
- Perform routine maintenance of administrative and clinical equipment
- Apply computer techniques to support office operations
- *Perform personnel management functions*
- *Negotiate leases and prices for equipment and supply contracts*

- *Denotes advanced skills.*

SOURCE: Reprinted by permission of the American Association of Medical Assistants from the AAMA Role Delineation Study: Occupational Analysis of the Medical Assisting Profession.

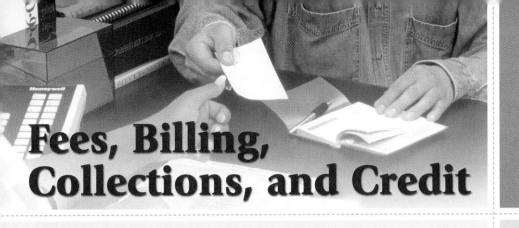

chapter 13

Fees, Billing, Collections, and Credit

Learning Objectives

After completing this chapter, you should be able to:

- Define and spell the terms to learn for this chapter.
- Discuss how fees are determined and be able to discuss this with patients.
- Discuss the patient information required at the time of registration and thereafter to maintain the records needed for billing.

- Discuss credit policy.
- Describe the various billing methods and preparation of billing statements.
- Discuss the collection process and the legalities involved.
- Understand the procedures for aging accounts.

Terms to Learn

accounting	ledger card	superbill
accounts receivable	post	third-party payer
age analysis	professional courtesy (PC)	Truth in Lending Act
assignment of benefits	statute of limitations	usual, customary, and
bookkeeping	subscriber	reasonable (UCR)

Case Study

A NEW PATIENT COMES INTO your office for a new patient evaluation. This patient is a referral from another doctor, and has never been to this office before. The office policy states that any deductibles and co-payments are collected at the time of the patient visit. After submission of the bill to an insurer, the balance owed is billed to the patient, and the patient is expected to pay within 30 days.

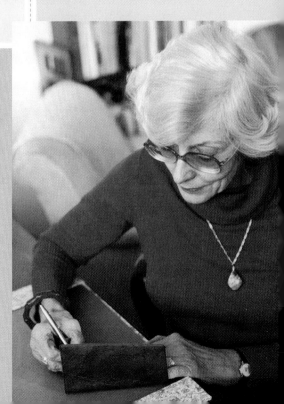

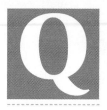

Quality service to the patient is the primary concern of any medical practice. However, revenue is also necessary to maintain a viable business. The process of setting up a fee schedule, extending credit, billing, and collection are an important part of the practice. To ensure and maintain a sound billing and collection system, the medical assistant must be aware of the importance that patients understand their financial responsibility to the doctor and to offer assistance in setting up financial arrangements.

Professional Fees

The fee is determined by the physician or the practice's partners as a result of taking into consideration the time and services involved as well as the prevailing rate fee in the community (Figure 13-1). The economic level of the community and the average fee charged will determine the prevailing rate fee.

Fees charged for medical services are referred to as usual, customary, and reasonable.

- The usual fee is what a physician usually charges for a procedure or service.

- Customary refers to the fee charged for the same procedure by the majority of physicians with the same or similar training to perform the same procedure. This fee is also based on the socioeconomic and geographical area.

- A reasonable fee is what a physician charges for a modified procedure or service that is more difficult and requires more time and effort.

Government sponsored insurance programs maintain a record of the usual charges submitted for specific services by individual doctors. The physician will make the final determination as to what the fees for services

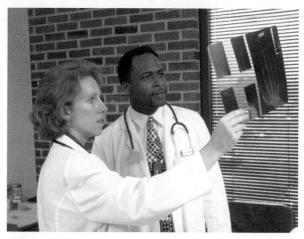

FIGURE 13-1 A physician's services frequently involve consultation with other staff members.

will be. It is the medical assistant's responsibility to convey this information to the patient in a positive, responsible manner.

It is necessary to initiate a discussion of fees with patients and inform them of costs, office financial policies, and credit procedures so they can plan for medical expenses. Patients are entitled to an accurate estimate of their obligations. The medical assistant must become comfortable with these discussions. It is suggested to provide all of this information prior to the patient's first visit. This can be accomplished through the initial telephone contact and by providing a hardcopy of the materials via the U.S. Postal Service. A thorough knowledge of the physician's practice and policies will help to handle any misunderstandings, and would minimize collection problems later. Patient Education discusses more on keeping the patient informed to financial matters.

Posted information regarding payment policies and fees helps patients become aware of office procedures. It also encourages discussion of such matters. Some medical offices have a statement displayed addressing the

Patient Education

The patient must have a thorough understanding of office policy with regards to financial matters. The initial visit to the office should include information on fees, payment, and financial arrangements. This can be addressed in a patient information booklet or pamphlet given to the patient. Patients who will require surgical or other medical procedures should be made aware of fees, insurance allowances, and methods of payment. The patient must understand that he or she has the ultimate responsibility for all charges.

The informed patient will have a clear understanding of all obligations to the office and will be more likely to discuss financial arrangements. This mutual understanding helps to minimize the problems of collection for delinquent accounts.

issue of fee policy. For example, a plastic surgeon's statement may include actual fees for services. A typed fee schedule should be available for quick reference. The medical assistant, if instructed by the physician, should be able to quote fees or a range of fees from this schedule. This schedule is approved by the physician and will be updated as needed. Medical offices should post a notification that states "Payment is due on the date of service" in a prominent area for patients to view.

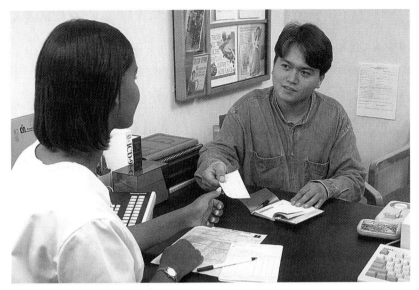

FIGURE 13-2 Payment at the time of medical service is the preferred method.

Billing

Payment of medical services can be achieved in one of three ways. First, there is payment at the time of the services, which is the preferred method (Figure 13-2). The second payment method is billing the patient for services and extending credit. The third, and usually the least desirable, is the use of outside collection assistance.

The medical assistant needs to become familiar with health insurance coverage and the differences in the various plans. As HMOs, IPAs, and PPOs become a major influence in medical practices, the levels of benefits, co-payments, and deductibles are important aspects of the fee and billing process. Patients can become easily confused about these matters, so health care providers and their staff need to be knowledgeable in these areas. See Chapter 15 for an explanation of HMOs, IPAs, and PPOs.

No matter which type of bill service is used in the medical office, each patient must sign a consent form that allows the medical office to bill the insurance carrier for services provided. This form should be placed on file and updated annually. Medicare requires specific wording on consent forms. For the most accurate wording, visit MedLearn at www.cms.gov. Each year the Center for Medicare and Medicaid Services (CMS) distributes a CD to health care providers that contains the updated fee schedule and general information on Medicare payment schedules and payment policies. The CD also provides an immediate gateway to the MedLearn Web site.

Billing Methods

The faster you bill a patient or insurance company, the faster you will receive payment. Billing methods depend on the preferences and policies of the medical office. Billing may be performed internally, generated by the physician's office, or externally, through the use of a billing service. External billing is used with large volume billing. Internal billing can include the use of the superbill, or encounter form, ledger card, and follow-up mailed statements.

Superbill/Encounter Form

The superbill (charge/encounter slip) is the document generated by the medical office and used as a charge slip, statement, and insurance reporting form (Figure 13-3). This document is a two- or three-part carbonized form that performs several functions. It provides a comprehensive list of patient services, with respective codes and fees, on which the physician indicates with a check mark the services that have been rendered. The superbill can be used to input computer information for billing, and it provides the patient with a record of the account activity (charges, payments, adjustments) for the day of service and, thus, can be used as a receipt. It also provides a record that can be used for insurance purposes. The third copy can be kept in the patient's file.

Ledger card

Statements may be handwritten, typewritten, or photocopies of the ledger card. The ledger card is used to record the charges, adjustments, and payments for the patient. The statement must be good quality and large enough to allow itemization of charges. Photocopied statements must be clear and legible and can be sent in a window envelope. Envelopes should be imprinted with ADDRESS CORRECTION REQUESTED under the return address.

Accurate information is absolutely necessary when billing patients. Good records are essential to follow-up with collections. The patient registration form is a

TEXAS CARDIOLOGY   877 555-1212

Patient Number	Ticket Number	Service Date	Prior Balance / Pat
Patient Name		Gender	Ins
Address		Phone	Other
SSN	Referring Dr.		Total
Primary Insurance Co.	Policy/Group ID		Paymt
Secondary Insurance Co.	Policy/Group ID		Bal Due

X	Code	Service
		New Patient
	99203	Limited/Simple (30m)
	99204	Comprehensive (45m)
	99205	Complex (60m)
		New Patient Consult
		(Need Referring MD)
	99243	Brief (40m)
	99244	Full Consult (60m)
	99245	Very Complex (80m)
		Established Patient
	99211	Nurse Visit
	99212	Very Brief FU (10m)
	99213	Limited/Simple FU (15m)
	99214	Comprehensive FU (25m)
	99215	Complex FU (40m)
		New Cons. 2nd Opin.
	99274	Moderate 2nd Opinion
	99275	Complex 2nd Opinion
		Home Health
	99375	Home Health 30 days
		Drugs:
	J3420	B-12 Injection
	J1940	Lasix
	90724	Flu (Dx V-04.8)
	G0008	MC Flu Admin Fee
		Misc Rx _____
	90782	IM Injections
	90784	IV Injections
	A4615	O2 Cannula

Location (checkboxes)   **Cardiologist** (checkboxes)

X	Code	Service
		Office Procedures
	93000	EKG w/ Interp
	93015	Stress Tread w/ Interp
	93040	Rhythm strip w/ Interp
	93307	2D Echo Compl.
	93320	Doppler Compl.
	93325	Color Flow Compl.
	93308	2D Echo F/U
	93321	Doppler F/U
	ES	Stress Echo
	BUB	Echo/Bubble/Doppler
		Event Monitor
	93268	Loop- Non MC
	G0005	Loop - Hookup - MC
	G0007	Loop - Interp - MC
	93012	Chest Plate Tech - Non MC
	93014	Chest Pl - Interp Non MC
	G0016	Chest Pl - Interp MC
		Holter Monitor
	93224	Holter w/ Interp Global
		Other
	92960	Cardioversion
	93734	Pacer Eval - Single
	93735	Pacer Eval - Sngl w/ Prg
	93731	Pacer Eval - Dual
	93732	Pacer Eval - Dual w/ Prg
	99499	Review outside records
	99080	Special Reports

X	Code	Service
		Diagnostic w/o Interp
		(Technical only)
	93005	EKG
	93017	Stress Tread
	93225	Holter Hookup
	93226	Holter Scan
	93307-TC	2D Echo
	93320-TC	Doppler Compl.
	93325-TC	Color Flow
	93308-TC	2D Echo F/U
	93321-TC	Doppler F/U
	93880-TC	Carotid Doppler
	Phys	**Interpretation-Supervision, Interpretation & Report Only**
	93010	EKG Interp & Reortt only
	TR	Regular Stress Test--S, I & R
	NU	Nuclear Stress Test--S, I & R
	ES-26	Stress Echocardiogram--S, I & R
	307	Echocardiogram 2-D
	320-26	Doppler Echocardiogram
	325-26	Color Flow
	308	Echocardiogram 2-D F/U
	321-26	Doppler F/U
	227	Holter Monitor - I & R only
	71250-26	UltraFast CT
	XXXXX	**LAB ORDERED** (see attached sheet)
	36415	VeniPuncture (non MC)
	99000	Specimen Collection (Lab)

Next Appointment:
Return in: _____ (Wks) (Mo) (Yr)

Before next appointment:
☐ Ekg ☐ Echo ☐ Doppler ☐ CXR ☐ Event Monitor
☐ TM ☐ Stress Echo ☐ CFD ☐ Holter ☐ Lab

BI:

Hospital Admission:
☐ Admit Cath
☐ Admit to _____ unit at: _____
☐ BAP ☐ WMC ☐ CMC ☐ SHMC
☐ Other:

Notes:

Cardiac Diagnoses

FIGURE 13-3   A superbill has multiple uses.

good way to establish an information base. The following information is needed to maintain a current billing file for each patient and should be included on the registration form:

Full name of patient (If the patient is a minor, then the full name and address of the parent or guardian is also needed)

Date of birth

Address (residence and mailing address, do NOT accept a post office box only)

Telephone number (home, work, and cell phone)

Occupation and employer (employer's address and telephone number)

Nearest relative (address and telephone number)

Insurance information (company name, address, and telephone number)

Designated insurance identification number and group number

Driver's license number

If the patient and the subscriber, or the person who holds the insurance policy, are the same, this information is taken only once. If the patient is covered under a policy held by another family member (the subscriber), then the complete information is taken from the subscriber. Patient billing information should be updated every six months to one year by having patients fill out new forms.

Once the account has been set up, the medical assistant must be made aware of any changes in information. Patients should be reminded at each visit of the need to inform the office of any changes in information with particular attention to changes of address, telephone number, employer, and insurance information. A notice can be posted at the reception desk as a reminder to patients. The receptionist should also ask if the patient has any changes in information at the time the patient checks in.

Manual Billing

Manual billing was used by physician offices prior to the use of computerized billing. The bookkeeping system was all manual and all billing was generated by the office. Most medical offices have converted to computerized billing because it is more cost effective and efficient. Lifespan Considerations addresses employees that may not be computer-prepared.

Computerized Billing

Computer software is available for internal billing purposes; however, many offices with regular, monthly,

Lifespan
Considerations

Since in recent years the medical office has become computerized, many older employees may not be computer-prepared. The office should provide training for these individuals so they can be a productive part of the team.

large-volume billing utilize outside computerized billing services. Many different computer programs exist and can be custom designed for the needs of the office (Figure 13-4). Database programs will include patient information, procedure and diagnosis codes, and insurance companies. Options are available to print statements, ledgers, and receipts. Professionalism has more on privacy of patient information stored on the computer.

The Billing Period: Frequency of Billing

Consistency with billing procedures is very important. The medical assistant must have a thorough understanding of office policy with regards to the timing of billing. When a billing date for an account has been established, it is extremely important not to vary the timing of the mailing statements.

There are two types of billing: once-a-month billing and cycle billing. Once-a-month billing requires that statements leave the office in time to reach the patient no later than the last day of the month. Cycle billing requires that certain portions of the accounts receivable are billed at given times during the month. For example, patients whose names begin with A-F would be billed on the first of the month, G-L on the seventh, and so on. The advantages of cycle billing over once-a-month billing are: the avoidance of once-a-month work overload, and stabilization of cash flow. The medical assistant can handle routine duties each day with the inclusion of statements, rather than intensive billing responsibilities once a month. By spacing the billing periods, more time can be given to each statement.

Patients must be made aware of the timing of billing statements. If a change is made, patients should be notified. This can be done by enclosing a notice of billing policy changes in each statement, two months prior to the change.

Billing Third-Party Payers and Minors

Third-party payers include a party or person other than the patient, such as an insurance company, who assumes responsibility for paying the patient's bill. Patient registration should include information regarding insurance. Patients should be asked to provide all insurance identification cards and copies should be made and kept in the patient's file.

A signed assignment of benefits form, can be used by the office to ensure that insurance payments are made directly to the physician. Legal and Ethical Issues has more on privacy policies and patients' rights.

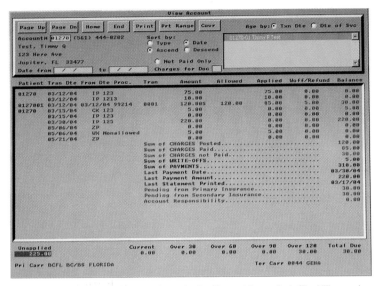

FIGURE 13-4 Computer programs can be customized to meet the medical office billing needs.

Bills for minors are addressed to parents or legal guardians (Figure 13-5). Minors are not responsible for bills unless they are declared emancipated. The parent or the subscriber to the primary insurance policy who brings the child for treatment is responsible for payment. Financial agreements between divorced or separated parents is the personal business of the parents. However, if documentation exists in the minor's file as to financial responsibility, then that party should be billed.

Credit Policy

Payment at the time of service is the ideal method of collection. The medical assistants at the front desk need to overcome any inhibitions regarding discussion of fees and payments. Patients can be informed when they call to schedule an appointment of office policies regarding payment. This is the first step in the collections process. Patients not prepared to pay at the time of service should receive a billing statement

Professionalism

Personal information about patients that is stored in the computer or on disks is just as private as information that is stored in paper files, and should be treated as such. Never allow the computer screen to be turned so that anyone but the operator can see it. Never leave the computer, even for a short time, without logging out and removing all patient information from the screen.

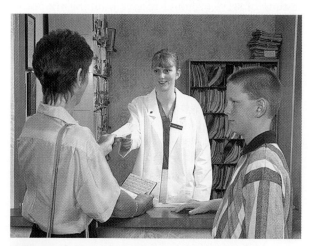

Legal and Ethical Issues

Financial information regarding the patient is confidential. All discussions whether in person or on the telephone should be conducted in an area that is out of view and hearing of other patients. Credit information about a patient is also confidential and may not be released without the patient's expressed permission. Statements outlining credit arrangements and interest charges must be in writing. If the responsibility for payment is to be handled by a person other than the patient, a signed statement by the third party is necessary to verify this obligation. In accordance with HIPAA, the physician is allowed to release a patient's outstanding balance to collection agencies.

when they leave the office with a request to send payment immediately.

The medical assistant must find out the policies the physician wants administered and consistently and fairly maintain them. A credit policy is an important part of any accounts receivable system.

Often payment is collected upon completion of the service. When payment is deferred, credit arrangements must be made. This is best done during the patient's initial visit. All necessary information should be gathered from the patient with regard to demographics, insurance, employment, and signatures.

The medical assistant must have an understanding of the federal laws affecting credit. One of the most important is Regulation Z of the Truth in Lending Act (formerly the Consumer Protection Act of 1968) that was

FIGURE 13-5 A parent or legal guardian is responsible for a minor's medical bills.

enacted to protect the consumer. This is an agreement between doctor and patient to accept payment in more than four installments. Under this act the physician must provide disclosure of information regarding finance charges. When there are to be no finance charges, the agreement form should be completed stating this fact. The original form is given to the patient and a copy is retained by the doctor. The disclosure must be very specific and the patient must sign it in the medical assistant's presence.

Credit bureaus operate as sources of credit data on individuals. Many of them specialize in medical and dental collections. They may supply data verifying a patient's employment, residence, and payment history. The medical office needs to be sure that it is working with a reputable credit bureau.

Collections

Every medical office should have a collection policy in place, as it is not advantageous to the office to have a haphazard method for collecting overdue accounts. The medical assistant must understand the collection policy of the medical practice and must administer it consistently and fairly according to the physician's directives. Most practices have a collection process in place that allows for timely and effective collections. Guidelines 13-1 are useful in creating and maintaining positive collection procedures.

Collection Process

Accounts that are extremely overdue become very difficult and costly to collect. Patients need to be educated on billing and collection procedures so that there is a clear understanding of the financial expectations. The patient information booklet given to new patients should have a section outlining office policy regarding billing and col-

13-1 GUIDELINES

Collections

- Seek immediate payment.
- Use charge slips or superbills.
- Secure accurate patient information and update as needed.
- Inform patient at the time of the appointment of possible fees and responsibility.
- Outline all fees and finance charges for the patient.
- Confirm third party responsibility.
- Bill consistently following office policy.
- Institute collection procedures as needed with personal interview, telephone calls, and letters.
- Follow up on all commitments by the patient.

lection. This information may be also distributed in a formal financial policy document. Patients need to be encouraged to openly discuss problems or questions they might have with respect to their bills.

The reasons a bill is outstanding will vary. Some reasons are:

- The patient does not feel that the bill is important.
- The patient is unable to pay (for varying reasons).
- The patient has a misunderstanding about the fee.

The medical assistant must determine, in a timely manner, the reason that payments are overdue in order to address it, and continue with the collection process. When all normal collection efforts are exhausted and the account is slated for collection, the medical office can consider a "written off" policy for a designated predetermined amount that may be forgiven and becomes lost revenue. This is only considered when the cost of the collection efforts is greater than the designated predetermined amount. For example if the patient's bill is $80.00 and the cost of collection efforts exceeds $80.00, there would be an office policy and procedure in the office manual stating the specific threshold amount for collection services.

Delinquent Accounts

Failure to collect delinquent accounts affects the medical practice in many ways. Patients who owe money may stay away from the office out of embarrassment due to their financial situation. Failure to collect delinquent accounts may imply guilt on the part of the physician as to the quality of care that the patient received. Ultimately, failure to collect delinquent accounts burdens the entire practice due to lost revenue.

Aging Accounts Receivable

It is extremely important to age all accounts receivable. Age analysis refers to the process of determining how long an account has been past due, and then instituting the necessary collection procedures. Computerized systems will allow the medical assistant to print out an aging report with a 30-day, 60-day, and 90-day and over analysis. This can be used to determine the next collection step. Manual systems may use a coding system to age accounts with various colors or flags to indicate the different ages. These may be attached directly to the patient's ledger card.

Collection Techniques

The medical office may employ several methods of collection. Reminder notices, telephone calls, collection letters, and finally a collection agency may be used. The physician decides office policy regarding collection of overdue payments; the medical assistant has responsibility to carry out the policy consistently and fairly.

A personal interview can be a very effective collection method. The patient who is seen in the office for an appointment and has an outstanding account is readily available for discussion with the office staff. This is the time to tactfully bring attention to the overdue account and to make arrangements with the patient for payment.

Reminder notices can be placed on bills when mailed to patients asking for their prompt attention to a past due bill. Other reminder notices may ask a patient to contact the office if there is a question about the past due bill. When no payment or contact is made, then a reminder letter is sent. It should not be a form letter but rather an individual letter that lets the patient know that his or her account is being reviewed and there is concern as to the unpaid debt. Tactful, professional telephone calls may also become part of the collection process and sometimes can be more effective than the letter. The last option may be the use of a collection agency when all other attempts at collection have failed.

Regulations

There are some general rules to follow when attempting to collect overdue accounts and there are laws that govern issues regarding collection such as the Fair Debt Collection Practices Act. Office staff involved with billing and collections need to be familiar with their particular state laws when applying collection techniques. Guidelines 13-2 provide basic rules to assist in the task of making collections.

13-2   GUIDELINES

Making Collections

- Never threaten an action that you do not intend to take. For example, do not tell the patient that his or her account will be handed over to a collection agency if full payment is not received by this afternoon.
- Do not make a collection telephone call before 8 A.M. or after 9 P.M., and do not call on Sundays and holidays.
- Do not make a collection call to the patient's workplace.
- Carefully identify the person accepting the telephone call. Do not discuss a delinquent account with anyone except the debtor.
- Never raise your voice, use profane language, or show anger in any way.
- Do not misrepresent yourself, by implying you are someone other than who you are.
- Do not charge interest unless the debtor has agreed to make 4 (or more) installment payments at a particular rate of interest.
- Do not harass or intimidate the debtor.

As previously stated, violation of these rules could be an offense under the Fair Debt Collection Practices Act, which is a federal law that protects debtors from harassment.

It is important not to make threatening statements that will not be pursued. Collection telephone calls must be between the hours of 8 A.M. and 9 P.M. Avoid calling debtors at their place of employment. Never use a postcard or put an overdue notice on the outside of an envelope.

Telephone Collections

A telephone call at the right time and in the right manner can be more effective than a letter. The medical assistant must be sure to make the call tactful, brief, and to the point. Make sure that all conversation is with the debtor. A firm commitment to make payment should be obtained before ending the conversation. If there is no result by the date mutually agreed upon,

then the next step in the collection process must be instituted. When calling and finding the debtor is not available, only a message should be left stating that the individual needs to contact the office.

Collection Letters

The personalized letter has many advantages over the form letter. Patients who receive the personalized letter will feel that their account has been reviewed individually rather than just another form letter that has been sent to every patient with an overdue balance. The letter may be inserted with the statement. The letter should inquire why the bill has not been paid. There should be an offer to assist the patient with making payment arrangements. The letter must convey the message that action will be taken to resolve the payment obligation. Figure 13-6 provides an example of a reminder letter.

Special Problems

Even with the best billing and collection system, problems will arise making collection a challenge for the medical assistant. A "skip" is a collection problem that requires immediate action because this individual has a balance due and has moved without leaving a forwarding address. The greater the amount of time it takes to locate the "skip," the less likely you will receive payment. Skips can be traced by checking the registration form to confirm addresses, calling telephone numbers, and calling references without divulging the nature of the call. "Address Correction Requested" on the returned statement envelope may help to get the patient's statement delivered. The post office may charge a fee for "Address Correction Requested," but it is a sound investment nonetheless.

Bankruptcy

A patient who files for bankruptcy is protected by the court. When notice is received of a patient's bankruptcy, all collection attempts must cease and the medical office must file a claim for payment with the courts.

Claims against Estates

When a patient dies, a bill should be sent to the estate of the deceased. Contacting next of kin will provide

WINDY CITY CLINIC
Beth Williams, M.D.
123 Michigan Avenue, Chicago, IL 60610
(312) 123-1234

Date

Patient Name
Street Address
City, State and ZIP Code

Dear Patient:

Your balance of $400.00 has been on our books for 18 months. Normally at this time, because your payment is long past due, your account would be handed over to our collection agency. However, we prefer to hear from you regarding your preference in this matter.

Please check one of the following options, and return this letter to our office:

☐ I would prefer to settle this account. Payment in full is enclosed.

☐ I would like to make regular weekly/monthly payments of $_____ until this account is paid in full. My first payment is enclosed.

☐ I don't believe that I owe this amount for the following reasons(s):

_____

_____

_____

_____
patient's signature

Failure to return this letter will result in turning this account over to a collection agency.

Sincerely Yours,

Beth A. Williams, M.D.

FIGURE 13-6 A reminder letter.

information regarding who is the administrator of the estate. It is important to follow up with the collection of bills to prevent any impression of physician's fault for medical care of the deceased patient.

Statute of Limitations

Statute of limitations refers to the amount of time a legal collection suit may be brought against a debtor. This will vary state to state and should be verified with state agencies. If you have aging accounts that are more than three years old, you should investigate the statute of limitations in your state before spending time, effort, and money to collect the debt.

Using a Collection Agency

Professional collection agencies are available for use when all other collection attempts fail. Be sure to review the account with the physician before turning it over for collection. The collection agency should be chosen carefully. Reputable agencies will have references that can be checked and will readily discuss their collection methods. Further checks can be done with the Better Business Bureau and national credit agencies. If possible, interview the collection agency prior to choosing one. The agency should be professional and willing to discuss collection procedures with you.

Collection agencies charge for their services either by a flat fee per account or a percentage of the amount collected. In either case, the physician's office needs to be aware of the costs involved when using this method to collect past due accounts. Be certain not to include the patient's diagnosis when turning over an account for collection. This is a violation of the patient's privacy and the HIPAA guidelines.

Once the patient is told his or her account is going to a collection agency, it must, by law, be turned over to collection. After the account has been turned over, no further collection attempts can be made by the physician's office. The collection agency will need copies of patient information, such as itemized statements showing the dates and amounts of all transactions. Again do not include the patient diagnosis. If the patient should contact the office after the account has been turned over for collection, the patient should be referred to the collection agency.

Accounting Systems

Accounting is the system of reporting the financial results of a business. The basis of accounting is the ability to make an analysis, statement, or summary about financial matters. Many physicians hire an accountant or accounting service to prepare tax returns and prepare financial statements that are used to obtain bank financing. If the physician is in a partnership with other physicians, the accountant's financial statements will assist in dividing the earnings among the partners. Providing accurate financial records to the accountant is one of the medical assistant's responsibilities.

Bookkeeping is the process of managing the accounts for a business. Bookkeeping is a continual process and should be done on a daily basis. The medical assistant or office manager may assume this duty, or the medical practice could hire a bookkeeper. All receipts and charges should be entered immediately into a daily journal, day sheet, or record. Receipts, in duplicate, must be written for all money received. One copy is given to the patient and one copy stays in the office file.

Bookkeeping is a precise skill requiring great attention to detail. Most offices use computer software for bookkeeping. However, the manual method is still used in some smaller offices. Guidelines 13-3 for manual bookkeeping provided here or those followed in your office offer sound, basic rules for the beginning or practiced bookkeeper. Preparing for Externship has more on bookkeeping and computer skills in a medical office.

13-3 GUIDELINES

Manual Bookkeeping

- Use a black pen and clear penmanship. Do not use pencil.
- Keep the columns straight with decimal points lined up.
- Check all arithmetic carefully for errors, such as misplaced decimal points or errors in adding and subtracting.
- Do not erase, write over, or use opaque correction fluid. Make all corrections by drawing a straight line through the incorrect figure and writing the correct figure above it.
- Try to work in a quiet place each day without interruptions. Bookkeeping should not be done at the front desk while answering the telephone and greeting patients.
- Pay close attention to detail.
- Form all numbers carefully to avoid errors in calculations. Use care to avoid transposing numbers (for example: 79 instead of 97).
- Always find errors as soon as they appear. Do not carry the error forward in the account books.
- Double check every entry.
- Do not discuss patient financial records with other staff members. They are confidential.

Before going into the externship, every medical assistant student should be able to stroke at least 35 words per minute. This should be the minimum, and more is better. Accuracy is of paramount importance. In addition, a basic mathematics or bookkeeping course is extremely helpful, if only for learning the basic language. A course in basic computer operation is also necessary.

Patient Accounts

The medical office is unique as a business because its services are not always paid for at the time of delivery, as would be the case in a business such as retailing. Patient accounts require careful bookkeeping. The bookkeeper or medical assistant must be sure that when insurance payments are received, they are correctly posted, or recorded, ensuring that patient's statements are accurate, and that the physician receives payments for services rendered. Most medical offices are run on a "cash" basis, which means that the charge for a medical service is entered in the financial records as income only when the payment is received. Many businesses, such as retailers and merchants, use the accrual basis of accounting for income, which enters income when the service is rendered, even if a payment has not been received. For an example of the components of a manual patient billing system, see Figure 13-7.

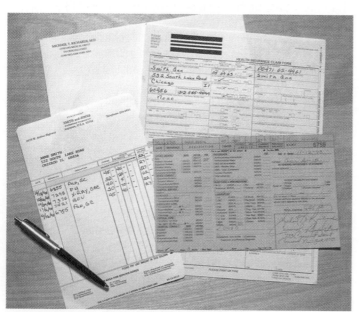

FIGURE 13-7 Components of the manual billing system.

The physician needs to be paid for the procedures done in the office. The medical assistant may need to ensure that patient accounts are in balance with financial obligations (See Procedure 13-1).

Accounts Receivable

Money owed to the physician is called accounts receivable. The accounts receivable ledger is a journal containing a record of all patients' accounts. Terms that relate to accounts receivable are:

- Credit—indicates that a payment has been received on an account or money paid. To credit an account means to record a payment to the account. A patient has a credit balance when a payment exceeds a charge.

- Debit—indicates that a charge has been entered into the account or money owed. To debit an account means to subtract from that account. In some methods of bookkeeping, debits are entered in red. If the balance of the account is negative (a debit balance), this can be indicated by placing the total in red ink or in brackets. A physician's practice usually operates with a debit balance since the total charges to patients exceed the amount paid by all the patients due to the lag time in payment from insurers and others.

- Adjustment—indicates entering a change into the account record such as a discount, write-off, or an amount not allowed by an insurance company (disallowance). A discount is entered as a credit since this amount will be subtracted from the total amount owed.

- Balance—indicates the difference between the debit (money owed) and the credit (money paid).

Accounts Receivable Insurance
Accounts receivable insurance may be purchased to protect against accounts receivable loss. The accounts receivable balance is reported each month and ledgers are kept in a secure place within the office.

Accounts Payable

Accounts payable are the amounts the physician owes to others for equipment and services that have not yet been paid. Examples of accounts payable expenditures in a medical office are:

- Office supplies, such as paper goods, day sheets, appointment cards, scheduling books.
- Medical supplies and equipment.
- Equipment repair and maintenance including housekeeping.
- Utilities such as telephone and electric.
- Taxes.
- Payroll.
- Rent.

Perform Accounts Receivable

OBJECTIVE: Demonstrate skills to ensure that patient accounts are in balance and financial obligations are met in a timely manner.

Equipment and Supplies
data; computer or ledger; telephone

Method
1. Review the accounts receivable account aging.
2. Determine if third party (insurance) payments have been received and posted to the patient accounts being reviewed.
3. Contact insurance carriers to resolve any outstanding payments, according to the facility policies.

4. Update patient account with appropriate notes.

Charting Example
Contacted Marty Shapiro at United Healthcare. He stated that check for $169 for services rendered to patient was sent on December 12, 2005. Have placed notice in tickler file to call again next week.

Records relating to accounts payable include the purchase orders, packing slips that come with the delivered goods, and the invoice requesting payment. The medical assistant, or bookkeeper, who is handling accounts payable payments must carefully document the payment made on the check stub and place the check number and date paid onto the retained invoice copy.

Bookkeeping Systems

Most medical practices today use computerized bookkeeping rather than manual. Manual bookkeeping, however, is still used in many offices where you may work. Manual bookkeeping means that an item is entered by hand and is calculated using a hand calculator. Computerized bookkeeping is most often utilized by medical practices for efficiency and accuracy. Many software programs are available for this purpose. Medical practices use two basic types of bookkeeping systems: single-entry and double-entry. The following are examples of manual bookkeeping.

Single-Entry Bookkeeping

In a single-entry system, the bookkeeper or medical assistant records all financial transactions into the bookkeeping system just once. He or she makes a single-entry. This is a simple system to learn, inexpensive, and requires only three key records:

- Journal, or day sheet, which is also called the daily journal, or log.
- The cash payment journal. (See Figure 13-8 for an illustration of one type of cash payment record—the checkbook and stubs.)
- The accounts receivable ledger contains a record of the money owed to the physician.

Some offices will also have a journal for payroll records and petty cash (Figure 13-9). Petty cash vouchers are used to identify petty cash expenses (Figure 13-10).

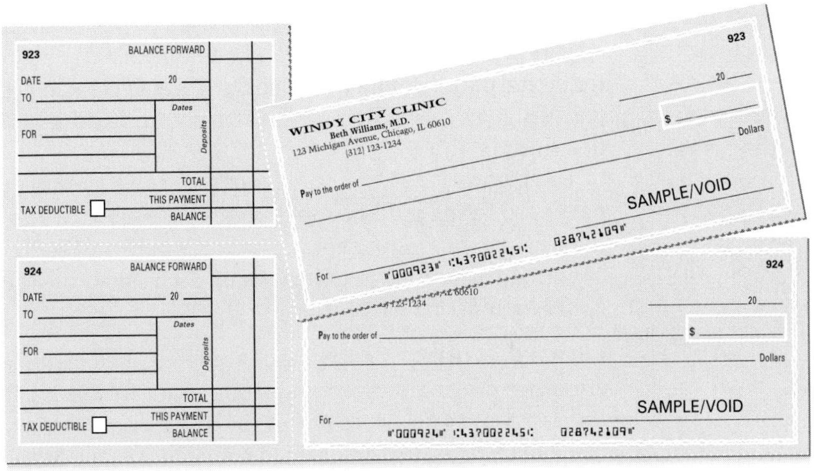

FIGURE 13-8 Cashbook and stubs are cash payment records.

Number	Date	Description	Amount	Office Expenses	Car	Misc.	Balance
	6-1	Fund established					75.00
1	6-2	Postage due	1.42	1.42			73.58
2	6-8	Taxi — (2)	8.00		8.00		65.58
3	6-10	Delivery charge	3.98			3.98	61.60
4	6-25	Supplies	11.62	11.62			49.98
		Total	25.02	13.04	8.00	3.98	
	7-1	Balance 49.98					
	ck #	790 25.02					
		75.00					

FIGURE 13-9 Petty cash record.

Double-Entry Bookkeeping

In double-entry bookkeeping, a financial transaction is recorded in two different places. This system is inexpensive but requires a trained bookkeeper.

The "double-entry" forces a balance since all accounting procedures require two entries to keep the accounting records in balance. For example, when a patient pays an outstanding bill, cash is recorded as an asset, and the receivable, which was the money owed or an asset, is eliminated.

Accounting is based on the premise that the assets of the business, less the liabilities of the business, equal the net worth of that business. This is expressed by the standard accounting formula: Assets = Liabilities + Net Worth. The double-entry system assures that the accounts are in balance.

Assets include everything owned by the medical practice such as cash, bank accounts, money owed to the physician, equipment, and real estate. Liabilities are money the medical practice owes to its creditors such as money owed for medical supplies to a vendor (supplier).

The Pegboard System (Write-It-Once System)

The Pegboard system is an old system that is rarely used. Computer software has replaced this style of bookkeeping in most physician offices, but a few offices may still utilize this system.

Amount $ _8.00_	No. _2_
RECEIVED OF PETTY CASH	
	June 8, 20 08
For _Dr. Williams — taxi_	
Charge to _Medical Conference_	
Approved by _B.F.F._	Received by _Mary King_

FIGURE 13-10 A petty cash voucher.

The pegboard system is used to document patient bills and payments. This system is also called the write-it-once method because a system of interrelated forms are placed onto the pegboard and used with the same master day sheet. It is an efficient system because the same data is entered on all the forms at one time. The pegboard system is inexpensive as long as all employees are trained in its use. However, be aware that the forms manufactured by one company are usually not compatible with forms from another company.

The actual pegboard is a firm-backed board that contains pegs along the left-hand side. These pegs hold the perforated edges of a day sheet (same as a daily journal) firmly onto the pegboard. Other forms can be held firmly by the pegs so when posting is done, the form, such as a superbill, will not slip.

Required Pegboard System Forms

There are four components of the pegboard system. These are

- Day sheets
- Ledger cards
- Superbill (charge/encounter slips)
- Receipt forms

These forms have a carbon ribbon attached or are on special paper which will permit entering charges, payments, and adjustments onto the master day sheet, the charge slip (superbill), and the patient's ledger card at the same time.

DAY SHEETS The day sheet component of the pegboard system is used to list or post each day's financial transactions: charges, payments, adjustments, and credits. The day sheet, one for each day of the month, must be balanced at the end of each day. The balance from the previous day is carried over to the present day's day sheet as part of the balancing process. In a large or busy practice, there may be more than one day sheet generated per day. The day sheet contains five basic sections that are described in Table 13-1.

See Figure 13-11 for an example of the accounting pegboard system. Remember that the pegboard system, using the double entry system based on the accounting equation, requires that each side of the equation must be balanced.

LEDGER CARDS Ledger cards are rarely used in modern office practice; however, it is important for the medical assistant to be aware of this form of record keeping.

Ledger cards are maintained for each patient or for a family as a whole. These provide a record of all

TABLE 13-1 Day Sheet Sections

Section	Description
Section 1	The individual transaction, such as patient charges, are posted in this column. The ledger card, charge slip, and receipt forms are used when posting in this row/column. Included in this column are: ■ Patient name ■ Description of transaction ■ Charges and credits ■ Previous and current balances
Section 2	This is the deposit portion of the day sheet. Some forms actually include a detachable slip that can be used as a deposit slip into a bank account. A payment made by the patient would also be listed under the appropriate right-hand column (cash, check, insurance).
Section 3	This is an optional column and depends on the needs of the practice. For example, it can be used to break down the type of service that was provided (office visit, office surgery, hospital visit).
Section 4	This is the totals column/row. Each of the columns feedings into the bottom section is totaled at the end of the day.
Section 5	This section is critical in checking that the accounts balance. It also keeps track of the cumulative accounts receivable figure owed by all the patients. This column is useful in determining how much money is still owed to the physician by looking at just one number.

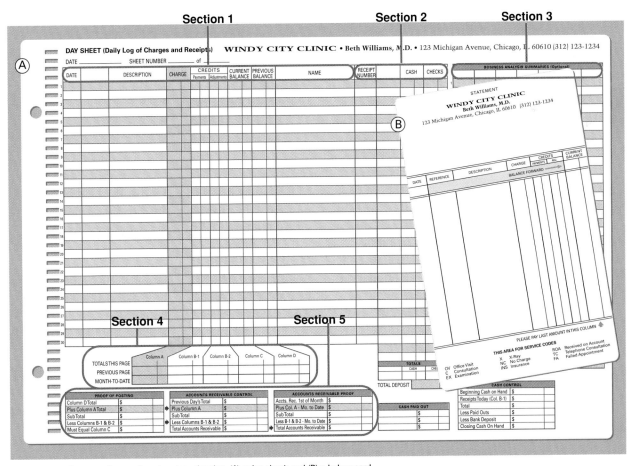

FIGURE 13-11 An accounting pegboard system showing: (A) a day sheet; and (B) a ledger card.

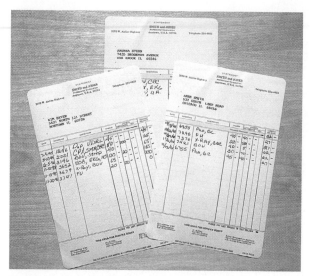

FIGURE 13-12 Examples of ledger cards.

services and charges pertaining to the patient and his or her family and can also be used as statements (Figure 13-12). The ledger card will contain all the charges for the entire family being seen by the physician. The correct charge for each individual family member must be placed next to the appropriate name so that insurance billings can be made correctly. The front of the ledger card will contain:

Name of patient

Mailing address

Description of the activity (office visit, post-op visit, prenatal visit)

Amount of the charge or payment

Adjustment(s), if any apply

Total balance due by that patient or family

The back of the ledger card includes space for information regarding the collection process. This includes the name, address, and telephone number of the employer of the person responsible for the bill, the spouse's name, address, and telephone number, the name and address of the nearest relative, and insurance information. There is also a space for additional comments such as the name of a secondary insurer.

When using the pegboard system, the ledger card is placed under the superbill (charge slip) and directly over the day sheet making sure to line up the entry line on the ledger card with the next available space on the day sheet. It is important not to miss any lines when entering information onto the day sheet.

Ledger cards can be copied and used as a statement that is sent to the patient. In offices using a computerized billing system, the bill is generated by the computer. Ledger cards are kept in a separate file container that is sized to fit them. This container is usually kept in an accessible spot close to the receptionist or person responsible for handling charges and billing.

RECEIPT FORMS A receipt form is used when a patient payment is made but no service is provided on that day. For example, a patient may come into the office or mail in a check to pay a bill. In some offices, this amount is entered onto the day sheet and ledger card, at the same time, the receipt form is completed for the patient. If the patient pays the bill with cash, a receipt is given. If the payment is made by check, the patient may use the canceled check as a receipt or may request a written receipt.

Using the Pegboard System

Every financial transaction, except the use of petty cash, is recorded on the day sheet. Each patient will have a ledger card on which individual financial activity is recorded. When the pegboard system is used, the patient's name, receipt number (the next chronological number on the day sheet), and previous balance are entered on the day sheet with a superbill attached when the patient arrives in the office. The superbill is then removed and attached to the patient's chart. After the patient is seen by the physician, the superbill is put back on the same line of the day sheet where it was originally written after placing the charge amounts next to the service rendered. Procedure 13-2 explains the pegboard system.

If the patient makes a payment in person, then issue a receipt by placing a receipt form on the pegboard in place of the superbill. Place the patient's ledger card onto the day sheet. Enter the previous balance owed on the day sheet, and calculate the new balance after this payment. On the ledger card, post the date, patient's name, a description of the transaction, such as ROA (received on account), and the amount of the payment.

If a payment is made through the mail, a receipt is not sent. The amount credited to the account will appear on the next bill sent to the patient.

Adjustments

Adjustments are any changes made that affect the patient's balance. They can occur when the physician reduces a fee, or agrees to write-off a portion of the charge and accept the insurance payment as full payment. For example, if the physician has charged $1,500 for a surgical procedure and agrees to accept the insurance payment of $1,200, then an adjustment is made for $300. The $300 appears in the adjustment column, and is subtracted from the previous balance to indicate that $1,200 is now currently owed. If the $300 was not added to the adjustment column, the totals in section 4 on the balance sheet would not balance. An adjustment or correction also has to be made to correct an error in posting.

PROCEDURE

Pegboard System

OBJECTIVE: Process patient accounts using the write-it-once system without error in posting or mathematics.

Equipment and Supplies

pegboard; superbills (charge slips); new day sheet; ledger cards for each patient scheduled during the day; calculator

Method

1. Place a new day sheet and a strip of superbills (charge slips) onto the pegboard making sure they are fastened securely into the pegs.
2. Complete all the information required at the top of the day sheet (date and page number)
3. Carry balances forward from the previous day sheet and enter it into section 4. These include "Previous Page" columns A-D, "Previous Day's Total," and "Accounts Rec. 1st of the Month," which are entered into the Accounts Receivable Control and Accounts Receivable Proof boxes. Step 3 is necessary before the day sheet is ready to use.
4. Remove the superbill from the pegboard and clip it to the front of the patient's chart. The physician will enter the procedure performed that day on the appropriate line of the superbill, fill in the diagnosis, and sign the form after he or she sees the patient. The insurance code number is included on the superbill for ease of processing. The superbill is then given to the receptionist by the medical assistant or the patient so that arrangements can be made for payment.
5. To record charges: place the ledger card under the next superbill and turn back the top two pages of the superbill. Turn back these pages to correctly line up the space for the amount to be posted on the charge slip, and through to the ledger card and day sheet. Write the amount charged, pressing firmly and evenly to press through to the forms and day sheet.
6. To record payments: When the superbill is received at the front desk, the medical assistant or receptionist will enter the correct charge next to every procedure or service and place this total on the front of the superbill. The superbill is then again placed back on the pegboard, using care to line it up on top of the correct patient's name. The ledger card is then placed under the last page of the charge slip aligning the first blank line of the ledger card with the carbonized entry strip on the superbill. On some types of superbills, you will turn back the first two pages of the superbill and enter the total charge and payment into the correct columns. Complete recording this transaction by filling in all the information that the office requires in the far right-hand columns (for example, method of payment such as cash or check).
7. To post adjustments: When an adjustment is made (for example a discount given to another health professional), the medical assistant/receptionist will enter the correct discounted amount into the computer system or subtract it from the balance due from the insurance company. If the adjustment is for non-sufficient funds, add the check amount and service fee charged by the bank to the patient balance. Always follow the facility's policy on adjustments.
8. To post collection agency payments: If the patient pays a collection agency and the collection agency forwards the money, credit that payment to the patient account and write "collection agency payment of $(amount received)" next to it.
9. If a credit balance then exists and the physician or office manager approves, issue a refund check to the patient.

Charting Example

Refunded $49 to patient for overpayment.

TABLE 13-2 Correcting Posting Errors

Date	Description	Debit	Credit Payments	Adjustments	Balance
06/19/XX	OV	25.00			25.00
06/19/XX	Error in pstg	(25.00)			0

Balancing the Day Sheets

To make sure that the accounts and entries are correct, the day sheet(s) need to be balanced at the end of the day. Use a calculator to balance day sheets and always double-check each total. When balancing the day sheet, use a calculator with paper tapes, if possible. This will allow a review of the tape for calculation errors if the figures do not balance.

When errors in posting are corrected, the corrections should be made in the same column as the original posting (Table 13-2).

The steps for balancing the day sheets are presented in Table 13-3.

Accounts Receivable Control

It is important to keep a running record of all money owed to the physician (accounts receivable). To make sure this number is accurate, an "Accounts Receivable Control" column and an "Accounts Receivable Proof" column are maintained at the bottom of the day sheet.

On the first day of the month, the day sheet being used will have a zero placed in the box marked "Previous Page." If the day sheet page is for the second of the month through the end of the month, a "Previous Page" number is brought forward from the accounts receivable total on the previous page (day before).

The columns A and B totals are brought straight across from the Proof of Posting boxes into the correct spaces in the Accounts Receivable Control section. These two figures are added together for a subtotal and then the sum of columns B1 and B2 are subtracted from this amount. This number is the new total accounts receivable figure.

The Accounts Receivable Proof is calculated in the same manner with the last box matching the last box on

---

TABLE 13-3 Balancing the Day Sheets

1. Total columns A, B1, B2, C, and D and place the total for each column in the boxes marked "Totals This Page." These column totals then need to be added to numbers brought forward and entered into the "Previous Page" column. This will provide the "Month to Date" total. The "Month to Date" totals are important since they indicate all the credits, charges, and transactions that have occurred from the first day of the month to the present day.

2. The Proof of Posting box is used to make sure that all entries and the totals columns are correct. The numbers used to calculate this figure are taken from the "Totals This Page" column box.
   a. Enter the amount from today's column D total, which is the sum of the previous balances into the appropriate box.
   b. Place the total for column A, which represents all the charges for this day, in the appropriate box ("Plus Column A Total") and create a subtotal by adding column D and column A totals.
   c. Add columns B1 and B2, which are both credit columns (payments and adjustments), then enter this amount in the box "Less Columns B1 and B2." This amount will then be subtracted (minus) from the subtotal of column D and column A.
   d. If the calculations have been correct, this new subtotal obtained after subtracting columns B1 and B2 should be equal to column C, which is the current balance.

   Note that when doing a proof of posting, column D is added to column A minus the sum of columns B1 and B2 and this must equal column C. Therefore, a proof of posting formula is:

   $$D + A - (B1 + B2) = C$$

   This means the previous balance (D) plus the charge (A) minus the sum of the payments and adjustments (B1 and B2) is equal to the current balance (C).

the Accounts Receivable Control for proof of posting. See Figure 13-13 for an illustration of accounts receivable control.

An accounts receivable ratio provides a measurement of how fast the outstanding accounts are being paid. The Accounts Receivable Ratio equals the Current Accounts Receivable Balance divided by the Average Gross Monthly Charges.

For example, if the current accounts receivable balance is $20,000 and the annual gross charges are $120,000, then the average monthly charges are $10,000 ($120,000 ÷ 12). The accounts receivable ratio would equal $20,000 ÷ $10,000 = 2 months.

Since a desirable accounts receivable ratio, or the amount of time it takes to have the uncollected debts paid, is two months or less, this example is at the high end of the limit. The medical assistant will have to work hard to get collections under two months.

Locating Errors

The key to error control is to prevent them in the first place. If there is a difference in the balances of the day sheet, there are several steps that can be taken to locate the error.

1. If the columns on the day sheet do not balance (using the proof of posting box at bottom of the day sheet), check all calculations. Ideally you will have saved the calculator tape. Find the difference in the balances and search for that identical amount on the ledger cards and superbill.

2. If an error is divisible by nine, it may be a transposition error. For example, if the difference in the balance is $63, you may find that you wrote $329 instead of $392.

3. Check all the columns, in particular the Previous Balance column to make sure you did not post the amount incorrectly.

4. Check the alignment of all digits to make sure a zero was not misaligned, for example in writing 200 instead of 20. One bookkeeping method for avoiding this type of error is to use a dash in the cents column instead of two zeros. Thus $45.00 would be written as $45.—.

Computerized Systems

Most offices perform the accounting function using a computer program. The computer system and program selected will depend on the needs of the office. Practice management software offers many services and can be modified to fit the needs of a particular office or specialty. When shopping for practice management software, offices often hire a consultant to evaluate the practice requirements. Specialized software is advertised in professional journals and is demonstrated at

ACCOUNTS RECEIVABLE CONTROL				
Month of March , 20 — —			Accounts receivable at end of preceding month: $22,500	
	Services Rendered	Received from Patients	Adjustments Increase/ (Decrease)	Accounts Receivable Balance
1	$ 800	$ 1000		$22,300
2	$ 700	$ 400		$22,600
3	$ 900	$ 1100	($100)	$22,300
4	$ 1000	$ 700		$22,600

FIGURE 13-13 Accounts Receivable Control.

professional meetings for physicians and medical office personnel. Prior to making a final decision concerning office software, ask physicians' offices or practices that have similar needs for their suggestions. Another concern in choosing new software is cost. New software may require the office hardware to be upgraded. A consultant will be able to advise the office concerning these needs. The new software should contain Current Procedural Terminology (CPT) and International Classification of Diseases (ICD). The software must have these capabilities; however, this data changes yearly and the system must be able to accommodate these updates.

When using a computerized system always back up data and information on a separate disk, such as a CD-ROM that is then stored separately. Some systems also keep the information on the hard drive. Some offices keep one hard copy of printed material to be kept on file in the event the computer system goes down or there is a power failure.

HIPAA mandated the use of the computer to submit bills to insurance companies electronically. Several comprehensive software systems are available for the computer that combines many office functions into one program. These software packages will make patient appointments, keep all patient records (including lab results and x-ray reports), maintain all insurance and billing information, and perform all bookkeeping functions including insurance payments, patient payments, and accounts due. In addition, there is a function within these programs that will electronically submit the bill to an insurance clearinghouse for dissemination to the payment centers.

Most comprehensive software programs are quite expensive, so before deciding which one to buy, careful attention should be given to the needs of the office, as well as which methods the office has chosen to comply with HIPAA regulations.

To access the information in these programs, every employee must have his or her own unique, login name and password. To be in compliance with HIPAA regulations, upon leaving employment, the employee's login name and password must be rendered unusable. Only those employees with a "need" to access the information may have login names and passwords. In addition, the person responsible for providing employees with access must keep records of who accesses the information, what information was accessed, and when (date and time) information is accessed. These logs must be kept for a designated period of time, usually at least two years.

A paper backup copy of the computer files is not necessary, but a disk backup file or an off-premises electronic backup file is necessary. The process by which the backup files can or should be accessed is written into the office's policy manual, along with the reasons and circumstances for granting access. One designated person has total access for the system and is responsible for the software, the passwords, and the backup files. This person is also documented in the office policy and procedure manual.

Professional Courtesy

Professional courtesy (PC) is typically offered by physicians to other physicians, staff, and family members, and clergy in addition to indigent patients. Professional courtesy may be rendered only at the discretion of the physician, must fall within federal guidelines, and insurance requirements, and must be recorded in the patient's record.

SUMMARY

The professional health care facility will have in place office policy regarding fee setting, billing, and collection. The medical assistant has the responsibility to carry out such policy with a professional, courteous attitude. Informed patients will have a better understanding of office expectations. This helps to lessen the problems encountered with accounts receivable. When an account does become a collection dilemma, a series of steps can be instituted to quickly and efficiently address any problems. The goal of such policy is to protect the financial well-being and goodwill of the medical practice.

Chapter Review

COMPETENCY REVIEW

1. Define and spell the terms to learn for this chapter.
2. With a fellow student, role-play a telephone conversation you would have with Samuel Jones, a patient who is unemployed, to collect an overdue bill of 60 days for $225.
3. Write a sample collection letter from Dr. Beth Williams to Samuel Jones identified in the previous question.
4. What statements can you make to a patient to encourage payment at the time of service?
5. Discuss the ethical considerations involved when making collections.

PREPARING FOR THE CERTIFICATION EXAM

1. A patient's detailed record of financial transactions at a medical office is called a/an
   A. ledger
   B. accounts payable record
   C. register
   D. reconciliation
   E. medical record

2. Once an account has been referred for collection, the medical office should
   A. discuss payment with the patient
   B. not attempt to collect payment
   C. call the patient's employer
   D. cancel the balance
   E. send a reminder letter

3. Which form serves as the documentation of services, a billing statement, and an insurance processing form?
   A. receipt
   B. ledger
   C. account
   D. superbill
   E. credit memo

4. A "skip" has/is
   A. forgotten to pay
   B. lost his or her job
   C. moved with no forwarding address
   D. not a collection problem
   E. skipped a monthly payment

continued on next page

5. If the computer system goes down, what method would NOT be used to store electronic data?
   A. separate disk
   B. CD-ROM
   C. print a hard copy
   D. hard drive
   E. file cabinet

6. Regulation Z of the Truth in Lending Act requires physicians to outline costs, including finance charges when payment arrangements are made in
   A. two or more installments
   B. four or more installments
   C. eight or more installments
   D. three or more installments
   E. five or more installments

7. The accounts receivable record tells you
   A. how much money is owed to the practice
   B. the effectiveness of the billing system
   C. total collections divided by gross changes
   D. total collections divided by net charges
   E. how fast overdue accounts are being paid

8. Claims against estates should be
   A. canceled
   B. sent to collection
   C. discounted
   D. sent to the administrator of the estate
   E. addressed to the next of kin

9. Good bookkeeping habits include
   A. using a blue pen
   B. using a pencil to easily make changes
   C. using opaque correction fluid
   D. checking the entry once
   E. use of clear penmanship

10. The pegboard system is the same as the
    A. single-entry bookkeeping system
    B. write-it-one system
    C. computerized system
    D. write-it-now system
    E. computerized program

CRITICAL THINKING

1. What and how should you advise the patient of your credit policies to ensure the patient will understand the practice policies?

ON THE JOB

Services were rendered to Jeffrey Boylan on October 1, 2005. It is now 45 days since Mr. Boylan's received care, and he has not yet made a payment on his outstanding balance of $150.00. At this point, the office's policy requires that a reminder letter be sent. Compose a collection letter to Mr. Boylan, in accordance with HIPAA and office guidelines. Address: Mr. Jeffrey Boylan, 14 Meadow Road, Anytown, State 12345

INTERNET ACTIVITY

Your office is considering between manual and computerized accounting systems. Search the Internet for the various accounting systems. Develop an excel spreadsheet and list the manual and computerized systems found online with all necessary equipment, components, warranties, and prices.

MediaLink More on fees, billing, collections, and credit in a medical office, including interactive resources, can be found in the Student CD-ROM accompanying this textbook.

Medical Assistant Role Delineation Chart

HIGHLIGHT indicates material covered in this chapter.

ADMINISTRATIVE

Administrative Procedures

- Perform basic administrative medical assisting functions
- Schedule, coordinate and monitor appointments
- Schedule inpatient/outpatient admissions and procedures
- Understand and apply third-party guidelines
- Obtain reimbursement through accurate claims submission
- Monitor third-party reimbursement
- Understand and adhere to managed care policies and procedures
- *Negotiate managed care contracts*

Practice Finances

- Perform procedural and diagnostic coding
- Apply bookkeeping principles
- Manage accounts receivable
- *Manage accounts payable*
- *Process payroll*
- *Document and maintain accounting and banking records*
- *Develop and maintain fee schedules*
- *Manage renewals of business and professional insurance policies*
- *Manage personnel benefits and maintain records*
- *Perform marketing, financial, and strategic planning*

CLINICAL

Fundamental Principles

- Apply principles of aseptic technique and infection control
- Comply with quality assurance practices
- Screen and follow up patient test results

Diagnostic Orders

- Collect and process specimens
- Perform diagnostic tests

Patient Care

- Adhere to established patient screening procedures
- Obtain patient history and vital signs
- Prepare and maintain examination and treatment areas
- Prepare patient for examinations, procedures and treatments
- Assist with examinations, procedures and treatments
- Prepare and administer medications and immunizations
- Maintain medication and immunization records
- Recognize and respond to emergencies
- Coordinate patient care information with other health care providers
- Initiate IV and administer IV medications with appropriate training and as permitted by state law

GENERAL

Professionalism

- Display a professional manner and image
- Demonstrate initiative and responsibility
- Work as a member of the health care team
- Prioritize and perform multiple tasks
- Adapt to change
- Promote the CMA credential
- Enhance skills through continuing education
- Treat all patients with compassion and empathy
- Promote the practice through positive public relations

Communication Skills

- Recognize and respect cultural diversity
- Adapt communications to individual's ability to understand
- Use professional telephone technique
- Recognize and respond effectively to verbal, nonverbal, and written communications
- Use medical terminology appropriately
- Utilize electronic technology to receive, organize, prioritize and transmit information
- Serve as liaison

Legal Concepts

- Perform within legal and ethical boundaries
- Prepare and maintain medical records
- Document accurately
- Follow employer's established policies dealing with the health care contract
- Implement and maintain federal and state health care legislation and regulations
- Comply with established risk management and safety procedures
- Recognize professional credentialing criteria
- *Develop and maintain personnel, policy and procedure manuals*

Instruction

- Instruct individuals according to their needs
- Explain office policies and procedures
- Teach methods of health promotion and disease prevention
- Locate community resources and disseminate information
- *Develop educational materials*
- *Conduct continuing education activities*

Operational Functions

- Perform inventory of supplies and equipment
- Perform routine maintenance of administrative and clinical equipment
- Apply computer techniques to support office operations
- *Perform personnel management functions*
- *Negotiate leases and prices for equipment and supply contracts*

- *Denotes advanced skills.*

SOURCE: Reprinted by permission of the American Association of Medical Assistants from the AAMA Role Delineation Study: Occupational Analysis of the Medical Assisting Profession.

BETH WILLIAMS, MD
123 MICHIGAN AVENUE
CHICAGO, IL 60610

STATEMEN
FROM
THRU
CUST #

For *Office furniture*

"000923" ⑈:437002245⑈: 028742109"

BALANCE FORWARD   727 18

10   20 05

van's

h Supply

DEPOSITS   35 00
            142 32

ges

COUNT - - - - - - - -
BALANCE $2,646.(
CREDITS $8,000.(
AID $.(
BITS $7,871.3
ARGES $5.0
ANCE $2,770.3
/CREDITS
EBITS

WINDY CITY CLINIC
Beth Williams, M.D.
123 Michigan Avenue, Chicago, IL 60610
(312) 123-1234

Pay to the order of *Jamie Young*

Fifty cents only

chapter 14

Financial Management

Learning Objectives

After completing this chapter, you should be able to:

- Define and spell the terms to learn for this chapter.
- State the correct procedure for writing a check and check stub.
- Describe the write-it-once check writing system.
- State the correct method for endorsing a check based on the guidelines issued by the federal government.
- Differentiate between the ABA number and the MICR on a check.
- State the risks associated with accepting a third-party check, cash, or check from an out-of-state bank.
- List the criteria for a negotiable instrument.
- State and describe three types of endorsements.
- List six recurring monthly expenses.
- Describe the five steps to follow when making a deposit.
- List and discuss nine steps for reconciling a bank statement.

Terms to Learn

accounts payable
accounts receivable
American Banker's Association (ABA) number
audit
canceled checks
cash disbursement

credits
debits
deposits
embezzlement
gross annual wage
Magnetic Ink Character Recognition (MICR)
negotiable instrument

payee
payer
reconciliation
signee
stop-payment order
tax withholding
third-party checks
warrant

Case Study

DR. EVERETT'S OFFICE HAS A PETTY CASH DRAWER in which Dr. Everett keeps fifty dollars to pay postage, due mail, and other incidentals. The office policy is to replace any cash taken out of the drawer with a receipt for the money taken. In this way, when the money is to be restocked, there is an account of where the fifty dollars was spent. It is the end of the month and time to get the cash for the petty cash drawer. When you count the money left and add the receipts, you find the total in the drawer is only forty dollars. Only you and Sarah, the clinic manager, have access to the drawer. You ask her about the ten missing dollars, and she says that she "borrowed" ten dollars a week ago and intends to repay the money on payday, which is a week away.

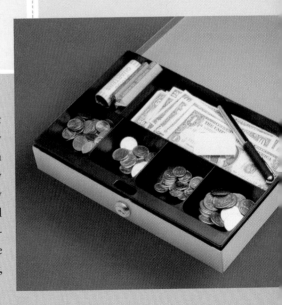

he medical assistant's responsibilities for maintaining control of the medical office's banking and accounting procedures are two-fold. First, absolute accuracy is necessary when working with bank deposits, reconciliation of funds, and all related bookkeeping activities. The second responsibility relates to the trust the physician has placed on the employee for handling cash, checks, and accounts. The medical assistant acts as the agent for the physician.

Function of Banking

The basic banking functions are depositing funds, writing checks, transferring funds between bank accounts, withdrawing funds, reconciling statements, and using banking services. Most of the funds that come into a medical office are from the collection of accounts receivable.

Money may need to be withdrawn from a checking or savings account to pay business-related expenses. Every time funds (money) are moved from one account to another or used as cash, it must be handled in a systematic manner and carefully documented. Monthly statements for both checking and savings accounts must be reconciled or balanced to determine what money or funds are available for use.

Bank records are subject to government examination since the federal government regulates banking practices. In addition, the accountant for the medical practice will need accurate records for preparation of federal tax returns. Since the medical assistant will not be present when the accountant reviews the books, all information must be clear and accurate.

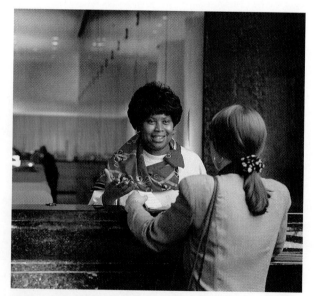

FIGURE 14-1 Bank teller assisting with customer service.

Types of Bank Accounts

Banks maintain both checking and savings accounts for their customers (Figure 14-1). A checking account allows the owner of the account to withdraw money from the account by writing checks, which are used as payment for outstanding debts (bills). Cash can also be withdrawn from a checking account. Checking accounts are not usually interest-bearing accounts. Some accounts earn interest only if there is a minimum balance in the account. Generally, the bank charges a fee, or service charge, (for example, $5.00 per month) to maintain the account.

A saving's account is an interest-bearing account in which funds not needed for daily expenses can be placed. Interest is earned monthly or quarterly. This means the bank will calculate a certain percentage (such as 3%) based on the average balance during a month and pay that amount to the account. Cash can be withdrawn from a savings account or transferred into a checking account. There is usually a limit to the number of monthly withdrawals without paying a fee.

A money market account is used more as an investment tool that usually pays a higher level of interest.

Online Banking

Most banks provide a service to their customers called "online banking." Online banking provides the customer access to his or her bank account 24-hours a day, seven days a week. By using the computer to access the World Wide Web, customers can enter the Web address for their bank's home page. This address can be obtained from the bank. Once on the bank's home page, the customer chooses "online banking." A sign-in or log-in page will appear that asks for a username and password. The username and password are usually set by the customer and are unique to each customer. Some banks also require the account number be entered.

Online banking lets customers reconcile their account, pay bills, see which checks have been processed, and check the total amount in their account. One advantage of online banking is that customers can see the bank's record of their account, and compare the bank's record to their own. Customers may see which checks have been processed and which deposits have been fully credited to their account. Another advantage of online banking is the ability to download data from the bank Web site directly to the customer's money management software program.

Online banking is a paperless system, so it is important that, when using online banking, records be kept in the office. If a bill is paid, it must be noted in the accounts payable records to ensure that the office's records always match the bank's records, and any money taken out of the account to pay a bill is posted in the office records.

Checks

A check is a written order to a bank to pay or transfer money. A check, which is payable on demand, is considered a negotiable instrument. A negotiable instrument is one that actualizes or permits the transfer of money to another person. In order to have a negotiable instrument, it must be:

- Written and signed by the maker (payer) of the check
- State a sum of money to be paid
- Payable on demand or at a fixed date in the future
- Payable to the holder (payee) of the check

Checks are supplied, for a slight charge, by the bank where the money is held or a company specializing in printing checks. These are referred to as blank checks since they contain only basic information, including the account number and name and address of the account owner.

Large medical offices that require a large supply of checks can request a business office checkbook that has several checks per page in a large bound checkbook. Medical offices can also request a duplicate or write-in-once check system. A carbon copy of the check is made when written to ensure accountability for each check.

There is standard information included on all checks regardless of the bank that issues them. This preprinted information includes:

- Name and address of the payer (person signing the check to release the money)
- Telephone number of payer (in some cases)
- Preprinted sequential number on each check
- Space to enter the full date
- American Bank Association (ABA) number
- "Pay to the order of" space in which to enter the name of the payee (the person or company to receive the money)
- Space to enter the amount of the check in writing
- Small box or space to enter the amount of the check in numbers
- Space for the signature of payer
- Preprinted name and address of bank
- Magnetic ink character recognition (MICR) figures used for bank processing of the check

The blank spaces must be completed before a bank will honor and cash the check.

Advantages of Checks

Checks are recommended for a variety of reasons, including safety of funds, convenience, ease of maintaining a record or documentation of money transfer,

reliability of records for tax purposes, summary of deposits from receipts, protection while money is in the bank account (banks carry insurance to cover loss), and stop-payment orders that can be issued by the payer to protect any lost or stolen checks.

Types of Checks

The various types of checks include cashier's checks, certified checks, bank drafts, limited checks, money orders, traveler's checks, voucher checks, and warrants. Box 14-1 lists definitions of the different types of checks. Preparing for Externship discusses the importance of knowing the different types of checks.

Warrant

A warrant is not actually a negotiable check. It is a statement issued to indicate that a debt should be paid. For example, an insurance adjuster may issue a warrant indicating that a fire insurance claim should be paid. This warrant then becomes authorization to the insurance company to issue a check as payment.

ABA Number

The American Banker's Association (ABA) number is always located in the upper right-hand corner of a printed check. It is printed as a fraction on a business check or as a straight series of numbers (1–109/210) on a personal check. The ABA originated this number to identify the area where the bank on which the check is written is located and to identify the individual bank.

Magnetic Ink Character Recognition (MICR)

Magnetic Ink Character Recognition (MICR) is a system of combining characters and numbers located at the bottom left side of checks and deposit slips. The MICR is read by high-speed machinery, increasing the speed and accuracy of processing bank statements and check sorting. It also facilitates the bookkeeping process within the bank. Printed on each check, the MICR is a form of identification for the bank and the account. The first series of numbers identifies the bank and its location. The second series of numbers identifies the individual account. During bank processing,

Prepare a Check

OBJECTIVE: Correctly prepare a check.

Equipment and Supplies
blank checks with stub or record; pen

Method

1. Move all the checks in the pad to the left so that the smallest numbered check will lay across the check register.
2. Fill in the check stub or check record before writing the check.
3. Use ink or a typewriter to complete check and stub.
4. Write the name of the payee on the "Pay to the order of" line.
5. Write out the full amount of the check on the "Pay" line.
6. Write the full date and check number in the designated boxes.
7. Write the amount of the check, using numbers in the designated area.
8. Fill in all blank spaces and leave no room for anyone to add anything. Always begin writing or figures at the extreme left of the space.
9. Date the check on the day it is written. Never postdate a check. Postdating a check means writing a future date on a check.
10. Use care when spelling the name of the payee. Do not use abbreviations or titles, such as MD. Leave no space either before or after the payee's name. If space remains after the name, draw a straight line from the name to the end of the space.
11. Make sure the dollar amount written on the second line agrees with numerical dollar amount entered in the space on the first line.
12. Use care when writing a check for less than one dollar. Write out the amount with the word "only" indicating to the reader that the amount should be noted as less than one dollar. Do not cross out the word dollars. It is not advisable to write checks for less than one dollar. In addition to the time spent bookkeeping such a small amount, many banks place a service charge for each check written. This can be costly.
13. Finally, subtract the amount of this check from the "Balance Brought Forward" line. Write this amount as the new balance forward.

---

additional numbers are printed across the bottom of the check to indicate the amount of the check.

Check Writing

The check writing process needs to be handled carefully to avoid errors. Methods for writing checks will vary from office to office depending upon the preferences of the physician and the accountant. Your office may use a traditional checkbook with individual checks on each page, a business office checkbook, a write-it-once system, or a computer generated check processing system. When writing a check, all the spaces must be filled in. At the top right corner is a space for the date. This is the date the check is written. The person or business to which the check is written is placed on the line following "Pay to the order of." At the end of that line is a block to put the amount of the check in numbers (for example, $100.00). The next line is the amount of the check written in words (for example, "One hundred and no/100 dollars"). A space to note what the check is

for appears on the bottom left corner of the check. You might note, for example, that this check was for "office supplies." The line on the bottom right is for the writer of the check to sign. This line must be signed by the owner of the bank account, or his or her authorized agent. In some offices, the office manager is designated to sign checks for the physician.

Write-it-once System

The write-it-once system is based on the use of a check with a carbon strip on the back that allows a record to be kept of the date, check number, payee, and net amount of the check. A pegboard system (see Chapter 13), check register sheet, and checks with a carbonized writing strip on the back are used for this method. The check register sheet is placed over the pegs of a pegboard. Checks with the carbonized strip on the back edge are then placed on top of the check register, lining up the first line of the check register with the writing line of the first check. Any information that is written

BOX 14-1
Types of Checks

- **Cashier's checks** are written using the bank's own check or form and are issued by the bank. A cashier's check guarantees the money is available since the bank checks the payer's account before issuing the check. The purchaser can also pay cash to have a cashier's check issued. The funds to pay the check are debited against the payer's account when the check is issued by the bank. Cashier's checks can be requested of a bank by savings account holders who do not have a checking account. There is usually a charge for this service.

- **Certified checks** are similar to a cashier's check since the bank guarantees the money is available. A certified check is actually written on the payer's own check form. The teller will verify this check by placing an official stamp directly on the check. The bank actually withdraws the money from the payer's account when it certifies the check.

- **Bank drafts** are checks that are drawn up by a bank against funds (money) that are deposited to its account in another bank.

- **Limited checks** are issued on special check forms that contain a preprinted maximum dollar amount for which the check can be written. There may also be a time limit during which the check is valid or must be cashed. Limited checks are used for payroll checks and insurance payments.

- **Money orders** are purchased for the cash value typed on the check. Money orders can be purchased from banks, the United States Postal Service, and other authorized agents. International money orders can be purchased to be cashed in foreign countries.

A money order is purchased with cash, and there is a charge for this service. Money orders are frequently used by individuals who do not have bank accounts since it is recommended that cash not be sent through the mail. Money orders are considered safe to accept as payment since they are redeemable at the value typed on the check.

- **Traveler's checks** are familiar to most people who travel. These checks are preprinted in certain dollar amounts ($10, $20, $50, $100, $500 and $1,000) and are prepaid. Considered a safe means for carrying money when traveling, traveler's checks are also convenient since most places will accept a traveler's check and only the payer can cash it. There is a space for two signatures of the payer: one at the time of purchase and another when the check is cashed. The payee is able to check the two signatures, thus protecting the payer in the event the check is stolen or lost. People purchasing traveler's checks are advised to always sign the checks at the time of purchase before leaving the bank.

- **Voucher checks** contain three detachable sections for transaction information. This type of check is frequently used for payroll checks since additional information can be supplied to the payee. The upper portion of the check contains the actual check; the lower portion provides details about the transaction, such as any payroll deductions, account to which the check is to be credited, or reason for issuing the check; the third portion is a carbon that remains with the payer as a record of the transaction. This copy can then be filed with any additional information that is available, such as invoices or receipts.

on the check (for example, payee, dollar amounts) will then appear on the check register sheet as a permanent record.

The user must press hard when writing on this type of check so that the impression will go through to the check register underneath. The check register has space for 25 checks to be recorded on one page. Procedure 14-1 describes the check writing process using a write-it-once system.

Checks must be handwritten in ink or typewritten so they cannot be altered. Pencil is not used for check writing. The signature cannot be typewritten. Correctly written checks require legible handwriting. No blank space should be left before the name of the payee, the written dollar amount, and the numbered dollar amount. This is to prevent another person from altering any of these items. See Figure 14-2 for a sample of correctly written checks.

In some cases, the net amount of the check is imprinted by machine. All the other information is entered by hand. Checks have to be handwritten when using the write-it-once method. Checks with stubs will have to be detached from the stub for typing. However, the stub must be completed immediately.

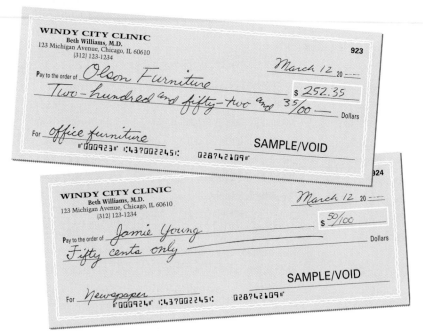

FIGURE 14-2 Correctly written checks.

Checks can be prepared ahead of time by the medical assistant and given to the physician to sign. Attach all materials, such as invoices and statements, to the check for the physician to sign. Writing a check payable to cash ("cash" checks) is not advised. These checks are easily cashed since they have no payee designated and have been signed by the payer. Banks will usually require that the person cashing this type of check endorse the check while in front of the teller. Review the guidelines for check writing to assure checks are written properly.

Errors in Writing Checks

Errors in writing checks can be handled in several ways. Do not erase on checks. They are printed on sensitive paper and erasures may not process correctly. In addition, banks are suspicious of all alterations on checks.

If there is a major error, such as writing out a different dollar amount than appears in the boxed space for the numerical amount or the payee name is written in the space meant for the handwritten dollar amount, the check is not valid. In this case, draw a line through the check and write VOID in ink in large letters on the face of the check. Keep the VOID check so that it is not considered missing when the reconciliation of the bank statement is done. If the check has already been signed, many people will tear off and discard just the signature and keep the remainder of the check for a record.

Not all errors will result in voiding the check. If the error is minor, such as writing the number "4" instead of "5," you may change the "4" to a "5" if it is still readable; the signee, the person signing the check, must then initial this change.

Accepting Checks

An office policy should be in place to guide staff about accepting checks from patients (Patient Education). It is acceptable for patients to pay for services with a personal check. Most of the accounts receivable, the outstanding bills, in a medical office are paid by checks written against the bank accounts of patients. Lifespan Considerations discusses an elderly patient's need, at times, to designate an agent to sign his or her checks.

There are some checks that most medical offices consider risky and avoid cashing. These include third-party checks, checks drawn on an out-of-town bank, overpayment of account checks, and "paid in full" checks.

Third-party checks refer to a check written by a party unknown to you. You are considered the third party in this process. The patient (the second party), the payee, has received a check from another person to pay his or her medical bill. The person who wrote the check is considered the first party. You are at risk in accepting this check since you do not know the payer who has signed the check and, thus, may have trouble collecting the money for which the check is issued.

Patient Education

The role of the medical assistant in educating the patient is twofold: to instruct the patient on the banking practices of the office and to safeguard the patient and the physician from loss of money through carelessness.

The patient may be given an informational pamphlet prepared specifically for your office with guidelines and options for payment of services. Patients should be instructed not to send cash through the mail.

In many cases, these checks will be for an amount greater than the amount of the bill and you would have to issue a refund in cash. This would require maintaining extra cash in the office, additional staff work, and may result in financial loss if the check turns out to be invalid. Therefore many offices do not accept these checks. Government checks (for example, tax refunds) and payroll checks are examples of third-party checks that are considered to be reliable.

Checks drawn on out-of-town banks are generally not accepted for payment unless identification is sought from the payee. It is difficult to collect payment if a check is not good, and it may not be easy to reach an out-of-town bank, concerning the validity of a check, prior to accepting it.

Occasionally, a patient writes a check for an overpayment of an account. This can happen accidentally if a patient has not maintained adequate records or if the patient's insurance company has also made a payment to the patient's account in the medical office. In this case, a refund needs to be made to the patient. This can be handled by issuing a refund check for the amount of overpayment or returning the incorrect check to the patient if it has not been deposited.

Checks written with the statement added "paid in full" are to be avoided. Patients sometimes write this on their check when they believe they no longer owe any money to the physician. If you deposit the check you acknowledge that this is correct. Therefore, if the patient still owes money on the bill and you deposit the check, you may have difficulty collecting any further payments.

Completing the Check Stub

A check stub can be used as a permanent record of the date, amount, payee of the check, and purpose of the check. The check stub has room to place the new balance, which is obtained by subtracting the current check from the previous balance. See Figure 14-3 for an illustration of a correctly completed check stub.

Endorsement of Checks

In order to transfer money from one person to another, the check must be endorsed. According to federal banking regulations, an endorsement is placed on the back of the check within the top one and one-half inches on the left side of the check as it is turned over. This upper left-hand corner is referred to as the "trailing edge" of a check. If the endorsement is not placed within this designated area or extends beyond the one and one-half inch mark, it can be refused by a bank. An endorsement can either be a payee's written signature or rubber-stamped. To prevent theft, checks should be endorsed "for deposit only" as soon as they arrive in the mail.

Lifespan
Considerations

Sometimes an elderly person who is physically unable to write a check, or who cannot see to write a check, will designate an agent to write and sign checks for him or her. Most often it is a family member. This is an arrangement the person has made with the bank and is a perfectly legitimate and legal way to handle finances. When money is owed to the doctor's office, it is usually the agent who will write the check for the patient, but it will be credited to the patient's account.

It is common procedure in a medical office to endorse checks at the time they are received. This is often done with an endorsement stamp that contains the doctor's name, account number, and the name of the bank.

Endorsements are regulated by the Uniform Negotiable Instrument Act. A check that has been transferred to more than one person (third-party payer) would have more than one endorsement on the back. Types of endorsements are discussed in Table 14-1.

Mailing Checks

Care should be used when mailing checks so that the check is not visible through the envelope. Special nontransparent envelopes can be purchased. Other methods are to place the check in a piece of folded paper or to actually fold the check in half.

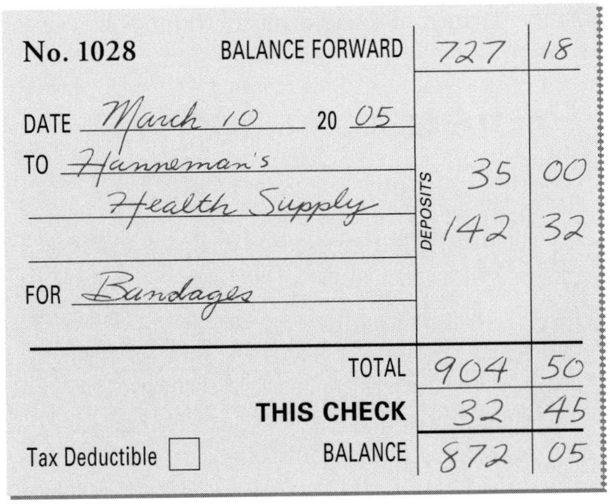

No. 1028	BALANCE FORWARD	727	18
DATE *March 10* 20 *05*			
TO *Hanneman's*		35	00
Health Supply	DEPOSITS	142	32
FOR *Bandages*			
	TOTAL	904	50
	THIS CHECK	32	45
Tax Deductible ☐	BALANCE	872	05

FIGURE 14-3 Correctly completed check stub.

TABLE 14-1 Endorsements

Endorsement	Description	Example
Blank	Signature of the payee. Check can be cashed by anyone. This is not used in the business office.	Beth Williams
Full	Indicates person's name, company, account number, bank name, and payee's name.	Pay to the order of First Town Bank Beth Williams, M.D. 123-123456
Restrictive	Specifies to whom money should be paid, and the money's purpose, such as "For Deposit Only." You can rubber-stamp the physician's signature. It is considered the safest endorsement.	Pay to the order of First Town Bank For Deposit Only Beth Williams, M.D. 123-123456

Returned Checks

A check may be returned by the bank for a variety of reasons. When this occurs, a returned item notice is also included with the check detailing the reason for the return. Checks are returned, for example, when the payee name, date, or signature of payer is missing. If a check is returned with the payee's name or date missing, it is acceptable for the medical assistant to fill in the date and physician's name. If the payer's signature is missing, then the check will have to be returned to the payer. It is always wise to place a telephone call to a patient with the reasons for returning his or her check. All checks should be reviewed for either a written or stamped endorsement before depositing.

More serious reasons for the return of checks include not sufficient funds (NSF) in the payer's account or a stop-payment order issued by the payer. In the case of NSF, the payer's account does not have enough money to cover the amount of the check. You will need to contact the writer of the check and ask how he or she wishes to make the payment (Professionalism). If funds have been added to the account, the patient (payer) may ask that the check be resubmitted. To resubmit a check, call the payer's bank to determine if there are sufficient funds, write the word resubmit on both the face and the back of the check, make out another deposit slip, and resubmit. Many banks charge the account if the deposited check is NSF. Offices will then charge the patient, in addition to the amount of the NSF check, the fee charged to them by the bank and a handling charge. See Procedure 14-2 on posting non-sufficient funds checks.

Some medical offices have a policy that if a check is returned for NSF, they will not resubmit the check. They request the payment be made immediately, with either cash, a cashier's check, or money order. The returned check should be held until payment has been made. If the patient has not taken care of the bill after notification and a sufficient time have elapsed, then advise the patient in writing that the bill will be turned over to a collection agency. Some offices also charge for returned checks.

If a stop-payment order has been issued by the payer, then the bank will not allow the funds to be disbursed. The bank will indicate that you should contact the payer with the terms "refer to maker" on the item notice. This procedure is used when a check has been lost or stolen.

Professionalism

For many patients, money owed is a "touchy" and uncomfortable subject. Remember to always address this topic in a calm, nonjudgmental way. If a patient requests to make payment arrangements, comply only if the office has a policy about payment arrangements. Always follow the office policy, and never veer from the policy. In this way, your honesty in dealing with money issues will never be questioned.

Paying Bills

All bills should be paid by check for documentation and control purposes. The only exception to this policy would be very small payments, such as daily newspaper delivery and public transportation costs. In these instances, the payments could be made from petty cash. However, it is advisable that all payments, even the daily newspaper, be paid from accounts established with appropriate vendors.

PROCEDURE

Post Non-sufficient Funds Checks

OBJECTIVE: Demonstrate the process for posting non-sufficient funds (NSF) checks.

Equipment and Supplies
data; computer or ledger card; pen

Method
1. Record amount of NSF check and service fee in adjustment column on day sheet and ledger card.
2. Accurately record the NSF check to show that the amount is added to the balance, instead of subtracted from it.

3. Note the reason for the adjustment to patient account.

Charting Example

$68 plus $20 NSF check fee = $88 added to patient balance

An office policy must be established regarding how often checks are written, for example weekly, biweekly, semimonthly, or monthly. This bill-paying schedule must match a schedule of when funds are available for payment of the office expenses. For instance, your office policy may be to send all invoices to patients at the end of the month for payments that are due on the first of the next month. In this case, you would not want to write checks against your account to pay office expenses during the last week of the month since the payments from patients will not have arrived to cover your check writing.

The office banking policy should indicate who is responsible for writing and signing all checks. A smart policy is to separate the responsibilities; one person (the medical assistant) should write the checks and another person should be authorized to sign them (office manager or physician). In some medical offices, two authorized signatures are required in order to transfer funds from one account to another or to write checks over a certain dollar amount, such as $1,000.

It is not recommended to pay bills on the day they arrive since they are generally not due for 30 days. During that 30-day period, the money that is used to pay bills can remain in an interest-bearing account. The incentive to paying bills as they arrive occurs when a supplier (vendor) offers a discount if payment is included with the order or paid within ten days. Since this discount could be as much as 10 to 20 percent, it is wise to take advantage of it. Examples of recurring monthly expenses may include:

- Insurance premium(s)
- Rent or mortgage
- Waste removal
- Utilities, including telephone charges

- Housekeeping and maintenance expenses
- Laundry
- Equipment rental, such as a copy machine
- Taxes
- Maintenance contracts for equipment
- Medical and office supplies
- Postage

A schedule for paying these expenses should be kept on a master calendar or in a tickler (reminder) file. If all checks for expenses are written on a particular day of the month, a planned transfer of funds can be made from a savings account to a checking account to cover these checks.

Some offices use a tickler file to remind the bookkeeper when each bill is due. The office will have some recurrent bills that are the same amount and paid at the same time each month. One example of a recurrent bill is the office rent. The rent for the office is typically the same amount each month and is due on the same day of each month. For some offices, there may be an annual, bimonthly, or quarterly lease arrangement. In this case, the lease money may be paid up to one year in advance. The bills for the electricity, the water, the telephone, and the gas will vary in amount from month to month, but will still be due on the same day each month. These bills should be paid early enough in the month that the actual payment for the service reaches the company to which it is owed before the actual "due" date listed on the bill. It is a good idea to file these bills for payment days earlier than the actual due date so the checks or payment for them will be sent several days in advance to give the post office time to deliver the payment by the due date.

Hiring an Accountant or Bookkeeping Firm

Larger medical practices may hire an accountant or bookkeeping firm to process all checks. This is an accurate means of handling banking procedures. However, these services can be too costly for smaller medical offices. In some firms, a computerized check-writing service system is used.

Deposits

Deposits, which refer to money (cash and checks) placed into a bank account, can be made to either checking or savings accounts. Offices will vary somewhat on specific methods of handling deposits, but the following procedures are usually followed:

- Prepare and make deposits daily.
- Maintain all records of daily receipts (for checks and cash) together in a safe location.

- Compare the total on the deposit slip against the total on the day sheet.
- Keep a duplicate copy of all deposits on file in the office. Photocopy a deposit slip before submitting it to the bank. Some offices copy checks for later reference.
- Keep bank receipts of all deposits on file in the office.
- Immediately note all deposits in the checkbook.

All deposits should be made to the bank as soon as possible. Until cash and checks can be deposited, they should be stored in a secure location that is not accessible to patients.

Always compare the total credited to the accounts receivable with the total on the deposit slip. Occasionally, a check is omitted from the accounts receivable record. Numbers may be transposed when completing the deposit slip or the accounts receivable total. Using the pegboard or write-it-once system, results in a du-

---

14-3 PROCEDURE

Prepare a Deposit Slip

OBJECTIVE: Complete a bank deposit slip.

Equipment and Supplies
pen; deposit slip; checks and currency to be deposited; endorsing stamp; calculator

Method
1. Using the endorsing stamp, endorse all checks to be deposited. This means stamp the back of each check to be deposited with the endorsing stamp.
2. Complete the information on the front of the deposit slip:
   - Account name
   - Account number
   - Date of the deposit
3. If there is cash to be deposited, enter the amount of the cash in the upper right box of the deposit slip beside the "CASH" indicator. In the "CURRENCY box," list the total amount of all cash paper money to be deposited. In the "COIN" box, list the total of all the coin money to be deposited.
4. List each check to be deposited on a different line. If there are more checks than will fit on the

front, list each additional check on the reverse side of the deposit slip.
5. Beside the numbers, list who wrote the check. In the box beside the numbered box, list the amount of the check.
6. List each check in a different numbered box.
7. When all the checks to be deposited are entered on the reverse side of the deposit slip, use a calculator to add all the checks, and enter the total of the checks in the space at the bottom of the deposit slip that reads "TOTAL." This amount is also placed on the front of the deposit slip in the space that reads "TOTAL FROM REVERSE SIDE."
8. Use the calculator to add the total amount of the cash and the checks being deposited. List this amount in the space labeled TOTAL and in the space labeled NET DEPOSIT on the front of the deposit slip.
9. Place the deposit slip and the cash and checks listed on the slip in an envelope for deposit to the bank.

plicate deposit slip. Maintain an accurate balance of all accounts on a daily basis.

Completing the Deposit Slip

A deposit slip is completed every time a deposit is made into a bank account. The slip indicates the total dollar amounts of cash and checks being deposited. Entries on the slip should be printed in black ink. Currency (coins and bills) is totaled separately from checks. Each check must be entered on a different line. If there are more checks than lines provided, the excessive checks can be entered on the back of the deposit slip. The currency and coin totals and check totals are added together. Then this amount, the total for the deposit, is entered on the bottom line of the deposit slip. Procedure 14-3 lists steps for preparing deposit slips. See Figure 14-4 for an example of a deposit slip.

Check all deposits on the deposit slip against the day sheet totals. If the two figures do not match, check for the error in several ways:

- Recheck addition.
- Check each item on the deposit slip.
- Check for transposed numbers.
- If the error is still not found, subtract the difference between the deposit slip and the day sheet, then search for an item with that number.
- Check for errors of omission.

The correct order for listing money on a bank deposit is as follows: currency, coins, checks, and money orders.

Deposit to Savings Accounts

All cash and checks can also be deposited into a savings account. When the amount in a checking account becomes greater than the amount needed to cover the checks written on the account, deposits can be made into a savings account, which will have a greater interest return on the money than a checking account. When transferring funds from a checking account to a savings account, it is advisable to do so by check. This provides a record of the transaction.

A savings account is set up using a statement or a passbook, which are for maintaining a record of deposits, withdrawals, interest earned, and account balance. The passbook should be kept in a safe place

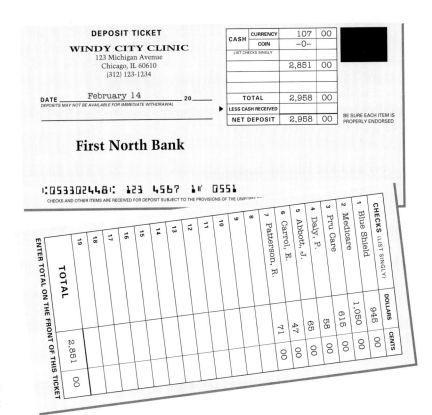

FIGURE 14-4 An example of the front and back side of a deposit slip.

designated for banking materials in the office. Statment savings accounts are sent monthly or quarterly.

Making the Deposit

Deposits can be made to both the checking and savings accounts in person, by mail, or by night depository. If a deposit is made in person, there will be an immediate receipt of deposit. A deposit by mail will result with a receipt by mail. However, cash should not be sent in the mail.

The night depository method can be set up for a business by obtaining a night depository key and depository bags with security locks. The deposit slip, cash, and checks are placed in the bag and then dropped off at the end of the day when the bank may be closed.

It is preferable that only one person be responsible for the deposits and another person be responsible for the receivable records. This separation of responsibilities is a critical method of fiscal or financial control.

Accepting Cash

Cash can be accepted as a form of payment, but this is not encouraged. Receipts must be given for all cash payments. Having large amounts of cash in an office poses a security risk and also holds the potential for the embezzlement of funds. Embezzlement is the taking of funds and involves a breach of trust. Large cash amounts may necessitate making bank deposits more than once a day.

Cash Disbursement

Cash disbursement refers to payments made to your creditors. The term "cash" is misleading since, in most cases, the disbursement is made by check, and not cash. Payment by check provides a permanent record as documentation for taxes and proof of payment.

Bank Hold on Accounts

Occasionally, a bank will place a "hold" on a checking account. A statement may appear that reads "Hold for Uncollected Funds (HCF)" when a deposit needs to "clear" so that the bank can make sure the funds (money) are present before allowing anyone to write a check on that account. This is called a "hold." The bank will not actually credit the account in which the money was deposited until the check has been processed and the funds paid to the payer's bank. These funds cannot be used by the depositor until the check or funds have cleared and the hold is removed. The bank will notify the depositor of the length of time for the hold.

Bank Statement

The purpose of a statement from the bank is to confirm the amount of funds that are in each account. The bank statement can uncover errors that have been made in either the office bookkeeping system or the bank bookkeeping system.

A monthly bank statement includes all debits and credits that have been processed. Debits are charges against an account; credits are additions to an account. The statement will include canceled checks—checks that have been processed and paid out to the medical practice's creditors by the bank. Many banks no longer return canceled checks, which indicates a further need to maintain excellent record keeping on the check stub when the check is written.

Figure 14-5 is an example of a typical bank statement.

Reconciliation of Bank Statements

Reconciliation of bank statements refers to the comparison of the figures on the bank statements with the records maintained in the medical office and the adjustment of banking records so that both are in agreement. The purpose of the reconciliation of bank statements is to match the account activity and totals against the medical office records. Bank statements include the following information:

- Account number
- Average collected balance
- Minimum balance
- Tax ID number (usually the Social Security number of the physician)
- Beginning balance
- Deposit history
- Interest/credits
- Checks and debits
- Service charges
- Ending balance

Bank statements should be reconciled as soon as they are received, and errors that are found should be corrected immediately. Office policy

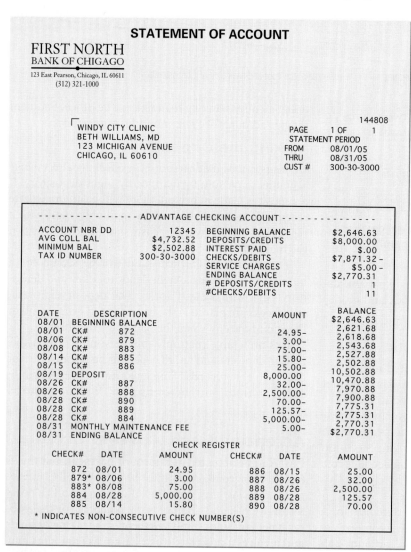

FIGURE 14-5 A typical bank statement.

PROCEDURE

Reconciling a Bank Statement

OBJECTIVE: Reconcile a bank statement for a checking account.

Equipment and Supplies

current and previous bank statements; cancelled checks (if returned by the bank); checkbook stubs

Method

1. Compare the beginning balance of the current statement with the ending balance of the previous statement. These should be the same.
2. Write the current ending balance in the appropriate space on the reverse side of the bank statement.
3. Compare deposits noted on the statement against your records or receipts by making a check mark next to each correct number.
4. List separately all outstanding deposits. These are deposits made toward the end of the month that have not been included in the current statement. Add these together and place the total on the reverse side of the statement in the space provided.
5. Add the ending balance to the total of deposits not already included and write this amount on the TOTAL line.
6. Compare the value of the checks listed on the statement with the value listed in the checkbook or check stubs and place a check mark next to each correct number.
7. Note all numbers missing from the sequential list of check numbers; these are checks that have not yet cleared your bank (outstanding checks). List all outstanding checks. Add the total for outstanding checks and place that figure on the line indicated on the back of the statement.
8. Subtract the total figure for checks outstanding from the previous total on the back of the statement to determine the current balance. This amount should agree with the amount in your check book or stub balance.

Example:

1. Bank balance shown on this statement: $ _____
   ADD (+)
2. Deposits not credited in this statement, (if any) $ _____
3. TOTAL $ _____
   SUBTRACT (−)
4. Checks outstanding $ _____
5. BALANCE $ _____

Summary of RULES:

#1 Note ending statement balance.

#2 Add all deposits not yet credited.

#3 Determine subtotal of step #1 and #2.

#4 Subtract total outstanding checks.

#5 Determine balance or final total.

---

may indicate an exact date when reconciliation should take place. For better fiscal control, the person reconciling the bank statement should be someone other than the person who prepares the checks and makes the deposits. This can prevent the embezzlement of funds.

If it is an interest-bearing account, the interest earned will be on the average collected balance. It is the average amount of money in that account during the period covered by the statement. Any interest credited to the account or any service fees charged to the account, as shown on the bank statement, should be recorded in the checking account records before beginning the reconciliation.

The processed checks will be listed by number. Any checks that are listed in non-consecutive order may be indicated with an asterisk (*).

The reverse side of the bank statement includes information on how to handle errors or questions about the statement, and a form to assist in reconciling the bank statement. Procedure 14-4 lists step-by-step instructions for reconciling a bank statement.

Saving Documentation

Documents relating to banking procedures should be saved in an organized manner. In addition to banking documents, such as copies of deposit slips and check stubs, your records must include the following for verification of business expenses:

- Receipts
- Vouchers for expenses and salaries

The medical assistant acts as the physician's agent when performing the banking procedures for the medical office. In this capacity, the medical assistant must exercise great care and integrity to protect all cash and check receipts that come into the office. Similarly, all disbursements, made by the medical assistant on behalf of the physician and the medical office, must be handled responsibly. Information relating to the banking practices or the total assets of the physician or the medical practice is confidential and should never be discussed outside of the office.

- Invoices
- Statements from suppliers
- Proof of payments

These supporting documents should be saved in a file with check numbers of payments written on the document. After the bank statement has been reconciled each month, it should be stored with the canceled checks as further documentation of business activity. Remember that business expenses are subject to auditing by the Internal Revenue Service (IRS). Good record-keeping is essential when providing documentation to the IRS. For more on the medical assistant's responsibilities when performing banking procedures, see Legal and Ethical Issues.

Petty Cash

Petty cash is available for small purchases, reimbursements, postage due or other miscellaneous expenses within the medical office. For example, petty cash is used for postage due on certified mail received in the office, or postage due on underpaid letters received. Petty cash must be tracked and recorded in a daily financial log. To replenish petty cash, a check is written for the predetermined amount. There is usually a designated amount of cash placed in a drawer or box at the beginning of each month for this purpose. This amount will vary from office to office, depending on the needs of the office, but is usually $50 to $100. At the end of a designated period (a week, or a month), all the receipts for money taken out of the petty cash drawer will be totaled and added to the money remaining in the drawer. This total should match the amount placed in the drawer at the beginning. The cash used during the period will then be replaced to make the total cash available in the drawer equal to the beginning amount. Petty cash is usually handled by one responsible office person and a designee in his or her absence and is kept in a secret place under lock and key.

Payroll

Payroll responsibilities include calculating payroll checks for all the staff. Some medical offices contract an independent payroll service. This may or may not include the physician, depending on how the payment system is set up. Payroll checks are generally issued weekly, biweekly, or monthly. These result in the following pay periods for a year:

Weekly—52 pay periods a year

Biweekly—26 pay periods a year

Monthly—12 pay periods a year

The physician determines the type of pay period the office will use. All employees will then be paid at the same time. Figure 14-6 is an example of an employee payroll record.

The employee's payroll check is determined by first calculating the gross annual wage before taxes and any withholdings that are taken out. Use the formula:

(Hourly wage $\times$ Number of hours worked per week) $\times$ 52 Weeks in a year = Gross pay (or Hourly wage $\times$ 2080 Full-time hours in a year = Annual pay)

The annual gross wage for an employee earning $9.00 per hour working a 40-hour week would be:

$$\$9.00 \times 40 \times 52 = \$18,720$$

annual gross wage

To determine the amount the employee earns per day, use the following formula:

(Annual gross pay $\div$ 52) $\div$ 5 = Day's pay

For the example above: ($18,720 $\div$ 52) = $360

$360 $\div$ 5 = $72

Therefore, if this employee missed a day of work, $72 would be deducted to arrive at the adjusted gross pay ($360 − $72 = $288). Occasionally, an employee will be requested to work overtime or to work more hours than normal for that pay period (a 40-hour week at 8 hours a day for 5 days per week). To calculate the overtime pay of time and a half (1 hour pay plus ½ hour pay) for an employee who worked one day of overtime at the hourly wage of $9.00, simply divide $9.00 in half ($4.50) and add that amount to the regular $9.00 hourly wage ($9.00 + $4.50 = $13.50). The payment for one hour of overtime for this employee would be $13.50 instead of the regular $9.00 payment.

Money is withheld from the employee's paycheck, depending on the taxes that must be paid by the employee and employer. This is referred to as tax withholding. For example, if the withholding tax is four percent, then this amount is calculated based on the employee's gross pay. The taxes are then subtracted from the gross or an adjusted gross pay. The amount after subtracting the withholdings is what appears on the employee's paycheck.

Government regulations require that records must be maintained for each employee relating to the following payroll items:

- Amount of gross pay
- Social Security number of the employee
- Number of exemptions of each employee (taken from W-4 form completed by the employee at the time of hire)
- Deductions for Social Security, federal, state, and city taxes
- State disability insurance and unemployment tax, where applicable

Methods for Calculating Payroll Checks

There are several systems for calculating and issuing payroll checks. They include manual, pegboard, and computer.

Manual

Meticulous recordkeeping is necessary when performing any payroll function. Procedure 14-5 lists steps for manually generating a payroll in a medical office. Separate records are needed for documentation of the gross income, tax withholdings, and each of the checks issued for all employees. This can mean that the records for payroll are kept in more than one record book or logbook. For example, the check stub will indicate the name, date, and amount of the payroll check, while a logbook is needed to track the gross income and withholdings, which are totaled monthly, quarterly, and annually.

Pegboard

The advantage of using a pegboard (write-it-once) method is that all or most of the payroll record is in one record.

Computer

There are several software packages available that are used to calculate payroll and tax withholdings and print payroll checks. Such software programs can save time for office staff over the traditional manual method. In

NAME Joyce Walker   SOCIAL SECURITY NO. 123-12-1234
ADDRESS 22 W. Elm Avenue, Apt 3C   DATE OF EMPLOYMENT 6-30-05
Goram City, MI 55555   TELEPHONE (010)123-4567
EXEMPTIONS 1   HOURLY RATE $10.00

| HOURS | | GROSS SALARY | DEDUCTIONS | | | | | NET SALARY | DATE | CHECK NO. |
REG.	O.T.		FWT	SWT	FICA					
80		800 –	72–	14–	61⁶⁰			652⁴⁰	7/14	276
80		800 –	72–	14–	61⁶⁰			652⁴⁰	7/28	414
72		720 –	64⁸⁰	12⁶⁰	55⁴⁵			587¹⁵	8/11	565
80	4	860 –	77⁴⁰	15⁰⁵	66²⁰			701³⁵	8/25	697
QUARTERLY TOTAL										
YEAR TO DATE										

FIGURE 14-6 An example of an employee payroll record.

addition, the amounts calculated for withholding can be performed more accurately with the computer than with the manual method. In some offices, an outside payroll service is hired to process all payroll checks, withholding payments, and keep records.

Income Tax Withholding

Federal, state, and city taxes are withheld from the paycheck of the employee. These tax payments are made directly to the government. Employers have an obligation by law to withhold a portion of their employee's earnings for tax purposes, and report and forward this amount to the government. To determine the amount of money to be withheld from each paycheck, each employee must complete a W-4 form when he or she is hired (Figure 14-7). The W-4 form must include:

- Employee's name and current address
- Social Security number
- Marital status
- The number of exemptions the employee claims that should be used when calculating withheld tax money

Tables used to determine the amount of withholding are provided in the Federal Employer's Tax Guide.

PROCEDURE

Generating Payroll in a Medical Office

OBJECTIVE: Manually generate payroll.

Equipment and Supplies
pen; calculator; checkbook; employee time card; employee payroll record; payroll register; tax tables

Method
1. Gather the above equipment.
2. Using the employee time card, calculate the total number of regular hours worked and then the total number of overtime hours worked. Enter the totals obtained on the payroll register.
3. In the employee payroll record, obtain the employee's pay rate. Calculate the pay rate times the total number of regular hours worked. Next, calculate the overtime pay rate times the total number of overtime hours. Enter the totals for each on the payroll register. Add the regular hours earned and overtime hours earned and place this amount on the payroll register under the heading total gross.
4. Gather the employee payroll record and tax tables. Determine how much to withhold for federal income tax. This depends on the marital status of the employee as well as the amount of exemptions. Next, calculate the total FICA tax to be withheld for Medicare and Social Security. Enter the amounts on the payroll register.
5. Determine how much to withhold for local and state taxes. This depends on the marital status of the employee and the amount of exemptions. Enter the amounts on the payroll register.
6. Compute employer's contributions to the unemployment fund of the state of residence and FUTA. Next, document these calculations on the employer's account.
7. Determine if there are any other deductions (i.e. stock purchase plans, insurance, flexible spending account, or 401K).
8. To calculate the net earnings subtract the total amount of deductions from the gross earnings.
9. Complete the check stub and check with the required information.

See Figure 14-8 for a sample federal tax-withholding table. Tables are available for married persons, single persons, and unmarried heads of households and cover weekly, biweekly, monthly, semimonthly, and daily periods.

Social Security, Medicare, and Income Tax Withholding

The federal government mandates, or requires, the following taxes be paid: Social Security (Federal Insurance Contribution Act or FICA), Medicare, and federal income tax. These taxes are based on a percentage of the employee's total gross income (see calculation on page 260 for determining gross income). The number of exemptions claimed on the W-4 form and the marital status of the employee are taken into account when calculating the tax. The employer has an obligation to match the employee's payment for Social Security and Medicare. This means that if the employee has $100 withheld for Social Security and Medicare, the employer must match the $100 and make a total payment to the government for that employee of $200. The employer does not have to match the federal, state, and local taxes.

Deposit Requirements

The federal tax money withheld and the FICA payment are placed into a federal deposit account in a Federal Reserve Bank or into an authorized banking institution, either at the end of each period or at the end of the month. The Internal Revenue Service (IRS) has a severe penalty for failure to deposit this money.

Employers must file a quarterly report (Form 941 Employer's Quarterly Federal Tax Return) before the last day of the first month after the end of the quarter. These dates are April 30, July 31, October 31, and January 31.

Federal Unemployment Tax

Every employer must contribute to the unemployment tax act as mandated under the Federal Unemployment Tax Act (FUTA). If the employer is making payments into a state unemployment fund, this can generally be applied as credit against the FUTA tax amount.

Form W-4 (20XX)

Purpose. Complete Form W-4 so that your employer can withhold the correct federal income tax from your pay. Because your tax situation may change, you may want to refigure your withholding each year.

Exemption from withholding. If you are exempt, complete only lines 1, 2, 3, 4, and 7 and sign the form to validate it. Your exemption for 20XX expires February 16, 20XX. See Pub. 505, Tax Withholding and Estimated Tax.

Note. You cannot claim exemption from withholding if (a) your income exceeds $800 and includes more than $250 of unearned income (for example, interest and dividends) and (b) another person can claim you as a dependent on their tax return.

Basic instructions. If you are not exempt, complete the **Personal Allowances Worksheet** below. The worksheets on page 2 adjust your withholding allowances based on itemized deductions, certain credits, adjustments to income, or two-earner/two-job situations. Complete all worksheets that apply. However, you may claim fewer (or zero) allowances.

Head of household. Generally, you may claim head of household filing status on your tax return only if you are unmarried and pay more than 50% of the costs of keeping up a home for yourself and your dependent(s) or other qualifying individuals. See line E below.

Tax credits. You can take projected tax credits into account in figuring your allowable number of withholding allowances. Credits for child or dependent care expenses and the child tax credit may be claimed using the **Personal Allowances Worksheet** below. See Pub. 919, How Do I Adjust My Tax Withholding? for information on converting your other credits into withholding allowances.

Nonwage income. If you have a large amount of nonwage income, such as interest or dividends, consider making estimated tax payments using Form 1040-ES, Estimated Tax for Individuals. Otherwise, you may owe additional tax.

Two earners/two jobs. If you have a working spouse or more than one job, figure the total number of allowances you are entitled to claim on all jobs using worksheets from only one Form W-4. Your withholding usually will be most accurate when all allowances are claimed on the Form W-4 for the highest paying job and zero allowances are claimed on the others.

Nonresident alien. If you are a nonresident alien, see the Instructions for Form 8233 before completing this Form W-4.

Check your withholding. After your Form W-4 takes effect, use Pub. 919 to see how the dollar amount you are having withheld compares to your projected total tax for 20XX. See Pub. 919, especially if your earnings exceed $125,000 (Single) or $175,000 (Married).

Recent name change? If your name on line 1 differs from that shown on your social security card, call 1-800-772-1213 to initiate a name change and obtain a social security card showing your correct name.

Personal Allowances Worksheet (Keep for your records.)

A Enter "1" for **yourself** if no one else can claim you as a dependent . . . . **A** _____

B Enter "1" if:
- You are single and have only one job; or
- You are married, have only one job, and your spouse does not work; or
- Your wages from a second job or your spouse's wages (or the total of both) are $1,000 or less.

. . **B** _____

C Enter "1" for your **spouse.** But, you may choose to enter "-0-" if you are married and have either a working spouse or more than one job. (Entering "-0-" may help you avoid having too little tax withheld.) . . . . **C** _____

D Enter number of **dependents** (other than your spouse or yourself) you will claim on your tax return . . . . . . **D** _____

E Enter "1" if you will file as **head of household** on your tax return (see conditions under **Head of household** above) . **E** _____

F Enter "1" if you have at least $1,500 of **child or dependent care expenses** for which you plan to claim a credit . . **F** _____
(**Note.** Do **not** include child support payments. See **Pub. 503,** Child and Dependent Care Expenses, for details.)

G **Child Tax Credit** (including additional child tax credit):
- If your total income will be less than $54,000 ($79,000 if married), enter "2" for each eligible child.
- If your total income will be between $54,000 and $84,000 ($79,000 and $119,000 if married), enter "1" for each eligible child plus "1" **additional** if you have four or more eligible children. **G** _____

H Add lines A through G and enter total here. (**Note.** This may be different from the number of exemptions you claim on your tax return.) ▶ **H** _____

For accuracy, complete all worksheets that apply.
- If you plan to **itemize or claim adjustments to income** and want to reduce your withholding, see the **Deductions and Adjustments Worksheet** on page 2.
- If you have **more than one job** or are **married and you and your spouse both work** and the combined earnings from all jobs exceed $35,000 ($25,000 if married) see the **Two-Earner/Two-Job Worksheet** on page 2 to avoid having too little tax withheld.
- If **neither** of the above situations applies, **stop here** and enter the number from line H on line 5 of Form W-4 below.

Cut here and give Form W-4 to your employer. Keep the top part for your records.

Form **W-4**

Department of the Treasury
Internal Revenue Service

Employee's Withholding Allowance Certificate

▶ Whether you are entitled to claim a certain number of allowances or exemption from withholding is subject to review by the IRS. Your employer may be required to send a copy of this form to the IRS.

OMB No. 1545-0010

20XX

1 Type or print your first name and middle initial	Last name	2 Your social security number

Home address (number and street or rural route)	3 ☐ Single ☐ Married ☐ Married, but withhold at higher Single rate.
City or town, state, and ZIP code	**Note.** If married, but legally separated, or spouse is a nonresident alien, check the "Single" box.
	4 If your last name differs from that shown on your social security card, check here. You must call 1-800-772-1213 for a new card. ▶ ☐

5 Total number of allowances you are claiming (from line **H** above **or** from the applicable worksheet on page 2) | **5** _____

6 Additional amount, if any, you want withheld from each paycheck . . . . | **6** $ _____

7 I claim exemption from withholding for 20XX, and I certify that I meet **both** of the following conditions for exemption.
- Last year I had a right to a refund of **all** federal income tax withheld because I had **no** tax liability **and**
- This year I expect a refund of **all** federal income tax withheld because I expect to have **no** tax liability.

If you meet both conditions, write "Exempt" here . . . . ▶ | **7** _____

Under penalties of perjury, I declare that I have examined this certificate and to the best of my knowledge and belief, it is true, correct, and complete.

Employee's signature
(Form is not valid unless you sign it.) ▶ _____   Date ▶ _____

8 Employer's name and address (Employer: Complete lines 8 and 10 only if sending to the IRS.)	9 Office code (optional)	10 Employer identification number (EIN)

For Privacy Act and Paperwork Reduction Act Notice, see page 2.   Cat. No. 10220Q   Form **W-4** (20XX)

FIGURE 14-7 An example of a W-4 required by the IRS.

2004 Tax Table

See the instructions for line 43 that begin on page 33 to see if you must use the Tax Table below to figure your tax.

Example. Mr. and Mrs. Brown are filing a joint return. Their taxable income on Form 1040, line 42, is $25,300. First, they find the $25,300–25,350 taxable income line. Next, they find the column for married filing jointly and read down the column. The amount shown where the taxable income line and filing status column meet is $3,084. This is the tax amount they should enter on Form 1040, line 43.

Sample Table

At least	But less than	Single	Married filing jointly*	Married filing separately	Head of a household
			Your tax is—		
25,200	25,250	3,426	3,069	3,426	3,274
25,250	25,300	3,434	3,076	3,434	3,281
25,300	25,350	3,441	(3,084)	3,441	3,289
25,350	25,400	3,449	3,091	3,449	3,296

If line 42 (taxable income) is— At least	But less than	Single	Married filing jointly*	Married filing separately	Head of a household
			Your tax is—		
0	5	0	0	0	0
5	15	1	1	1	1
15	25	2	2	2	2
25	50	4	4	4	4
50	75	6	6	6	6
75	100	9	9	9	9
100	125	11	11	11	11
125	150	14	14	14	14
150	175	16	16	16	16
175	200	19	19	19	19
200	225	21	21	21	21
225	250	24	24	24	24
250	275	26	26	26	26
275	300	29	29	29	29
300	325	31	31	31	31
325	350	34	34	34	34
350	375	36	36	36	36
375	400	39	39	39	39
400	425	41	41	41	41
425	450	44	44	44	44
450	475	46	46	46	46
475	500	49	49	49	49
500	525	51	51	51	51
525	550	54	54	54	54
550	575	56	56	56	56
575	600	59	59	59	59
600	625	61	61	61	61
625	650	64	64	64	64
650	675	66	66	66	66
675	700	69	69	69	69
700	725	71	71	71	71
725	750	74	74	74	74
750	775	76	76	76	76
775	800	79	79	79	79
800	825	81	81	81	81
825	850	84	84	84	84
850	875	86	86	86	86
875	900	89	89	89	89
900	925	91	91	91	91
925	950	94	94	94	94
950	975	96	96	96	96
975	1,000	99	99	99	99

1,000

At least	But less than	Single	Married filing jointly*	Married filing separately	Head of a household
1,000	1,025	101	101	101	101
1,025	1,050	104	104	104	104
1,050	1,075	106	106	106	106
1,075	1,100	109	109	109	109
1,100	1,125	111	111	111	111
1,125	1,150	114	114	114	114
1,150	1,175	116	116	116	116
1,175	1,200	119	119	119	119
1,200	1,225	121	121	121	121
1,225	1,250	124	124	124	124
1,250	1,275	126	126	126	126
1,275	1,300	129	129	129	129

If line 42 (taxable income) is— At least	But less than	Single	Married filing jointly*	Married filing separately	Head of a household
			Your tax is—		
1,300	1,325	131	131	131	131
1,325	1,350	134	134	134	134
1,350	1,375	136	136	136	136
1,375	1,400	139	139	139	139
1,400	1,425	141	141	141	141
1,425	1,450	144	144	144	144
1,450	1,475	146	146	146	146
1,475	1,500	149	149	149	149
1,500	1,525	151	151	151	151
1,525	1,550	154	154	154	154
1,550	1,575	156	156	156	156
1,575	1,600	159	159	159	159
1,600	1,625	161	161	161	161
1,625	1,650	164	164	164	164
1,650	1,675	166	166	166	166
1,675	1,700	169	169	169	169
1,700	1,725	171	171	171	171
1,725	1,750	174	174	174	174
1,750	1,775	176	176	176	176
1,775	1,800	179	179	179	179
1,800	1,825	181	181	181	181
1,825	1,850	184	184	184	184
1,850	1,875	186	186	186	186
1,875	1,900	189	189	189	189
1,900	1,925	191	191	191	191
1,925	1,950	194	194	194	194
1,950	1,975	196	196	196	196
1,975	2,000	199	199	199	199

2,000

At least	But less than	Single	Married filing jointly*	Married filing separately	Head of a household
2,000	2,025	201	201	201	201
2,025	2,050	204	204	204	204
2,050	2,075	206	206	206	206
2,075	2,100	209	209	209	209
2,100	2,125	211	211	211	211
2,125	2,150	214	214	214	214
2,150	2,175	216	216	216	216
2,175	2,200	219	219	219	219
2,200	2,225	221	221	221	221
2,225	2,250	224	224	224	224
2,250	2,275	226	226	226	226
2,275	2,300	229	229	229	229
2,300	2,325	231	231	231	231
2,325	2,350	234	234	234	234
2,350	2,375	236	236	236	236
2,375	2,400	239	239	239	239
2,400	2,425	241	241	241	241
2,425	2,450	244	244	244	244
2,450	2,475	246	246	246	246
2,475	2,500	249	249	249	249
2,500	2,525	251	251	251	251
2,525	2,550	254	254	254	254
2,550	2,575	256	256	256	256
2,575	2,600	259	259	259	259
2,600	2,625	261	261	261	261
2,625	2,650	264	264	264	264
2,650	2,675	266	266	266	266
2,675	2,700	269	269	269	269

If line 42 (taxable income) is— At least	But less than	Single	Married filing jointly*	Married filing separately	Head of a household
			Your tax is—		
2,700	2,725	271	271	271	271
2,725	2,750	274	274	274	274
2,750	2,775	276	276	276	276
2,775	2,800	279	279	279	279
2,800	2,825	281	281	281	281
2,825	2,850	284	284	284	284
2,850	2,875	286	286	286	286
2,875	2,900	289	289	289	289
2,900	2,925	291	291	291	291
2,925	2,950	294	294	294	294
2,950	2,975	296	296	296	296
2,975	3,000	299	299	299	299

3,000

At least	But less than	Single	Married filing jointly*	Married filing separately	Head of a household
3,000	3,050	303	303	303	303
3,050	3,100	308	308	308	308
3,100	3,150	313	313	313	313
3,150	3,200	318	318	318	318
3,200	3,250	323	323	323	323
3,250	3,300	328	328	328	328
3,300	3,350	333	333	333	333
3,350	3,400	338	338	338	338
3,400	3,450	343	343	343	343
3,450	3,500	348	348	348	348
3,500	3,550	353	353	353	353
3,550	3,600	358	358	358	358
3,600	3,650	363	363	363	363
3,650	3,700	368	368	368	368
3,700	3,750	373	373	373	373
3,750	3,800	378	378	378	378
3,800	3,850	383	383	383	383
3,850	3,900	388	388	388	388
3,900	3,950	393	393	393	393
3,950	4,000	398	398	398	398

4,000

At least	But less than	Single	Married filing jointly*	Married filing separately	Head of a household
4,000	4,050	403	403	403	403
4,050	4,100	408	408	408	408
4,100	4,150	413	413	413	413
4,150	4,200	418	418	418	418
4,200	4,250	423	423	423	423
4,250	4,300	428	428	428	428
4,300	4,350	433	433	433	433
4,350	4,400	438	438	438	438
4,400	4,450	443	443	443	443
4,450	4,500	448	448	448	448
4,500	4,550	453	453	453	453
4,550	4,600	458	458	458	458
4,600	4,650	463	463	463	463
4,650	4,700	468	468	468	468
4,700	4,750	473	473	473	473
4,750	4,800	478	478	478	478
4,800	4,850	483	483	483	483
4,850	4,900	488	488	488	488
4,900	4,950	493	493	493	493
4,950	5,000	498	498	498	498

(Continued on page 61)

* This column must also be used by a qualifying widow(er).

FIGURE 14-8 An example of a federal tax witholding table.

FUTA is the sole responsibility of the employer. It is based on the employee's gross income, but must not be deducted from the employee's wage.

FUTA deposits are calculated quarterly and the amount due must be paid by the last day of the first month after the quarter ends. Therefore, for the first quarter of the year ending on March 31st, the payment must be made by April 30th. An annual FUTA report must be filed to the federal government using Form 940 each year.

State Unemployment Tax

All states have unemployment compensation laws. Most states require only the employer to make payments toward this fund. However, a few states require both the employer and employee to make a payment. In this case, the employer would withhold a certain calculated amount from the employee's paycheck.

In some states, the employer does not have to make a payment to unemployment compensation if there are very few employees (four or less). Each state's regulation concerning tax requirements should be checked carefully before preparing the payroll.

State Disability Insurance

Some states require a certain amount of money be withheld from the employee's check to cover a disability insurance plan. This insurance coverage assists employees in the event they become injured or disabled and unable to work. Money may also be withheld, as requested by the employee, for health, life, and disability insurances, and pension plan contributions.

Annual Tax Returns

W-2 forms must be completed at the end of each year and given to each employee. The amount of wages that were taxable under Social Security and Medicare must be listed separately on the W-2 form. The employer must provide three copies of the W-2 form to each employee from whom these taxes were withheld (one each for federal and state filing and one for the employee's file). According to the law, this form must be received by the employee by January 31. The W-2 form (Figure 14-9) lists the total gross income, total federal, state, and local taxes that were withheld, taxable fringe benefits, such as tips, and the employee's total net income for the year.

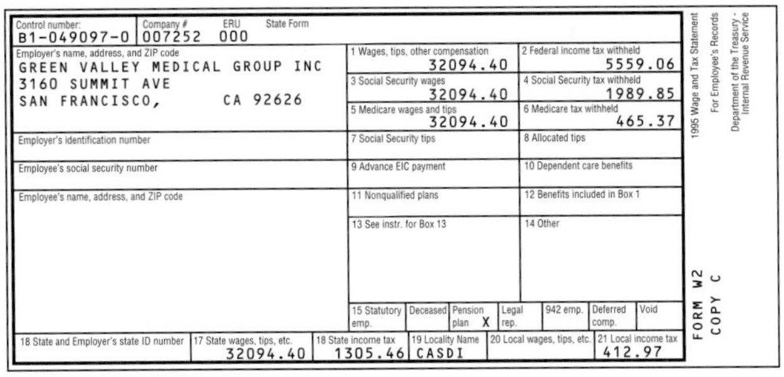

Control number: B1-049097-0
Company # 007252 ERU 000 State Form
Employer's name, address, and ZIP code: GREEN VALLEY MEDICAL GROUP INC, 3160 SUMMIT AVE, SAN FRANCISCO, CA 92626
1 Wages, tips, other compensation: 32094.40
2 Federal income tax withheld: 5559.06
3 Social Security wages: 32094.40
4 Social Security tax withheld: 1989.85
5 Medicare wages and tips: 32094.40
6 Medicare tax withheld: 465.37
Employer's identification number
7 Social Security tips
8 Allocated tips
Employee's social security number
9 Advance EIC payment
10 Dependent care benefits
Employee's name, address, and ZIP code
11 Nonqualified plans
12 Benefits included in Box 1
13 See instr. for Box 13
14 Other
15 Statutory emp. | Deceased | Pension plan X | Legal rep. | 942 emp. | Deferred comp. | Void
18 State and Employer's state ID number
17 State wages, tips, etc.: 32094.40
18 State income tax: 1305.46
19 Locality Name: CASDI
20 Local wages, tips, etc.
21 Local income tax: 412.97
1995 Wage and Tax Statement
For Employee's Records
Department of the Treasury - Internal Revenue Service
FORM W2
COPY C

FIGURE 14-9 An example of a W-2 form required by the IRS.

The preparation of reports to the federal government and the W-2 forms for the employees can be time-consuming and requires some training. Many offices that do not have a bookkeeper or medical assistant assigned to this duty, use the services of an accountant. The records and reports the accountant will use need to be prepared ahead of time. The pegboard system, if used, can provide summaries of the income, expenses, and payroll for the office. If a manual system is used, the totals for all the tax payment periods should be calculated for the accountant. The accountant will then audit or reexamine all the financial statements for accuracy.

SUMMARY

Banking is one of the critical office procedures, since it requires careful handling of money and records. A thorough understanding of banking procedures and terminology is vital to running on efficient medical office. Great trust is placed upon the medical assistant by the physician to handle his or her banking needs with accuracy.

Chapter Review

COMPETENCY REVIEW

1. Define and spell the terms to learn for the chapter.
2. Using your own bank statement, reconcile it to your checkbook records.
3. Create and complete a check and check stub in the amount of 65 cents drafted to Bill Jay.
4. Call a local bank and request information regarding the various options for checking and savings accounts.
5. Create a bank deposit slip for $23.10 in cash and checks for $54.00, $21.25, $110.00, $29.00, and $9.25.

1. A check that will become void if written over a certain amount is a
   A. certified check
   B. limited check
   C. cashier's check
   D. warrant
   E. deposit

2. The person who signs the check is the
   A. maker
   B. payee
   C. payer
   D. teller
   E. depositor

3. The code number found in the upper and sometimes lower right-hand corner of a printed check is the
   A. MICR
   B. withdrawal number
   C. registration number
   D. ABA number
   E. Social Security number

4. Future-dated checks are referred to as
   A. postdated
   B. old
   C. traveler's
   D. voucher
   E. predated

5. Which of the following is petty cash NOT available for?
   A. small purchase
   B. payroll
   C. postage due
   D. reimbursements
   E. other miscellaneous expenses

6. Which of the following is a FALSE statement about check stubs?
   A. stubs should have the purpose of check
   B. stubs should have the name of payee
   C. stubs should have the name of payer
   D. stubs should be filled out after removing from checkbook
   E. stubs should be retained

7. Third-party checks that are safe to accept are those that are
   A. from patients
   B. from insurance companies
   C. from vendors
   D. never to be accepted
   E. from out-of-town patients

8. Reconcile the bank statement and checkbook balance for the following: bank statement $1,200, checkbook balance $1,350, bank fees $20, outstanding checks $140 and $200. What is the correct checkbook balance?
   A. $1,200
   B. $1,310
   C. $1,330
   D. $1,350
   E. $1,430

9. What information is NOT listed on an employee's W-4 form?
   A. marital status
   B. number of exemptions
   C. salary
   D. employee's Social Security number
   E. current address

10. By law, the employer must match employee contributions on what tax?
    A. disability insurance
    B. workmans' compensation
    C. Social Security
    D. state
    E. self-employment tax

CRITICAL THINKING

1. What effect will Sara's decision to "borrow" money from petty cash have on the funds?

2. What could Sara have done differently if she wished to borrow money from petty cash?

ON THE JOB

Your office has decided that all payroll should be handled through direct deposit into the employee bank accounts. Call your bank, ask them how that procedure would be handled for a medical office. There are forms to complete and information on other bank account numbers and ABA numbers that you will need to collect and complete, according to the bank's procedures.

INTERNET ACTIVITY

Call your bank and get its online address. Then go to the Internet and access the bank's home page. If you do not have a bank account, call several local banks and go to their home pages. List the steps in setting up an online banking account.

MediaLink More on financial management, including interactive resources, can be found on the Student CD-ROM accompanying this textbook.

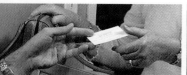

Medical Assistant Role Delineation Chart

HIGHLIGHT indicates material covered in this chapter.

ADMINISTRATIVE

Administrative Procedures

- Perform basic administrative medical assisting functions
- Schedule, coordinate and monitor appointments
- Schedule inpatient/outpatient admissions and procedures
- Understand and apply third-party guidelines
- Obtain reimbursement through accurate claims submission
- Monitor third-party reimbursement
- Understand and adhere to managed care policies and procedures
- *Negotiate managed care contracts*

Practice Finances

- Perform procedural and diagnostic coding
- Apply bookkeeping principles

- Manage accounts receivable
- *Manage accounts payable*
- *Process payroll*
- *Document and maintain accounting and banking records*
- *Develop and maintain fee schedules*
- *Manage renewals of business and professional insurance policies*
- *Manage personnel benefits and maintain records*
- *Perform marketing, financial, and strategic planning*

CLINICAL

Fundamental Principles

- Apply principles of aseptic technique and infection control
- Comply with quality assurance practices
- Screen and follow up patient test results

Diagnostic Orders

- Collect and process specimens
- Perform diagnostic tests

Patient Care

- Adhere to established patient screening procedures
- Obtain patient history and vital signs
- Prepare and maintain examination and treatment areas
- Prepare patient for examinations, procedures and treatments

- Assist with examinations, procedures and treatments
- Prepare and administer medications and immunizations
- Maintain medication and immunization records
- Recognize and respond to emergencies
- Coordinate patient care information with other health care providers
- Initiate IV and administer IV medications with appropriate training and as permitted by state law

GENERAL

Professionalism

- Display a professional manner and image
- Demonstrate initiative and responsibility
- Work as a member of the health care team
- Prioritize and perform multiple tasks
- Adapt to change
- Promote the CMA credential
- Enhance skills through continuing education
- Treat all patients with compassion and empathy
- Promote the practice through positive public relations

Communication Skills

- Recognize and respect cultural diversity
- Adapt communications to individual's ability to understand
- Use professional telephone technique

- Recognize and respond effectively to verbal, nonverbal, and written communications
- Use medical terminology appropriately
- Utilize electronic technology to receive, organize, prioritize and transmit information
- Serve as liaison

Legal Concepts

- Perform within legal and ethical boundaries
- Prepare and maintain medical records
- Document accurately
- Follow employer's established policies dealing with the health care contract
- Implement and maintain federal and state health care legislation and regulations
- Comply with established risk management and safety procedures
- Recognize professional credentialing criteria
- *Develop and maintain personnel, policy and procedure manuals*

Instruction

- Instruct individuals according to their needs
- Explain office policies and procedures
- Teach methods of health promotion and disease prevention
- Locate community resources and disseminate information
- *Develop educational materials*
- *Conduct continuing education activities*

Operational Functions

- Perform inventory of supplies and equipment
- Perform routine maintenance of administrative and clinical equipment
- Apply computer techniques to support office operations
- *Perform personnel management functions*
- *Negotiate leases and prices for equipment and supply contracts*

- *Denotes advanced skills.*

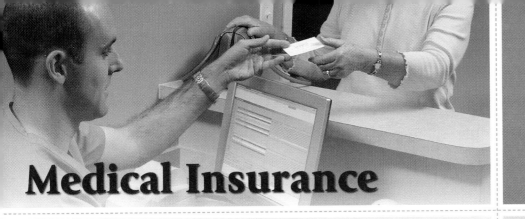

Medical Insurance

Learning Objectives

After completing this chapter, you should be able to:

- Define and spell the terms to learn for this chapter.

- Describe group, individual, and government-sponsored (public) health benefits and explain the differences between them.

- Explain the differences between health maintenance organizations (HMOs), preferred provider organizations (PPOs), and traditional insurance programs.

Terms to Learn

benefit period

claim

closed-panel HMO

crossover claim

deductible

exclusive provider organization (EPO)

fee schedule

health maintenance organization (HMO)

integrated delivery system (IDS)

medical foundation

open-panel HMO

point-of-service plan (POS)

preauthorization

preferred provider organization (PPO)

premium

prepaid plan

primary care physician (PCP)

referral

self-referral

subscriber

Case Study

MIRIAM JONES IS THE CMA WORKING at the front desk today at Dr. Johnson's office. She is responsible for checking in patients and verifying their insurance. Jessie is a patient who arrives for an appointment. She is 16 years old and the oldest of three children in a single parent family. Jessie's mother cannot afford the insurance plan at her job. However, Jessie is able to receive medical care because she and her siblings qualify for government medical coverage.

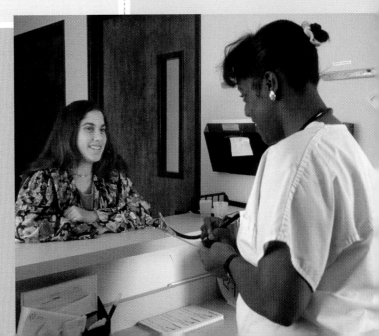

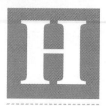ealth insurance was originally designed to help patients with catastrophic medical expenses that occurred as a result of an unexpected illness or injury. Health benefits have existed as a contract between the subscriber (insured) and the carrier (insurance company or third party payer). The first medical or health insurance plans were not intended to cover all costs associated with health care. Over the years, insurance plans for medical and health care have expanded. As the cost of medical care has escalated, new and different types of health care plans and many regulations have also come into being. In today's medical practices, as much as 85 percent of a physician's income is paid by some form of medical insurance.

The successful medical assistant understands the importance of insurance to both the patient and the practice. He or she keeps current with regulations governing the health insurance industry and how these regulations affect the practice's reimbursements as well as the patients who are insured under the various policies available. This means the medical assistant must be able to process a written and documented request for reimbursement, or claim, for an eligible expense in a correct and timely manner.

Purpose of Health Insurance

Generally, insurance is something that provides protection against or compensation for specific types of risk, loss, or ruin. It is a contract in which an insurance company or agency agrees to pay a sum of money to the insured in the event of some contingency such as death, accident, or illness, in return for the payment of a premium by the insured. Medical insurance was not designed to cover all costs associated with health care, but to assist the patient with expenses incurred for medical treatment.

Health Insurance and Availability of Health Insurance

Health insurance includes all forms of insurance against financial loss resulting from illness or injury. These losses may include the expenses of hospitalization, surgery, and other medical services. Commercial insurance companies sell various types of medical policies. Both commercial and nonprofit programs offer essentially the same types of coverage, which are divided into four categories: regular medical expenses, hospitalization, surgery, and major medical expenses.

Hospitalization insurance includes expenses such as the cost of the hospital room and meals, use of the operating room, x-ray and laboratory fees for tests done while the insured patient is in the hospital as well as some medications and supplies. Hospitalization benefits, under insurance plans, are usually limited to a total monetary amount or a maximum number of days.

Insurance covering surgical procedures may change according to the city or state where the surgery is performed. These limits are based on "reasonable and customary" charges for various types of surgery within the region. A general statement regarding the insurers co-payment and deduction may be required by the patient as designated by the insurance carrier.

Relatively new types of insurance are the fixed payment plans. These are offered by organizations that operate their own health care facilities or that have made arrangements with a hospital or health care provider within a city or region. The fixed-payment plan offers subscribers, or members, complete medical care in return for a fixed monthly fee or semi-monthly fee. This fee is called a premium. When the premium is paid, certain benefits become available for reimbursement. Some contracts specify a maximum lifetime benefit. For example, health maintenance organizations (HMOs) base their operations on fixed prepayment plans.

Health care insurance today is available in these three common options, each having subset options discussed below:

- Managed Care—fixed, prepaid-fee plans with contracted health care providers obtained either independently or as a group.

- Group-sponsored or individual policies—purchased through commercial insurance companies.

- Government-sponsored programs—financed and regulated by federal or state governments for specific groups of people. Some examples of government-sponsored insurance include Medicare, Medicaid, workers' compensation, and military plans such as TRICARE and CHAMPVA.

Any of these plans will help with the cost of health care, but they do not cover all expenses. For any of the insurance options, the insured pays a monthly fee, or premium, for specific coverage. Often, the insured also has a deductible, or a sum of money that must be paid before the insurance plan pays benefits for services rendered. Patient Education has more on handling covered and non-covered insurance services.

Managed Care Organizations (MCOs)

Managed care organizations offer options that are available through private insurance carriers and through some government programs. This type of plan is referred

Most patients have difficulty understanding the details of health insurance. Practicing medical assistants often encounter patients who are convinced that, because they have paid premiums to the insurance company, they should pay nothing further to the provider of service. Tact and patience are essential in educating patients about covered and non-covered services.

to as a prepaid plan in that a group of physicians will have a contractual agreement to provide services to subscribers on a negotiated fee-for-service basis. A fee schedule lists the amount to be paid by the insurance company for each procedure or service subject to the managed care contract.

In some managed care situations, the patient is assigned a primary care provider (PCP), who is responsible for the overall management of the patient's health. This PCP acts as a gatekeeper, determining the medical necessity of services by specialist providers. At the same time, the managed care organization stresses the concept of wellness, often paying higher benefits for routine health maintenance (physical examinations, routine immunizations, etc.). In this manner, the managed care organization tries to decrease the number of visits a patient needs to make per calendar year for health care services of an acute nature.

The History of Managed Care Systems

America's first privately owned, prepaid medical group was founded in 1929 in Southern California. The Ross-Loos Medical Group was composed of several medical group locations and provided services to Los Angeles Department of Water and Power employees. In the 1970s, Ross-Loos merged with a health plan group in Philadelphia to become CIGNA Healthplans of California. The federal Health Maintenance Organization Act of 1973 allowed this to occur. The act:

- Provided funds (loans and grants) to assist in the development of new federally qualified HMOs.
- Required most employers with more than 25 employees to offer HMO benefits as an alternative to traditional health insurance plans.
- Established federal standards for HMOs.

In 1985, the Preferred Provider Health Care Act impacted the preferred provider organizations (PPOs). This act allowed subscribers to utilize providers outside the defined network. A 1988 amendment to the HMO Act of 1973 made similar changes to the HMO system.

Advantages and Disadvantages of Managed Care

How has managed care impacted the cost of health care? Costs have been contained by who, what, and where. This means the manage care organization has a limited number of physicians and facilities from which the patient receives services. The manage care organization also chooses the types of services the patient can or will receive. Box 15-1 lists advantages and disadvantages of managed care.

Health Maintenance Organizations (HMOs)

A health maintenance organization (HMO) is type of managed care plan in which a range of health care services by a limited group of providers (such as

---

BOX 15-1
Advantages and Disadvantages of Managed Care

Advantages
- Smaller out-of-pocket expenses for the patient.
- Patient pays a nominal co-payment.
- Some plans do not have a deductible.
- Contains health care cost.
- Payment for authorized services.
- Fee schedules are established.
- Preventive medical treatment is usually covered.

Disadvantages
- Increased amount of paperwork.
- Preauthorization requirements.
- Lower reimbursement rates.
- Limited physician choices.
- Coverage is not guaranteed to be renewed.
- Specialized care is limited at times.
- Referrals are limited at times.
- Limited flexibility.
- Non-approved or non-authorized treatments are not covered.

physicians and hospitals) are made available to plan members for a predetermined fee (the capitation rate). The HMO concept was started to control the cost explosion in health care as a result of over utilization of services. Before HMOs became so widespread, insurance companies reimbursed providers for all their charges without questioning whether the services were necessary. There was little incentive for providers to control costs. HMOs operate on a budget that is the total of their member patients' fees. For this reason, HMOs attempt to control the length of hospital stays or unnecessary surgery for their members. Two important components of an HMO are:

- All medical services are provided based upon a predetermined (per capita) fee and not on a fee-for-service basis. If the actual cost of services exceeds this predetermined (or capitation) amount, then the provider must absorb the excess in costs. This provides the incentive for the provider to control costs.

- A member patient must use the physicians and hospitals that are identified by the HMO. The HMO will pay for any covered services that are provided by designated providers, hospitals, durable medical equipment, and pharmacies. Therefore pre-approval must be granted through the primary care physician (PCP) when and if a patient has to seek consultation or medical services out of the network. The exception to this is in the case of recognized emergency services.

HMOs place an emphasis on maintaining health. Regular physical examinations and patient education are encouraged. The advantage of HMOs is the control of health costs by encouraging providers to limit unnecessary tests and procedures. Premiums therefore, are lower. The disadvantage is that providers may decide not to provide services patients need in order to cut costs.

A member patient who joins an HMO may either choose a personal physician from a list of provider physicians or be assigned a primary care physician (PCP) who is generally an internist, family practitioner, gynecologist, or pediatrician. The PCP must provide all primary care services since the HMO will not pay for the costs of a non-member provider, except in the case of an emergency. HMOs are required to tell members, in the documents regarding their coverage, of the patient's right to ask for an investigation of any problems concerning care or coverage under the HMO.

HMO Models
There are two categories of HMO models: Closed-panel HMO and open-panel HMO. In the closed-panel HMO, the clinic is owned by the HMO and the physicians are employees of the HMO. There are two types of closed-panel models: the group model HMO

and staff model HMO. In the group model, the HMO may contract with physicians who are part of an independent group practice. The HMO reimburses the physician group for providing care to subscribers. The group is responsible for reimbursing the treating physician. In the staff model, the physicians are employees of the HMO. All premiums are paid to the HMO.

In the open-panel HMO, the health care providers are not employees of the HMO and do not belong to a medical group owned or managed by the HMO. There are three models under this category: direct contract model, individual practice association (IPA) model, and the network model. Individual physicians in the community provide contracted health care services to subscribers in the direct contract model. The individual practice association (IPA) model is similar to the direct contract model in that the physicians are not employees of the HMO. The difference is that the IPA can negotiate contracts and manage the capitation payment from the HMO. With the network model HMO, contracted services are provided by more than one physician group practices.

Preferred Provider Organizations (PPOs)
The "preferred provider option" means that the patient must use a medical provider (physician or hospital) who is under contract with the insurer for an agreed-on-fee. A preferred provider organization (PPO) is similar to an HMO but differs in two main areas:

- The PPO is a fee-for-service program and not based on a prepayment or capitation program such as with the HMO. Thus the physicians and hospitals, designated as a PPO, are reimbursed for each medical service they provide.

- The PPO members or enrollees are not restricted to certain designated physicians or hospitals. The PPO member may receive care from a non-PPO provider, however they will generally have to pay more when they do this.

PPOs manage cost containment in the following ways:

- They negotiate fees with providers that are less than the current market fees.

- There are financial incentives for PPO members to use a PPO provider.

- The quality and type of services offered by PPO providers are carefully monitored to maintain cost containment.

Point-of-Service Plan (POS)
To allow for more flexibility, some HMOs and PPOs have created a point-of-service plan (POS). Within this plan, patients may choose to use the panel of providers within the HMO network or to utilize the services of non-HMO providers. If the enrollee chooses to use a

provider within the network, the enrollee is only responsible for the regular co-payment and no deductible amount applies. The same benefits apply if the patient is referred by a physician to a specialist outside the network (with authorization from the HMO). If an enrollee chooses to see an out-of-network provider without authorization, the enrollee may be responsible for greater out-of-pocket expenses. This is known as self-referral. The enrollee may be subject to larger deductible and coinsurance charges.

Exclusive Provider Organizations (EPOs)

Exclusive Provider Organizations (EPOs) are a combination of concepts developed by HMOs and PPOs. The EPO, a managed care system, allows the patient to only select from a defined panel of providers. This system reimburses these providers on a modified fee-for-service method, not on the basis of capitation, as in an HMO. The EPO differs from a PPO since no insurance reimbursement is made if there is a non-emergency service provided by a non-EPO provider.

Integrated Delivery System (IDS)

An organization of provider sites (e.g. ambulatory centers, clinics, or hospitals) with a contracted relationship that offer services to subscribers is known as an integrated delivery system (IDS). One such organization is a physician-hospital organization (PHO). PHOs are composed of hospital(s) and physician groups, or clinics. The PHO obtains managed care plan contracts. In this organization, the physicians are able to maintain their own practices while providing care to contracted plan members. A nonprofit IDS is a medical foundation. This type of organization contracts and acquires assets of physician practices. The foundation manages the business and clinical aspects of the practice. Other examples of IDS organizations are: management service organization (MSO), group practice without walls (GPWW), and integrated provider organization (IPO).

Commercial Plans

Group-sponsored or individual policies can be purchased through commercial insurance companies. Commercial health insurance carriers are usually for-profit organizations. These companies may offer traditional fee-for-service insurance as well as a managed care option to their subscribers. Generally, the insured pays a premium and receives coverage for specific services. Figure 15-1 shows a member insurance card, listing the name of the insured, the effective date of the coverage, and other information of importance to the health care provider.

Always ask to see your patient's insurance card. Make a copy of both sides of the card and then return

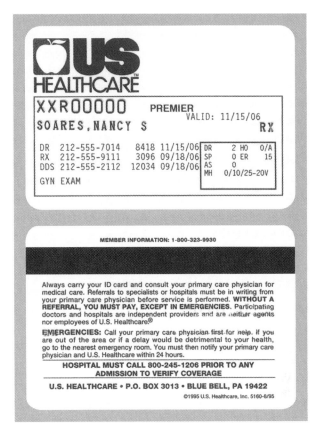

FIGURE 15-1 An insurance card front and back.

it immediately to the patient. You may also wish to write information regarding the insurance plan number on the patient's chart in addition to placing a copy of the card in the chart. Verify the patient's name with a form of photo identification. Compare the name on the insurance card with the name on the photo ID.

Become familiar with the insurance representatives who serve your area. The representatives are knowledgeable, conduct office seminars, and can answer many questions over the telephone. Professionalism has more on sources for insurance information.

Professionalism

A professional medical assistant will make every effort to stay current with health insurance procedures. There are many sources available from which you can obtain the most up-to-date information. There are also seminars and other professional development events that may address changes in insurance plans. Another source is a representative from the actual health care plan. Establish a relationship with someone at each major insurance company so that you can get accurate information.

Blue Cross/Blue Shield

Perhaps the most well known insurance plans are Blue Cross/Blue Shield plans that operate in all states and have become the largest prepayment medical insurance system in the country. These Blue plans date back to the 1930s when Blue Cross was introduced to provide coverage for hospital costs. Then in 1939, Blue Shield was sponsored by state medical societies in Michigan and California to provide medical and surgical coverage. Both plans cover all services now and offer various types of health care plans similar to other commercial carriers. Blue Cross and Blue Shield plans exist in every state and operate locally under each individual state's laws.

Government Programs

Federal and state governments provide health care benefits for specific groups of people through various programs such as Medicare, Medicaid, workers' compensation, and military plans.

Medicare

Perhaps the best known government plan is Medicare. Medicare is health insurance for the elderly that is provided by the United States government. The Medicare

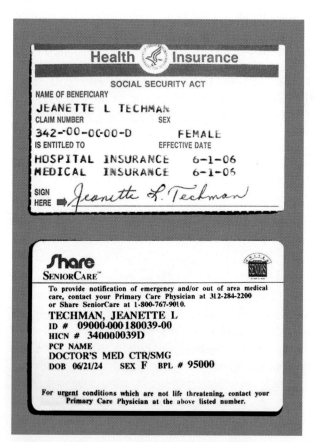

FIGURE 15-2 Medicare and supplemental private insurance cards.

system is operated by the Social Security Administration and paid for largely through Social Security funds. It is designed for persons 65 years old and older and for the severely disabled. Medicare covers approximately 32 million elderly citizens as well as two million permanently disabled persons. Eligible patients are issued a Medicare card (Figure 15-2).

Medicare is actually a two-part health care benefit system: Part A for hospital insurance and Part B for medical insurance.

Part A, which covers hospital expenses, provides coverage automatically when an insured becomes eligible for Social Security benefits. The patient must apply to receive Medicare benefits from the Social Security Administration.

Part B covers medical expenses for doctors, medical services, outpatient hospital care, durable medical equipment, and some medical services not covered by Part A. In order to qualify for Part B Medicare coverage, the insured must pay a monthly premium. This coverage is not automatic, nor does the coverage pay for all services. The patient pays a yearly deductible. After this deductible is met, Medicare will pay for 80 percent of the approved amount of covered services and the insured is liable for the 20 percent co-insurance. The 80 percent reimbursement rate of Medicare is based on their Resource-Based Relative Value Scale (RBRVS), which was developed using values for every medical and surgical procedure based on the work, practice, and malpractice expenses while accounting for regional differences. Some supplies may also be covered if found to be medically necessary for the patient.

Medicare covers all expenses for the first 60 days of hospitalization, except for an initial amount, or deductible, that is paid by the patient. Medicare will also pay for a portion of hospital costs for an additional 30 days. Medicare does not cover extended nursing-home care, or the costs of lengthy or chronic illnesses. Prescription drugs are covered under a separate medical policy.

Medicare supplements are policies that pay benefits on the co-payments and deductibles required and not paid by Medicare. Co-pay or co-payment is an amount of money the patient must pay before the insurance plan will pay. This amount can be as little as $10. Some policies require special forms to be filed before benefits can be paid to the insured. It is important for the medical assistant to check coverage with the individual carrier of the supplement policy, as the coverage provided varies widely from carrier to carrier.

Medicare deductibles, covered services, and co-payments change, so it is important to understand which services are covered under Medicare and which are not. Medical assistants should maintain their knowledge of Medicare coverages and be knowledgeable regarding the benefit period, or period of time that payments for Medicare hospital benefits are available. Lifespan Considerations has more on keeping up-to-date on Medicare guidelines.

Medicaid

While not directly a federal program, Medicaid also qualifies as government insurance. Some of the cost of the Medicaid program, designed for the medically indigent, or persons without funds, comes from state funds, with some federal money to offset costs. Federal funds may assist by supplying 50 percent to 80 percent of the cost of the state's Medicaid program. Since Medicaid is administered by individual states, the rules for eligibility and for payment vary from state to state. In most instances, however, the patient must qualify for benefits on a monthly basis. Some services require preauthorization (prior approval from the Medicaid administrator) or the cost of services will not be paid. When dealing with Medicaid patients, the medical assistant should verify coverage at each and every visit and become familiar with the policies and procedures covering Medicaid in his or her individual state.

Eligibility for Medicare does not automatically confer Medicaid eligibility. In some cases in which a person is eligible for both Medicare and Medicaid, a crossover claim is filed.

Military

Military medical benefits are also part of United States government programs. TRICARE is the U.S. Department of Defense's worldwide health care program for active duty and retired uniformed services members and theirs families. Box 15-2 shows TRICARE plans' coverage.

A spouse, widow, widower, children of veterans with total or permanent service-connected disabilities, and surviving spouse or dependents of veterans who have died as a result of service-connected disabilities are covered under a program called CHAMPVA (Civilian Health and Medical Program of the Veterans Administration).

Providers of service must be approved in order for the patient to receive benefits for services. Special forms are required for claim filing. Certain services require approval from the government agency responsible for administering these programs before payment can be made.

Workers' Compensation

Another type of government mandated insurance is called workers' compensation. This particular insurance is for injuries directly related to work. Payment of premiums is the employer's responsibility; the employee pays nothing. In workers' compensation cases, the provider of services must complete a report called a Surgeon's Report and must submit further reports at pre-determined intervals. In addition, if the patient re-

Lifespan
Considerations

Patients enrolled in Medicare may not be abreast of the changes that occur with their coverage. Some do not understand the difference between Medicare Part A and Part B. With changes in prescription drug coverage, your patients may be even more confused about what is covered and what is not. As a professional medical assistant, it is your responsibility to stay aware of changes that occur and explain the changes to the patients. Use the Internet and refer to the Federal Register to develop a good working knowledge of Medicare guidelines.

ceives regular care in the same practice that treats the work injury, any information connected to the injury or illness being treated under workers' compensation must be kept separate from all other patient information. Billing is to be done separately and the patient will not be billed for services. Billing statements are sent to the employer or insurer, instead. Because of the special type of documentation required for workers' compensation claims, some providers of service will not see workers' compensation patients. In some states, the patient must see physicians who specialize in these types of cases.

Disability Insurance

Disability insurance is a particular type of insurance that usually begins paying the patient (not the doctor or the hospital) after the insured has been disabled

---

BOX 15-2
Tricare

- TRICARE Prime—a managed care option similar to a civilian health maintenance organization.
- TRICARE Extra—a preferred provider option in which beneficiaries choose a doctor, hospital, or other medical provider within the TRICARE provider network.
- TRICARE Standard—a fee-for-service option.
- TRICARE For Life—an option available to Medicare-eligible beneficiaries age 65 and over.

Information is courtesy of http://www.tricareonline.com.

(unable to work) for a specific period of time. A waiting period of weeks or months before benefits are paid is not uncommon with these policies. The benefit period is the amount of time the insured will receive a monthly check after the policy begins to pay. This can be from six months to life. The payment is paid directly to the insured. This type of insurance coverage is not used for the purpose of paying medical bills. It is to be used for the income that patient has lost due to his or her disability. Most disability insurance also requires special forms to be completed by the attending physician before benefits can be paid to the insured. Before the medical assistant has the physician sign the disability insurance form, he or she needs to proofread it very carefully. After the physician has signed the disability insurance form, the medical assistant will make a copy of it and place it in the patient's medical record.

Types of Health Insurance Benefits

Many patients (and medical assistants) find the proliferation of health care policies confusing. It is important to understand what type of insurance coverage the patient has and what types of services this insurance covers. Remember, insurance is a contract between the insured (the patient or the patient's family) and the insurance company. Questions about specific coverage should be directed to the insurance carrier, as policies vary widely, even with the same carrier. Many health care providers file insurance forms for patients as a courtesy, but this service is usually not required by the insurance companies.

Legal and Ethical Issues

When dealing with insurance, confidentiality and honesty are major issues. The patient's right to confidentiality with regard to sensitive medical information must be scrupulously respected. Insurance reimbursement, as it is currently structured, provides a constant temptation to do what is necessary to recover the full amount of charges. As a successful medical assistant, be careful to release only information authorized by the patient, and avoid becoming involved with insurance fraud in any manner.

Legal and Ethical Issues has more about information released for insurance reimbursement.

The most basic insurance policies cover doctor office visits, hospitalization, emergency room, surgery, and wellness examinations. For coverage to be effective, the services must be performed on an inpatient basis, except surgeries may be performed as an outpatient. There may also be an annual deductible, which is the portion the patient must pay before the insurance company will pay any benefits. This type of coverage is usually the least expensive. Additionally, a fixed percentage of covered charges beyond the deductible, called coinsurance, may be required. To reduce unnecessary patient visits to the physician, insurance companies frequently require a small fee be paid at each visit, called a co-payment.

Major medical insurance covers expenses related to catastrophic illnesses or injuries. It also covers prolonged illnesses. Major medical is usually a supplemental policy to basic insurance policies. Adding this type of policy increases the premium rate the insured will pay.

Surgical insurance is just what its name implies—an insurance policy covering surgical services. These policies are not as common today as they once were; most surgical services are now covered under basic medical coverage.

Long-term care is an insurance policy designed to cover nursing home care costs. Other insurance policies have very limited coverage if any for long term care.

Dental insurance covers the dental examination, cleaning, polishing, fillings, and certain extractions. Most insurance carriers require a deductible. Depending on the insurance carrier, most procedures are covered from 50 percent to 100 percent.

Vision insurance covers the cost of an eye examination, contact lens or prescription frames and lenses. Some vision insurance policy also covers laser corrective eye surgery. The percent covered by the insurance carrier depends on the insured's policy.

International health and medical insurance covers the insured while outside of the United States in countries where the policy applies.

Student health insurance is important when the parent's insurance policy may no longer cover a child or children that are attending school. Basic insurance, major medical, or both are available. This type of coverage is usually at a reasonable rate that is affordable for the student.

Payment of Benefits

When a covered service has been rendered, the insurance carrier is obligated to pay its portion of the cost. How is this portion calculated? Many insurance carriers use the UCR (usual, customary, reasonable) method (also see Chapter 13). The URC method allows the carrier to establish a payment base for allowed or covered services. In this model, payment is set by determining:

- The usual fee a provider charges the majority of patients for a particular service.
- The geographic location of the practice and the provider's specialty.
- Any complications or unusual services or procedures.

Indemnity schedules, another means of determining the amount of payment made by an insurance carrier, are based on a maximum amount for a specific service. Payment to the provider of service is based on the lower of either the provider's submitted charge or the fee schedule. This method of payment is very common in managed care situations.

To communicate effectively and efficiently with providers of medical care, insurance companies have adopted several methods of standardizing information received. Many insurance companies, working together and separately, developed a means of calculating pricing factors in reimbursement. The results of these efforts are called Relative Value Studies (RVS). In each instance, the system takes into account the time, skill, and overhead expense of the provider as required for each service. These factors are then turned into unit counts applied to a specific service, allowing for the most efficient and effective method of calculating payment.

Since 1992, Medicare has established payment on a resource-based Relative Value Scale, which incorporates the RVS, but also allows for increases in charges tied to economic changes and other factors.

Each insurance carrier has a certain deadline for submitting insurance claims. Claims must be submitted in a timely manner in order to be processed, and if the deadline for filing has passed, no money can be recovered from the insurance carrier. It is extremely important to become familiar with these filing deadlines that vary from carrier to carrier. It is also important that the appropriate form be used for filing charges. Most carriers accept the CMS-1500 (see Chapter 16); some require forms specific to that carrier. Some carriers require supporting documentation (such as reports) that must be submitted in a timely manner.

If a patient has more than one insurance carrier, it is crucial that the primary carrier be determined for proper billing to occur. The claim must be submitted first to the primary carrier for processing, the claim must be processed, and a statement of remittance completed before the information can be sent to any secondary carrier.

Coverage for some expenses such as cosmetic surgery is excluded from policies, and are called exclusions. Payments for some medications are excluded if they are not on an approved list, called a formulary.

As with all aspects of insurance processing, accuracy and attention to detail are the primary concerns. The successful medical assistant keeps abreast of rules, regulations, and changes about insurance claims processing to prompt insurance reimbursement for the practice that is as high as is allowed for services rendered. The medical assistant will need to bill the third party payer for the patient and collect the fees owed to the physician from them. See Procedure 15-1 for performing billing and collection procedures.

Preauthorization and Precertfication

It may be necessary to seek preauthorization from the health insurance provider for certain services. Remember that part of the patient registration process is gathering all pertinent information including the insurance plan requirements. The medical assistant will need to obtain the required prior approval known as precertification or preauthorization.

Preauthorization is obtaining the permission from the insurance plan before performing a procedure or providing certain services to subscribers. It is important to find out if preauthorization is necessary prior to the patient's scheduled appointment. Involve the patient in this process; he or she may not be aware that preauthorization is necessary for the particular plan. Failure to have this permission may delay treatment. The insurance carrier may not pay all or part of the procedure or service if preauthorization is not granted beforehand. Precertification or preauthorization is usually obtained a minimum of 24 hours before a patient arrives for an office visit, hospitalization, certain procedures and treatments, and referrals to a specialist. To aquire prior authorization, the medical assistant will contact the insurance carrier, provide all of the patient information and procedure. The medical assistant should have the following information before contacting the insurance carrier:

- Patient's medical record with insurance information.
- Percertification form.
- Specific procedure or service requested, number of treatments, and period of time necessary for the treatments.
- Specific documentation by the physician in the patient's medical record supporting the requested procedure or service.
- Name, address, telephone number, and fax number of the provider who will perform the procedure or service that has been requested.

The insurance carrier will provide precertification or preauthorization information (usually a number) that will be necessary to include on the insurance

Perform Billing and Collection Procedures

OBJECTIVE: Demonstrate the ability to record payments received from a patient, to record patient information using a patient ledger card and day sheet, and to generate an insurance bill using a charge slip. Demonstrate the ability to then record a payment and provide receipt to the patient.

Equipment and Supplies
day sheet; ledger card; co-payment check; receipt book

Method
1. Pull the appropriate ledger card and place it directly on the day sheet.
2. Temporarily remove the strip of charge slips from the pegboard.
3. Enter the patient's previous balance on the day sheet. The ledger card does not extend to this column.
4. Post the date, patient's name, descriptions, and co-payment amount.
5. Calculate the new balance by subtracting the payment from the previous balance.
6. Generate an insurance bill for the remaining balance.
7. Create a receipt for the patient.

Charting Example
$20 co-pay paid by pt. at time of office visit. Allied insurance billed for balance of $79 on March 12.

---

claim. The medical assistant should make a copy of the completed precertification form and place it in the patient's medical record.

In case an insurance plan rejects the request, it may be necessary for the physician to write a letter to the carrier. With the consent of the patient, the physician should state the patient's diagnosis and professional rationale for prescribing a particular treatment. It may be helpful to recommend that the subscriber send a letter of appeal as well. A copy of the letter to the carrier must also be kept in the patient's medical record. If possible, obtain a copy of the letter of appeal from the patient to also place in the patient's medical record. The third party payers, usually insurance companies, expect medical assistants to follow their guidelines for precertification and preauthorization. See Procedure 15-2 for how to apply third party payer guidelines.

Referrals and Authorization

A patient often needs more specialized care than the family physician can provide. The patient will be referred to another physician or facility.

A referral is used to send a patient for treatment to another facility or physician. There are three types of referrals: regular, urgent, and STAT. Regular referrals are requested when the primary care physician has determined the need for a specialist to continue quality care. Regular referrals can take up to a week to obtain the authorization from the insurance plan. An urgent referral is granted for a non-life threatening need for quality of care and may take up to 48 hours to aquire prior authorization. A STAT referral is approved for life threatening quality of care. Whether the referral is regular, urgent, or STAT, it will require prior authorization direct from the insurance carrier. Prior authorization may be obtained by telephone, fax, e-mail, or in writing on specific insurance carrier forms (Figure 15-3). A medical assistant will need to always have the referral

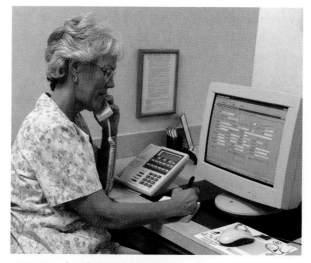

FIGURE 15-3 A medical assistant may obtain a referral over the telephone.

Apply Third Party Guidelines

OBJECTIVE: To apply knowledge of third party guidelines to obtain prior approval for a procedure.

Equipment and Supplies

physician's report recommending procedure; telephone; notepad; pen

Method

1. Gather information about the patient
2. Locate insurance carrier's number.
3. Call carrier and introduce yourself, indicating your office.
4. Instruct carrier that physician recommends procedure, but that third party carrier requires preauthorization for the procedure.
5. Give carrier necessary information, as requested.
6. Document in patient chart preauthorization number for procedure.

Charting Example

Michelle Kimenhour preauthorized hysterectomy for pt. on September 26. Preauthorization number GAQ3498.

---

authorization prior to patient treatment and must maintain all information for insurance billing and utilization review purposes.

When a physician requests that a patient be referred to a specialist, it is important that this is documented in the patient's medical record. The appropriate paperwork must be sent to the referring physician. Referral recommendations should be in writing. When submitting the request to the health insurance plan, be sure to follow the appropriate procedures for that plan. The medical assistant should have the following information before contacting the insurance carrier:

- Patient's medical record with insurance information.
- Referral form.
- Specific procedure or service requested, number of treatments, and period of time necessary for the treatments.
- Specific documentation by the physician in the patient's medical record supporting the reason for the referral.
- Name, address, telephone number, and fax number of the provider who will be providing the procedure or service.
- Appointment date, time, and location.
- Diagnosis and procedure codes.

If certain forms are required, make sure that you have the current form and that it is filled out properly. Some requests are rejected due to incorrect or incomplete paperwork. The medical assistant should make a copy of the completed referral form and place it in the patient's medical record.

Verification of Insurance Benefits

A medical assistant will always need to confirm or verify the patient's eligibility for insurance benefits prior to the office visit for services. Verification may take time but, by performing the following guidelines, will be more effective for the insurance process.

Guidelines for insurance verification:

- Initial contact with the patient—obtain all insurance information (i.e. insurer name, guarantor name, insurance identification number, patient's address, telephone number, and birth date).
- Insurance company name, address, telephone number, fax number, co-payment fees, deductibles, and preauthorizations.
- Provide patient with written information regarding medical office policies and procedures for dealing with his or her insurance carrier.
- Discuss insurance benefits with the patient prior to services rendered.

As a medical assistant, you will need to apply managed care policies and procedures in the office as presented in Procedure 15-3. Preparing for Externship has more on working with insurance.

Apply Managed Care Policies and Procedures

OBJECTIVE: Demonstrate knowledge of managed care policies.

Equipment and Supplies
insurance card; patient record

Method
1. Greet patient and request insurance card.
2. Check card to see if coverage is current.

3. Correctly enter card information into data base.
4. Photocopy card.
5. Return card to patient.

Fee Schedules

Health care insurance providers determine fees based on several components. Determining factors include time, location of practice, type of practice, value of services, and the allowable charge. Allowable charge is the highest amount that third party payers will make for services rendered.

Health Care Cost Containment

The cost of medicine has risen steadily throughout the years. As new advances are discovered to treat and cure disease, heal injuries, and prolong life, the costs are passed on to the consumer or patient. Traditionally, medical care has been rendered on a fee-for-service

Preparing for
Externship

Part of your training as an extern *will involve working with the insurance process. You may have to verify coverage, obtain preauthorizations, and request permission for referrals. Understanding the policies and procedures regarding the different plans is an on-going process. Ask questions about unfamiliar plans. Make sure you have the most current information available. Both the physician and the patient rely on those who are responsible for handling insurance in the office. The physician wants to be correctly reimbursed, and the patient does not want any unexpected costs.*

basis, which was a separate charge or fee set up by individual physicians for every service. Insurance carriers initially set up their policies on this basis, as well. However, as medical care costs rose, the insurers, carriers, patients, and medical community began to offer cost-saving alternatives to higher medical costs and the escalating costs of medical premiums.

The first cost containment measure, the Peer Review Organization (PRO), was initiated when Congress amended the Social Security Act of 1972 and established the Professional Standards Review Organization (PSRO). This was a voluntary group of physicians who monitored the necessity of hospital admissions and reviewed the treatment costs and medical records of hospitals. Unfortunately, the cost of operating this system was greater than the savings that the program could generate each year. In order to establish stricter controls over Medicare reimbursement for inpatient costs, Congress created control peer review organizations (PROs). These PROs were intended to determine whether proposed services were reasonable and medically necessary and whether or not the services provided on an inpatient basis could be provided more efficiently on an outpatient basis.

As part of the cost containment process, a patient classification system was developed, which provides a means of relating the type of patients a hospital treats to the costs incurred by the hospital. Yale University developed the design of diagnosis-related groups (DRGs) in the late 1960s. The initial idea was to provide a means of monitoring the quality of care and the utilization of services in a hospital setting. Payment rates based on DRGs have now been established as the basis for a hospital's Medicare reimbursements. While DRGs have an effect on hospital reimbursements, they are not used to calculate payments made to outpatient providers. Physicians now have contracts with managed care companies and insurance companies.

The Federal Register

The *Federal Register* is a daily legal publication of the National Archives and Records Administration (NARA). The medical assistant would use this register for seeking information on Federal rules, regulations, notices, executive orders, proclamations, and Presidential documents. The *Federal Register* may be accessed through the World Wide Web, microfiche, or as a daily newspaper.

SUMMARY

Most patients coming into the medical office have some form of health care insurance. These include commercial insurers, and government plans such as Medicare, Medicaid, workers' compensation, and military insurance (TRICARE AND CHAMPVA). Many patients are members of health care plans, such as health maintenance organizations (HMOs), and preferred provider organizations (PPOs). The medical assistant should have a working knowledge of each type of insurance in order to be able to quickly and accurately process insurance forms.

Chapter Review

COMPETENCY REVIEW

1. Define and spell the terms to learn for this chapter.
2. List the three insurance options currently available.
3. What are the two important components of an HMO?
4. How does a PPO differ from an HMO?
5. What is the purpose of the peer review organization (PRO)?

PREPARING FOR THE CERTIFICATION EXAM

1. What is the term for a written and documented request for reimbursement?
   A. premium
   B. co-payment
   C. claim
   D. referral
   E. fee schedule

2. Which BEST describes health maintenance organizations?
   A. They are prepaid plans.
   B. Patients are only allowed to see physicians within the network.
   C. All HMOs are government-sponsored.
   D. Patients pay no premiums to HMOs.
   E. There is only one type of managed care plan.

3. Which government insurance provides coverage for citizens over 65 years old and the severely disabled?
   A. Medicaid
   B. TRICARE
   C. Workers' compensation
   D. Medicare
   E. Disability

4. Preauthorization is necessary in the following situations EXCEPT:
   A. referral to a specialist
   B. new treatment prescribed by the PCP
   C. making a PCP appointment for a regular physical
   D. hospital admission
   E. a medical procedure by a specialist

continued on next page

5. What is the term for an amount specified by an insurance plan that the patient must pay before the plan pays for medical services?
   A. rider
   B. deductible
   C. premium
   D. reimbursement
   E. co-payment

6. Medicare Part A covers:
   A. doctor visits
   B. hospital costs
   C. prescription drugs
   D. visits to specialists
   E. extended nursing-home care

7. Which is NOT considered a primary care physician?
   A. Chiropractor
   B. Internist
   C. Family practitioner
   D. Gynecologist
   E. Pediatrician

8. Which type of benefit begins paying the patient after the insured has been disabled and unable to work for a specific period of time?
   A. Medicaid
   B. TRICARE
   C. Medicare
   D. Workers' compensation
   E. Disability insurance

9. Which factor is NOT considered when using the UCR method to determine reimbursement rates for physicians' services?
   A. any complications or unusual services or procedures
   B. the geographic location of the practice and the provider's specialty
   C. the usual fee a provider charges the majority of patients for a particular service
   D. the subscriber's deductible amount
   E. the type of practice and its address

10. Which are NOT types of referrals?
    A. STAT and regular
    B. urgent and STAT
    C. regular and urgent
    D. regular, urgent, and life-threatening
    E. regular, urgent, and STAT

CRITICAL THINKING

1. Jessie and her siblings are eligible for what type of insurance coverage?

2. What group or groups of people qualify for this type of coverage?

3. Two years later, Jessie gets pregnant. She is not employed and her significant other does not have medical benefits. Jessie and her unborn child are able to qualify for what type of services?

INTERNET ACTIVITY

Most health insurance providers have Web sites to provide information to their members and the public. Because changes occur so quickly, important information regarding health plans is posted to keep those who are interested up to date. Conduct a search to find the Web sites for Medicare, Medicaid, a commercial insurance company, and TRICARE. List the Web site addresses and list the different plans offered by each.

ON THE JOB

Lisa Medina, CMA, processes insurance claims for a large internal medicine practice. You have recently been hired as Lisa's assistant and she has asked you to verify insurance coverage for the patients who have appointments to see Dr. Williams in the next two days. Lisa "advises" you to be careful when having to obtain preauthorizations. She hands you a list of "approved" services and tells you to use this information when calling the insurance companies.

1. Name some of the options that are possible for handling this situation.
2. For what types of services might you have to obtain preauthorizations?
3. Would Lisa's "advice" be considered fraud? Explain your response.
4. What is the proper procedure for obtaining preauthorizations?

MediaLink More on medical insurance, including interactive resources, can be found in the Student CD-ROM accompanying this textbook.

Medical Assistant Role Delineation Chart

HIGHLIGHT indicates material covered in this chapter.

ADMINISTRATIVE

Administrative Procedures

- Perform basic administrative medical assisting functions
- Schedule, coordinate and monitor appointments
- Schedule inpatient/outpatient admissions and procedures
- Understand and apply third-party guidelines
- Obtain reimbursement through accurate claims submission
- Monitor third-party reimbursement
- Understand and adhere to managed care policies and procedures
- *Negotiate managed care contracts*

Practice Finances

- Perform procedural and diagnostic coding
- Apply bookkeeping principles

- Manage accounts receivable
- *Manage accounts payable*
- *Process payroll*
- *Document and maintain accounting and banking records*
- *Develop and maintain fee schedules*
- *Manage renewals of business and professional insurance policies*
- *Manage personnel benefits and maintain records*
- *Perform marketing, financial, and strategic planning*

CLINICAL

Fundamental Principles

- Apply principles of aseptic technique and infection control
- Comply with quality assurance practices
- Screen and follow up patient test results

Diagnostic Orders

- Collect and process specimens
- Perform diagnostic tests

Patient Care

- Adhere to established patient screening procedures
- Obtain patient history and vital signs
- Prepare and maintain examination and treatment areas
- Prepare patient for examinations, procedures and treatments

- Assist with examinations, procedures and treatments
- Prepare and administer medications and immunizations
- Maintain medication and immunization records
- Recognize and respond to emergencies
- Coordinate patient care information with other health care providers
- Initiate IV and administer IV medications with appropriate training and as permitted by state law

GENERAL

Professionalism

- Display a professional manner and image
- Demonstrate initiative and responsibility
- Work as a member of the health care team
- Prioritize and perform multiple tasks
- Adapt to change
- Promote the CMA credential
- Enhance skills through continuing education
- Treat all patients with compassion and empathy
- Promote the practice through positive public relations

Communication Skills

- Recognize and respect cultural diversity
- Adapt communications to individual's ability to understand
- Use professional telephone technique

- Recognize and respond effectively to verbal, nonverbal, and written communications
- Use medical terminology appropriately
- Utilize electronic technology to receive, organize, prioritize and transmit information
- Serve as liaison

Legal Concepts

- Perform within legal and ethical boundaries
- Prepare and maintain medical records
- Document accurately
- Follow employer's established policies dealing with the health care contract
- Implement and maintain federal and state health care legislation and regulations
- Comply with established risk management and safety procedures
- Recognize professional credentialing criteria
- *Develop and maintain personnel, policy and procedure manuals*

Instruction

- Instruct individuals according to their needs
- Explain office policies and procedures
- Teach methods of health promotion and disease prevention
- Locate community resources and disseminate information
- *Develop educational materials*
- *Conduct continuing education activities*

Operational Functions

- Perform inventory of supplies and equipment
- Perform routine maintenance of administrative and clinical equipment
- Apply computer techniques to support office operations
- *Perform personnel management functions*
- *Negotiate leases and prices for equipment and supply contracts*

- *Denotes advanced skills.*

Medical Insurance Claims

chapter 16

Learning Objectives

After completing this chapter, you should be able to:

- Define and spell the terms to learn for this chapter.
- Define and discuss various health insurance forms.
- Explain the differences among the discussed insurance policies.
- List the information required on a medical claim form and explain why each piece of information is needed.

- Discuss legal issues affecting medical claims submission.
- Discuss tracking insurance claims.
- Discuss insurance claims processing.
- List the reasons for insurance claims being rejected.
- Explain why insurance claim security is so important.

Terms to Learn

assignment of benefits
benefit period
breach of confidentiality

nonparticipating
provider
participating providers

preauthorization
superbill

Case Study

LEWIS JORDAN, RMA, WORKS AS DR. MILLER'S insurance clerk. His duties include verifying insurance and processing claims. Mary Free is a new patient and has an appointment to see Dr. Miller next week. She has Blue Cross/Blue Shield insurance. Mark Flannery is also a patient. He was in to see Dr. Miller last month and the claim for his care was rejected. The codes, quantities, and modifiers were all correct on the CMS-1500.

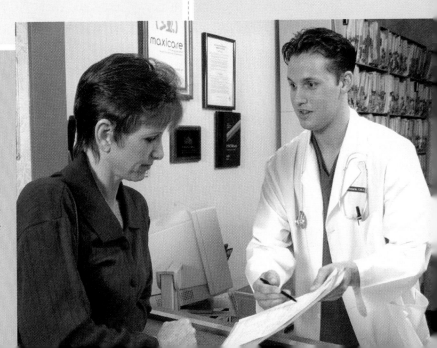

The health insurance claim form provides communication between the insurance company and physician for the patient. There are three main points to this communication process that are critical in order to receive proper reimbursement from the insurance carrier. First, the correct health insurance claim form must be used. Second, the information provided in the health insurance claim form must be accurate. One little mistake can cause the claim to be rejected. The medical assistant must always proofread the claim form before submitting it. Third, the health insurance claim form is mailed or e-mailed to the correct insurance carrier.

Types of Health Insurance Claim Forms

The CMS-1500 is the most common health insurance claim form. This form is used to file claims for physicians' services. It may be sent to the insurance carrier by standard mail or electronically. Another type of health insurance claim form is the CMS-1450 or the UB-92 (Figure 16-1). This type of form is used for services related to hospitalization. Since this type of health insurance claim form is used in a hospital setting, most medical assistants are less likely to encounter it. Most commercial insurance carriers utilize the CMS-1500 form.

Blue Cross/Blue Shield

Many Blue Cross/Blue Shield plans provide their own type of health insurance claim form. These forms are provided at the Web sites of various Blue Cross/Blue Shield plans. Depending on the type of service, the CMS-1500 or the CMS-1540 may also be used.

Managed Care

When the medical assistant is submitting a claim, he or she must find out which health insurance claim form to use. Most managed care organizations use the CMS-1500 and the CMS-1540. Using the incorrect form may cause the claim to be rejected. This will then delay payment to the physician for services rendered. Preparing for Externship has more about being familiar with the CMS-1500 form.

Medicare

Medicare deductibles, covered services, and co-payments change, so it is important to understand which services are covered under Medicare and which are not. Wise medical assistants maintain their knowledge of Medicare coverage and the benefit period, or period of time for which payments of Medicare hospital benefits are available.

The medical assistant working in a medical office needs to be familiar with the CMS-1500 claim form. This claim is used when a patient has Medicare (Figure 16-2). If the CMS-1500 claim form is not used, it will be rejected. Remember when claims are rejected, it delays payment to the physician. This claim form can be sent by standard mail or electronically.

Medicaid

Since Medicaid is administered by individual states, the rules for eligibility and for payment vary from state to state. In most instances, however, the patient must qualify for benefits on a monthly basis. Some services require preauthorization (prior approval from the Medicaid administrator) or the cost of services will not be paid. When dealing with Medicaid patients, the medical assistant should verify coverage at each and every visit and become familiar with the policies and procedures covering Medicaid in his or her individual state.

Eligibility for Medicare does not automatically confer Medicaid eligibility. In cases where a person is eligible for both Medicare and Medicaid (Medi/Medi), a crossover claim is filed.

After the patient has checked out of the office, the medical assistant will complete a CMS-1500 form. This form can be sent by standard mail or electronically depending upon the medical office.

Military

Military medical benefits are also part of government programs. There are three types of health insurance claim forms used to submit services to Tricare.

DD Form 2642 is completed and sent by the patient or a family member. This form is completed when the patient or family member is requesting payment for medical services.

CMS-1500 is completed and sent by the physician's office. Payment will be sent to the physician's office.

Preparing for
Externship

It may be helpful to practice manually filling out CMS-1500 forms. Get familiar with each section and find out what information is needed to complete the forms. If you have the opportunity, use the different software packages available to submit claims. Most have tutorial software on which you can train.

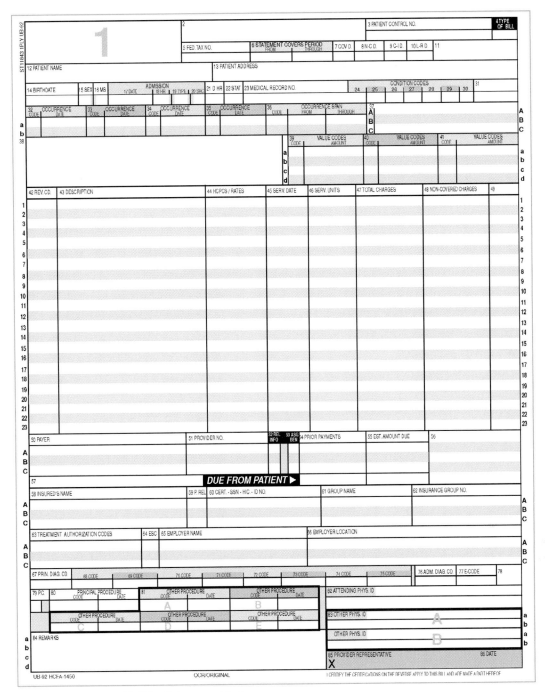

FIGURE 16-1 A CMS-1450/UB-92 health insurance claim form.

UB-92 is completed and sent by the hospital. Payment will be sent to the hospital.

Workers' Compensation

Workers' compensation is an insurance set up specifically for injuries that are related directly to work. Payment of premiums is the employer's responsibility; the employee pays nothing. Because of the particular type of documentation required for workers' compensation claims, some providers of service will not see workers' compensation patients. In some states, the patient must see physicians who specialize in these types of cases.

The most frequently used claim form is the CMS-1500, but some states or insurance carriers have a specifically designed form that must be completed. Before the medical assistant completes a claim form, he or she must investigate which claim form to use. This can be accomplished by calling the insurance carrier or checking the insurance carrier's Web site.

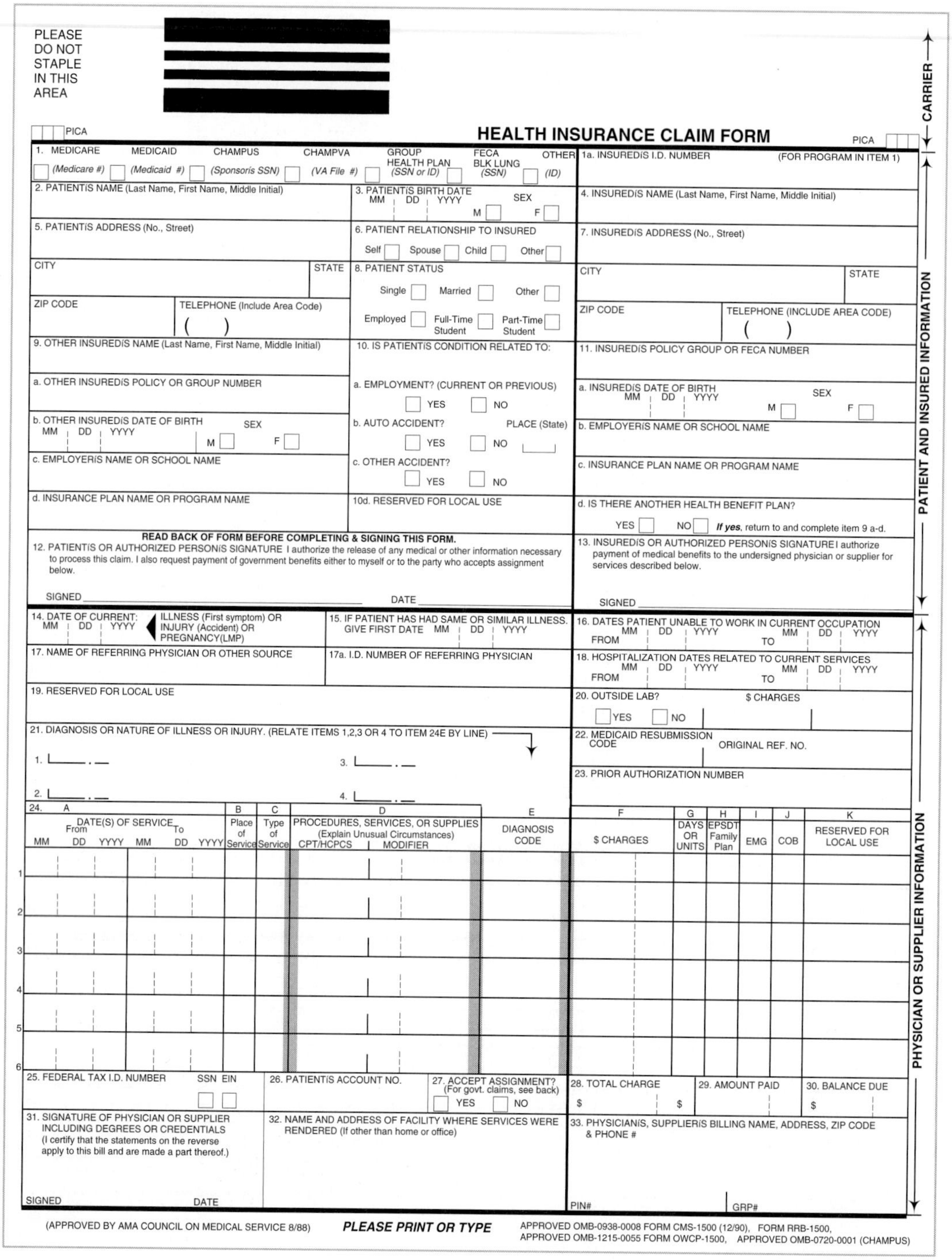

FIGURE 16-2 A blank CMS-1500 form.

Type of Claims

There are two methods for a medical assistant to submit claims to an insurance carrier or third-party payer. The traditional way to submit claims is by completing information on a paper claim form and mailing it to the insurance carrier. The more current and faster way to submit claims is done by using a computer to complete an electronic claim form and sending the claim electronically. The same information is provided when submitting a claim by paper or electronically.

Paper

There are only a small amount of providers who are able to submit paper claims. Paper claims are completed by the medical assistant manually. When this type of claim form is submitted, it often has errors. This means there is a greater chance for the insurance carrier to reject the claim form. The types of errors include omissions, as well as typographical, and mathematical. When a claim form has one or more errors, the claim form must be resubmitted correctly for payment. This increases the turnaround time for the medical office to receive payment and means a delayed cash flow. The patient can also be concerned when the insurance carrier has taken long to make a payment because of delays in processing a claim.

Advantages and Disadvantages of Paper Claims

The cost involved with using paper claims is minimal. The equipment and supplies needed to complete the claim forms include the claim forms and coding books. As long as the office has sufficient amount of forms, they can be accessed at any time.

The disadvantages, however, are in the cost to complete a paper claim process that includes storage space, postage, mailing, resubmission, follow-up, and copies of claim forms that are submitted and resubmitted. When the medical assistant completes a claim form manually, it must be on an original claim form. It must be legible, completed in dark ink, and printed in capital letters. This can be very time consuming. Never use punctuation, decimals, dollar signs, or correction aids. Do not tape, staple, or clip items to the claim form. Always place the necessary documentation required with the completed claim form in an envelope to be mailed and make sure the insurance address is correct.

Electronic Media Claim (EMC)

All medical offices were mandated to be in compliance with electronic filing by October 2003. Electronic claims are a way to send claims and communicate from computer to computer rather than on paper. Electronic Media Claims have fewer errors because there are fewer omissions and they are legible.

Advantages of Electronic Claims

The electronic process speeds claims processing on both the provider's end and at the insurance carrier's end. Many plans make direct electronic deposits of payments for insurance claims into the provider's bank account. Processing claims electronically decreases payment turnaround time. It also shortens the payment cycle, thereby increasing cash flow into the medical office. Sending claim forms electronically instead of by mail saves postage and labor cost for the medical office. Errors may still occur on electronic claims, so it is very important for the medical assistant to proofread all claims before submitting them.

Electronic claims submission requires the same information as on the CMS-1500 form, but instead of sending the claim form by mail, all information is sent directly to the insurance carrier's computer server. This type of submission is referred to as a paperless claim. To send a claim electronically, the medical assistant must do the following:

- Collect all information needed about the patient, including diagnostic and procedure codes as though you were completing a manual CMS-1500 form. The claim form on the screen may not be identical to a hard copy of the CMS form.

- Connect your computer to the insurance company's computer server, using instructions provided by the insurance company. Type in your identification number and password and follow the instructions and prompts on the screen.

- Fill out the claim form as you would the CMS-1500. When the insurance carrier recognizes the physician's identification number, it will automatically assign a processing number to the claim. Keep track of this number for future reference; it is your confirmation that the claim has been received. The best place to document this information is in the insurance claims log.

Software programs are available that allow claim processing without the need to re-enter some of the data more than once. It is important to be familiar with the procedures and software used to prevent delay of payment.

Disadvantages of Electronic Claims

One of the disadvantages of submitting claims electronically is the initial start-up expense. Initially, the medical office would require an Internet service provider, computer, software, printer, and backup or storage devices. Glitches may occur with the computer that delays processing time, transmission, and payments.

Transmitting Claims Electronically

Claims can be transmitted electronically in three ways. The first method is sending the transmission directly to the payer. To communicate electronically between the payer and the medical office, an electronic data exchange (EDI) information system must be utilized.

The second method is transmitting claims through a clearinghouse. The clearinghouse does not modify any of the data. It is responsible for putting the data in a format appropriate for EDI use. Clearinghouses eliminate the need for medical offices to have specific software that may be required by different carriers. The clearinghouse also checks each claim form for accuracy, and returns it to the medical office for correction, thereby reducing the incidence of claim rejection.

The last method is direct data entry (DDE) which is an online service provided by some carriers. The data from the claim is keyed in a specific format and then transmitted directly to the carrier.

Status of Insurance Claims

The status of insurance claims is a concern of every medical office. Lost, incomplete, or rejected claims cause delays in reimbursement to the practice. Over time, this is costly to any medical office. Errors or omission on a health care insurance claim form can cause a claim to be rejected. If this occurs, the medical assistant must investigate the reason and resubmit the claim.

Clean Claims

A health insurance claim form that has been completed correctly without any errors or omissions is called a clean claim. Clean claims are also submitted on time to the insurance carrier. The first time this claim is submitted to the insurance carrier, it is processed and payment is sent to the provider.

Dirty Claims

When a health insurance claim form is incorrect by having missing data or errors, this is considered to be a dirty claim. This will cause the claim to be rejected and when claims are rejected, payment is delayed. Delayed payments become costly to a medical office because the form must be resubmitted taking the time of a medical assistant to complete the insurance form again.

Invalid Claims

A health insurance claim form that has been completed but has some type of incorrect information is considered an invalid claim.

Denied Claims

Denied claims can occur when procedures or services are not covered by the patient's insurance policy or when the patient has not met his or her deductible. Ineligible procedures or services can also cause a claim to be denied. Patient Education discusses reviewing insurance details with patients who are not familiar with their coverage.

The Claim Form

Each time a patient is seen for services, the medial assistant must verify the insurance information in the patient's medical record. For a new patient or a patient with a new insurance card or cards, the medical assistant needs to copy the front and back of the patient's insurance card(s). After making a copy of each insurance card, the medical assistant will file it in the patient's medical record. Then, the medical assistant will verify that the patient has signed the assignment of benefits form. This form allows physicians to be paid directly from the insurance carrier. After the patient has been seen by the physician, the medical assistant can complete the CMS-1500 form. The CMS-1500 has 33 blocks of information to complete. Blocks 1 to 13 represent information about the patient's demographics and insurance carrier. Blocks 14 to 33 represent information about the patient's diagnosis, procedure(s) performed, the amount of each procedure, and the total charge. It also represents information about the physician. Procedure 16-1 reviews each step for correctly completing the CMS-1500 form.

Claims Processing

Claims are processed at insurance companies by a claims administrator. The claim form is a critical item in claims processing. While there are several forms used for claims processing, the most commonly used form was designed by the Health Care Financing Administration and is called a CMS-1500. For a claim to be processed, this form must be filled out completely and correctly. The following information is required for all claims:

- The name of the insured's insurance company
- The name of the insured
- The insured's identification number
- The address of the insured
- The telephone number of the insured

Data about the patient is also required. In general, the upper portion of the form describes the patient and the lower half of the form (separated by a heavy line) refers to the provider of services, the services provided to the patient, and the medical necessity of those services.

As with all patient information, all rules of confidentiality apply. Professionalism warns about consequences for failure of confidentiality. Therefore, the patient must sign a release of information for a claim form to be completed. To make this process simpler, many offices have a standard release form for this purpose. Once the form has been signed and is on file in the patient's record, a notation of "SIGNATURE ON FILE" may be written or typed in box 12 of the CMS-1500 form. Box 13 deals with payment of benefits. If this box

Professionalism

The professional medical assistant has access to all patient records. The records contain confidential information that only a few designated people should have access to. It is against the law to reveal any information concerning a patient or even talk about a patient's condition to the patient anywhere but in a professional setting. Be aware that neighbors, friends, may ask you about patients who have had appointments with the doctor. By law, you cannot reveal this information. HIPAA is very specific concerning confidentiality. You can be fined up to $250,000 per incident or be jailed up to 10 years for violation of HIPAA laws.

is signed, payment will frequently be made directly to the provider of services. If the box is not signed, or for a contract that cannot be assigned, payment is made to the insured. Many insurance carriers, including Medicare, allow for lifetime assignment of benefits

---

16-1 | **PROCEDURE**

Completing the CMS-1500 Form

OBJECTIVE: Correctly complete a CMS-1500 form.

Equipment and Supplies
patient's medical record; patient's insurance information; patient's ledger card; superbill; CMS-1500 form; black ink pen; computer with a printer; or typewriter

Method
1. Box 1 refers to government medical plans. Place an "X" in the appropriate box to indicate type of coverage if applicable.
   a. Enter the identification number listed on the insurance card.
2. Enter the patient's name in the order requested on the form.
3. Enter the patient's 8-digit birth date. Place an "X" in the appropriate box that indicates patient's gender.

4. Enter the insured's name in the order requested on the form. Enter the word "SAME" if the patient and insured are the same.
5. Enter the patient's complete address and telephone number.
6. Place an "X" in the box that indicates the patient's relationship to the insured.
7. Enter the insured's complete address and telephone number.
8. Place an "X" in the box that indicates the patient's marital status. Place an "X" in the appropriate box to indicate if the patient is employed or a full-time or part-time student.

(continued)

Completing the CMS-1500 Form (continued)

9. Enter the other insured's name in the order requested on the form.
   a. Enter the other insured's policy or group number.
   b. Enter the other insured's 8-digit birth date. Place an "X" in the box that indicates the other insured's gender.
   c. Enter the other insured's employer's name or school name.
   d. Enter the other insured's insurance plan name or program name.
10. Place an "X" in either the YES or NO boxes to indicate if the patient's condition is related to:
    a. employment,
    b. auto accident, or
    c. other accident.
    d. Reserved for local use. Leave blank.
11. Enter the insured's policy group or FECA number.
    a. Enter the insured's 8-digit birth date. Place an "X" in the box that indicates the insured's gender.
    b. Enter the insured's employer's name or school name.
    c. Enter the insured's insurance plan name or program name.
    d. Place an "X" in either the YES or NO box to indicate if there is another health benefit plan. If YES, 9a to 9d must be completed.
12. In order to release and use the patient's medical information to process the claim, have the patient or authorized person sign and date in the appropriate area, or if applicable, note SIGNATURE ON FILE.
13. In order to authorize payment for the claim dispersed to the provider, have the insured or authorized person sign in the appropriate area, or if applicable, note SIGNATURE ON FILE.
14. Enter the 8-digit date of current illness, injury, or pregnancy.
15. Enter dates if patient has had same or similar condition.
16. Enter 8-digit from and to dates the patient is unable to work in his or her current occupation.
17. Enter the name of the referring physician or other source.
    a. Enter the I.D. number of the referring physician.
18. Enter the 8-digit from and to hospitalization dates related to the current services.

19. Reserved for local use. Leave blank.
20. Place an "X" in either the YES or NO box to indicate if an outside laboratory was used. Enter the amount of the charges.
21. Enter the correct ICD-9-CM code related to the diagnosis or nature of the illness or injury. Each ICD-9-CM code must be entered in priority order. Each form can only contain four ICD-9-CM codes.
22. Enter the Medicaid resubmission code and original reference number.
23. Enter the prior authorization number.
24. Enter information into columns A through K.
    A. Enter the 8-digit from and to dates the patient had services.
    B. Enter the 2-digit code for place of service.
    C. Leave blank.
    D. Enter the correct CPT/HCPCS code and modifier for procedures, services, or supplies.
    E. Enter the correct diagnosis code (1, 2, 3, or 4) that corresponds with the correct service that was rendered.
    F. Enter the charges for the service rendered.
    G. Enter the number days or units of service.
    H. Leave blank.
    I. Leave blank.
    J. Leave blank
    K. Leave blank.
25. Enter the federal tax I.D. number or Social Security Number.
26. Enter the patient's account number.
27. Place an "X" in either the YES or NO box to indicate if assignment will be accepted.
28. Enter total charges.
29. Enter amount paid.
30. Enter balance due.
31. Enter signature of physician or supplier including degrees or credentials.
32. Enter the complete name and address of the facility where the services were rendered.
33. Enter the physician's, supplier's billing name, address, zip code, and telephone number.
34. Proofread the CMS-1500 form for accuracy.
35. Make a copy of the CMS-1500 form to keep in the patient's medical record—for paper claim submissions only.
36. Enter required data into the insurance claims log.
37. Send the completed CMS-1500 form (Figure 16-3) and required documentation to the insurance carrier.

HEALTH INSURANCE CLAIM FORM

						PICA

| PICA | | | | | | |

1. MEDICARE (Medicare #) [X] **MEDICAID** (Medicaid #) **CHAMPUS** (Sponsor's SSN) **CHAMPVA** (VA File #) **GROUP HEALTH PLAN** (SSN or ID) **FECA BLK LUNG** (SSN) **OTHER** (ID)

1a. INSURED'S I.D. NUMBER (FOR PROGRAM IN ITEM 1)

2. PATIENT'S NAME (Last Name, First Name, Middle Initial)
Jones, Jill

3. PATIENT'S BIRTH DATE MM 12 DD 04 YYYY 1932 **SEX** M [ ] F [ ]

4. INSURED'S NAME (Last Name, First Name, Middle Initial)

5. PATIENT'S ADDRESS (No., Street)
555 High Street

6. PATIENT RELATIONSHIP TO INSURED
Self [X] Spouse [ ] Child [ ] Other [ ]

7. INSURED'S ADDRESS (No., Street)

CITY Anycity   **STATE** CA

8. PATIENT STATUS
Single [X] Married [ ] Other [ ]
Employed [X] Full-Time Student [ ] Part-Time Student [ ]

CITY   **STATE** CA

ZIP CODE 12345   **TELEPHONE** (Include Area Code) (805) 555-1234

ZIP CODE 12345   **TELEPHONE** (INCLUDE AREA CODE) (805) 555-1234

9. OTHER INSURED'S NAME (Last Name, First Name, Middle Initial)

10. IS PATIENT'S CONDITION RELATED TO:

11. INSURED'S POLICY GROUP OR FECA NUMBER

a. OTHER INSURED'S POLICY OR GROUP NUMBER

a. EMPLOYMENT? (CURRENT OR PREVIOUS) YES [ ] NO [X]

a. INSURED'S DATE OF BIRTH MM DD YYYY **SEX** M [ ] F [ ]

b. OTHER INSURED'S DATE OF BIRTH MM DD YYYY **SEX** M [ ] F [X]

b. AUTO ACCIDENT? **PLACE (State)** YES [ ] NO [X]

b. EMPLOYER'S NAME OR SCHOOL NAME

c. EMPLOYER'S NAME OR SCHOOL NAME

c. OTHER ACCIDENT? YES [ ] NO [X]

c. INSURANCE PLAN NAME OR PROGRAM NAME

d. INSURANCE PLAN NAME OR PROGRAM NAME

10d. RESERVED FOR LOCAL USE

d. IS THERE ANOTHER HEALTH BENEFIT PLAN? YES [ ] NO [ ] *If yes*, return to and complete item 9 a-d.

READ BACK OF FORM BEFORE COMPLETING & SIGNING THIS FORM.
12. PATIENT'S OR AUTHORIZED PERSON'S SIGNATURE I authorize the release of any medical or other information necessary to process this claim. I also request payment of government benefits either to myself or to the party who accepts assignment below.

SIGNED Signature on file   DATE 01/01/2005

13. INSURED'S OR AUTHORIZED PERSON'S SIGNATURE I authorize payment of medical benefits to the undersigned physician or supplier for services described below.

SIGNED

14. DATE OF CURRENT: ILLNESS (First symptom) OR INJURY (Accident) OR PREGNANCY(LMP) MM DD YYYY

15. IF PATIENT HAS HAD SAME OR SIMILAR ILLNESS. GIVE FIRST DATE MM DD YYYY

16. DATES PATIENT UNABLE TO WORK IN CURRENT OCCUPATION FROM MM DD YYYY TO MM DD YYYY

17. NAME OF REFERRING PHYSICIAN OR OTHER SOURCE

17a. I.D. NUMBER OF REFERRING PHYSICIAN

18. HOSPITALIZATION DATES RELATED TO CURRENT SERVICES FROM MM DD YYYY TO MM DD YYYY

19. RESERVED FOR LOCAL USE

20. OUTSIDE LAB? YES [ ] NO [ ] **$ CHARGES**

21. DIAGNOSIS OR NATURE OF ILLNESS OR INJURY. (RELATE ITEMS 1,2,3 OR 4 TO ITEM 24E BY LINE)
1. V58.1
2. 787.XX
3. 105.2
4.

22. MEDICAID RESUBMISSION CODE **ORIGINAL REF. NO.**

23. PRIOR AUTHORIZATION NUMBER

24. A DATE(S) OF SERVICE					B Place of Service	C Type of Service	D PROCEDURES, SERVICES, OR SUPPLIES (Explain Unusual Circumstances) CPT/HCPCS | MODIFIER	E DIAGNOSIS CODE	F $ CHARGES		G DAYS OR UNITS	H EPSDT Family Plan	I EMG	J COB	K RESERVED FOR LOCAL USE
From MM	DD	YYYY	To MM	DD	YYYY											
1 MM	DD	YYYY	MM	DD	YYYY	11		J2469	1	XXXX	XX	10				
2 MM	DD	YYYY	MM	DD	YYYY	11		J9XXX	X	XXXX	XX	X				
3 MM	DD	YYYY	MM	DD	YYYY	11		GXXXX 59	1	XXXX	XX	1				
4																
5																
6																

25. FEDERAL TAX I.D. NUMBER SSN [ ] EIN [X]
123-45-6789

26. PATIENT'S ACCOUNT NO.
987654321

27. ACCEPT ASSIGNMENT? (For govt. claims, see back) YES [X] NO [ ]

28. TOTAL CHARGE $ **29. AMOUNT PAID** $ **30. BALANCE DUE** $

31. SIGNATURE OF PHYSICIAN OR SUPPLIER INCLUDING DEGREES OR CREDENTIALS (I certify that the statements on the reverse apply to this bill and are made a part thereof.)
SIGNED On file   DATE

32. NAME AND ADDRESS OF FACILITY WHERE SERVICES WERE RENDERED (If other than home or office)

33. PHYSICIAN'S, SUPPLIER'S BILLING NAME, ADDRESS, ZIP CODE & PHONE #
Martin Smith, MD
51 Provider Dr.
Anycity, CA 12345
PIN#   GRP#

(APPROVED BY AMA COUNCIL ON MEDICAL SERVICE 8/88)   **PLEASE PRINT OR TYPE**   APPROVED OMB-0938-0008 FORM CMS-1500 (12-90), FORM RRB-1500, APPROVED OMB-1215-0055 FORM OWCP-1500, APPROVED OMB-0720-0001 (CHAMPUS)

CARRIER — PATIENT AND INSURED INFORMATION — PHYSICIAN OR SUPPLIER INFORMATION

FIGURE 16-3   A completed CMS-1500 form.

Assignment of Lifetime Medicare Benefits

Name of Beneficiary ________________________________

Medicare Number ________________________________

I, the undersigned, request that all authorized Medicare benefits be paid to me or on my behalf to ____________________ (Name of Physician or Supplier) for all services rendered to me by the aforementioned provider. I hereby authorize any holder of my medical records to release to the Health Care Financing Administration and its agents any information necessary to determine and secure the payment of all benefits.*

Signed ________________________ (Signature of Beneficiary) Date ____________

* If you are a patient in a hospital or skilled nursing home, this authorization is in effect for the period of your confinement. Otherwise, this authorization is in effect until you choose to revoke it.

FIGURE 16-4 A Health Care Insurance Claim Form—Assignment of Lifetime Medicare.

(Figure 16-4). With a signature on one form, the notation "SIGNATURE ON FILE" can also be made in box 13. This saves the medical assistant the time required for a patient to sign an insurance claim form for each office visit. The forms, however, must be kept in the patient record and must be available at all times.

One confusing element in insurance processing is the concept of "participating" and "nonparticipating" providers. Most insurance companies will make special incentives available to those who choose to become participating providers, who can be the physician or medical facility that will accept the insurance company's allowed amount for services rendered to be payment in full (less patient co-payments). To become a participating provider, the physician completes a form and is assigned a number that is unique to the physician or practice.

With most insurance plans, payment is made directly to participating providers, while payment is made to the patient for claims of a nonparticipating provider. The nonparticipating provider bills the patient and the patient is expected to pay the charges.

There are advantages to both ways of handling insurance claims. Often, insurance companies reimburse at a lower rate than the physician bills. In this case, the physician must "write off" or agree to forfeit the amount the insurance company does not authorize. It is an expense to any practice when administrative staff (medical assistant or insurance claims processing clerk, for example) is on the payroll and need to spend time submitting and tracking insurance claims. However, payment is made directly to the physician's practice, often within a few days (especially with electronic claim submission), ensuring that large charges do not accumulate on the physician's accounts receivable. Each practice must weigh the advantages and disadvantages carefully before making a decision to become either a participating or nonparticipating practice.

Many medical offices now use a single sheet to speed the process of reimbursement. This form is called a superbill and lists the patient's name, diagnoses and treatments with additional space to fill in claim information. Some insurance carriers will accept a superbill in lieu of a claim form, although this depends on the specific carrier. Originally, superbills were created to allow patients to file their own claims; however, as insurance rules and regulations have become more complex and coding and documentation requirements more stringent, most medical practices file insurance claims for their patients as a courtesy. Lifespan Considerations has more about completing insurance claim forms.

It is important for the medical assistant to verify if a patient has primary and secondary medical insurance coverage. A patient who has health insurance coverage with more than one medical insurance plan will have one primary insurance coverage and the other insurance as secondary coverage. If the patient has coverage with his or her employer as well as his or her spouse's employer, then the patient's employer's medical insurance plan

Lifespan Considerations

Some insurance plans *require that the subscriber fill out the claim forms. To someone, especially an older patient, who has never worked with filing claims, this can be very confusing. Because the physician cannot receive payment for services until claims are filed, it can be helpful to assist the patient in filling out the appropriate forms. Some offices do this for a small fee, while others do it at no charge. Remember to have the patient sign an authorization to release medical information before submitting any claim.*

would be primary, while the spouse's employer's medical insurance plan would be secondary. This is to prevent a person from profiting on his or her medical insurance. It also prevents double payment on services provided.

The "birthday rule" is used by insurance claims administrators to determine which parent's benefit plans will pay for the medical bills of a dependent child when the child is covered by the plans of both parents. The plan of the parent whose birthday falls earliest in the year (not the oldest parent) will be the primary plan. When parents have the same birthday, the primary medical insurance will be the one with the earliest date of inception. This rule only applies to parents who are legally married.

If the parents are divorced, the court will determine which parent's medical insurance will be primarily responsible. Just because a parent has legal custody does not mean that his or her medical insurance will be primary.

Claim Security

Confidentiality is an important issue in regards to the sensitive information that is found in a patient's medical record. Care must be taken when processing insurance claims that appropriate information is only released to the appropriate person. Security involves protection of patient information. Security is the responsibility of all who have access to patients' records. Care must be taken in the work area not to leave records unattended. When discussing patient information with insurance carriers over the telephone, it is best to be in an area where you cannot be easily overheard. It is considered to be a breach of confidentiality, or failure to keep something confidential, when patient information is released to others without authorization from the patient (Legal and Ethical Issues).

Before releasing any information regarding a patient to anyone, you must obtain a signed "Authorization for Release of Medical Information" statement. Authorization can be given by having the patient sign block 12, Patient's or Authorized Person's Signature, on the CMS-1500. A practice can also create its own release form. It is good routine to have the patient renew this authorization annually.

Another element of claim security is making sure electronic data containing health information about a patient is secure when stored on a computer network. A firewall is used to prevent unauthorized access from another computer system to the data stored on the computer network.

Tracking Claim Forms

When a medical assistant is submitting paper claims, he or she must have a tracking system in place to follow up on claims that have been submitted. An insurance claims log is used for this purpose. An insurance claims log can be documented manually or it may be kept on a computerized spreadsheet. It gives the medical assistant the status of a claim quickly. After the medical assistant completes a claim form, he or she then enters data into the insurance claims log. The data entered at this time includes the patient's name, date of service, insurance carrier, date the claim was submitted, and amount of the claim submitted. When the medical assistant follows up on the claim, the date must be documented on the insurance claims log. Once the medical assistant receives payment on the claim, this date must also be documented on the insurance claims log. The difference between the submitted and paid amounts is also documented on the insurance claims log. After the claim is paid in full, the medical assistant can highlight that section of the insurance claims log to indicate that the claim is completely processed.

Claim Form Rejection

Occasionally, if a claim is not correct in some way, the insurance company will reject the claim. Some of the most common reasons for claim rejection include:

- Incorrect or missing patient registration information (name, address, insurance number)
- Incorrect or missing name of a referring physician
- Incorrect or missing diagnosis code
- Overlapping, incorrect, or duplicate dates of service
- Incorrect place of service
- Invalid, incorrect, or missing procedure code
- Incorrect or missing number of days or units
- Incorrect or missing modifier

If a claim is rejected for any reason, it must be corrected and resubmitted to the insurance carrier. There are usually time limits for refiling rejected claims, so the medical assistant must be very aware of these deadlines and resubmit the claims before the time has expired. Expired claims will not be processed by the insurance carrier and will ultimately cost the practice money.

As a precaution, the medical assistant must review every claim for accuracy prior to submitting it. While no one process or procedure can guarantee that a claim will never be rejected or reviewed, a careful, studious approach to the claims process can ensure greater accuracy.

Preventing Claim Form Rejection

To prevent a claim from being rejected, the medical assistant must have all the books and equipment readily available. When he or she is filing insurance claim forms, the medical assistant must carefully review each claim before it is submitted. Limiting distractions that occur in the medical office can also help the medical assistant ensure the claim form is correct and complete. Having time to focus on claims processing is not always possible, but if the office team works together, it can be accommodated. Having a certain time period each day set aside for working on claims and not doing other tasks, can help the medical assistant complete the forms correctly and, most of the time, faster. Lastly, have another medical office staff member review each insurance claim form before it is submitted. A second set of eyes may notice errors or omissions not detected by the person processing the forms.

SUMMARY

The health insurance claim form provides communication between the insurance company and physician for the patient. When the medical assistant is submitting a claim, he or she must find out which health insurance claim form to use. The most commonly used form is the CMS-1500 claim form. Claims are submitted in paper form or electronically. The medical assistant must be familiar with how to complete the CMS-1500 form.

Chapter Review

COMPETENCY REVIEW

1. Define and spell the terms to learn for this chapter.
2. Explain the "birthday rule."
3. What is the name of the standardized form used to submit insurance claims? What information must be included on this form?
4. List the reasons a claim may be rejected.
5. Use the health insurance claim forms shown in Figures 16-4 and 16-5 to complete the forms for: Jane Doe, address 123 Main Street, Anytown, ST 60000, U.S.A., telephone 444-555-1234, S/S # 123-45-6789, DOB (date of birth) 1/15/1973. She is single and self-insured. Jane Doe's insurance number is the same as her social security number. Jane saw Dr. Brent Smith for the first time on May 27, 2005 and he diagnosed her with primary hypertension. Jane paid $40.00 for the office visit. Jane's account number is 00321. Dr. Smith is located at 555 Frances Street, Anytown, ST 60000, U.S.A., telephone 444-555-1111, Federal Tax ID # 000000000.

PREPARING FOR THE CERTIFICATION EXAM

1. What information is not required for completing a CMS-1500?
   A. the number of people in the household
   B. the name of the insured
   C. the name of the insured's insurance company
   D. the insured's identification number
   E. the telephone number of the insured

2. Once a patient has signed a release of information statement, what may be written in box 12 of the CMS-1500?
   A. BENEFITS ASSIGNED
   B. CONFIDENTIAL
   C. SIGNATURE ON FILE
   D. PERMISSION GRANTED
   E. the patient must sign each time

continued on next page

3. Which form allows a medical office to use a single sheet that lists the patient's name, diagnoses, treatments, and claim information?
   A. charge sheet
   B. CMS-1500
   C. superclaim
   D. reimbursement form
   E. superbill

4. Which is NOT a reason a claim may be rejected?
   A. overlapping dates of service
   B. missing name of a referring physician
   C. incorrect place of service
   D. incorrect patient telephone number
   E. correct diagnosis is given

5. The CMS-1500 claim form
   A. is accepted by every insurance company.
   B. must be filled out by the patient
   C. must be filled out by the provider
   D. is accepted as a standard submission (claim) form by most carriers
   E. is never used

6. Which is filed when a patient is eligible for both Medicare and Medicaid?
   A. CMS-1500   D. crossover claim
   B. HCFA-1500   E. DD form 2642
   C. superbill

7. Which insurance is mandated by the federal government to cover those who have received injuries directly related to work?
   A. Blue Cross/Blue Shield
   B. disability insurance
   C. workers' compensation
   D. Medicaid
   E. CHAMPUS

8. Which is a reason a claim might be rejected?
   A. appropriate diagnosis code
   B. missing procedure code
   C. correct place of service
   D. correct date of service
   E. correct social security number

9. When a health insurance claim form has missing data or errors, this is considered to be a?
   A. clean claim
   B. invalid claim
   C. dirty claim
   D. denied claim
   E. rejected claim

10. Electronic claim submission
   A. is difficult and costly
   B. cannot be completed by a medical assistant
   C. is referred to as a paperless claim
   D. increases the time it takes to pay a claim
   E. frequently have errors

CRITICAL THINKING

1. What steps should Lewis take to verify Mary Free's insurance?
2. List some reasons the claim for Mark's care could have been rejected.

ON THE JOB

Drake Scott, CMA, is responsible for processing insurance claims for a large medical clinic. You have just hired Anne Obermark, CMA to work with Drake in processing insurance claims. You determined that Anne will be responsible for tracking claims.

1. Why is it important for Anne to track insurance claims processed through the clinic?
2. What kind of information should the insurance claim log contain?
3. When Anne checks the insurance claim log, she finds five claims that have not been paid in the past three months. What should Anne do?

INTERNET ACTIVITY

There are many software packages available to help complete and submit insurance claims. Conduct a search to find 5 such packages. List the unique features, similar features, and cost.

MediaLink More on medical insurance claims, including interactive resources, can be found on the Student CD-ROM accompanying this textbook.

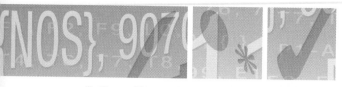

Medical Assistant Role Delineation Chart

HIGHLIGHT indicates material covered in this chapter.

ADMINISTRATIVE

Administrative Procedures

- Perform basic administrative medical assisting functions
- Schedule, coordinate and monitor appointments
- Schedule inpatient/outpatient admissions and procedures
- Understand and apply third-party guidelines
- Obtain reimbursement through accurate claims submission
- Monitor third-party reimbursement
- Understand and adhere to managed care policies and procedures
- *Negotiate managed care contracts*

Practice Finances

- Perform procedural and diagnostic coding
- Apply bookkeeping principles

- Manage accounts receivable
- *Manage accounts payable*
- *Process payroll*
- *Document and maintain accounting and banking records*
- *Develop and maintain fee schedules*
- *Manage renewals of business and professional insurance policies*
- *Manage personnel benefits and maintain records*
- *Perform marketing, financial, and strategic planning*

CLINICAL

Fundamental Principles

- Apply principles of aseptic technique and infection control
- Comply with quality assurance practices
- Screen and follow up patient test results

Diagnostic Orders

- Collect and process specimens
- Perform diagnostic tests

Patient Care

- Adhere to established patient screening procedures
- Obtain patient history and vital signs
- Prepare and maintain examination and treatment areas
- Prepare patient for examinations, procedures and treatments

- Assist with examinations, procedures and treatments
- Prepare and administer medications and immunizations
- Maintain medication and immunization records
- Recognize and respond to emergencies
- Coordinate patient care information with other health care providers
- Initiate IV and administer IV medications with appropriate training and as permitted by state law

GENERAL

Professionalism

- Display a professional manner and image
- Demonstrate initiative and responsibility
- Work as a member of the health care team
- Prioritize and perform multiple tasks
- Adapt to change
- Promote the CMA credential
- Enhance skills through continuing education
- Treat all patients with compassion and empathy
- Promote the practice through positive public relations

Communication Skills

- Recognize and respect cultural diversity
- Adapt communications to individual's ability to understand
- Use professional telephone technique

- Recognize and respond effectively to verbal, nonverbal, and written communications
- Use medical terminology appropriately
- Utilize electronic technology to receive, organize, prioritize and transmit information
- Serve as liaison

Legal Concepts

- Perform within legal and ethical boundaries
- Prepare and maintain medical records
- Document accurately
- Follow employer's established policies dealing with the health care contract
- Implement and maintain federal and state health care legislation and regulations
- Comply with established risk management and safety procedures
- Recognize professional credentialing criteria
- *Develop and maintain personnel, policy and procedure manuals*

Instruction

- Instruct individuals according to their needs
- Explain office policies and procedures
- Teach methods of health promotion and disease prevention
- Locate community resources and disseminate information
- *Develop educational materials*
- *Conduct continuing education activities*

Operational Functions

- Perform inventory of supplies and equipment
- Perform routine maintenance of administrative and clinical equipment
- Apply computer techniques to support office operations
- *Perform personnel management functions*
- *Negotiate leases and prices for equipment and supply contracts*

■ *Denotes advanced skills.*

SOURCE: Reprinted by permission of the American Association of Medical Assistants from the AAMA Role Delineation Study: Occupational Analysis of the Medical Assisting Profession.

Medical Coding

Learning Objectives

After completing this chapter, you should be able to:

- Define and spell the terms to learn for this chapter.
- Describe the purpose of diagnosis coding.
- Correctly apply the principles of ICD-9-CM coding.

- Describe the purpose of CPT coding.
- Correctly apply the principles of CPT coding.
- Discuss basic coding rules for CPT.

Terms to Learn

Current Procedural Terminology (CPT)

Evaluation and Management (E/M)

International Classification of Diseases, Ninth Revision Clinical Modification (ICD-9-CM)

International Classification of Diseases, Tenth Revision (ICD-10)

modifier

principal diagnosis

procedural coding

symbol

World Health Organization (WHO)

Case Study

CASEY ALLEN, A 5-MONTH OLD MALE, WAS seen by Dr. Adams for chronic otitis media. This was the child's third bout in the last 10 months. Dr. Adams recommended bilateral myringtomies and tube placement. The physician also ordered an audiogram. The insurance company denied the claim, stating the procedure code was wrong for the diagnosis.

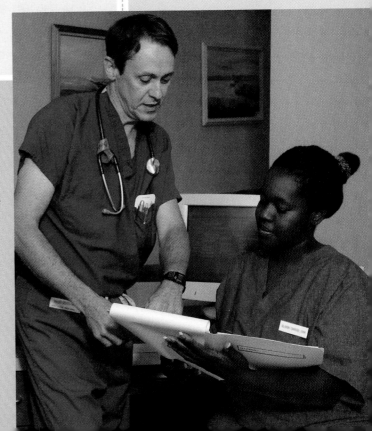

The process of insurance billing includes the accurate identification of the diagnostic, procedure, and service codes on the medical insurance claim form. The diagnostic code is located in the International Classification of Disease, Ninth Revision Clinical Modifications (ICD-9-CM) listing. The procedure and service codes are located in the Current Procedural Terminology (CPT) listing. Each individual code specifically represents a numeric or alphanumeric identification for insurance carriers and aids in obtaining the maximum reimbursement. The medical assistant will need to identify the appropriate codes, which reflect the correct diagnosis and the procedure or service performed, in order to maintain sound billing practices.

Insurance Coding

Proper coding of insurance claims is the basis of the practice income. Incorrect coding will cause delays or denials in reimbursement. Anytime the medical assistant does not observe clear and concise documentation in the patient's medical record to support the ICD-9-CM or CPT code, he or she must consult the physician for further clarification. To be proficient in coding, the medical assistant must also have a good understanding of medical terminology, diseases, procedures, as well as anatomy and physiology. Having a medical dictionary is a handy resource for any medical assistant who is coding. Another helpful resource is the Internet. Having access to the Internet allows the medical assistant to research a disease or procedure he or she does not understand. The Health Insurance Portability and Accountability Act of 1996 (HIPAA) requires correct coding of services and may sanction providers who do not comply with the rules. It is important for the medical assistant to understand how to code and bill with accuracy. In addition, HIPAA requires the use of the CMS-1500 form for Medicare billing, and for most providers, for all medical billing, as well as electronic submission of all bills. In many ambulatory care settings, the process of insurance coding begins with identifying and recording the appropriate diagnosis, procedure, or service codes on the superbill (Figure 17-1). The superbill is a document generated by the medical office and used as a charge slip, statement, and insurance reporting form. It is important for the codes on the superbill to be updated each year when the medical office receives the newest published coding books.

This document provides a comprehensive list of patient procedures, services, and diagnoses with respective codes and fees on which the physician indicates the services rendered. The superbill is used as a reference base for traditional paper insurance forms and electronic claims (Figure 17-2). Lifespan Considerations emphasizes the importance of understanding the superbill to advise patients, especially the elderly.

History of Coding

In 1937, the *International List of Causes of Death* was introduced. Then in 1948, the World Health Organization (WHO) published the *International Classification of Diseases*. This provided a revised list of the first classification system. In the United States, the Department of Health and Human Services published the ICD-9-CM (International Classification of Diseases, Ninth Clinical Modification) in 1979. By 1988, the Medicare Catastrophic Coverage Act was passed. This law made it a requirement for physicians to use diagnosis codes to receive Medicare reimbursement. Coding has gradually grown from a new office task to a career that requires extensive training and knowledge of both the medical and insurance professions. Coding is so important to proper fee reimbursement that an office may offer a bonus payment to its insurance coders if their insurance processing results in increased and accurate collections for the physician's practice. For information about becoming a certified medical coding specialist, contact the American Health Information Management Association (AHIMA) and the American Academy of Professional Coders (AAPC).

Lifespan
Considerations

Elderly patients and caregivers *of patients may not understand the diagnosis as stated on the superbill. The medical assistant can help the patient or patient's parent with any questions he or she may have concerning the superbill.*

Understanding the ICD-9-CM

Upon the physician evaluation, each patient will be diagnosed in medical terms. These medical terms are converted into numeric and alphanumeric diagnosis codes. The diagnosis codes are systematically classified in the International Classification of Disease, published by a specialized agency for health of the United Nations known as the World Health Organization (WHO).

UROLOGIC GYNECOLOGY
GENERAL GYNECOLOGY
OBSTETRICS

WINDY CITY CLINIC
Beth Williams, M.D.
123 Michigan Avenue, Chicago, IL 60610
(312) 123-1234

ID.# 20-1342846

No. 4815

PATIENT INFORMATION

| PATIENT'S LAST NAME | | FIRST | INITIAL | BIRTHDATE | SEX ☐ MALE ☐ FEMALE | TODAY'S DATE / |

| ADDRESS | CITY | STATE | ZIP | RELATION TO SUBSCRIBER | REFERRING PHYSICIAN |

| SUBSCRIBER or POLICY HOLDER | | | | INSURANCE |

| ADDRESS | CITY | STATE | ZIP | INSURANCE ID.# | COVERAGE CODE | GROUP |

OTHER HEALTH COVERAGE?
☐ NO
☐ YES IDENTIFY _____

DISABILITY RELATED TO:
☐ ACCIDENT ☐ PREGNANCY
☐ INDEPENDENT ☐ OTHER

DATE SYMPTOMS APPEARED, INCEPTION OF PREGNANCY, OR ACCIDENT OCCURED: _____

ASSIGNMENT and RELEASE: *I hereby assign my insurance benefits to be paid directly to the undersigned physician. I am financially responsible for noncovered services. I also authorize the physician to release any information required to process this claim.*

SIGNATURE OF PATIENT (or Parent, if Minor) _____ DATE / /

PROCEDURES	CPT-Mod	AMOUNT
A. OFFICE VISITS		
1 New GYN, Limited	90010	
2 New GYN, Intermediate	90015	
3 New GYN, Extensive	90017	
4 New GYN, Comprehensive	90020	
5 Return GYN, Minimal	90030	
6 Return GYN, Brief	90040	
7 Return GYN, Limited	90050	
8 Return GYN, Intermediate	90060	
9 Return GYN, Extended	90070	
10 Return GYN, Comprehensive	90080	
11 Return GYN, Post-Operative	99024	
B. CONSULTATION		
12 GYN Consultation, Limited	90600	
13 GYN Consultation, Intermed.	90605	
14 GYN Consultation, Compreh.	90620	
15 GYN Consultation, Complex	90630	
16 Second Opinion Surgery	90653	
C. TELEPHONE CONSULTATION		
17 Telephone Consult., Simple	99013	
18 Telephone Consult., Intermed.	99014	
19 Telephone Consult., Compreh.	99015	
D. SPECIAL SERVICES		
20 ER Service after Office Hrs.	99064	
21 ER Service during Office Hrs.	99065	
22 Night Call before 10 pm	99050	
23 Night Call after 10 pm	99052	
24 Sunday or Holiday Service	99054	
25 Office Non-Schedule	99058	
E. OB CARE		
26 Prenatal Dx, Consultation	90620	
27 Initial OB, NOrmal	59400	
28 Initial OB, High Risk	59400.22	
29 Return OB, Normal	59420	
30 Return OB, High Risk	59420.22	

PROCEDURES	CPT-Mod	AMOUNT
31 Post-Partum	59430	
F. GYN PROCEDURES		
32 Irrigation of Vagina	57150*	
33 Insert Pessary	57160*	
34 Pessary Supplies	99070	
35 Colposcopy	57452	
36 Biopsy, Cervix	57500	
37 Biopsy, Vagina	57100	
38 Biopsy, Vulva	56600	
39 Biopsy, Endometrium	58100	
40 Biopsy, Skin		
0.5 cm.	11420	
0.6 to 1.0 cm.	11421	
1.1 to 2.0 cm.	11423	
41 Cryotherapy, Cervix	57511	
42 Destruct. Condyloma	56501	
43 Diaphragm Fitting	57170	
44 Diaphragm Supplies	99070	
45 IUD Insertion	58300	
46 IUD Supplies	99070	
47 IUD Removal	58301	
G. UROLOGIC PROCEDURES		
48 Urethral Dilation	53660	
49 Urethral Dilation, Repeat	53661	
50 Bladder Instillation	51700	
51 Periurethral Injection	53665	
52 Simple Catheterization	53670	
53 Manual Electric Stimulation	97118	
H. LAB		
54 Urine Analysis	81000	
55 Urine Culture	87068	
56 Hematocrit	85015	
57 Hemogram	85021	
58 Commercial-Lat.	87087	
59 Wet Mount	87210	

PROCEDURES	CPT-Mod	AMOUNT
60 PG Test, Urine	86006	
61 Antigen Test	86006	
62 Cytopathology Smear	88155	
63 Specimen Handling	99000	
I. MISCELLANEOUS		
64 Surgical Tray	99070	
65 Therapeutic Injection	90782	
66 Injection, Kenalog	J1870	
67 Injection, Xylocaine	J3480	
68 Injection, Estrogen	J2655	
69 Injection, Progesterone	J2675	
70 Injection, Vitamin B12	P4320	
71 Special Reports	99080	

TODAY'S TOTAL FEE $

DIAGNOSIS	CODE
Abortion:	
Threatened	640.0
Incomplete	637.1
Habitual	646.3
Abnormal Urination	788.6
Abnormal PAP Smear	795.0
Adenomyosis	617.0
Adnexal MAss	625.8
Amenorrhera	626.0
Anemia	285.9
Arthritis	716.9
Artificial Menopause	627.4
Asthma-Hayfever	493.0
Atrophic Vaginitis	627.3
Bartholin Abscess	616.3
Benign Neoplasm:	
Cervix	219.0
Uterus	219.1
Ovary	220
Vagina	221.1
Vulva	221.2
Benign Neoplasm of Skin:	
Buttocks	216.5
Abdomen	216.5

DIAGNOSIS	CODE
Breasts	216.5
Vulva	221.1
Breast Disorder (Mass)	611.72
Bronchitis	491
Carcinoma In Situ:	
Cervix	233.1
Uterus	233.2
Female Genital Organs	233.3
Cervical Dysplasia	622.1
Cervicitis	616.0
Contraceptive Management	V25.0
Cystocele	618.0
Cystourethritis	595.0
Diabetes Mellitus	250.0
Thyroid Disorder	246.9
Dysmenorrhea	625.3
Dyspareunia	625.0
Dysuria	788.1
Ectopic Pregnancy	617.0
Endometriosis	617.9
Enuresis-Unstable Bladder	788.3
Frequency of Urination	788.4
Functional Disorder:	
Bladder Instability	596.5

DIAGNOSIS	CODE
Galactorrhea	676.6
Hemorrhoids	455.0
Hypertension	401
Incontinence of Urine	788.3
Interstitial Cystitis	595.1
Irritable Colon	564.1
Irregular Menstrual Cycle	626.4
Malignant Neoplasm:	
Cervix	180.9
Uterus	182.0
Ovary	183.0
Vagina	184.0
Vulva	184.4
Menopausal Syndrome	627.2
Menometrorrhagia	626.2
Oligomenorrhea	626.1
Obesity	278.0
Ovarian Cyst	620.2
Pelvic Inflammatory Disease	614.9
Pelvic Peritoneal Adhesions	614.6
Polycystic Ovaries	256.4
Postmenopausal Bleeding	627.1
Post-Op Wound Infection	998.5
Pregnancy Prenatal	V22

DIAGNOSIS	CODE
Pregnancy Postpartum	V24.2
Rectocele	618.0
Retention of Urine	788.2
Stress Incontinence	625.6
Urethral Stricture	598
Urethral Syndrome	597.81
Uterine Leiomyoma	218
Uterine Prolapse:	
Incomplete	618.2
Complete	618.3
Vaginal Discharge-Non Specific	623.5
Vaginal Enterocele	618.6
Vaginal Prolapse	618.0
Vaginal Vault Prolapse Post	
Hysterectomy	618.5
Vulvovaginitis:	
Non Specific	616.1
Candida	112.1
Trichomonas	131.01

MISCELLANEOUS DIAGNOSIS

DOCTOR'S SIGNATURE _____ DATE / /

SERVICES PERFORMED AT: ☐ Office ☐ Emergency Room
☐ WINDY CITY CLINIC
123 Michigan Avenue, Chicago, IL 60610
(312) 123-1234
☐ Hospital Calls at $ _____ per Visit

ADMITTED _____ / /
DISCHARGED _____ / /

RETURN VISIT INFORMATION
15 • 30 • 45 • 60
_____ DAYS _____ WEEKS _____ MONTHS ☐ WILL CALL
Procedure: _____

ACCEPT ASSIGNMENT
☐ YES
☐ NO

INSTRUCTIONS TO PATIENT FOR FILING INSURANCE CLAIMS

1. Complete patient information portion of this form.
2. Sign and date.
3. Mail this form directly to your insurance company with your own insurance company's form.
4. Patients with health care insurance please remember:
   A. Professional services are charged to the patient, and not to the insurance company.
   B. Insured patients are expected to take care of their fees as services are rendered.
   C. This office cannot accept responsibility for collecting your insurance claim or for negotiating a settlement on a disputed claim.
   D. You are responsible for payment of your account.

TODAY'S FEE	$
OLD BALANCE	$
ADJUSTMENTS	$
TOTAL DUE	$
AMOUNT RECEIVED TODAY	$
☐ CASH ☐ CHECK ☐ C.C.	
NEW BALANCE	$

FIGURE 17-1 An example of a superbill.

WHO accumulates all of the diagnoses reported on claim forms and places the diagnostic codes into a computerized database. This database tracks statistical information, such as morbidity data.

Every year ICD-9-CM codes are updated. The newly published codes are available to the public on or before October 1st. Every medical office should use the newest published copy of the ICD-9-CM (Figure 17-3)

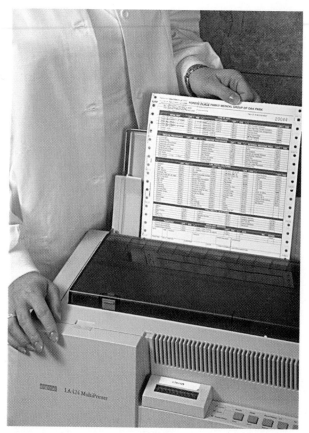

FIGURE 17-2 A computer generated superbill.

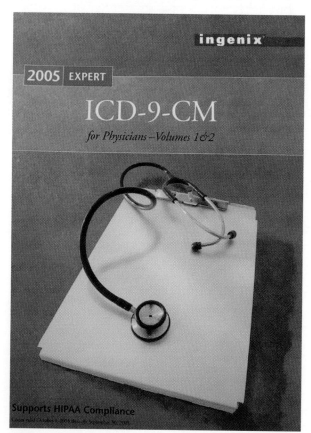

FIGURE 17-3 ICD-9 Code Book.

to perform coding. If the newest published copy of the ICD-9-CM is not used, this could cause the claim to be rejected because of incorrect coding.

Formats and Conventions of ICD-9-CM

ICD-9-CM (International Classification of Diseases, Ninth Clinical Modification) provides numeric and alphanumeric codes for patient diagnoses. In order for an insurance payment to be processed appropriately, the diagnosis code must appear on a claim form and must support the medical necessity of the procedure code (service rendered).

The ICD-9-CM coding manual contains three volumes of information. Volume III deals with inpatient diagnosis and treatment and is used to code inpatient hospital-billed procedures. It is not used in most ambulatory care settings. Therefore, we will concentrate on Volumes I, the Tabular List, and Volume II, the Alphabetic Index.

Volume I (the Tabular List) contains 17 chapters of disease and injury codes and supplementary classifications for V and E codes. It also contains five appendices. In the Tabular List, codes are arranged in numerical order.

Volume II or the Alphabetic Index, lists the disease and injuries that are in the Tabular List in alphabetical order. In addition, Volume II contains an index of poisoning and adverse effects of chemicals and drugs and an index of injuries caused by external efforts, such as accidents.

Steps in ICD Coding

To understand how to code diagnoses, it is important that the medical assistant understand the organization of the ICD-9-CM. Diagnoses are given a three-digit main code, with fourth and fifth digits when required for certain conditions that define the code to the highest level of specificity. To code properly, it is necessary to begin with Volume II, the Alphabetic Index. Diagnoses and conditions are located alphabetically by condition, not body system. Therefore, when trying to find a code for a closed fracture of the right arm, the coder would begin by looking for the key word "fracture." This term is listed in bold type. The coder would next locate the word "arm." A code number of 818.0 is given. Next, the coder would turn to the numeric index (Volume I, Tabular List) and find the code number 818.0. After reading the description, the code 818.0 is determined to be the correct one. However, the diagnosis may need greater specification that requires an additional fifth digit to designate the specific bone of the arm that contains the fracture. Special notes and symbols used in ICD-9-CM coding, such as not otherwise specified (NOS), are listed as reference material in the code books and should be used only when a higher level of specificity is not available.

When coding for claim reimbursement, the medical assistant must also understand the significance of a principal diagnosis. The principal diagnosis is the reason the patient sought care on a particular date. Principal diagnosis is used when performing coding in the hospital setting and when a final diagnosis was unable to be determined without further patient follow-up. The primary diagnosis represents the patient's major health problem for that particular claim. This is important when you file a claim for a patient who has more than one diagnosis, for example cancer and a urinary tract infection (UTI). If the UTI is unrelated to the cancer, and the cancer will not affect the treatment or recovery from the UTI, then the code used for that claim would be UTI. Any other diagnoses treated at that time (up to four) must also be listed. For example, if a diabetic patient is seen for an ear infection, the ear infection is the primary diagnosis, while diabetes is a secondary diagnosis.

Special Codes

The ICD-9-CM coding system also allows for visits (V codes) not directly related to illness or injury or to add supportive information to patient family or personal history. The codes are used to describe a person who may not have a current illness, but uses the health care system for some specific purpose, such as well-baby care, birth control advice, pregnancy test, or immunizations. The codes are also used as supportive information when some circumstance or problem is present that may influence the patient's health, but is not in itself a current illness or problem, such as an allergy to penicillin.

The ICD-9-CM manual also uses tables for certain diseases and conditions. A diagnosis of hypertension, for example, must be coded from the hypertension table. A neoplasm, whether benign or malignant, must be coded from the neoplasm table, and the morphology (behavior) of the neoplasm is coded from a morphology table (M code). Additionally, adverse reactions or poisoning are listed in a section listing various drugs and other agents. Again, the medical assistant should become familiar with the organization of the ICD-9-CM manual in order to code diagnoses properly and correctly. Procedure 17-1 provides steps on how to assign the correct ICD-9-CM codes.

E codes (Figure 17-4) are used to describe external causes of injury and poisoning or adverse effect. These codes may not be used as primary or principal diagnoses (they do not stand alone). E codes are used as additional information regarding a particular diagnosis and to further define the cause of a poisoning or adverse effects, such as therapeutic use, attempted suicide, or accidental. For example, a drug overdose can be either accidental or taken as a suicide attempt. The use of E codes (E930–E949) is mandatory when coding the use of drugs.

Abbreviations, Symbols, and Other Conventions

Instructional notes are included in the listings to guide the user on how to accurately code. Following are some examples:

NEC—Not elsewhere classifiable

NOS—Not otherwise specified

[]—Brackets enclose synonyms, alternative terminology, or explanatory phrases

()—Parentheses enclose supplementary words, called nonessential modifiers, that may be present in the narrative description of a disease without affecting the code assignment

}—The brace encloses a series of terms, each of which is modified by the statement appearing to the right of the brace

● bullet—Indicates a new code

▲—Indicates a revision in the Tabular List and a code change in the Alphabetic index

►◄—Indicates revised text

Boldface type—Used for all codes and titles in the Tabular List

Italicized type—Used for all exclusion notes and to identify codes that should not be used for describing the primary diagnosis

ICD-10

The diagnosis codes in the International Classification of Diseases, Tenth Revision (ICD-10) contain increased specificity and include recently discovered or diagnosed diseases. The ICD-10 has more codes as well as organizational and content modifications and new features.

Procedure Coding

Required elements for reimbursement from insurance carriers are based on a coding system that converts uniform descriptions of medical, surgical, and diagnostic services into numbers. This system, developed by the American Medical Association (AMA) in 1966, allows providers to communicate the procedures and services provided to the patient with increased accuracy. Reimbursement is based on codes submitted for services rendered. The process of transferring a narrative description of procedures into numbers is referred to as procedure coding.

SUPPLEMENTARY CLASSIFICATION OF EXTERNAL CAUSES OF INJURY AND POISONING (E800-E999)

This section is provided to permit the classification of environmental events, circumstances, and conditions as the cause of injury, poisoning, and other adverse effects. Where a code from this section is applicable, it is intended that it shall be used in addition to a code from one of the main chapters of ICD-9-CM, indicating the nature of the condition. Certain other conditions which may be stated to be due to external causes are classified in Chapters 1 to 16 of ICD-9-CM. For these, the "E" code classification should be used as an additional code for more detailed analysis.

Machinery accidents [other than those connected with transport] are classifiable to category E919, in which the fourth-digit allows a broad classification of the type of machinery involved. If a more detailed classification of type of machinery is required, it is suggested that the "Classification of Industrial Accidents according to Agency," prepared by the International Labor Office, be used in addition. This is reproduced in Appendix D for optional use.

Categories for "late effects" of accidents and other external causes are to be found at E929, E959, E969, E977, E989, and E999.

DEFINITIONS AND EXAMPLES RELATED TO TRANSPORT ACCIDENTS

(a) A **transport accident** (E800-E848) is any accident involving a device designed primarily for, or being used at the time primarily for, conveying persons or goods from one place to another.

> INCLUDES   accidents involving:
> aircraft and spacecraft (E840-E845)
> watercraft (E830-E838)
> motor vehicle (E810-E825)
> railway (E800-E807)
> other road vehicles (E826-E829)

In classifying accidents which involve more than one kind of transport, the above order of precedence of transport accidents should be used.

Accidents involving agricultural and construction machines, such as tractors, cranes, and bulldozers, are regarded as transport accidents only when these vehicles are under their own power on a highway [otherwise the vehicles are regarded as machinery]. Vehicles which can travel on land or water, such as hovercraft and other amphibious vehicles, are regarded as watercraft when on the water, as motor vehicles when on the highway, and as off-road motor vehicles when on land, but off the highway.

> EXCLUDES   accidents:
> in sports which involve the use of transport
> but where the transport vehicle itself
> was not involved in the accident
> involving vehicles which are part of industrial
> equipment used entirely on industrial
> premises
> occurring during transportation but unrelated
> to the hazards associated with the
> means of transportation [e.g., injuries
> received in a fight on board ship;
> transport vehicle involved in a
> cataclysm such as an earthquake]
> to persons engaged in the maintenance or
> repair of transport equipment or vehicle
> not in motion, unless injured by
> another vehicle in motion

(b) A **railway accident** is a transport accident involving a railway train or other railway vehicle operated on rails, whether in motion or not.

> EXCLUDES   accidents:
> in repair shops
> in roundhouse or on turntable
> on railway premises but not involving a train
> or other railway vehicle

(c) A **railway train** or **railway vehicle** is any device with or without cars coupled to it, designed for traffic on a railway.

> INCLUDES   interurban:
> electric car ⎫ (operated chiefly on its
> streetcar ⎬ own right-of-way,
>   ⎭ not open to other
>   traffic)
> railway train, any power [diesel] [electric]
> [steam]
> funicular
> monorail or two-rail
> subterranean or elevated
> other vehicle designed to run on a railway
> track

> EXCLUDES   interurban electric cars [streetcars] specified to
> be operating on a right-of-way that forms
> part of the public street or highway
> [definition (n)]

(d) A **railway** or **railroad** is a right-of-way designed for traffic on rails, which is used by carriages or wagons transporting passengers or freight, and by other rolling stock, and which is not open to other public vehicular traffic.

(e) A **motor vehicle accident** is a transport accident involving a motor vehicle. It is defined as a motor vehicle traffic accident or as a motor vehicle nontraffic accident according to whether the accident occurs on a public highway or elsewhere.

> EXCLUDES   injury or damage due to cataclysm
> injury or damage while a motor vehicle, not
> under its own power, is being loaded on,
> or unloaded from, another conveyance

(f) A **motor vehicle traffic accident** is any motor vehicle accident occurring on a public highway [i.e., originating, terminating, or involving a vehicle partially on the highway]. A motor vehicle accident is assumed to have occurred on the highway unless another place is specified, except in the case of accidents involving only off-road motor vehicles which are classified as nontraffic accidents unless the contrary is stated.

(g) A **motor vehicle nontraffic accident** is any motor vehicle accident which occurs entirely in any place other than a public highway.

(h) A **public highway** [**trafficway**] or **street** is the entire width between property lines [or other boundary lines] of every way or place, of which any part is open to the use of the public for purposes of vehicular traffic as a matter of right or custom. A **roadway** is that part of the public highway designed, improved, and ordinarily used, for vehicular travel.

> INCLUDES   approaches (public) to:
> docks
> public building
> station

> EXCLUDES   driveway (private)
> parking lot
> ramp
> roads in:
> airfield
> farm
> industrial premises
> mine
> private grounds
> quarry

✓ 4th Fourth-digit Required   ▶◀ Revised Text   ● New Code   ▲ Revised Code Title

FIGURE 17-4   An E-code section of the ICD-9-CM. Printed with permission from Ingenix, Inc. Copyright © 2004.

PROCEDURE

ICD-9-CM Coding

OBJECTIVE: Accurately assign an ICD-9-CM code.

Equipment and Supplies

patient's medical record; patient's insurance card; computer with printer or typewriter; medical billing software; current ICD-9-CM coding book; medical reference material; superbill with the doctor's diagnosis

Method

1. Locate the condition or diagnosis on the superbill or in the patient's medical record.
2. In Volume II (Alphabetic Index) of the ICD-9-CM book, locate the condition or diagnosis. (A condition may be expressed as: a noun, an adjective, or an eponym)
3. Examine the diagnostic statement to determine if the main term specifically describes that disease. If it does not, then look at the modifiers listed under that main term to find a more specific code. Also read any notes or cross references that may apply.
4. Then, locate the code in Volume I (Tabular Index).
5. Match the code description in the Tabular Index with the diagnosis in the patient's medical record.
6. Any of the codes from 0021.0 through V 82.9 in ICD-9-CM can be used to describe the main reason for the patient's office visit.
7. First list the ICD-9-CM code for the condition, problem, or diagnosis that is the main reason for the visit. Then, list coexisting conditions under additional codes.

8. Use codes at their highest level—5th digit codes first, then 4th digit, 3rd digit, and so on.
9. Do not code questionable or probable diagnoses, or the rule-out (R/O) diagnosis. One of the signs or symptoms of the R/O diagnosis will have to be identified by the physician as the reason for the office visit. For example, in R/O cystic fibrosis, the symptom of dyspnea would be coded until a definitive diagnosis of cystic fibrosis is made.
10. V codes describe factors that influence the health status of the patient, such as pregnancy test or vaccination, and are not used to code current illnesses. V codes are located in Volume II.
11. E codes are used for identifying external environmental events or conditions as the cause of injury, some adverse effect, or poisoning. For example, a drug overdose, either accidental or taken as a suicide attempt. The use of E codes (E 930-E 949) is mandatory when coding the use of drugs.
12. M codes, in Appendix A of Volume I, relate to the morphology of neoplasms. Morphology codes are not used as the primary diagnosis code; they are listed after the ICD-9-CM code. Each M code begins with the letter "M." The M codes cannot be used on claims for patient billing.
13. List all diagnosis codes (up to four) on the insurance claim form.

Healthcare Common Procedure Coding System (HCPCS) Sections

To report services and procedures for Medicaid and Medicare patient, the Healthcare Common Procedure Coding System (HCPCS) is used. There are two coding levels (Level I and Level II) available in HCPCS. Level I provides the same codes from the Current Procedural Terminology (CPT) manual, which provides procedure and service codes. Level II has codes that are not available in the CPT. This part has twenty-two sections that contain five-digit alphanumeric codes (Figure 17-5). These codes are for items that Medicare covers, such as

materials, supplies, and injections. Each Level II code begins with a letter with four numbers behind it. E1280 is an example of a Level II HCPCS code. HCPCS also has modifiers. Each modifier consists of two letters. These can also be used in addition to the modifiers from the CPT manual.

Getting to Know the CPT

In order to maximize reimbursements for a particular practice, the medical assistant must be familiar with CPT codes and how they are used. Codes are reviewed

Durable Medical Equipment

E1231 — E1520

Y **E1231** Wheelchair, pediatric size, tilt-in-space, rigid, adjustable, with seating system   🦽
MED: 100-3, 280.1

Y **E1232** Wheelchair, pediatric size, tilt-in-space, folding, adjustable, with seating system   🦽
MED: 100-3, 280.1

Y **E1233** Wheelchair, pediatric size, tilt-in-space, rigid, adjustable, without seating system   🦽
MED: 100-3, 280.1

Y **E1234** Wheelchair, pediatric size, tilt-in-space, folding, adjustable, without seating system   🦽
MED: 100-3, 280.1

Y **E1235** Wheelchair, pediatric size, rigid, adjustable, with seating system   🦽
MED: 100-3, 280.1

Y **E1236** Wheelchair, pediatric size, folding, adjustable, with seating system   🦽
MED: 100-3, 280.1

Y **E1237** Wheelchair, pediatric size, rigid, adjustable, without seating system   🦽
MED: 100-3, 280.1

Y **E1238** Wheelchair, pediatric size, folding, adjustable, without seating system   🦽
MED: 100-3, 280.1

● **E1239** Power wheelchair, pediatric size, not otherwise specified

WHEELCHAIR — LIGHTWEIGHT

A **E1240** Lightweight wheelchair; detachable arms, desk or full-length, swing-away, detachable, elevating legrest   🦽 ⃠
MED: 100-3, 280.1

A **E1250** Lightweight wheelchair; fixed full-length arms, swing-away, detachable footrests   ⃠
MED: 100-3, 280.1
See code(s): K0003

A **E1260** Lightweight wheelchair; detachable arms, desk or full-length, swing-away, detachable, footrests   ⃠
MED: 100-3, 280.1
See code(s): K0003

A **E1270** Lightweight wheelchair; fixed full-length arms, swing-away, detachable elevating legrests   🦽 ⃠
MED: 100-3, 280.1

WHEELCHAIR — HEAVY-DUTY

A **E1280** Heavy-duty wheelchair; detachable arms, desk or full-length, elevating legrests   🦽 ⃠
MED: 100-3, 280.1

A **E1285** Heavy-duty wheelchair; fixed full-length arms, swing-away, detachable footrests   ⃠
MED: 100-3, 280.1
See code(s): K0006

A **E1290** Heavy-duty wheelchair; detachable arms, desk or full-length, swing-away, detachable footrests   ⃠
MED: 100-3, 280.1
See code(s): K0006

A **E1295** Heavy-duty wheelchair; fixed full-length arms, elevating legrests   🦽 ⃠
MED: 100-3, 280.1

Y **E1296** Special wheelchair seat height from floor   🦽 ⃠
MED: 100-3, 280.3

Y **E1297** Special wheelchair seat depth, by upholstery   🦽 ⃠
MED: 100-3, 280.3

Y **E1298** Special wheelchair seat depth and/or width, by construction   🦽 ⃠
MED: 100-3, 280.3

WHIRLPOOL — EQUIPMENT

E **E1300** Whirlpool, portable (overtub type)   ⃠
MED: 100-3, 280.1

Y **E1310** Whirlpool, nonportable (built-in type)   🦽 ⃠
MED: 100-3, 280.1

REPAIRS AND REPLACEMENT SUPPLIES

Y ☑ **E1340** Repair or nonroutine service for durable medical equipment requiring the skill of a technician, labor component, per 15 minutes   ⃠
Medicare jurisdiction: local carrier if repair of implanted DME.
MED: 100-2, 15, 110.2

ADDITIONAL OXYGEN RELATED EQUIPMENT

Y **E1353** Regulator   ⃠
MED: 100-3, 240.2

Y **E1355** Stand/rack   ⃠
MED: 100-3, 240.2

Y **E1372** Immersion external heater for nebulizer   🦽 ⃠
MED: 100-3, 240.2

Y **E1390** Oxygen concentrator, single delivery port, capable of delivering 85 percent or greater oxygen concentration at the prescribed flow rate   🦽 ⃠
MED: 100-3, 240.2

Y ☑ **E1391** Oxygen concentrator, dual delivery port, capable of delivering 85 percent or greater oxygen concentration at the prescribed flow rate, each   🦽 ⃠
MED: 100-3, 240.2

N **E1399** Durable medical equipment, miscellaneous   ⃠
Determine if an alternative HCPCS Level II or a CPT code better describes the service being reported. This code should be used only if a more specific code is unavailable. Medicare jurisdiction: local carrier if repair or implanted DME.

Y **E1405** Oxygen and water vapor enriching system with heated delivery   🦽 ⃠
MED: 100-3, 240.2; 100-4, 20, 20; 100-4, 20, 20.4

Y **E1406** Oxygen and water vapor enriching system without heated delivery   🦽 ⃠
MED: 100-3, 240.2; 100-4, 20, 20; 100-4, 20, 20.4

ARTIFICIAL KIDNEY MACHINES AND ACCESSORIES

For glucose monitors, see A4253–A4256. For supplies for ESRD, see procedure codes A4651–A4929.

A **E1500** Centrifuge, for dialysis   ⃠

A **E1510** Kidney, dialysate delivery system kidney machine, pump recirculating, air removal system, flowrate meter, power off, heater and temp control with alarm, IV poles, pressure gauge, concentrate container   ⃠

A **E1520** Heparin infusion pump for hemodialysis   ⃠

| Special Coverage Instructions | Noncovered by Medicare | Carrier Discretion | ☑ Quantity Alert | ● New Code | ○ Reinstated Code | ▲ Revised Code |

FIGURE 17-5   HCPCS Level II sections. Printed with permission from Ingenix, Inc. Copyright © 2004.

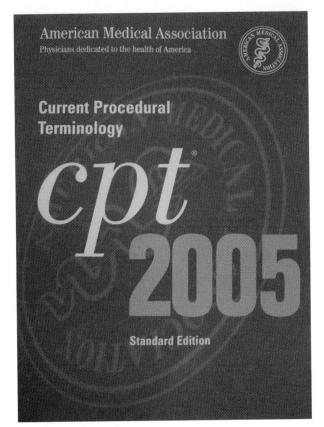

FIGURE 17-6 CPT coding book.

follow. Several appendices follow, including a complete list of all modifiers used in CPT with descriptions, as well as a quick reference summary of codes that have been added, deleted, or revised. Patient Education discusses the need for the medical assistant to understand the codes to inform patients of the codes' meanings.

Understanding Evaluation and Management

For a beginning coder, the most complex section of the CPT coding system is the Evaluation and Management Services. E/M, as it is referred to, is based on the following criteria: history of the patient, complexity of the examination, and the degree of difficulty in medical decision-making. Of these three factors, the medical decision-making factor can be the most complex.

Levels of Evaluation and Management

The four levels of decision-making are: straightforward, low complex, moderate complex, and high complex. The E/M codes are service oriented and were designed to link the procedure or diagnosis with the amount of time it takes the physician to diagnosis and treat the patient. For coding purposes, all patients are either an established patient or a new patient. It is important to understand the difference between a new and established patient, a consultation and a referral, and to be sure the proper place of service (office, hospital, skilled nursing facility, emergency department) is coded. Take a few moments to look through the CPT manual to become familiar with its structure and how codes are presented. Commonly accepted descriptions of services or procedures are presented after the code number. There are two types of codes listed. One type stands alone; the other is indented. Only the codes that stand alone have full descriptions. Indented codes include only that portion of the stand-alone code before the semicolon. This is an extremely important concept to remember.

and updated on a yearly basis. Coding from the most current edition of the CPT manual is essential (Figure 17-6). The CPT manual is available for purchase from the AMA.

The CPT manual is organized numerically or alphanumerically in sections according to classified types of service (Table 17-1). The most commonly used codes for Evaluation and Management (E/M) services (office visits, consultations, the physician's component for emergency services and inpatient hospital care, etc.) are located in the front of the book. Codes for anesthesia, surgery, radiology, pathology and laboratory, and miscellaneous medical services

Patient Education

Procedure and diagnosis coding is required for billing purposes and physician orders of extended services. The diagnosis code reflects detailed information about the illness or injury converted to numeric form. The procedure code reflects detailed information about the service provided utilizing levels of care. Patients may have questions concerning "all those numbers" and their meaning. The medical assistant can explain the codes used and that they are used for billing purposes.

Procedures and services are listed by name of service or procedure, anatomic site, condition or disease, synonym, eponym, or abbreviation. In order to code services correctly, locate the desired procedure in the index at the back of the CPT manual. Often a single code is given, although ranges of possible codes (joined with a hyphen) are presented and should be utilized, if necessary.

Modifiers

There are times when it is necessary to report a service not contained in the CPT manual. These procedures may be reported using the "unlisted procedure" code for that particular section, or by use of a modifier—a two-digit code preceded by a hyphen that clarifies the procedure. This is used in circumstances when the procedure code does not accurately describe the procedure. The two-digit modifier provides additional information about services provided to a patient. For example, the most common modifier is "50," which indicates the procedure was bilateral and done at the same time, such as bilateral myringotomies and tube insertion. The two-digit code for this procedure would be listed followed by a hyphen and the number 50. When using multiple modifiers always list the modifier -99 first. This indicates to the person checking the claim that multiple modifiers are being used (Figure 17-7).

Medical Coding

The medicine section of the CPT manual is organized according to body system, not disease. This section of the manual also includes codes for noninvasive procedures and treatment procedures. Included in this section are many diagnostic tests, such as an EKG, and many procedures (noninvasive) performed in a physician's office. If the procedure is invasive, meaning that it enters the skin (other than by injection) or a body cavity, it is found in the surgical section of the manual. Procedure 17-2 reviews examples for assigning CPT codes.

Symbols

Symbols are used in the CPT manual to distinguish changes or give instructions to be used when coding. These symbols add additional information or instructions for proper coding of certain procedures. It is imperative that the coder be familiar with the symbols and their meaning in order to accurately code procedures.

Insurance Fraud

Unfortunately, insurance fraud occurs on a regular basis. The Centers for Medicare and Medicaid Services Web site (http://www.cms.hhs.gov/providers/fraud/) has information to help you better understand insurance fraud. Even though this information comes strictly from the Centers for Medicare and Medicaid Services Web site, it can also apply to other insurance carriers.

Medicare Definition of Fraud

As a medical assistant, it is important to understand insurance fraud. Insurance fraud is often committed within the Medicare system. "Fraud" is an intentional representation that an individual knows to be false or does not believe to be true and makes, knowing that the representation could result in some unauthorized benefit to him or herself or some other person.

The most frequent kind of fraud arises from false statements or misrepresentations that claim to provide proof to entitlement or payment under the Medicare program. The violator may be a physician or other practitioner, a hospital or other institutional provider, a clinical laboratory or other supplier, an employee of any provider, a billing service, a beneficiary, a Medicare carrier employee, or any person in a position to file a claim for Medicare benefits. Under the broad definition of fraud are other violations, including the offering or acceptance of kickbacks and the routine waiver of co-payments.

Fraud schemes range from those perpetrated by individuals acting alone to broad-based activities by institutions or groups of individuals, sometimes employing sophisticated telemarketing and other promotional techniques to lure consumers into serving

TABLE 17-1	CPT Manual: Examples of Sections and Codes	
CPT Section	**Code**
Evaluation and Management	99200–99499
Anesthesia	00100–01999
Surgery	10000–69999
Radiology	70000–79999
Pathology and Laboratory	80000–89999
Medical Services	90700–99999

Symbols

▲   Revised Code

●   New Code

►◄   New or Revised Text

⊃   Reference to *CPT Assistant, CPT Changes Book*

✚   Add-on Code

⊘   Exemptions to Modifier 51

⊙   Conscious Sedation

Modifiers (See Appendix A for Definitions)

21   Prolonged Evaluation and Management Services

22   Unusual Procedural Services

23   Unusual Anesthesia

24   Unrelated Evaluation and Management Service by the Same Physician During a Postoperative Period

25   Significant, Separately Identifiable Evaluation and Management Service by the Same Physician on the Same Day of the Procedure or Other Service

26   Professional Component

32   Mandated Services

47   Anesthesia by Surgeon

50   Bilateral Procedure

51   Multiple Procedures

52   Reduced Services

53   Discontinued Procedure

54   Surgical Care Only

55   Postoperative Management Only

56   Preoperative Management Only

57   Decision for Surgery

58   Staged or Related Procedure or Service by the Same Physician During the Postoperative Period

59   Distinct Procedural Service

62   Two Surgeons

63   Procedure Performed on Infants

66   Surgical Team

76   Repeat Procedure by Same Physician

77   Repeat Procedure by Another Physician

78   Return to the Operating Room for a Related Procedure During the Postoperative Period

79   Unrelated Procedure or Service by the Same Physician During the Postoperative Period

80   Assistant Surgeon

81   Minimum Assistant Surgeon

82   Assistant Surgeon (when qualified resident surgeon not available)

90   Reference (Outside) Laboratory

91   Repeat Clinical Diagnostic Laboratory Test

99   Multiple Modifiers

Physical Status Modifiers

P1-A normal healthy patient

P2-A patient with mild systemic disease

P3-A patient with severe systemic disease

P4-A patient with severe systemic disease that is a constant threat to life

P5-A moribund patient who is not expected to survive without the operation

P6-A declared brain-dead patient whose organs are being removed for donor purposes

Modifiers Approved for Hospital Outpatient Use Level I (CPT)

25   Significant, Separately Identifiable Evaluation and Management Service by the Same Physician on the Same Day of the Procedure or Other Service

27   Multiple Outpatient Hospital E/M Encounters on the Same Date

50   Bilateral Procedure

52   Reduced Services

58   Staged or Related Procedure or Service by the Same Physician During the Postoperative Period

59   Distinct Procedural Service

73   Discontinued Out-Patient Procedure Prior to Anesthesia Administration

74   Discontinued Out-Patient Procedure After Anesthesia Administration

76   Repeat Procedure by Same Physician

77   Repeat Procedure by Another Physician

78   Return to the Operating Room for a Related Procedure During the Postoperative Period

79   Unrelated Procedure or Service by the Same Physician During the Postoperative Period

91   Repeat Clinical Diagnostic Laboratory Test

Level II (HCPCS/National)

LT   Left side (used to identify procedures performed on the left side of the body)

RT   Right side (used to identify procedures performed on the right side of the body)

E1   Upper left, eyelid

E2   Lower left, eyelid

E3   Upper right, eyelid

E4   Lower right, eyelid

FA   Left hand, thumb

F1   Left hand, second digit

F2   Left hand, third digit

F3   Left hand, fourth digit

F4   Left hand, fifth digit

F5   Right hand, thumb

F6   Right hand, second digit

F7   Right hand, third digit

F8   Right hand, fourth digit

F9   Right hand, fifth digit

LC   Left circumflex, coronary artery (Hospitals use with codes 92980-92984, 92995, 92996)

LD   Left anterior descending coronary artery (Hospitals use with codes 92980-92984, 92995, 92996)

RC   Right coronary artery (Hospitals use with codes 92980-92984, 92995, 92996)

QM   Ambulance service provided under arrangement by a provider of services

QN   Ambulance service furnished directly by a provider of services

TA   Left foot, great toe

T1   Left foot, second digit

T2   Left foot, third digit

T3   Left foot, fourth digit

T4   Left foot, fifth digit

T5   Right foot, great toe

T6   Right foot, second digit

T7   Right foot, third digit

T8   Right foot, fourth digit

T9   Right foot, fifth digit

FIGURE 17-7   Modifier page from the CPT. Printed with permission by the American Medical Association. Copyright © 2004.

PROCEDURE

Assigning a CPT Code

OBJECTIVE: Accurately assign a CPT code.

Equipment and Supplies

patient's medical record; computer; medical billing software; current CPT coding book; superbill with procedure marked

Method

1. Locate the completed procedure on the superbill.
2. If the only procedure done was a physician visit, locate CPT codes 99200–99499 in the front of the CPT coding book.
3. Determine by the patient's medical record whether this office visit was a first time visit or a follow-up visit.
4. Also determine by the patient's medical record whether this visit was done by the patient's attending physician, or whether it was done by a consulting physician.
5. Note where the visit took place (nursing home, hospital, emergency room, office, etc.).
6. After locating the place of service set of codes in the CPT book, locate the level of the visit within the place of service set of codes. It may be necessary to study the patient's personal, family, and social history, the physical examination, and determine which and how many tests were done in order to determine the correct level of service. This is one of the most important codes you can list because improper level of service billing can result in nonpayment of the bill, and can also result in very large monetary fines.
7. If there was a surgical procedure, these will be in the code section between 10000 and 69999 of the CPT book. For these codes, locate the surgical procedure and read the operative report. For some situations, the anesthetic for the surgery is included in the surgery code. In other cases, the anesthesia must be billed as a separate code. In addition, some surgical procedure groups are billed under one code, while others are billed as separate procedures. It will usually be necessary to read the operative report to determine which situation applies.
8. Some equipment used in surgery is billable under the 10000 to 69999 codes, while other equipment is billed separately.
9. Any radiological procedure is billed under the codes 70000 to 79999, including x-rays, diagnostic ultrasound, angiography, and computerized tomography.
10. Locate the procedure done in the section 70000 to 79999.
11. In the appropriate section, locate the part of the body to which the procedure was done.
12. Last, locate the correct procedure, being careful to note if the test was bilateral, unilateral, or if there were two different views done.
13. If a laboratory test was run, or if a specimen was sent to the laboratory for pathology inspection, the code will be under 80000 to 89999.
14. If the test was a laboratory test, it will be in the first part of this section. It is necessary to know what test was done, and whether the test is a "panel," which contains many tests within one ordered block, or if the test is organ-specific or disease-specific.
15. In addition, if the test was actually done by an outside laboratory, then the test itself cannot be billed. However, the cost of the venipuncture to obtain the specimen and the cost of transporting the specimen to the laboratory, if it was transported by the physician's staff, may be billed.
16. In some cases, some medicines can be billed to insurance. Some general rules apply to most billable medicines.
17. Usually billed medicines must be injected, not administered orally.
18. Many specialized procedures, such as ophthalmology services and pulmonary tests and services, can be billed under the CPT codes.
19. Always compare the final CPT codes with the ICD codes before finalizing the bill. There must be a logical "match." For example, if the patient was seen in the physician's office for removal of a foreign body in the ear, the visit can be billed, but the blood sugar done at the same time cannot be billed under a diagnosis of foreign body in the ear.

as the unwitting tools in the schemes. Seldom do perpetrators target only one insurer or either the public or private sector exclusively. Rather, most are defrauding several private and public sector victims, such as Medicare, simultaneously. According to a 1993 survey by the Health Insurance Association of America for private insurers' health care fraud investigations, overall health care fraud activity broke down as follows:

- 43%—Fraudulent diagnosis
- 34%—Billing for services not rendered
- 21%—Waiver of patient deductibles and co-payments
- 2%—Other

In Medicare, the most common forms of fraud include:

- Billing insurance companies for services not furnished
- Misrepresenting the diagnosis to justify payment
- Soliciting, offering, or receiving a kickback
- Billing for separate services that are usually bundled in a single procedure code
- Falsifying certificates of medical necessity, plans of treatment, and medical records to justify payment
- Billing for a service not furnished as billed; i.e., "upcoding"

Fraud Tips

The Centers for Medicare and Medicaid Services Web site also offers consumers and patients information to help them identify fraud. The medical assistant can also watch for the following items, whether the provider is telling the patient, or you are asked to relay this information to the patient:

- The test is free; he only needs your Medicare number for his records.
- Medicare wants you to have the item or service.
- They know how to get Medicare to pay for it.
- The more tests they provide, the cheaper they are.
- The equipment or service is free; it won't cost you anything.

Consumers should also be suspicious of medical offices or employers who do the following:

- Routinely waive co-payments without checking on ability to pay
- Advertise "free" consultations to Medicare beneficiaries

Professionalism

The medical record must reflect all services and care for which the insurance company is billed. If a provider is found to have billed for services not received, or if a provider is found to have billed for a more complicated or expensive service than was actually received, the penalty will be denial of the claim, or worse, monetary sanctions and even prison. If the medical assistant believes that such a bill is being submitted, he or she should discuss the situation with the physician in order to be assured that the care being delivered is, in fact, the service being billed.

- Claim they represent Medicare
- Use pressure or scare tactics to sell high priced medical services or diagnostic tests
- Bill Medicare for services the patient does not recall receiving
- Use telemarketing and door-to-door selling as marketing tools

Professionalism discusses the importance of reflecting correct billing practices in the medical record. Box 17-1 lists information on how to report suspected fraud.

Compliance Plan

Each medical office should have a compliance plan. A medical office without a compliance plan may be at risk for liability issues. It also demonstrates to the physician, fraud investigators, or insurance carriers that the medical office is attempting to locate and correct errors. Having a compliance plan gives the staff members of the medical office a process of locating, correcting, and preventing practices that are illegal. Health and Human Services Office of Inspector General provides compliance guidance for fraud prevention and detection. The following are basic components for an effective compliance plan:

- Conducting periodic audits of billing and coding practices
- Developing written standards and procedures for compliance
- Training and educating staff members on procedures

BOX 17-1
How to Report Suspected Fraud

Before you get in touch with your state Medicaid agency, contact or call the National Fraud Hotline and be ready to provide as much information as possible, including:

- The name of the Medicaid client
- The client's Medicaid card number
- The name of the doctor, hospital, or other health care provider
- The date of service
- The amount of money that Medicaid approved and may have paid
- A description of the acts that you suspect involve fraud or abuse

Who to Contact

Contact Your State Agency Directly—Medicaid is a joint Federal and State-funded program. Although the Federal Government requires that certain persons be eligible for Medicaid benefits and sets standards for quality of care, the States carry out most of the day-to-day business of Medicaid. If you suspect that fraud is being committed against Medicaid, first get in touch with the Program Integrity contact at your State Medicaid Agency. A list of *State Medicaid Contacts* has the names of the Program Integrity contact that you should use to report suspected fraud, whether it involves a person, a company, or an agency.

Call the OIG National Fraud Hotline—A second way to report suspected fraud in Medicaid is to call the Office of Inspector General's (OIG) *National Fraud Hotline* **1-800-HHS-TIPS (1-800-447-8477)**. This hotline handles calls about both Medicaid and Medicare, but it is not as direct as calling your state contact.

- Investigating violations and disclosing incidents to appropriate government agencies
- Discussing in staff meetings how to avoid erroneous or fraudulent conduct

As a medical assistant, it is important to research and understand practice standards so that the medical office is in compliance with various regulations.

Legal and Ethical Issues

Federal regulations on coding are specific and require full compliance. Coding of procedures and diagnoses must be supported by the documentation in the patient record. Providers as well as medical staff may be sanctioned with fines or prison terms if improper coding is discovered to increase reimbursement.

Coding Compliance

Reasonability of accurate documentation, completion of health insurance claim forms, and regulation compliance falls ultimately on the physician. It is the medical assistant's responsibility to make certain these responsibilities are followed (Legal and Ethical Issues).

Code Linkage

When the medical assistant is completing the health insurance claim form, it is critical for the diagnosis to be related to the procedure. An example of code linkage would be a diagnosis of diabetes mellitus and a glucose tolerance test. However, a diagnosis of hypertension and a procedure to remove five skin tags cannot be linked in a health insurance claim form because there is no connection between the patient's diagnosis and the procedure the physician performed. Coding inaccuracies such as this can result in minor to severe penalties.

SUMMARY

Most patients coming into the medical office have some form of health care insurance. The medical assistant should have a general overview of the coding process, using the procedure coding process (CPT codes) and diagnostic coding (ICD-9-CM) in order to be able to assist the medical coder if necessary.

Chapter Review

COMPETENCY REVIEW

1. Define and spell the terms to learn for this chapter.
2. Describe what steps you would take to determine if a patient has insurance coverage.
3. What code book is used to code a diagnosis?
4. What code book is used to code an office visit and procedure?
5. Explain the difference between a primary and secondary diagnosis, using the example of stroke and hypertension.

PREPARING FOR THE CERTIFICATION EXAM

1. Which describes transforming verbal descriptions into numerical designations?
   A. grouping
   B. coding
   C. classifying
   D. modifying
   E. rider

2. In ICD-9-CM coding conventions, E codes
   A. stand alone
   B. are required for all diagnoses
   C. give external causes or factors for illness or injury
   D. should never be used with V codes
   E. are the same as CPT codes

3. CPT stands for
   A. current physician's terminology
   B. current procedure terminology
   C. current procedural terminology
   D. current procedural term
   E. current procedural timetable

4. In CPT coding conventions, modifiers are used to
   A. explain unusual circumstances
   B. list a patient's treatment options
   C. frustrate a medical assistant
   D. communicate with the insurance company via electronic billing
   E. make the coding statement grammatically correct

5. The CMS-1500 claim form
   A. is accepted by most insurance companies in the United States
   B. must be filled out by the patient
   C. must be filled out by the provider
   D. is accepted as a standard submission (claim) form by most carriers
   E. is never used

continued on next page

6. In CPT coding conventions,
   A. both inpatient and outpatient visits use the same code
   B. inpatient visit codes are different from outpatient visit codes
   C. a complicated system is used to determine whether services were rendered on an inpatient or outpatient basis
   D. a call to the insurance company is required to determine which code to use
   E. all codes are the same as ICD-9-CM

7. ICD-9-CM codes
   A. may require a fifth digit for detail
   B. never require a fifth digit for detail
   C. always require a V code to support the diagnosis
   D. may be coded directly from Volume II
   E. should always be initialed by the physician

8. Which of the following is NOT true of diagnoses coding?
   A. the medical assistant needs to understand the ICD-9-CM
   B. diagnosis are given in three, four, or five digits
   C. always code to the highest level of specificity
   D. to code properly, start with Volume II
   E. Volume II is the numeric index

9. Which of the following is NOT true of CPT coding?
   A. the CPT coding book is updated yearly
   B. the CPT coding book is organized numerically
   C. CPT codes can be obtained from outdated CPT coding books
   D. the CPT coding book is organized alphanumerically
   E. E/M codes are located in the front of the CPT coding book

10. Electronic claim submission
    A. is difficult and costly
    B. is mandated by HIPAA for most medical providers
    C. is only done on rare occasions in most medical practices
    D. increases the time it takes for an insurance carrier to pay a claim
    E. does not require diagnosis codes

CRITICAL THINKING

1. What would the CPT code be for an audiogram?
2. How can a medical assistant made sure a diagnosis code is correct on the CMS-1500 before submitting it to the insurance carrier?
3. What is the diagnosis code for chronic otitis media?

ON THE JOB

Lisa Medina, certified medical coding specialist, processes insurance claims for a large internal medicine practice. You have recently been hired as Lisa's assistant and she has asked you to verify the accuracy of a group of claim forms. As you review the forms, you notice that one of the doctors regularly checks the superbill used in the office at one evaluation/management code level higher than the actual level of service provided.

1. Name some of the options that are possible for handling this situation.
2. Tell which option you would select.
3. Give three reasons for your selection of this particular option.
4. Whose advice might you seek before acting on your choice?

INTERNET ACTIVITY

There are many places to purchase ICD-9-CM and CPT coding books. Search the Internet to find the cost of the ICD-9-CM and CPT coding books and coding software. What month are the new editions of the ICD-9-CM and CPT coding books available?

MediaLink More on medical coding, including interactive resources, can be found on the Student CD-ROM accompanying this textbook.

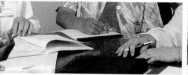

Medical Assistant Role Delineation Chart

HIGHLIGHT indicates material covered in this chapter.

ADMINISTRATIVE

Administrative Procedures

- Perform basic administrative medical assisting functions
- Schedule, coordinate and monitor appointments
- Schedule inpatient/outpatient admissions and procedures
- Understand and apply third-party guidelines
- Obtain reimbursement through accurate claims submission
- Monitor third-party reimbursement
- Understand and adhere to managed care policies and procedures
- *Negotiate managed care contracts*

Practice Finances

- Perform procedural and diagnostic coding
- Apply bookkeeping principles

- Manage accounts receivable
- *Manage accounts payable*
- *Process payroll*
- *Document and maintain accounting and banking records*
- *Develop and maintain fee schedules*
- *Manage renewals of business and professional insurance policies*
- *Manage personnel benefits and maintain records*
- *Perform marketing, financial, and strategic planning*

CLINICAL

Fundamental Principles

- Apply principles of aseptic technique and infection control
- Comply with quality assurance practices
- Screen and follow up patient test results

Diagnostic Orders

- Collect and process specimens
- Perform diagnostic tests

Patient Care

- Adhere to established patient screening procedures
- Obtain patient history and vital signs
- Prepare and maintain examination and treatment areas
- Prepare patient for examinations, procedures and treatments

- Assist with examinations, procedures and treatments
- Prepare and administer medications and immunizations
- Maintain medication and immunization records
- Recognize and respond to emergencies
- Coordinate patient care information with other health care providers
- Initiate IV and administer IV medications with appropriate training and as permitted by state law

GENERAL

Professionalism

- Display a professional manner and image
- Demonstrate initiative and responsibility
- Work as a member of the health care team
- Prioritize and perform multiple tasks
- Adapt to change
- Promote the CMA credential
- Enhance skills through continuing education
- Treat all patients with compassion and empathy
- Promote the practice through positive public relations

Communication Skills

- Recognize and respect cultural diversity
- Adapt communications to individual's ability to understand
- Use professional telephone technique

- Recognize and respond effectively to verbal, nonverbal, and written communications
- Use medical terminology appropriately
- Utilize electronic technology to receive, organize, prioritize and transmit information
- Serve as liaison

Legal Concepts

- Perform within legal and ethical boundaries
- Prepare and maintain medical records
- Document accurately
- Follow employer's established policies dealing with the health care contract
- Implement and maintain federal and state health care legislation and regulations
- Comply with established risk management and safety procedures
- Recognize professional credentialing criteria
- *Develop and maintain personnel, policy and procedure manuals*

Instruction

- Instruct individuals according to their needs
- Explain office policies and procedures
- Teach methods of health promotion and disease prevention
- Locate community resources and disseminate information
- *Develop educational materials*
- *Conduct continuing education activities*

Operational Functions

- Perform inventory of supplies and equipment
- Perform routine maintenance of administrative and clinical equipment
- Apply computer techniques to support office operations
- *Perform personnel management functions*
- *Negotiate leases and prices for equipment and supply contracts*

■ *Denotes advanced skills.*

SOURCE: Reprinted by permission of the American Association of Medical Assistants from the AAMA Role Delineation Study: Occupational Analysis of the Medical Assisting Profession.

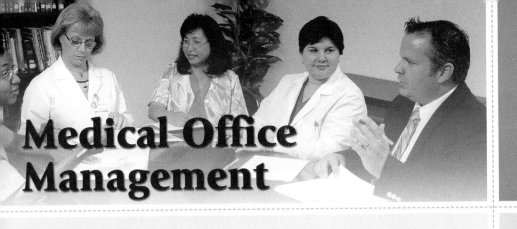

Medical Office Management

chapter 18

Learning Objectives

After reading this chapter, you should be able to:

- Define and spell the terms to learn for this chapter.
- Define the systems approach to management.
- List and discuss the personnel management duties as they relate to the medical office.
- Discuss the elements of monthly planning including holding staff meetings.
- Describe time management principles and how a TO DO list would enhance office organization.

- Differentiate between the employee policy manual and the office procedures manual.
- Describe ten responsibilities in assisting the physician to set up a medical meeting.
- Discuss how to perform basic library research to assist the physician in a medical paper development.
- List five items that belong in a patient information booklet.

Terms to Learn

colleague	grievance	seniority
discriminatory	probationary	solvent

Case Study

MARSHA BROWN IS AN OFFICE MANAGER at the Main Street Clinic. The clinic's business has been growing steadily, and the office is in need of a new medical assistant. Marsha decided to put an advertisement in the local newspaper and received many resumes in response to the ad. She took a couple of days to sort through the resumes, removing all that did not have appropriate backgrounds for the position. On Monday, she called several individuals who had the best resumes and set up interviews for the week.

Her first interview went very well, but it was difficult to read the application form that was completed. The second applicant was wearing a tongue ring during the interview, and at times, it was very difficult to understand her speech. The third applicant had the least experience, but looked very professional, wrote neatly, and spoke well. The next week, Marsha called the third applicant and offered her the position.

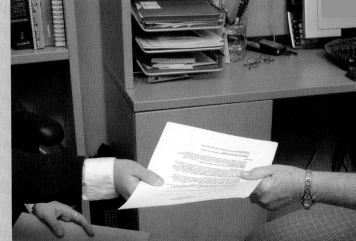

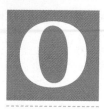

ffice management requires special administrative and people skills. Office management cannot be discussed without discussing time management. Careful planning of activities, delegation of tasks, and effective use of all personnel involve careful attention to how time is managed. Several documents are important for a smooth running medical office. These include the personnel policy manual, a procedures manual, and patient information booklets.

Systems Approach to Office Management

Current management philosophy recommends a systematic approach when managing a medical office. Under this approach, the functions of an office are categorized into systems that must function simultaneously and be integrated into a whole system, the medical office. For example, the administrative component of a medical office can be divided into the following systems:

- Personnel management
- Financial management (including banking, billing, collections, and insurance)
- Scheduling
- Facility and equipment management (including computers)
- Communications (written and oral including patient education)
- Legal concepts

The clinical component of managing an office can be considered a system by itself. Brief descriptions of the various systems that form the medical practice follow.

Personnel Management Responsibilities

Personnel management duties include recruitment and selection, probation, performance and salary review, discipline, and maintenance of employee records.

The recruitment and selection process is used when a medical practice needs to replace a staff member who has left or when more staff is needed for an expanding practice. All new employees are entitled to an orientation to their new position and duties. Large offices and clinics often have formal orientation training sessions that employees attend before beginning their day-to-day assignments.

Personnel management usually requires an annual salary review of each employee at which time, if the employee's performance has been acceptable, a merit raise in salary is granted. However, there will be times when it is necessary to discipline an employee during these reviews. These topics will be discussed in greater detail further in the chapter.

Employee Records

There are records that are required by law to be maintained for every employee. These include the following payroll records.

- Social Security number of the employee
- Number of exemptions claimed by the employee (W-4 form)
- Gross salary amount (salary before taxes are removed)
- Deductions for Social Security taxes, federal, state, and city withholding taxes, state disability tax, and state unemployment tax, if applicable.

Payroll is discussed further in Chapter 14.

Financial Management

Financial management includes banking, billing, collections, and insurance collections. This critical area is responsible for generating the income necessary to keep the practice solvent or capable of paying its bills and salaries. Fees, billings, collections, and credit are discussed in Chapter 13. Financial management, including employee record keeping, is discussed in Chapter 14.

Scheduling

The scheduling process involves using a systematic method for patient appointments. This is discussed in Chapter 8. Scheduling also includes managing staff work hours and vacation periods.

Facility and Equipment Management

Facility and equipment management includes facility layout and planning, inventory, maintaining safety and OSHA standards, and equipment replacement. This is discussed in Chapter 5. Computer use in the medical office is presented in Chapter 11.

Clinical Office Management

Apart from the administrative aspects of medical office management, there is also the clinical aspect. Managing the clinical aspect of a medical office requires a wide variety of duties, including the training of any new clinical personnel, keeping track of medical supplies and purchasing supplies when the stock is low, and making sure that the physician's requests are met and that proper procedures are followed. It is often within the clinical office duties that the office manager will have to handle safety issues and OSHA regulations. Because of the many duties required in managing the clinical aspect of the office, it is not uncommon to find that an office has a separate supervisor who will take on those duties to reduce the workload of the general office manager.

Communication

Written communication skills are presented in Chapter 4, oral communication, including verbal and nonverbal, in Chapter 10, and patient education in Volume III, Chapter 50.

Legal Concepts

Physicians have their own personal attorney to assist with handling legal documents and issues. However, medical assistants must have an understanding of legal terminology. Legal and ethical issues are discussed fully in Chapter 3.

The Office Manager

The office manager acts as a coordinator for the business activities conducted in the office. Each office varies somewhat; however, the general duties include:

- Acting as liaison between staff and physician/employer.
- Conducting performance and salary reviews.
- Delegating responsibilities to staff.
- Developing and training staff.
- Improving office efficiency.
- Maintaining office procedure manual.
- Planning and conducting staff meetings.
- Preparing patient education materials.
- Providing guidelines for patient education.
- Recruiting, hiring, and firing.
- Supervising cash, banking, and payroll operations.
- Supervising employees on a day-to-day basis.

- Supervising the purchase and storage of equipment and supplies.
- Training new personnel.

Along with knowledge of the clinical skills needed to run an efficient medical office, an office manager needs effective administrative and people skills. Medical assistants who have demonstrated these skills may seek to be promoted into this position. Other qualities or skills observed in good managers are:

- Ability to enforce policy, when necessary
- Ability to organize
- Ability to resolve conflicts
- Creativity
- Diplomacy
- Excellent judgment
- Flexibility
- Leadership/take charge initiative
- Objectivity
- Sense of fairness
- Willingness to continue to learn

The office manager's time is generally spent on administrative and employee issues. The employees, on the other hand, spend most of their time working with patients. A good office manager does not strive to become "the boss" but, rather, to establish and implement a team approach to management by including all staff in the decision-making process. Ultimately, the manager must make the final decision in conjunction with the physician/employer, but compliance with decisions is much greater when employees have had the opportunity to participate. Table 18-1 describes responsibilities

TABLE 18-1 Manager's Responsibilities to Employee and Physician/Employer

Employee	Physician/Employer
Interview	Increase efficiency of office.
Hire/terminate	Meet with physician to discuss problems/plans.
Orientate/train	Manage calendar for physician.
Arrange work schedules	Assist with meetings.
Arrange vacation coverage	Update physician on insurance changes related to Medicare fee schedules.
Conduct performance evaluations	Order CPT and ICD code books and current pharmacology books annually.
Consult with physician regarding salary increases	Renew insurance policies and pay premiums.

Professionalism

the office manager has to the employees and to the physician. Professionalism discusses more on being an office manager.

Many office managers are promoted based on seniority—a status gained by being the individual who has worked for the physician the longest. This is not always a wise practice since not everyone is a skilled manager. When no internal candidate is available with the necessary skills or interest for the office manager position, then the physician/employer will have to seek an outside candidate. This is usually handled by placing an advertisement in the medical help wanted sections of the local newspaper. In some cases, the physicians' colleagues (fellow members of the profession) will recommend a qualified candidate for the position.

Monthly Planning

The office manager may wish to develop a system in which the entire month is laid out on a calendar. All physicians' conferences, staff meetings, vacations, accountant meetings, and other vendor visits should be noted. One of the office manager's tasks will be to approve and decline vacation requests from staff members. It is important to list staff vacations on a

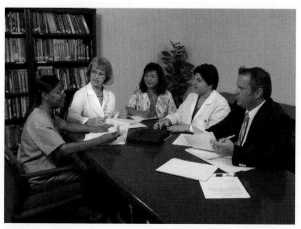

FIGURE 18-1 Regular staff meetings will help the efficiency of the medical office staff.

calendar because it helps to prevent overlapping of vacations, which can leave an office short-staffed. This calendar should be placed in an accessible location. It may be helpful to purchase an erasable-style wall calendar so that corrections and changes can be made easily.

The manager will create and update the physician's own calendar. It is not necessary to include staff vacations on the physician's calendar. However, the office manager's own vacation schedule and days off should be included in the physician's calendar.

Many physicians carry a personal pocket or electronic calendar in which they enter all patient hospital visits and meetings. It is wise to compare the office calendar with the physician's calendar on a periodic basis so that the office's master calendar can be updated.

Staff Meetings

Lack of communication between the staff and management is a common complaint in a medical office. Staff members wish to have direct communication with the physician, but this is often not possible in a large practice. The office manager can help to resolve this problem by requesting the physician(s) to attend all or part of the regularly scheduled staff meetings, if this is not already being done. Many of the best ideas for office improvement are a result of suggestions made at staff meetings (Figure 18-1).

Staff meetings should be held on a regular basis. If it is necessary to hold weekly meetings because of the nature of the practice, then the physician(s) should be invited monthly to accommodate his or her busy schedule.

Meetings may need to be scheduled during a time period in which the staff's hours overlap, either due to shift changes or staggered hours. For instance, if the practice is open from 9:00 A.M. to 9:00 P.M. on Thursdays, the meetings could be scheduled for 4:30 P.M. or 5:00 P.M. when all staff would be present. Generally, staff members are compensated when they arrive before or remain after working hours to attend staff meetings.

The office manager usually conducts staff meetings and facilitates team interaction. The office manager determines the time and date for the meeting, and also prepares the agenda, frequently with input from the physician and other staff. The key to a good meeting is a concise agenda that identifies items for discussion, such as staff responsibilities, and limits the time allotted. Focusing staff meetings and discussions in this way limits the amount of time wasted. Generally, minutes are recorded for future reference and distributed for review prior to the next meeting. See Box 18-1 for an example of an office staff meeting agenda. Procedure 18-1 shows how to prepare and hold a staff meeting.

Motivating Employees

Motivating employees is vital to maintaining a positive working environment and an efficiently run medical office. Respect, ownership of personal space or environment, a sense of affiliation with the practice, fair compensation, acknowledgement, recognition, emotional rewards, honesty, visibility at the top, empathy, trust, safety, and equal treatment of all staff are a few items that employees expect from management.

Respect from their management is a basic need of all employees. As their manager, greet them with a pleasant manner and always acknowledge their hard work. Listen to them when they need to talk and take their suggestions into consideration. Satisfied employees are one of the best resources that the office manager has in running an efficient medical office.

In the medical office, it is often that many people share one space. If possible, provide some personal space for each employee. This would preferably be a desk, but it may just be a small table or a locker located somewhere in the office. Allow employees to place pictures in the area in which they work most often. This makes the employee feel settled, and in turn, tends to produce a greater level of productivity.

Creating a sense of affiliation to the medical office is often achieveable by making simple considerations. Sharing in the highlights of staff member's lives, such as throwing a small birthday celebration or recognizing a special event (marriage or birth of a child),

BOX 18-1

Staff Meeting Agenda

Windy City Clinic
Staff Meeting Agenda
Date: December 19, 20XX
Time: 4:30–5:30 P.M.
Place: Staff Conference Room

Time	Agenda	Person Responsible
4:30	Introduction of new staff	M. King/ Office Manager
	Review of last meeting's minutes	
4:35	Discussion of new policies	
4:45	Problems with insurance	L. Turner/Insurance Coding Clerk
4:55	OSHA protocol for needlesticks	K. Wall/Lab Tech
5:05	Vacation schedules	M. King
5:10	New office location	Dr. Williams
5:20	New business meeting adjourned	Mary King

18-1 PROCEDURE

Staff Meeting Procedures

OBJECTIVE: Explain and present the necessary steps to preparing and running a staff meeting.

Equipment and Supplies
agenda items received from staff; meeting agenda; means of keeping time (watch, clock, stopwatch, etc.); room for the meeting; any audio/visual equipment that may be needed

Method
1. One week before the meeting, request agenda items from the staff.
2. Before the meeting, create a meeting agenda with all topics that need to be discussed. On the agenda include the date, time, and place of the meeting. List who will be running (facilitating) the meeting. This is most often the office manager. Assign a length of time to each topic and who will be responsible for that topic.
3. On the day of the meeting, start the meeting on time.
4. Begin by briefly covering the last meeting.
5. Try to keep each topic to its allowed amount of time.
6. Allow for time at the end of the meeting to have open discussion of any new business.
7. Adjourn the meeting. Try to stay on schedule as much as possible.
8. After the meeting, the minutes of the meeting should be typed and distributed to all involved.

help employees feel part of the office community or "family." Bringing the staff together outside of the office with special events, such as a company picnic, can also increase the sense of affiliation.

Generally, employees will want to feel that they are being compensated sufficiently for the amount of work they produce. If an employee feels that he or she is doing the quality and quantity of work that is required and that it is not reflected in his or her pay, the employee will most likely seek a position elsewhere. As an office manager, one of your responsibilities will be to make sure that your staff is being appropriately compensated.

There are other awards beyond pay. Employees need encouragement and recognition. Present them with items that praise their work, such as awards for meeting or exceeding set goals.

Communication is key to managing an efficient office and maintaining a cohesive work atmosphere. Employees like honest, straight talk from their employers. It is important to realize that in an office, secrets breed distrust. It is always best for employees to receive news from their manager rather than through rumors. Keep your staff informed of the good and the bad issues affecting the practice.

It is essential as the manager to be available to the employees. Being visible to your employees creates a positive rapport and any problems that may arise can often be dealt with swiftly and efficiently. Do not hide in the manager's office, staying busy with business affairs.

An office manager can often gain a great deal of loyalty from his or her employees through empathy. Though the office manager is a figure of authority to the employee, honest communication and a sincere regard for the employee's well being goes a long way in creating a comfortable and productive work place.

Leadership Styles

The ability to make appropriate calls of judgment, the willingness to learn new ideas, staying calm during stressful situations, and good listening skills are all attributes of good leaders. As an office manager, you will be the team leader of the medical office. Think back to good managers that you have had in the past. What attributes made them good managers? Was it their knowledge, or was it that they were easy to approach? If you think back, you may find traits in former managers that you can incorporate to create your version of an office manager.

The four standard types of leaders are authoritarian, democratic, permissive, and bureaucratic. Each type of leader has different distinctions and motivators. Knowledge of different management styles may help you fine-tune your own management style and give you ideas on how to benefit your employees.

Authoritarian leaders tend to be very direct. They will make most of their decisions on their own without the input of others. They will probably not be team players so much as solid leaders. Authoritarian leaders tend to want respect and obedience from their staff members and may even use fear to achieve staff obedience. The need for power and absolute authority often drives this type of leader. Authoritarian leaders work best in times of great stress and crisis situations.

A democratic leader will concentrate more on the relations between staff members and emphasize teamwork within the office. He or she tends to be motivated from within to provide a comfortable work environment for all. With a leader of this style, you will often find very open communication. Democratic leaders are more receptive to new ideas from staff members, which helps create an atmosphere of cooperation among the staff, instituting greater participation in the decision-making process. This style of leadership often leads to a contented staff.

Permissive leaders are very open with the staff. They are not strict with rules and policies. Like the democratic leader, the permissive leader is self-motivated. In many situations, he or she will let the staff make their own decisions and will not interfere with staff processes. However, medical offices need to keep an ordered environment and at times, permissive leadership can lead to disorganization and even hazardous conditions.

Bureaucratic leaders are very strong at enforcing rules. Their motivation comes from external means. They prefer to rely on established management methods for office matters. Bureaucratic leaders tend to be rigid and set in their ways. There is a level of insecurity in bureaucratic leaders because they do not trust themselves in making decisions that will affect the office. The staff often will find the bureaucratic leader to be very distant and formal.

Each type of leadership style has its benefits and its downfalls. The best leaders will use a combination of styles, depending upon the situations that they must face.

For any manager to do a proper job, he or she must establish a level of power to enact and enforce the rules necessary to run an efficient medical office. There are several different types of authoritative power that a manager may establish. One type uses the power of rewards. This type of power incorporates rewards or some type of enticement in exchange for better job performance and teamwork. When managers use rewards to exact better productivity from their employees, they are exercising a form of power over their employees. The degree to which this works will depend on the level of reward that the employee receives.

There are other types of power used by individuals in authoritative positions. Legitimate power is given to people based upon their title. The president of a company will hold legitimate power, the power of the title of president. Expert power is given to those who have a great deal of knowledge. This is earned through experience and education. Referent power is given out of high regard and respect. It comes with a person's likeability and even his or her success in the field. Informative power is a type of power that most individuals have experienced at some point in their lives. It is the power wielded by those with information that others want or need. Connective power—the idea that if you know the right people you can get what you need—is one reason to network at local organizations. As a student, it is never too early to start making connections.

With all power comes the ability to abuse or overuse it. The effects of overuse of power will depend on the type of power wielded by the individual. With reward power, one downfall is that the employees can become reliant upon rewards. Once this happens, the power becomes coercive, which is a negative power because it uses fear to motivate employees. The employee may be afraid of punishment or the manager may withhold certain rewards to gain cooperation. Also there is the possibility of jealousy among the employees; they may have the perception that someone is getting more attention or rewards than someone else. With coercive power, a misuse can lead to distrust and fear of the manager and of other employees. Misused legitimate power leads to fear of the person with the title or even the title itself. In the misuse of informative power, you will often see avoidance, a sense of unfairness, and a bit of hostility. Expert, referent, and connective powers all tend to lead to the same effects when misused. There is a perceived level of manipulation and intrusion among those affected.

Creating a Team Atmosphere

For a medical office to run at its most efficient level, the staff must work as a team. This can be difficult to manage on the part of the office manager. The office manager is in charge of strengthening and enhancing the team atmosphere. The following are some factors that must come together to create a successful office team:

- Size—the smaller a team, the better it will work together.
- Team personalities—it is inadvisable to put together a team made of the same personalities.

- Responsible team members—all members of the team must be accountable for their actions.
- Unified team approach—team members must come together to face the project with the same purpose and goals.

Every team must have its leader. It is important that the office manager realize that he or she is the team leader. Managers should treat all members of a team equally. Showing favoritism to one or two employees can easily break down the team atmosphere that has been created.

Managers also need to show that they are an integral part of the team. It will make employees more confident and content in their jobs to know that their manager is willing to help out with employee duties when assistance is needed.

In some medical offices, it may also be necessary to have several levels of leaders in the office team. There may be a leader of the front desk part of the team and a leader of the clinical part of the team. All leaders within the team must be highly organized and have a good deal of energy to help to keep the team unified and productive.

Team Size

The size of a group can greatly affect the dynamics of how it will work. Small groups often will be very intimate. Close bonds may form, but because of the small group dynamics, they also tend to be very unstable. However, as groups grow larger, they tend to become more stable, but at a loss of group intimacy. This information is important to know when assembling a team. You will find that the smaller a group, the more relaxed the atmosphere will be, whereas a larger group will have a more rigid structure. Similar to group size and structure, the smaller the office, the easier going it may be. Larger multi-physician offices tend to be much more formal and systematic.

Team Personality and Skills

Creating a team atmosphere will begin as early as the hiring process. Staff who feel they have no say in the people being hired tend to have a harder time adjusting to the presence of a new staff member. One way to minimize staff frictions would be to allow some staff members to help in the hiring process. It is important that the staff understand what you, as the office manager, are looking for in potential employees. They may be able to provide same insight into the personality of the job candidate, which would be helpful in maintaining a cohesive team atmosphere. Ultimately, the office manager and physician will have the final say in the hiring of the candidate, but this process lets the staff know that their opinion also matters.

It takes the right mix of people to create a strong team. It is never a good idea to fill an office with

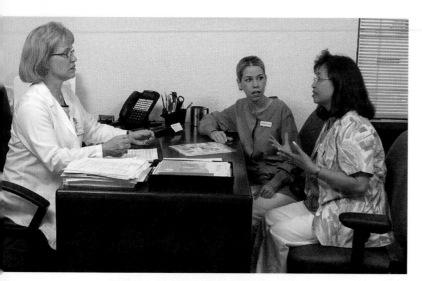

FIGURE 18-2 A medical office requires teamwork.

people who are of similar personality types and leadership styles. Often, similar weaknesses will manifest in the day-to-day business of the office, which defeats the goal of efficiency and teamwork. A manager should look for staff members who complement each other's talents and traits. For example, one member of the staff who is really good with computers but is weak in filing will be complemented by a staff member who is weak in computers but an excellent filer. Creating this mix will give you the foundation for a strong team (Figure 18-2).

You will find that within any given team, the different team members will take on various roles. These roles can be of a task-oriented nature, or they may be more nurturing. Some of the task-oriented roles include the information seeker, the information giver, the coordinator, the energizer, the evaluator/critic, and the recorder. These roles all focus on the goal that the team is working towards. The nurturing roles may include the encourager, the harmonizer, the compromiser, and the follower. A team member may take on one or many roles within the team.

Team Accountability

As a team, members must hold each other accountable for their actions. If something goes wrong, the team must come together to locate and fix the problem. This means that the team should not attack or try to blame a problem on any one member, but that they must find where, as a team, they lost track and how they can prevent a similar problem from reccuring.

Team Purpose and Goals

The team must find a way to work together. Ensuring that you have the correct personalities and talents matched up is a good start. Encourage team members to concentrate on a single goal. Successful teams work with the same purpose in mind and approach a problem or task using similar means. That way there is little conflict among the team as they work out problems that may get in the way of achieving their goal.

Any team will have some weaknesses. It is important for the office manager to monitor the progress of the team. You may find in a medical office that has employees who are strictly clinical and employees who are strictly clerical, that instead of working as one whole team, the tendency for these groups to divide themselves into two separate teams. The employees may feel comfortable with this, but this type of division usually puts strains on running the practice. As the office manager, you will need to prevent this from happening. When possible, it is a good idea to have staff members who are strictly front office employees switch places occasionally with those who are only accustomed to back office duties. This will help them to reexperience the duties and responsibilities of the office as a whole. When other options aren't working toward the goal of a cohesive team, the manager may wish to use team-building exercises. There are many companies that specialize in helping office managers pull their team together.

Hiring Procedures: Selecting the Right Staff Members

There will be times when the office manager will need to hire new staff. It may be that someone has left the office or that a new position has been created. Recruitment can begin in-house, which means that the job vacancy is posted within the medical office before the position is advertised elsewhere. An existing employee may apply for the vacant positions. If there are no interested or qualified internal candidates, several methods may be used to seek applicants.

Advertising the Position

There are many ways of advertising for open positions. These include placement of newspaper and trade journal ads, professional organizations, the Internet, formal training programs, and employment agencies, which charge a fee to be paid by the employer to the agency if an agency's candidate is hired. Local training programs in colleges are also excellent resources.

In most cases, the newspaper will often be the best way to reach your local population. However, Internet resources are becoming increasingly popular. There are many online providers that offer options for job advertisements. Remember to describe the position accurately. This will prevent the office from receiving too many resumes that do not pertain to the advertised position. If you are too general in your description, you may receive an excess of applicants. However, being too specific can cause the opposite problem: you may receive very few individuals applying for the position.

Once you have advertised and received resumes, then you will begin the task of sorting through the applicants' resumes. Each office manager has his or her own way of doing this, but some of the most commonly used sorting methods include first removing any resumes that have obvious errors, such as poor grammar and spelling errors. Next, many office managers will remove all resumes that do not show the appropriate background for the position that has been advertised. Once those resumes have been weeded out, office managers are usually left with the candidates that they believe show the most promise for the position. At this point, the interview process begins.

The Interview

Before each interview, it is good practice to have all applicants fill out a job application form (Figure 18-3). You may choose to send this to the applicant by mail and have them bring it with them to the interview. However, there are benefits to having the applicant fill out the form at the time of the interview. You will be able to see how the applicant handles filling out forms under a time constraint. You will also get a visual of the applicant's handwriting. It is important to see whether or not they have legible handwriting since most of these potential employee's will be writing directly into charts and must have legible handwriting. The last thing that you will learn from this process is how adept they are at completing a requested task. Do they take shortcuts, or do they complete every line? This can be an indication of how they handle on-the-spot tasks that may need to be resolved quickly and efficiently.

While interviewing, it is important to remember what you can and cannot ask an applicant. When interviewing, remember to assess important aspects of the applicant. How is he or she dressed? Does he or she reflect a professional appearance? Is the resume neatly prepared? This will give you insight into the type of employee

the applicant will make and whether he or she will fit into your current team. You will need to keep in mind the fair-employment practice (FEP) laws that affect hiring. Title VII of the Civil Rights Act of 1964, later amended as the Equal Employment Opportunity Act of 1972 (and further amended in 1990), prohibits asking applicants questions about their race, color, sex, religion, and national origin both during the interview and on the application. For example, asking a female applicant questions such as, "Did you have difficulty finding a baby-sitter today?" or "Do you plan to have children?" is considered discriminatory or prejudicial treatment and is therefore against the law.

Learning important information about applicants is key to making sure that they would be a good fit for your practice. You may want to ask them about past office experience, and want to know what types of physicians the applicant has worked with before.

EMPLOYMENT APPLICATION FORM

Directions: Answer all questions using black ink (print).

PERSONAL NAME

(LAST)	(FIRST)	(MI)
ADDRESS-STREET	CITY	STATE ZIP

PHONE NUMBER: SOCIAL SECURITY NUMBER:

POSITION DESIRED:

EXPECTED SALARY OR HOURLY WAGE:

EDUCATION

NAME OF SCHOOL	ADDRESS	DATE(S)	DEGREE/CERTIFICATE
HIGH SCHOOL			
VOCATIONAL/TECHNICAL			
COLLEGE			
OTHER			

WORK EXPERIENCE – Give present position (or last position held first).

JOB TITLE:	EMPLOYER	ADDRESS	DATES
DUTIES PERFORMED:			
JOB TITLE:	EMPLOYER	ADDRESS	DATES
DUTIES PERFORMED:			
JOB TITLE:	EMPLOYER	ADDRESS	DATES
DUTIES PERFORMED:			

REFERENCES – List three persons (other than relatives) who have known you for at least 2 years

NAME/TITLE	ADDRESS	TELEPHONE NUMBER

APPLICANT'S SIGNATURE _____

Date

FIGURE 18-3 A standard employment application form may be used.

Another good idea is to test applicants' ability to think on their feet. It has been an increasing practice to give applicants off-the-cuff questions to see how they respond. You are not looking for a correct answer, but only wish to see how they reason through the question. Do they give up and guess, or do they try to make a logical guess by thinking through the possibilities? Many managers will also give applicants situational questions. You may wish to ask how they would handle a patient that is upset about a test result.

As discussed in team building, it is sometimes a good idea to allow certain staff members to ask questions of the applicant. Again, staff members can give input whether or not the applicant will fit with the other staff.

It is important to find the right employee for the position. Always remember to look beyond experience and knowledge to the personality that will come with the applicant's experience. Sometimes it is better to hire someone with a little less experience to maintain a positive team atmosphere.

References

The next step in the selection process is to check references of the applicants. This is done by conducting a brief telephone interview with the person(s) referenced by the applicant. After interviewing all the applicants that interest you and checking their references, it will be time to decide whom to hire. You may choose to have your top applicants come back for second interviews. During this time, you may wish to have the physician in or other staff members interview the applicant.

Hiring

Once you have verified the references of your applicants, you can begin the process of selecting your top choices for the position. It may be that you call your top choice and offer them the position, but find that they decline your offer. You would then need to offer the position to your next choice.

After an applicant has accepted the position, all other applicants should be notified, either by telephone or in writing, that the position is filled. The new employee should receive a written confirmation of the job offer along with the salary. The office manager will usually sign this letter.

The first three months (90 days) is usually a probationary or trial period for all new employees. This time frame allows the supervisor to observe the new employee at work and to determine if the new employee is suited to the position for which he or she was hired. During this probationary period an employee can be terminated without cause. After 90 days, the employer must show just cause, or reason, to dismiss an employee. Absenteeism, poor performance, or

violations of OSHA and safety standards are examples of just cause.

Orientation and Training

If you were to take a poll of new employees and ask what was most frustrating about their first days on the job, they would reply "lack of orientation." An effective manager will have an organized, efficient method of orientation and training for all new hires. The time and effort will pay off in the long run.

What issues should be covered in orientation? The following list shows the minimum subjects that should be covered for all new hires.

- Work hours and schedule
- Office layout (include the locations of the restrooms and breakrooms)
- Dress code
- Lunch break
- Job description
- All employment records—including I-9's (Figure 18-4), emergency contact information, insurance enrollment, etc.
- OSHA Bloodborne Pathogens Standards and Universal Precautions—including request for a waiver form for Hepatitis B vaccine
- Fire safety—locations of fire extinguishers (Figure 18-5), exit procedures, stairwell locations (Figure 18-6)
- Confidentiality—signature on confidentiality statement
- Policy and Procedure Manual—employee should read and sign a statement that the document has been read and understood
- Physician's work preferences—explain the way the physician prefers to work; if a team approach is used, examples should be provided to help the medical assistant understand his or her role

Smaller offices with fewer employees may conduct orientation sessions on-the-job as the new employee begins working. This is not ideal but often necessary. Orientation materials and a schedule can be developed to assist in this training process.

While some of these issues should have been covered during the interview process, many new employees need to be reminded. The pressure of the interview often causes applicants to forget important issues. Reiterating these issues during orientation can prevent confusion and errors. A confident employee is an efficient employee. Legal and Ethical Issues discusses the importance of confidentiality in the workplace.

OMB No. 1115-0136

U.S. Department of Justice
Immigration and Naturalization Service

Employment Eligibility Verification

Please read instructions carefully before completing this form. The instructions must be available during completion of this form. ANTI-DISCRIMINATION NOTICE: It is illegal to discriminate against work eligible individuals. Employers CANNOT specify which document(s) they will accept from an employee. The refusal to hire an individual because of a future expiration date may also constitute illegal discrimination.

Section 1. Employee Information and Verification. To be completed and signed by employee at the time employment begins.

Print Name: Last	First	Middle Initial	Maiden Name
Address (Street Name and Number)		Apt. #	Date of Birth (month/day/year)
City	State	Zip Code	Social Security #

I am aware that federal law provides for imprisonment and/or fines for false statements or use of false documents in connection with the completion of this form.

I attest, under penalty of perjury, that I am (check one of the following):
- [ ] A citizen or national of the United States
- [ ] A Lawful Permanent Resident (Alien # A_____)
- [ ] An alien authorized to work until ___/___/___
  (Alien # or Admission #) _____

Employee's Signature

Date (month/day/year)

Preparer and/or Translator Certification. (To be completed and signed if Section 1 is prepared by a person other than the employee.) I attest, under penalty of perjury, that I have assisted in the completion of this form and that to the best of my knowledge the information is true and correct.

Preparer's/Translator's Signature	Print Name
Address (Street Name and Number, City, State, Zip Code)	Date (month/day/year)

Section 2. Employer Review and Verification. To be completed and signed by employer. Examine one document from List A OR examine one document from List B and one from List C, as listed on the reverse of this form, and record the title, number and expiration date, if any, of the document(s)

List A	OR	List B	AND	List C
Document title: _____		_____		_____
Issuing authority: _____		_____		_____
Document #: _____		_____		_____
Expiration Date (if any): ___/___/___		___/___/___		___/___/___
Document #: _____				
Expiration Date (if any): ___/___/___				

CERTIFICATION - I attest, under penalty of perjury, that I have examined the document(s) presented by the above-named employee, that the above-listed document(s) appear to be genuine and to relate to the employee named, that the employee began employment on (month/day/year) ___/___/___ **and that to the best of my knowledge the employee is eligible to work in the United States. (State employment agencies may omit the date the employee began employment.)**

Signature of Employer or Authorized Representative	Print Name	Title
Business or Organization Name	Address (Street Name and Number, City, State, Zip Code)	Date (month/day/year)

Section 3. Updating and Reverification. To be completed and signed by employer.

A. New Name (if applicable)	B. Date of rehire (month/day/year) (if applicable)

C. If employee's previous grant of work authorization has expired, provide the information below for the document that establishes current employment eligibility.

Document Title:_____   Document #:_____   Expiration Date (if any): ___/___/___

I attest, under penalty of perjury, that to the best of my knowledge, this employee is eligible to work in the United States, and if the employee presented document(s), the document(s) I have examined appear to be genuine and to relate to the individual.

Signature of Employer or Authorized Representative	Date (month/day/year)

Form I-9 (Rev. 11-21-91)N Page 2

FIGURE 18-4 A standard I-9 form.

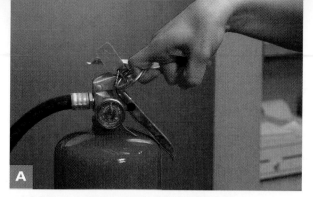

(A) Pull the pin on the upper handle of the fire extinguisher.

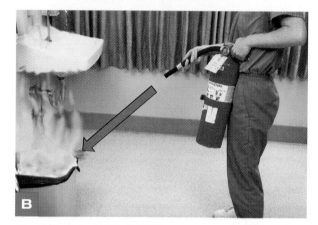

(B) Aim low toward the base of the fire.

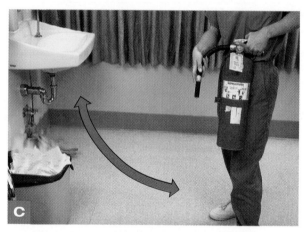

(C) Sweep the area from side to side.

FIGURE 18-5 It is important for new employees to know the location of all fire extinguishers.

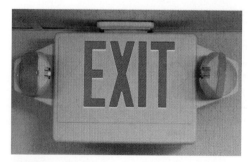

FIGURE 18-6 New employees should be shown all exits in case of an emergency.

Using Performance Evaluation Effectively

All employees need feedback on how well they are performing in their assigned positions. In addition, management needs opportunities to introduce new goals for their staff. The employee, in return, can have the chance to voice concerns and suggestions for increasing the morale and productivity of the staff. Regular evaluations offer the chance for a productive give-and-take beyond the day-to-day interactions.

When it comes to any evaluation, preparation is the key. As the office manager, you do not want to go into an evaluation unprepared. This will only set you up for problems. The appraisal should be given in a nonjudgmental manner. The manager should not take the stance of "the boss" versus the employee, but rather be open to understanding any problems the employee may be experiencing. Discussion of the job description and required duties should allow the employee to voice any frustration. At the same time, the manager should reinforce what is expected of the staff member. Teamwork should be emphasized.

The manager needs to sit down and look at the employee's performance as a whole. Reexamine the employee's job description and identify the most important aspects of the position. You will then want to rate the employee on those points. Look at whether the employee's performance was outstanding, good, average, poor, or unacceptable. Once you have evaluated these particulars, you can examine the whole of the employee's performance. How does he or she get along with the other members of the office team?

In this general evaluation of the employee, it is also important to give him or her goals to meet before the next evaluation. Mention areas in which the employee may want to improve work performance. If possible, you will always want to end the evaluation meeting on a good note. It is ideal that the employee leave the meeting with the feeling that something valuable was gained from the review.

In situations where employees are not performing up to the standard set for them, the performance evaluation may satisfy the legal requirements for documentation for rightful termination. If you are giving an employee a poor evaluation, it is a good idea to warn the employee at the start of the meeting. This will prevent the employee from being surprised when you begin to explain the problems with his or her performance.

Most employees look at an evaluation as the chance to ask for a raise in pay. When writing a personnel manual, there should be a delineation of the types of reviews and the time intervals at which they will be given. Following is a list of different types of reviews.

- Orientation or training—Every few days ask the employee how the training is going. Make sure he or she has the materials, equipment and supplies needed to perform the job. Ask the employee if he or she has any questions regarding policy and if supervision is being provided.

- Routine performance review—Reviews are normally performed at 90-day, six-month and yearly intervals. Approximately one hour should be devoted to this meeting. These reviews should not come as a surprise to the employee. They should be stated in the policy manual. Many offices offer the staff member the opportunity to do a self-evaluation prior to the meeting. This allows the employee the chance to think about his or her performance thus far. Figure 18-7 is an example of a form that may be used in a routine evaluation.

- Poor performance reviews—These are held when there have been obvious deficiencies in the performance of the employee. They offer the opportunity to help the employee improve. Conversely, they document the poor performance and set the stage for dismissal.

Should salary reviews be tied to the performance evaluation? There are several schools of thought regarding this issue. Whatever the policy of the office, fair and equal standards should be set.

What should the manager hope to accomplish with the meeting? It is important to target specific areas of performance. Following are some questions to ask in order to achieve effective management goals.

- How can improvement be achieved?
- How can you as the manager help the improvement?
- How can you remain fair and even in your opinion?
- How will you handle the possibility of a negative response from the employee?

Box 18-2 is a list of possible topics to cover during the review. Finally, as in all aspects of medical office management, document all that is said during the evaluation. Be mindful to document only objective facts and statements made and leave personal opinions aside.

Discipline and Probation

Occasionally it is necessary to discipline an employee. Due to the sensitive nature of medical work, there are certain situations that can result in immediate discharge. These include intoxication, drug use, breach of confidentiality, and sleeping on the job. The employee must be sent home on suspension while the incident is investigated. If the facts prove to be true, then the employee is dismissed.

BOX 18-2
Topics of Review for Front Office Personnel

Telephone technique

Balance of cash box daily

Accurate filing

Appointment scheduling

General

Treats patients with respect

Prioritizing of tasks

Makes efficient use of time

Works neatly

Follows directions

Cheerful and interested in the patient's comfort

Is punctual and has achieved good attendance

Uses good grammar

Appropriate appearance and hygiene

Works as a team member

Additional Topics for Medical Assistant's Review

Charts accurately

Anticipates the needs of the doctor

Is knowledgeable about procedures

PERFORMANCE EVALUATION AND DEVELOPMENT PLAN
(OFFICE AND CLERICAL)

NAME: _____ DATE OF EVALUATION: _____
DATE OF HIRE: _____ DEPARTMENT: _____
JOB TITLE: _____ SUPERVISOR: _____
DATE APPOINTED THIS JOB: _____ MANAGER: _____
LAST REVIEW DATE: _____ LAST REVIEW RATING: _____
NEXT REVIEW DATE: _____ CURRENT REVIEW RATING: _____

PURPOSE

The purpose of this evaluation is to:

1. SET GOALS WITHIN SCOPE OF PRESENT JOB.
2. COMMUNICATE OPENLY ABOUT PERFORMANCE.
3. EVALUATE PAST PERFORMANCE.
4. DISCUSS FUTURE DEVELOPMENT PLANS FOR GROWTH.

INSTRUCTIONS

1. Supervisor to review form prior to completion. If specific item they should be left blank.
2. Supervisor and employee to review job description prior to
3. In "COMMENTS" section supervisor may indicate which fac more heavily weighted in this particular evaluation.
4. Comments should be specific and job-related. All appropri should be commented on to some degree.

I. POSITION OBJECTIVES AND MAJOR RESPONSIBILITIES: Summ

II. ACCOMPLISHMENTS AND/OR IMPROVEMENTS: What specific a has employee made since last review with respect to set goals?

PLEASE CONSIDER THE EMPLOYEE'S DEMONSTRATED PERFORMANCE A CLOSELY DESCRIBES THAT PERFORMANCE.

4 - Performance consistently far exceeds expectations and requirements.
3 - Performance consistently exceeds normal expectations and job require
2 - Performance consistently meets expectations and job requirements.
1 - Performance usually meets expectations and minimum job requireme
0 - Performance does not meet job requirements.

– CONTINUED, NEXT PAGE –

ORDER # 72-119 • PERSONNEL RECORDS SYSTEM • © 1987 BIBBERO SYSTEMS, INC. • PETALUMA, CA • TO REORDER CALL TOLL FREE: (800)

7. DEPENDABILITY: Consider attendance, punctuality, idle time and reliance which can be placed on employee to persevere and carry through to completion all assigned tasks.

○ 0   ○ 1   ○ 2   ○ 3   ○ 4

8. COMPLIANCE WITH COMPANY POLICIES: Does the employee comply with rules and regulations which apply to safety, fair employment practices and general administrative procedure?

○ 0   ○ 1   ○ 2   ○ 3   ○ 4

9. SPECIFIC PERFORMANCE

	0	1	2	3	4	COMMENTS
A. Ability to handle scheduling:						
B. Willingness to work OT when necessary:						
C. Handling of calls and follow-up:						
D. Maintenance of equipment:						
E. Ability to handle patient complaints:						
F. Tact in dealing with patients:						
G. Speed (in specific technical procedures):						
H. Secretarial accuracy:						
I. Professional terminology:						
J. Assisting procedures:						
K. Laboratory techniques:						
L. X-ray techniques:						
M. Physical therapy:						
N. Collections:						
O. Medical Insurance:						
P. Bookkeeping:						

10. PERSONAL

	0	1	2	3	4	COMMENTS
A. Grooming:						
B. Professional conduct:						
C. Energy, enthusiasm:						
D. Ability to handle stress:						

ADDITIONAL COMMENTS: _____

– CONTINUED, NEXT PAGE –

ORDER # 72-119 • PERSONNEL RECORDS SYSTEM • © 1987 BIBBERO SYSTEMS, INC. • PETALUMA, CA • TO REORDER CALL TOLL FREE: (800) BIBBERO (800 242-2376) OR FAX (800) 242-9330

FIGURE 18-7 There are standard employee performance evaluation forms that may be used.

For frequent tardiness or absenteeism, an employee may be placed on probation and told that if the situation occurs again, the employee will be discharged. In some facilities, both verbal and written warnings are issued before corrective action is taken. Investigating every employee incident prevents someone being falsely fired. For instance, diabetic employees may appear to be on drugs when they are, in fact, having a diabetic reaction.

Any employee incident must be carefully documented with the time, date, and an objective statement about what happened and then placed into the employee's file. Document the incident immediately after it has occurred. It is always better to have a witness present when dismissing an employee.

Time Management

One of the greatest attributes of an effective office manager is the ability to successfully manage time. If the manager is organized, the office is usually organized. Time management requires the ability to prioritize the important tasks and to complete them on schedule. This is quite different from doing every task as it comes along. The office manager generally has little control over the tasks presented. The control is in how the tasks are handled and delegated.

One of the main responsibilities of the office manager/medical assistant is to manage all the peripheral office functions so that the physician is free to concentrate on practicing medicine. It is possible for the physician to gain an hour each day to devote to administrative and patient related tasks that only he or she can do, because tasks, such as opening the daily mail, searching for a drug sample to give to a patient, and dealing with pharmaceutical and other sales representatives, are handled by the office manager.

Before establishing a time management system, it is important to define the office goals with the physician. Physicians' goals vary from complex to simple and from long-term to short-term. These goals may include collecting all payments at the time of delivery of services, re-organizing or computerizing billing, limiting the practice, adding a partner or new service, writing a textbook, or plans for early retirement.

One of the dangers of strictly adhering to time management and goal-setting practices is that by totally concentrating on organizing the office, the patient may be forgotten in the process. The main concern should be to always take care of a patient who is waiting at the reception desk before straightening up the work area.

After the goals have been established, priorities can be set. The office manager/medical assistant can establish a priority list of the goals. A priority list is a composite of all the tasks that need to be accomplished to actualize each goal. These can be placed on a TO DO list as they come to the office manager's attention. Each item is assigned a priority designation of 1, 2, or 3, depending on how critical the item is to complete the task. For example, ordering supplies that are running out is a number 1, while rearranging a linen cupboard or a file drawer might be a number 3. Number 1 priority items must be done first and number 3 last. It is often tempting to do the easier tasks first since they take less time and show an immediate accomplishment. Good use of time management would determine that the inventory order should be placed immediately and the number 3 priority items be delegated to someone else or completed later, if necessary. It is a good idea to date a TO DO list and to cross off or check items as they are accomplished. Box 18-3 shows an example of one type of TO DO list.

Make every attempt to complete each task, such as handling paper, only once. As mail is opened, it needs to be quickly sorted according to importance, handled, and processed. Mail should be handled immediately, if possible.

<table>
<tr><td colspan="3">BOX 18-3
Medical Office TO DO List</td></tr>
<tr><td>**Priority**</td><td>**TO DO** _____</td><td>**Date:** ____</td></tr>
<tr><td>2</td><td colspan="2">Order paper supplies</td></tr>
<tr><td>1</td><td colspan="2">Arrange Dr. Williams' air transportation to medical convention next week</td></tr>
<tr><td>2</td><td colspan="2">Prepare performance appraisal for J. Jones</td></tr>
<tr><td>3</td><td colspan="2">Reorganize storeroom</td></tr>
<tr><td>1</td><td colspan="2">Type convention speech</td></tr>
<tr><td>1</td><td colspan="2">Place ad for new medical assistant</td></tr>
<tr><td>3</td><td colspan="2">Ask Janet to remove old magazines from reception room</td></tr>
<tr><td>1</td><td colspan="2">Call for PAP test report for Ms. Kohut</td></tr>
<tr><td>2</td><td colspan="2">Block out schedule book for next quarter</td></tr>
<tr><td>1</td><td colspan="2">Prepare agenda for Thursday's staff meeting</td></tr>
</table>

When leaving a telephone message, it is advisable to record detailed voice mail messages, whenever possible, since it can actually save time. Leaving a detailed message during the first call can prevent having to make another telephone call. An exception would be when calling a patient. The patient's confidentiality should be protected. See Chapter 6 for more information regarding voice messaging.

Never trust anything to memory in the medical office. Always write down all instructions from the physician, information from the patient, another employee, or supplier. It is better to maintain one small record book and keep all notations in that book rather than have several pieces of paper with information that can be misplaced. Many medical assistants carry a small notepad and pen in their pocket at all times.

Some offices require that the in-basket of the day's mail and incoming laboratory reports be emptied before the end of the day. This is a good time management technique to develop.

Personnel Policy Manual

The personnel policy manual, also known as the employee handbook, contains information for the employee about the employer-employee relationship, the work environment, and the expectations of the particular medical facility. This manual contains general information about office policies relating to dress and behavior codes, punctuality, office safety, and the role of the employee in an emergency, such as a fire. OSHA guidelines and Standard Precautions are included. It usually describes the circumstances or grounds for dismissal, such as sleeping, drinking, or swearing on the job.

Employees may be given specific information about the following issues or benefits.

- Compensation and reimbursement for work-related activities, such as attending conventions and courses (CEU/degree), and parking fees
- Emergency leave
- Grievance (complaint) process
- Health benefits
- Holidays
- Jury duty
- Overtime policy
- Pension plan
- Performance review and evaluation
- Probationary period
- Sick leave
- Termination of employment
- Vacation
- Work hours, including flex time

An office manager will find that an updated policy manual can be a useful tool when providing employee counseling. A well-designed policy manual remains flexible enough in its design to allow for revisions, if and when policies change. Small office policy manuals consist of several pages that are copied on-site. In large practices, the manual may be bound and copied at a printing service.

The employee handbook is often the first piece of office literature that the employee is asked to read. Employees should be asked to sign a statement indicating they have read and understood the information contained in it.

Office Procedures Manual

All offices should have a procedures manual describing how to carry out tasks within a particular medical practice. The office procedures manual varies in content from the personnel policy manual. Detailed descriptions of the standard operating procedure (SOP) and how to perform both administrative and clinical tasks are included in this manual.

Policy refers to a plan of action, such as "It is office policy that all employees receive hepatitis B (HBV) vaccination." The procedure will describe the steps to be performed to carry out the policy. For example, "a

series of three injections of HBV will be administered over a seven-month period of time, free of charge, to the employee." The terms policy and procedure are used interchangeably in many office.

The primary functions of a procedures manual are: (1) list the tasks to be performed within the office; (2) standardize the procedure for each task; and (3) describe job responsibilities and titles. The procedures manual, when properly updated, is an excellent reference tool for the new employee since it provides guidelines for performing specific tasks. Temporary or substitute employees also find it valuable.

Ideally, the procedure manual is contained in a loose-leaf binder that allows the addition of new pages for ease of updating. Each policy is numbered and dated. As the policy is updated, the number remains the same but the date changes to indicate the revision. The manual should be clearly labeled and available for employees to read.

New policies and procedures are usually distributed or posted for employees in addition to being added to the policy and procedures manuals. In some offices, staff are asked to initial the corner of the policy indicating they have read it.

Table 18-2 contains a list of information that should be included in a procedure's manual. Completing and updating a procedures manual is often a job function of the medical assistant or the office manager. While one person may have responsibility for development of the manual, good manuals are the result of the input from a variety of personnel. The physician should always provide the final review of all policies and procedures.

Medical Meetings and Speaking Engagements

The medical assistant may be asked to assist the physician in the travel arrangements for medical meetings or in the preparation of medical speaking engagements. Travel arrangements may include making hotel, flight, and car reservations, and sometimes typing a travel itinerary for the trip. Preparation for medical speaking engagements may require the medical assistant to do research for a physician's speech or to create certain documents such as handouts and computer presentations.

When making the travel arrangements, the physician may wish to use a local travel agent or one of the many Internet sites available for booking flights and hotels. It is important to find out what the physician's preferences are before making any plans. The physician may prefer a non-smoking hotel room and only business class flight tickets. Make sure the reservations are what he or she wants.

TABLE 18-2 Contents of an Office Procedure Manual

Content	Description
Job Description	Every position including office manager, medical assistant, nurses, technician, housekeeping personnel, and custodian.
Routine Office Tasks	Clinical tasks such as venipuncture, taking vital signs, EKGs, assisting with physical examinations, assisting with PAP test and other laboratory tests.
Special Procedures	Surgical tray set-up for individual physicians, assisting with special exams such as proctological exams, using specialized equipment such as ultrasound.
Emergency Procedures	Protocol for handling telephone and office emergencies, description of equipment used for emergency care such as mouth shield for CPR, proper sequence for alerting physician and 911 emergencies.
Quality Assurance	Procedures for maintaining quality control over all laboratory testing and procedures.
OSHA Compliance	Compliance regarding needles, other sharps, specimens, personal protective equipment, regulated waste control, HBV vaccine, laundry disposal, and contaminated equipment.

When putting together the travel itinerary, obtain all of the flight, hotel, car rental, and meeting or engagement information. Flight information includes travel dates, airline name, flight number, and departure and arrival times. The hotel information includes the hotel name, address, telephone number, reservation dates and confirmation number. Also assemble car rental reservations and any information pertinent to the meeting that the physician is attending. Keep a copy of the itinerary at the office and give a copy to the physician.

When helping a physician to prepare for a speaking engagement, you can help in a variety of capacities. It may include doing research. Be sure to provide all source material with any research that you reference and cite. The physician may ask you to create handouts for his or her presentation. The physician may also ask you to create a computer presentation. There are different software programs that will assist you in creating a presentation.

Patient Information Booklet

Many medical practices use a professional advertising service to develop informational brochures as a marketing tool. However, a patient information booklet or a variety of patient teaching materials can be developed in-house. These materials should provide patient information regarding office hours, payment guidelines, appointment and cancellation policy, the telephone answering service, information about the physician(s), directions to the facility, and parking information. A good patient information booklet can reduce the number of questions by telephone from patients, enhance the office's image, and reduce the number of patients who fail to follow instructions.

Instruction booklets for patients with special needs or to teach methods of disease prevention can be developed using a format and design described in Procedure 18-2. The patient information booklet should be handed to each new patient at the time of registration or mailed prior to the first appointment. Patient information materials never replace the need for personal instructions to the patient. They augment or reinforce patient teaching. Patient Education includes more about patient information booklets.

Medical Practice Marketing and Customer Service

Marketing is a subject that most office managers do not think much about when running a medical office. Marketing a medical practice involves various activities to promote the services of a physician or group of physicians to a population of patients. Marketing can promote a new office and improve the image of an established office to compete with the new offices and

Developing a Patient Information Booklet

OBJECTIVE: Develop a booklet to inform patients about services provided by your medical office.

Equipment and Supplies
computer; design software (if including images); high quality paper; printer (or an independent printing service)

Method

1. Make the booklet as appealing as possible. Allow white space around all the edges. Use large print for the elderly reader's benefit. The booklet should be small enough that it will fit easily into a pocket or purse.

2. Write the booklet with the reader in mind. Avoid the use of technical medical terms. Never use medical abbreviations in patient literature.

3. Avoid long paragraphs of explanation. Keep the sentences short and concise.

4. Provide a listing of the regular office hours.

5. List any special services offered by the practice or clinic such as patient education classes or blood pressure testing programs.

6. Explain the procedure for having a prescription refilled.

7. Explain the procedure for processing medical insurance forms.

8. Include a general statement about payment of fees, especially if payment is expected at the time of delivery of services. Specific fees are not discussed in patient brochures.

9. Provide information about the physician and the staff. For example, "Dr. Williams is in general practice specializing in family practice. Our pediatrician is Dr. Conway. Our physicians are on staff at two hospitals: Northwestern Memorial Hospital and Children's Memorial Hospital." The name and telephone number of the office manager, the personnel responsible for insurance processing and the patient educator should be included.

10. State what procedure to follow in case of an emergency. For example, instruct the patients to call 911 if the emergency is life threatening. Also provide a 24-hour emergency telephone number. Request the patient to keep this number near his or her telephone.

11. Include a telephone number at the end of the brochure in the event there are additional questions.

12. End the brochure by thanking the patient for taking the time to read the literature.

---

to retain patients. There are many ways that marketing can impact a medical office. Customer service can be a valuable marketing tool.

The Target Market

In marketing a medical office or facility, one of the first things to look at is the target market of the physician(s). What kinds of services are being offered? This can affect the physician's office location. A new geriatric medical practice has a better chance of doing well if it is located near retirement communities rather than with young families. The services of the office should match the area in which it is located.

After assessing the target market and the needs of the target group, types of services the practice could offer can be determined. Services may include new procedures that could benefit patients' needs.

Once you have determined your services, then a plan must be developed and put into place. The first step will be to look for any problems or opportunities that may come about in the execution of the plan. The plan should describe what steps need to be implemented, who is responsible, and a time frame. A plan must be thought through and in place before you begin to follow and execute it. Many ventures have failed due to poor planning. When the plan has been executed, it is a good idea to go back and review if the plan met expectations or not. Make note of any particular problems that may have arisen and positives that may have been learned in the process.

Patients need an introduction to all the caregivers they come into contact with in the office. Employees should always identify themselves to patients. Many patients need further education about the functions that individual employees are able to perform.

Patient information booklets are one of the best ways to educate the patient about the functions of the staff and medical office. While verbal instructions are still necessary, the booklets can enhance learning. Medical assistants need to involve the entire staff in the production of patient literature.

Marketing the Practice

There are many ways to promote a medical practice. Some marketing plans may require budgets for expenses to implement the plan. However, some marketing tools available to physicians and medical practices are free or at low-cost

Free Marketing and Public Relations

One of the best ways of promoting a practice is by word of mouth, which is completely free. Many patients choose their physician based upon friends and family recommending their own physician. Word of mouth is built upon a base of good customer service, which will be discussed later in the chapter.

Another method of promoting a practice is through public relation activities such as local charities and events. Involvement in the community will spread the office's name and show that you are a participating member of the community. Goodwill in the community can translate into growing the practice.

Web Sites

Building a practice Web site is a relatively new marketing tool for medical professionals. This can be done using simple Web site building software or hiring a Web site firm. It is important to plan what should be included on the Web site. The main objective of the site needs to be determined. What is the site's function? Is it only providing information regarding the practice? Would the patient to be able to access different forms and procedure instructions? Will patients be able to request appointments online? Remember to keep the site easy to use. Graphics and colors need to be simple and pleasing to the eye.

You will then have to choose a Web server to support your site. There are many options that will need to be researched. Some are free, but they will add advertisements to your site. Others will require a fee.

Customer Service

One of your most potent marketing tools will depend entirely upon your customer service. Just as word of mouth can bring you many customers, it can also drive them away if poor services are provided.

The patient, like a customer, will respond positively or negatively to his or her experience at the medical office. What impression does the patient have? Is the staff helpful? Is the staff attentive and considerate of the patient's time and condition? It is important that all patients are treated with respect and concern. Box 18-4 includes phrases that will leave the patient with a poor view of a medical office's customer service abilities.

BOX 18-4
Phrases that Decrease Customer Service Level

"I don't know."

"It's not my fault."

"What do you want?"

"I can't."

"It's not my job."

"You're wrong."

"It's not my problem."

SUMMARY

A smooth running office requires attention to many factors, including staff training, good time management skill, up-to-date policy and procedure manuals, and careful attention to detail. A medical office requires the same management skills that any business organization uses. Maintaining good customer service is key to keeping a contented patient base while enhancing the possibility of growing the practice.

COMPETENCY REVIEW

1. Define and spell the terms to learn for this chapter.
2. Prepare an office procedure for any one of the following tasks: appointment scheduling, patient reception process, taking vital signs, OSHA guidelines.
3. Prepare a monthly calendar for the month of December showing staff vacations and office coverage.
4. Develop a patient information booklet for your own physician's practice.
5. Prepare an employee policy for taking vacation days.

PREPARING FOR THE CERTIFICATION EXAM

1. Which of the following is a purpose of the procedure manual?
   A. standardization of procedures
   B. listing of job descriptions
   C. listing of tasks to perform within the office
   D. marketing tool
   E. listing of hospitals and clinics

2. An employee policy describing the grievance process should be contained in the
   A. general policy manual
   B. personnel policy manual
   C. employee handbook
   D. patient information booklet
   E. physician/employer file

3. What law affects the hiring of a new employee?
   A. OSHA
   B. EEOA
   C. Title VII of the Civil Rights Act
   D. EEOC
   E. AMA

4. A systems approach to office management is
   A. using outside consultants for all financial and business operations
   B. performing individual office functions in isolation
   C. integrating functions
   D. not advisable in the office setting
   E. is the only way to manage

5. Arranging staff vacation coverage is usually the responsibility of the
   A. physician
   B. individual who is going on vacation
   C. office manager
   D. medical assistant
   E. nurse

6. The purpose of a performance evaluation is to
   A. positively encourage the continued improvement of the employee's performance
   B. negotiate a salary increase
   C. find any fault(s) in an employee's performance
   D. provide a document to compare one employee's performance with another employee's performance
   E. improve office moral

7. Employee records must be kept for all of the following EXCEPT
   A. Social Security Number
   B. net salary
   C. gross salary
   D. number of claimed exemptions (W-4 form)
   E. deductions

8. Patient instruction booklets should be used
   A. in place of individual instructions
   B. to avoid contact with difficult patients
   C. to prevent lawsuits
   D. to standardize instructions
   E. only with hearing-impaired patients

9. A new employee's probationary period is usually
   A. 30 days
   B. 2 months
   C. 3 months
   D. 6 months
   E. 1 year

10. Seniority refers to the person in the organization who
    A. is the oldest
    B. is in the highest position of power
    C. has been recognized the most for achievement
    D. has been with the company the longest
    E. will be the first to leave the office

CRITICAL THINKING

1. Where else could Marsha have advertised the job opening?
2. How could she have sorted the resumes further?
3. Why was it important for Marsha to know about the applicant's handwriting?
4. Was it appropriate for the second interviewee to wear a tongue ring? Why or why not?
5. Do you think that Marsha made the right choice from the three applicants?

ON THE JOB

Sarah Egan is the office manager in Dr. Williams' practice. Nell Jacobs, who has worked as a medical assistant in the office for one year, has frequently been absent or tardy on Mondays. Sarah suspects that Nell has a drinking problem. However, Nell has never arrived at the office intoxicated—until today. Sarah has just observed Nell stumbling in the parking lot when getting out of her car. Her speech is slurred and her breath has a fruity odor that Sarah thinks could be alcohol. Nell doesn't appear to understand anything that Sarah is saying to her.

1. Given the situation, as the office manager, what should Sarah do immediately regarding Nell?
2. If Sarah decides to send Nell home, should she call Nell's husband to come and get her, or, perhaps, insist that Nell go home in a cab?
3. Does Sarah have an obligation to tell Dr. Williams about her suspicions regarding Nell?
4. Should this incident become part of Nell's employment record?
5. Is this incident grounds for firing an employee?
6. Because Nell is a medical assistant and works with patients, is it within Sarah's rights to demand a blood and urine screening for alcohol and drugs?
7. Should the police be notified of the incident?
8. If Nell is indeed intoxicated or under the influence of drugs, is Sarah obligated to refer Nell to counseling at an alcohol and drug rehabilitation facility?

INTERNET ACTIVITY

Research the different methods that the Internet provides for advertising job opportunities available at your medical office.

MediaLink More on medical office management, including interactive resources, can be found on the Student CD-ROM accompanying this textbook.

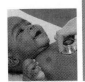

APPENDIX I:
Abbreviations and Symbols

a	ampere; anode; anterior; aqua; area; artery
AB, Ab	abortion; abnormal; antibody
ABC	aspiration biopsy cytology
ABG	arterial blood gases
ABLB	alternate binaural loudness balance
ABO	blood group
ABR	auditory brainstem response
AC	air conduction; anticoagulant
a.c.	before meals
ACAT	automated computerized axial tomography
Acc.	accommodation
ACG	angiocardiography
Ach	acetylcholine
ACL	anterior cruciate ligament
ACLS	advanced cardiac life support
ACR	American College of Rheumatology
ACS	American Cancer Society
ACTH	adrenocorticoptropic hormone
AD	right ear (O) (auris dexter); Alzheimer's Disease; advance directive
ADA	American Diabetes Association
ad lib	as desired; freely
adeno-CA	adenocarcinoma
ADH	antidiuretic hormone
ADHD	attention-deficit hyperactivity disorder
ADL	activities of daily living
ADP	adenosine diphosphate
AE	above the elbow
AF	atrial fibrillation
AFB	acid-fast bacillus (TB organism)
AFP	alpha-fetoprotein
A/G	albumin/globulin ratio
Ag	antigen
AGN	acute glomerulonephritis
AH	abdominal hysterectomy
AHF	antihemophilic factor VIII
AHG	antihemophillic globulin factor VIII
AI	aortic insufficiency; artificial insemination
AIDS	acquired immune deficiency syndrome
AIH	artificial insemination homologous
AK	above knee

AKA	above-knee amputation
alk phos	alkaline phosphatase
ALD	aldolase
ALL	acute lymphocytic leukemia
ALS	amyotropic lateral sclerosis
ALT	argon laser trabeculoplasty; alanine aminotransferase
AMA	American Medical Association
AMD	age-related macular degeneration
AMI	acute myocardial infarction
AML	acute myelogenous leukemia
Angio	angiogram
ANS	autonomic nervous system
A&P	auscultation and percussion; anatomy and physiology
AP, AP view	anterior-posterior; anteroposterior view
APB	atrial premature beat
APTT	activated partial thromboplastin time
ARC	AIDS-related complex
ARD	acute respiratory disease
ARDS	acute respiratory distress syndrome
ARF	acute respiratory failure; acute renal failure
ARMD	age-related macular degeneration
AROM	active range of motion
AS	aortic stenosis; arteriosclerosis; left ear (X)
ASCVD	arteriosclerotic cardiovascular disease
As, Ast, astigm	astigmatism
Ascus	atypical squamous cells of undetermined significance
ASD	atrial septal defect
ASH	asymmetrical septal hypertrophy
ASHD	arteriosclerotic heart disease
ASL	American Sign Language
Astigm.	astigmatism
AST	aspartate aminotransferase
ATN	acute tubular necrosis
ATP	adenosine triphosphate
AU	both ears (auris unitas)
AV, A-V	atrioventricular; arteriovenous
AVMs	arteriovenous malformations
AVR	aortic valve replacement

Ba	barium
BAC	blood alcohol concentration
BaE	barium enema
baso	basophil
BBB	bundle branch block (L for left; R for right)
BBT	basal body temperature
BC	bone conduction
BE	barium enema
BG, bG	blood glucose; blood sugar
b.i.d.	twice a day
BIN, bin	twice a night
BK	below knee
BKA	below-knee amputation
BM	bowel movement
BMD	bone mineral density (test)
BMR	basal metabolic rate
BNO	bladder neck obstruction
BP	blood pressure
BPH	benign prostatic hypertrophy
Broncho	bronchoscopy
BRP	bathroom privileges
BS	breath sounds; bowel sounds; blood sugar
BSE	breast self-examination
BSI	body systems isolation
BSP	bromsulphalein
BT	bleeding time
BUN	blood urea nitrogen
BX, bx	biopsy
c̄	with (cum)
C1, C2, etc.	first cervical vertebra, second cervical vertebra, etc.
C&S	culture and sensitivity
CA	cancer; carcinoembryonic antigen
Ca	calcium; cancer
CABG	coronary artery bypass graft
CAD	coronary artery disease
CAM	complementary and alternative medicines
cap	capsule
CAPD	continuous ambulatory peritoneal dialysis
CAT, CT	computerized axial tomography
cath	catheterization
CBC	complete blood count
CBD	common bile duct
CBS	chronic brain syndrome
cc	cubic centimeter
CC	clean-catch urine specimen; cardiac catheterization; chief complaint

CCU	coronary care unit; cardiac care unit	CWP	childbirth without pain	ELISA	enzyme-linked immunosorbent assay
CD4	protein on T-cell helper lymphocyte	Cx	cervix	EM	emmetropia (normal vision)
CDC	Centers for Disease Control and Prevention	CXR	chest x-ray	EMG	electromyography
		cyl.	cylindrical lens	ENG	electronystagmography
CDH	congenital dislocation of the hip	cysto	cystoscopic exam	ENT	ear, nose, and throat
CEA	carcinoembryonic antigen	/d	per day	EOM	extraocular movement
CF	cystic fibrosis	D	diopter (lens strength)	eosin, eos	eosinophil
CGL	chronic granulocytic leukemia	dB, db	decibel	ERCP	endoscopic retrograde cholangiopancreatography
c.gl.	correction with glasses	DBS	deep brain stimulation	ERT	estrogen replacement therapy; external radiation therapy
CGN	chronic glomerulonephritis	D/C	discontinue		
CHD	congestive heart disease	D&C	dilatation and curettage		
chemo	chemotherapy	D&E	dilation and evacuation	ERV	expiratory reserve volume
CHF	congestive heart failure	dc	discontinue	ESR, SR	erythrocyte sedimentation rate
CHO	carbohydrate	DC	discharge		
chol	cholesterol	DCIS	ductal carcinoma in situ	ESL, ESWL	extracorporeal shock-wave lithotripsy
Ci	curie	DDS	Doctor of Dental Surgery; dorsal cord stimulation	ESR, SR, sed rate	erythrocyte sedimentation rate; sedimentation rate
Cib	food (cibus)				
CIC	coronary intensive care	decub	decubitus	ESRD	end-stage renal disease
CIN	cervical intraepithelial neoplasia	Derm	dermatology	EST	electroshock therapy
		DES	diethylstilbestrol	ET	endotracheal; endotracheal
CIS	carcinoma in situ	DHT	dihydrotestosterone	ETF	eustachian tube function
CK	creatine kinase	DI	diabetes insipidus; diagnostic imaging		
CL, Cl	chloride			F	Fahrenheit
CLL	chronic lymphocytic leukemia	diff	differential	FACP	Fellow, American College of Physicians
		dil	dilute; diluted		
cm	centimeter	DJD	degenerative joint disease	FACS	Fellow, American College of Surgeons
CMG	cystometrogram	DM	diabetes mellitus		
CML	chronic myelogenous leukemia	DNA	deoxyribonucleic acid	FBS	fasting blood sugar
		DNR	do not resuscitate	FDA	Food and Drug Administration
CMP	cardiomyopathy	DO	doctor of osteopathy		
CNS	central nervous system	DOA	dead on arrival	FEF	forced expiratory flow
c/o	complains of	DOB	date of birth	FEKG	fetal electrocardiogram
CO	cardiac output	DOE	dyspnea upon exertion	FEV	forced expiratory volume
CO_2	carbon dioxide	DPT	diphtheria, pertussis, tetanus injection	FH	family history
COLD	chronic obstructive lung disease			FHR	fetal heart rate
		DRE	digital rectal examination	FHS	fetal heart sound
COPD	chronic obstructive pulmonary disease	DRGs	diagnostic related groups	FHT	fetal heart tone
		DSA	digital subtraction angiography	FMS	fibromyalgia syndrome
CP	cerebral palsy; chest pain			FROM	full range of motion
CPD	cephalopelvic disproportion	DTaP	diphtheria, tetanus and pertussis (vaccine)	FS	frozen section
				FSH	follicle-stimulating hormone
CPK	creatine phosphokinase	DTR	deep tendon reflex		
CPM	continuous passive motion	DT's	delerium tremens	FTA-ABS	fluorescent treponemal antibody absorption
CPR	cardiopulmonary resuscitation	DUB	dysfunctional uterine bleeding		
				FTND	full-term normal delivery
CPS	cycles per second	DVA	distance visual acuity	5-FU	5-fluorouracil
CR	computerized radiography	DVT	deep vein thrombosis	FUO	fever of undetermined origin
CRF	chronic renal failure	Dx	diagnosis		
CS,		EBV	Epstein-Barr virus	FVC	forced vital capacity
C-section	cesarean section	ECC	endocervical curettage	FX, fx	fracture
C&S	culture and sensitivity	ECCE	extracapsular cataract extraction		
C-section	cesarean section (surgical delivery)			g	gram
		ECF	extracellular fluid; extended care facility	Ga	gallium
CSF	cerebrospinal fluid			GB	gallbladder
C-spine	cervical spine film	ECG; EKG	electrocardiogram	GC	gonorrhea
CT	computed tomography	ECHO	echocardiogram	GCSF	granulocyte colony-stimulating factor
CTA	clear to auscultation	E. coli	Escherichia coli		
CTS	carpal tunnel syndrome	ECSL	extracorporeal shockwave lithotriptor	GERD	gastroesophageal reflux disease
CUC	chronic ulcerative colitis				
CV	cardiovascular	ECT	electroconvulsive therapy	GGT	gamma-glutamyl transferase
CVA	cerebrovascular accident	ED	erectile dysfunction		
CVD	cardiovascular disease	EDC	estimated date of confinement	GH	growth hormone
CVP	central venous pressure	EEG	electroencephalogram	GI	gastrointestinal
CVS	chorionic villus sampling	EENT	eyes, ears, nose, throat		
		EGD	esophagogastroduodenoscopy		

GIFT	gamete intrafallopian transfer	HTN	hypertension	kg	kilogram
GnRF	gonadotropin-releasing factor	Hx	history	KS	Kaposi's sarcoma
		hypo	hypodermic	KUB	kidneys, ureters, bladder
GOT	glutamic oxaloacetic transaminase	Hz	Hertz	kV	kilovolt
				kW	kilowatt
Gpi	globus pallidus	IBD	inflammatory bowel syndrome		
GPT	glutamic pyruvic transaminase			L, l	liter
		IBS	irritable bowel syndrome	L1, L2, etc.	first lumbar vertebra, second lumbar vertebra, etc.
gr	grain	IC	intracardiac; interstitial cystitis		
grav I	first pregnancy			LA	left atrium
GSW	gunshot wound	ICCE	intracapsular cataract cryoextraction	L&A	light and accommodation
gtt	drops (guttae)			lab	laboratory
GTT	glucose tolerance test	ICF	intracellular fluid	LAC	laceration; long arm cast
GU	genitourinary	ICP	intracranial pressure	LAK	lymphokine-activated killer (cells)
gyn, gyne	gynecology	ICSH	interstitial cell-stimulating hormone		
				LAT, lat	lateral
h	hour	ICU	intensive care unit	lb	pound
H	hypodermic; hydrogen	ID	intradermal	LB	large bowel
H&L	heart & lungs	I&D	incision and drainage	LBBB	left bundle branch block
HAA	hepatitis-associated antigen	IDDM	insulin-dependent diabetes mellitus	LBW	low birth weight
HAV	hepatitis A virus			LCIS	lobular carcinoma in situ
HBIG	hepatitis B immune globulin	Ig	immunoglobins (IgA, IgD, IgE, IgG, IgM)	LD	lactate dehydrogenase
HBOT	hyperbaric oxygen therapy			LDH	lactic dehydrogenase
HBP	high blood pressure	IH	infectious hepatitis	LDL	low-density lipoproteins
HBV	hepatitis B virus	IHSS	idiopathic hypertropic subaortic stenosis	LE	left eye; lupus erythematosus; lower extremity
HCG	human chorionic gonadotropin				
HCl	hydrochloric acid	IL-2	interleukin-2		
HCO_3	bicarbonate	IM	intramuscular	LEDs	light-emitting diodes
HCT, Hct, crit	hematocrit	inj	injection	LES	lower esophageal sphincter
		I&O	intake and output	LGI	lower gastrointestinal series
HCV	hepatitis C virus	IOL	intraocular pressure	LH	luteinizing hormone
HD	hemodialysis; Hodgkin's disease	IOP	intraocular pressure	LH-RH	luteinizing hormone-releasing hormone
		IPD	intermittent peritoneal dialysis		
HDL	high-density lipoproteins			LIF	left iliac fossa
HDN	hemolytic disease of the newborn	IPPB	intermittent positive pressure breathing	liq	liquid; fluid
				L K & S	liver, kidney, and spleen
HDS	herniated disk syndrome	IQ	intelligence quotient	ll	left lateral
HEENT	head, eyes, ears, nose and throat	IR	interventional radiologist	LLC	long leg cast
		IRDS	infant respiratory distress syndrome	LLE	left lower extremity
HF	heart failure			LLL	left lower lobe
Hg	mercury	IRT	internal radiation therapy	LLQ	left lower quadrant
HgB, Hb, Hgb, HGB	hemoglobin	IRV	inspiratory reserve volume	LMP	last menstrual period
		IS	intercostal space	LOM	limitation of motion
HGH	human growth hormone	ITP	idiopathic thrombocytopenia purpura	LP	lumbar puncture
HIV	human immunodeficiency virus (causes AIDS)			LPE	laser peripheral iridotomy
		IU	international unit	LPF	low-power field
HLA	human leukocyte antigen	IUD	intrauterine device	LRQ	lower right quadrant
HMD	hyaline membrane disease	IUGR	intrauterine growth rate; intrauterine growth retardation	L, lt	left
HNP	herniated nucleus pulposa (herniated disk)			LTH	lactogenic hormone
		IV	intravenous	LUE	left upper extremity
H_2O	water	IVC	intravenous cholangiogram; inferior vena cava; intraventricular catheter	LUL	left upper lobe
Hpd	hematoporphyrin derivative			LUQ	left upper quadrant
				LV	left ventricle
H. pylori	Heliocobacter pylori	IVCD	intraventricular conduction delay	LVAD	left ventricular assist device
HPV	human papillomavirus			lymph	lymphocyte
HRT	hormone replacement therapy	IVF	in vitro fertilization		
		IVP	intravenous pyelogram	M	molar; thousand; muscle
h.s.	at bedtime	IVS	interventricular septum	m	male; meter; minim
HSG	hysterosalpingography	IVU	intravenous urogram	mA	milliampere
HSO	hysterosalpingoophrectomy			mAs	milliampere second
HSV	herpes simplex virus	J	joule	MBC	minimal breathing capacity
HSV-2	herpes simplex virus-2	JNC	Joint National Committee	MCH	mean corpuscular hemoglobin
Ht	height	JVP	jugular venous pulse		
HT	hypermetropia (hyperopia)			MCHC	mean corpuscular hemoglobin concentration
HTLV	human T-cell leukemia-lymphoma virus	K	potassium		
		KB	knee bearing	mCi	millicurie
		KD	knee disarticulation	MCV	mean corpuscular volume
				MD	medical doctor; muscular dystrophy

mEq	milliequivalent	NPUAP	National Pressure Ulcer Advisory Panel	Pe tube	polyethylene tube placed in the eardrum
mets	metastases	NSAIDs	nonsteroidal anti-inflammatory drugs	PFT	pulmonary function test
MG	myasthenia gravis			PGH	pituitary growth hormone
mg	milligram (0.001 gram)	NSR	normal sinus rhythm	pH	acidity or alkalinity of urine
MH	marital history	n&v	nausea and vomiting	PH	past history
MI	myocardial infarction; mitral insufficiency	NVA	near visual acuity	PID	pelvic inflammatory disease
MICU	mobile intensive care unit	O	pint	PIF	prolactin release-inhibiting factor
MIF	melanocyte-stimulating hormone release-inhibiting factor	O_2	oxygen	PKU	phenylketonuria
		OA	osteoarthritis	PM, pm	afternoon, evening
mix astig	mixed astigmatism	OB	obstetrics	PMH	past medical history
mL, ml	milliliter	OB-GYN	obstetrics and gynecology	PMI	point of maximal impulse
mm	millimeter (0.001 meter; 0.039 inch)	OC	oral contraceptive	PMN, seg, poly	polymorphonuclear neutrophil
		OCD	obsessive-compulsive disorder		
mmHg	millimeters of mercury	OCG	oral cholecystography	PMP	previous menstrual period
mMol	millimole	OCPs	oral contraceptive pills	PMR	physical medicine and rehabilitation
MMR	measles, mumps, and rubella (vaccine)	od	once a day		
		OD	right eye (oculus dexter); overdose	PMS	premenstrual syndrome
mol wt	molecular weight			PND	paroxysmal nocturnal dyspnea; postnasal drip
mono	mononucleosis; monocyte	OHS	open heart surgery		
MR	mitral regurgitation	OM	otitis media	PNS	peripheral nervous system
MRI	magnetic resonance imaging	O&P	ova and parasites	P.O.	per os (by mouth)
MS	musculoskeletal; mitral stenosis; multiple sclerosis	ophth.	ophthalmology	PP	postprandial (after meals)
		OR	operating room	PPD	purified protein derivative (tuberculin test)
MSH	melanocyte-stimulating hormone	ortho	orthopedics		
		os	mouth opening; bone	PPI	proton pump inhibitors
MTX	methotrexate	OS	left eye (oculus sinister)	pr	per rectum
mV	millivolt	OTC	over the counter	PRF	prolactin-releasing factor
MV	minute volume	Oto	otology	prn	as required; as needed
MVA	motor vehicle accident	OU	both eyes (oculi unitas); each eye (oculus uterque)	PROM	passive range of motion
MVP	mitral valve prolapse			prot.	protocol
MVV	maximal voluntary ventilation	OV	office visit	PSA	prostate specific antigen
		oz	ounce	pt	patient; pint
MY	myopia			PT	prothrombin time
		P	pulse; phosphorus	PTC	percutaneous transhepatic cholangiography
n	nerve	PA	posteroanterior view (radiology); pernicious anemia		
Na	sodium			PTCA	percutaneous transluminal coronary angioplasty
NAD	no apparent distress				
NANBH	non-A, non-B hepatitis virus	PAC	premature arterial contraction	PTH	parathyroid hormone
				PTS	permanent threshold shift
NB	newborn	PAP	pulmonary arterial pressure; Papanicolaou test	PTT	partial thromboplastin time
nCi	nanocurie			PUD	peptic ulcer disease
NCU	nongonococcal urethritis	para I	first delivery	PUL	percutaneous ultrasonic lithotropsy
NCV	nerve conduction velocity	PAT	paroxysmal atrial tachycardia		
NED	no evidence of disease			PVC	premature ventricular contraction
NIDDM	non-insulin-dependent diabetes mellitus	Path	pathology		
		PBI	protein bound iodine	PVD	peripheral vascular disease
NG	nasogastric (tube)	p.c.	after meals (post cibum)		
NGU	nongonococcal urethritis	PCL	posterior cruciate ligament	q	every
NH_4	ammonia	PCP	Pneumocystis carinii pneumonia	qam, qm	every morning
NHL	non-Hodgkin's lymphoma			q.d.	daily
NHLBI	National Heart, Lung and Blood Institute	PCV	packed cell volume (hematocrit)	qh	every hour
				q2h	every 2 hours
NICU	neonatal intensive care unit	PD	peritoneal dialysis	q.i.d.	four times a day
NIDDM	non-insulin-dependent diabetes mellitus	PDR	Physicians' Desk Reference	qns	quantity not sufficient
		PE	physical examination; pulmonary embolism	qpm, qn	every night
NIH	National Institute of Health			qs	quantity sufficient
		PEEP	positive end-expiratory pressure	qt	quart
NMR	nuclear resonance imaging				
NPDL	nodular, poorly differentiated lymphocytes	PEG	percutaneous endoscopic gastrostomy; pneumoencephalogram	R	roentgen; respiration; right
				RA	rheumatoid arthritis; radium; right arm
NPH	neutral protamine Hegedorn (insulin)	PERLA	pupils equal, react to light and accommodation		
				rad	radiation absorbed dose
NPO	nothing by mouth (nil per os)	PET	positron emission tomography	RAI	radioactive iodine
				RAIU	radioactive iodine uptake
NPT	nocturnal penile tumescence			RBC	red blood cell

RD	respiratory disease
RDA	recommended daily allowance (dietary allowance)
RDS	respiratory distress syndrome
RE	right eye
REM	rapid eye movement
Rh	Rhesus (factor)
RIA	radioimmunoassay
RIF	right iliac fossa
RL	right lateral
RLL	right lower lobe
RLQ	right lower quadrant
RML	right middle lobe; right mediolateral (episiotomy)
RNA	ribonucleic acid
R/O	rule out
ROM	range of motion; read only memory
RP	retrograde pyelogram
RPM	revolutions per minute
RQ	respiratory quotient
RT	radiation therapy
RUL	right upper lobe
RUQ	right upper quadrant
RV	right ventricle
Rx	take thou; prescribe; treatment; therapy
s̄	without
S1	first heart sound
S2	second heart sound
SA, S-A	sinoatrial
SAC	short arm cast
SAD	seasonal affective disorder
SAH	subarachnoid hemorrhage
SALT	serum alanine aminotransferase
SARS	severe acute respiratory syndrome
SAST	serum aspartate aminotransferase
SBE	subacute bacterial endocarditis
SBFT	small-bowel follow-through
SC, sc, subq	subcutaneous
SCD	sudden cardiac death
SCLE	subacute cutaneous lupus erythematosus
SD	shoulder disarticulation; standard deviation
SEE-2	Signing Exact English
seg, poly	polymorphonuclear neutrophil
segs	segmented (mature RBCs)
SG	skin graft; specific gravity
s.gl.	without correction or glasses
SGOT	serum glutamic oxaloacetic transaminase
SGPT	serum glutamic pyruvic transaminase
sh	shoulder
SH	serum hepatitis
SIDS	sudden infant death syndrome
SK	streptokinase

SLE	systemic lupus erythematosus
SMBG	self-monitoring of blood glucose
SMD	senile macular degeneration
SOB	shortness of breath
SOM	serous otitis media
sono	sonogram, sonography
SOP	standard operating procedure
sp gr, SG	specific gravity
SPP	suprapublic prostatectomy
SR	sedimentation rate
ss	one half
st	stage (of disease)
ST	esotropia
staph	staphylococcus
stat	immediately
STD	skin test done; sexually transmitted diseases
STH	somatotropin hormone
strep	streptococcus
STS	serologic test for syphilis
STSG	split-thickness skin graft
Subcu, Subq	subcutaneous
SVC	superior vena cava
SVD	spontaneous vaginal delivery
SVT	supraventricular tachycardia
Sx	signs, symptoms
syr	syrup
T	temperature
T1, T2, etc.	first thoracic vertebra, second thoracic vertebra, etc.
T_3	triiodothyronine; third thoracic vertebra
T_3RU	triiodothyronine resin uptake
T_4	thyroxine; fourth thoracic vertebra; T-cell lymphocyte
T_7	free thyroxine index; seventh thoracic vertebra
T_8	T-cell lymphocyte (cytotoxic or killer cell)
T&A	tonsillectomy and adenoidectomy
tab	tablet
TAH	total abdominal hysterectomy
TB	tuberculosis
TBW	total body weight
TENS	transcutaneous electrical nerve stimulation
TFS	thyroid function test
THA	total hip arthroplasty
THR	total hip replacement
TIA	transient ischemic attack
t.i.d.	three times a day
TIMS	topical immunomodulators
TIPS	transjugular intrahepatic portosystemic shunt
TJ	triceps jerk
TKA	total knee arthroscopy
TKR	total knee replacement
TLC	total lung capacity
TMJ	temporomandibular joint

TNF	tumor necrosis factor
TNM	tumor, nodes, metastases
TNS	transcutaneous nerve stimulation
top	topically
TPA	*Treponema pallidum* agglutination (test)
TPA, tPA	tissue plasminogen activator
TPN	total parenteral nutrition
TPR	temperature, pulse, respiration
tr, tinct	tincture
TSE	testicular self-exam
TSH	thyroid-stimulating hormone
TSS	toxic shock syndrome
TTH	thyrotropic hormone
TTS	temporary threshold shift
TUIP	transurethral incision of the prostrate
TUMP	transurethral microwave thermotherapy
TUNA	transurethral needle ablation
TUR, TURP	transurethral resection of the prostate
TV	tidal volume
TX, Tx	traction; treatment; transplant
U	units
U/A	urinalysis
UC	urine culture; uterine contractions
UCHD	usual childhood diseases
UE	upper extremity
UG	urogenital
UGI	upper gastrointestinal (x-ray) series
U&L, U/L	upper and lower
ULQ	upper left quadrant
ung	ointment
URI	upper respiratory infection
URQ	upper right quadrant
u/s	ultrasound
USP	United States Pharmacopeia
UTI	urinary tract infection
UV	ultraviolet
UVR	ultraviolet radiation
v	vein
VA	visual acuity
VC	vital capacity
VCD	vacuum constriction device
VCG	vectorcardiogram
VCU, VCUG	voiding cystourethrogram
VD	venereal disease
VDRL	Venereal Disease Research Laboratory (syphilis test)
VF	visual field
VHD	ventricular heart disease
VLDL	very low-density lipoproteins
vol	volume
vol %	volume percent

VMA	vanillylmandelic acid	WNL	within normal limits	XRT	radiation therapy
VP	vasopressin	WPW	Wolff-Parkinson-White	XT	exotropia
VPB	ventricular premature		syndrome	XX	female sex chromosomes
	beat	wt	weight	XY	male sex chromosomes
VS	vital signs	w/v	weight by volume		
VSD	ventricular septal defect			YAG	yttrium-aluminum-garnet
VT	ventricular tachycardia	x	multiplied by		(laser)
		XM	cross match for blood (type	YOB	year of birth
WBC	white blood cell		and cross match)	yr	year
WDWN	well developed, well	XP	xeroderma pigmentosum		
	nourished	XR	x-ray	z	atomic number

CHARTING ABBREVIATIONS AND SYMBOLS

aa	of each	FHT	fetal heart tones	qm	every morning (quaque mane)
ac	before meals (ante cibum)	GB	gallbladder		
AD	right ear (auris dextra)	GI	gastrointestinal	qn	every night (quaque nocte)
ADL	activities of daily living	GU	genitourinary	R	right; respiration
ad lib	as desired	h, hr	hour	RBC	red blood cell; red blood
adm	admission	hpf	high power field		(cell) count
AE	above elbow	hs	hour of sleep; bedtime	Rh	Rhesus blood factor (Rh +
AJ	ankle jerk		(hora somni)		or Rh −)
AK	above knee	hypo	hypodermic injection	RLQ	right lower quadrant
alt dieb	every other day	ICU	intensive care unit	R/O	rule out
alt hor	every other hour	IM	intramuscular	ROM	range of motion
alt noc	every other night	I&O	intake and output	RUQ	right upper quadrant
AM, am	before noon (ante	IU	international unit	SC, sc, subq	subcutaneous
	meridiem); morning	IV	intravenous	SOB	shortness of breath
AMA	against medical advice	L	left	SOS	if necessary (si opus sit)
AMB	ambulate; ambulatory	L&A	light and accommodation	stat	immediately
ant	anterior	LAT	lateral	Sx	signs, symptoms
AP	anteroposterior	L&W	living and well	T, temp	temperature
A-P	anterior-posterior	LLQ	left lower quadrant	tabs	tablets
approx	approximately	LMP	last menstrual period	TC&DB	turn, cough, deep breathe
AQ, aq	water	LOA	left occipitoanterior	tid	three times a day
ASAP	as soon as possible	LPF	low power field (10x)	tinct	tincture
AS or LE	left ear (auris sinistra)	LUQ	left upper quadrant	TPN	total parenteral nutrition
AV	atrioventricular	MTD	right ear drum (membrana	trans	transverse
BE	below elbow		tympani dexter)	ULQ	upper left quadrant
bid	twice a day	MTS	left ear drum (membrana	ung	ointment
bin	twice a night		tympani sinister)	URQ	upper right quadrant
BK	below knee	neg	negative	VS	vital signs
BM	bowel movement	NG	nasogastric	WBC	white blood cell; white
BMR	basal metabolic rate	NPO	nothing by mouth		blood (cell) count
BRP	bathroom privileges	NS	normal saline	WM, BM	white male, black male
C	Centigrade, Celsius or	OD	right eye (oculus dexter)	WF, BF	white female, black
	calorie (kilocalorie)	OP	outpatient		female
caps	capsules	OR	operating room	×	times, power
CBR	complete bed rest	OS or OL	left eye (oculus sinister,	−	negative
CC	chief complaint; clean catch		oculus laevus)	+	positive
	(urine)	OU	each eye (oculus uterque)	F	female
CCU	cardiac (coronary) care	P	pulse	M	male
	unit	PA	posteroanterior	+/−	positive or negative
c/o	complains of	pc	after meals (post cibum)	*	birth
cont	continue	PI	present illness	†	death
dc	discontinue	po	by mouth (per os)	%	percent
DC	discharge from hospital	PO	postoperative	#	number; pound
DNA	does not apply	PM, pm	afternoon or evening (post	&	and
DNR	do not resuscitate		meridiem)	<	less than
DNS	did not show	prn	as necessary, as required,	=	equal
Dr	doctor		when necessary	>	greater than
D/W	dextrose in water	q	every (quaque)	?	question
Dx	diagnosis	qd	every day (quaque die)	@	at
EOM	extraocular movement	qh	every hour (quaque hora)	^	increase
ER	emergency room	q2h	every 2 hours	™	trade mark
Ex	examination	q4h	every 4 hours	©	copyright
F	Fahrenheit	qid	four times a day (quarter	®	registered
FHS	fetal heart sounds		in die)	¶	paragraph

APPENDIX II:
Glossary of Word Parts

PREFIXES

a	no, not, without, lack of, apart	end	within, inner	neo	new
ab	away from	endo	within, inner	nulli	none
ad	toward, near	ep	upon, over, above		
ambi	both	epi	upon, over, above	olig	little, scanty
an	no, not, without, lack of	eso	inward	oligo	little, scanty
ana	up	eu	good, normal		
ant	against	ex	out, away from	pan	all
ante	before	exo	out, away from	par	around, beside
anti	against	extra	outside, beyond	para	beside, alongside, abnormal
apo	separation			per	through
astro	star-shaped	hemi	half	peri	around
auto	self	heter	different	poly	many, much, excessive
		hetero	different	post	after, behind
bi	two, double	homo	similar, same	pre	before
bin	twice	homeo	similar, same, likeness, constant	primi	first
brachy	short			pro	before
brady	slow	hydr	water	proto	first
		hydro	water	pseudo	false
cac	bad	hyp	below, deficient	pyro	fire
cata	down	hyper	above, beyond, excessive		
centi	a hundred	hypo	below, under, deficient	quadri	four
chromo	color			quint	five
circum	around	in	in, into, not		
con	with, together	infra	below	re	back
contra	against	infer	below	retro	backward
		inter	between		
de	down, away from	intra	within	semi	half
deca	ten	ir (in)	into	sub	below, under, beneath
di (a)	through, between			supra	above, beyond
dia	through, between	macro	large	super	above, beyond
dif	apart, free from, separate	mal	bad	sym	together
dipl	double	mega	large, great	syn	together, with
di (s)	two, apart	meso	middle		
dis	apart	meta	beyond, over, between, change	tachy	fast
dys	bad, difficult, painful			tetra	four
		micro	small	trans	across
ec	out, outside, outer	milli	one-thousandth	tri	three
ecto	out, outside, outer	mon (o)	one		
em	in	mono	one	ultra	beyond
en	within	multi	many, much	uni	one

WORD ROOTS/COMBINING FORMS

abdomin	abdomen	aden	gland	alveol	small, hollow air sac
abort	to miscarry	aden/o	gland	ambyl	dull
absorpt	to suck in	adhes	stuck to	ambul	to walk
acanth	a thorn	adip	fat	amni/o	lamb
acetabul	vinegar cup	agglutinat	clumping	ampere	ampere
acid	acid	agon	agony	amputat	to cut though
acoust	hearing	agor/a	market place	amyl	starch
acr	extremity, point	albin	white	anastom	opening
acr/o	extremity, point	albumin	protein	andr	man
act	acting	alimentat	nourishment	andr/o	man
actin	ray	all	other	ang	vessel

ang/i	vessel
angin	to choke, quinsy
angi/o	vessel
anis/o	unequal
ankyl	stiffening, crooked
an/o	anus
anter/i	toward the front
anthrac	coal
aort	aorta
aort/o	aorta
append	appendix
arachn	spider
arche	beginning
arter	artery
arter/i	artery
arteri/o	artery
arthr	joint
arthr/o	joint
artific/i	not natural
aspirat	to draw in
atel	imperfect
atel/o	imperfect
ather	fatty substance, porridge
ather/o	fatty substance, porridge
atri	atrium
atri/o	atrium
aud/i	to hear
audi/o	to hear
auditor	hearing
aur	ear
aur/i	ear
auscultat	listen to
aut	self
axill	armpit
bacter/i	bacteria
balan	glans penis
bartholin	Bartholin's glands
bas/o	base
bil	bile, gall
bil/i	bile, gall
bi/o	life
blast/o	germ cell
blephar	eyelid
blephar/o	eyelid
bol	to cast, throw
brach/i	arm
bronch	bronchi
bronch/i	bronchi
bronchiol	bronchiole
bronch/o	bronchi
bucc	cheek
burs	a pouch
calc	lime, calcium
calc/i	calcium
calcan/e	heel bone
cancer	crab
capn	smoke
capsul	a little box
carcin	cancer
carcin/o	cancer
card	heart
card/i	heart
cardi/o	heart
carp	wrist
carp/o	wrist

cartil	gristle
castr	to prune
caud	tail
caus	heat
cavit	cavity
celi	abdomen, belly
cellul	little cell
centr	center
centr/i	center
cephal	head
cept	receive
cerebell	little brain
cerebell/o	little brain
cerebr/o	cerebrum
cervic	cervix, neck
cheil	lip
chem/o	chemical
chlor/o	green
chol	gall, bile
chole	gall, bile
chol/e	gall, bile
choledoch/o	common bile duct
chondr	cartilage
chondr/o	cartilage
chord	cord
chori/o	chorion
choroid	choroid
choroid/o	choroid
chromat	color
chrom/o	color
chym	juice
cine	motion
cinemat/o	motion
circulat	circular
cirrh	orange-yellow
cirrh/o	orange-yellow
cis	to cut
claudicat	to limp
clavicul	little key
cleid/o	clavicle
coagul	to clot
coagulat	to clot
coccyg/e	tailbone
coccyg/o	tail bone
cochle/o	land snail
coit	a coming together
col	colon
coll/a	glue
collis	neck
col/o	colon
colon	colon
colon/o	colon
colp/o	vagina
concuss	shaken violently
condyle	knuckle
con/i	dust
conjunctiv	to join together
connect	to bind together
constipat	to press together
continence	to hold
cor	pupil
coriat	corium
corne	cornea
corpor	body
corpor/e	body
cortic	cortex
cortis	cortex

cost	rib
cost/o	rib
cox	hip
cran/i	skull
crani/o	skull
creat	flesh
creatin	flesh, creatine
crine	to secrete
crin/o	to secrete
crur	leg
cry/o	cold
crypt	hidden
cubit	elbow, to lie
culd/o	cul-de-sac
curie	curie
cutane	skin
cyan	dark blue
cycl	ciliary body
cycl/o	ciliary body
cyst	bladder, sac
cyst/o	bladder, sac
cyt	cell
cyth	cell
cyt/o	cell
dacry	tear
dactyl	finger or toe
dactyl/o	finger or toe
defecat	to remove dregs
dem	people
dendr/o	tree
dent	tooth
dent/i	tooth
derm	skin
derm/a	skin
dermat	skin
dermat/o	skin
derm/o	skin
dextr/o	to the right
diast	to expand
didym	testis
digit	finger or toe
dilat	to widen
disk	a disk
dist	away from the point of origin
diverticul	diverticula
dors	backward
dors/i	backward
duct	to lead
duoden	duodenum
dur	dura, hard
dur/o	dura, hard
dwarf	small
dynam	power
ech/o	echo
ectop	displaced
eg/o	I, self
ejaculat	to throw out
electr/o	electricity
eme	to vomit
embol	to cast, to throw
emulsificat	disintergrate
encephal	brain
encephal/o	brain
enchyma	to pour

enter	intestine	gon/o	genitals	lacrim	tear
enucleat	to remove the kernel of	granul/o	little grain, granular	lamin	lamina, thin plate
eosin/o	rose-colored	gravida	pregnant	lamp (s)	to shine
episi/o	vulva, pudenda	gryp	curve	lapar/o	flank, abdomen
equ/i	equal	gynec/o	female	laryng	larynx
erget	work			laryng/e	larynx
erg/o	work	halat	breathe	laryng/o	larynx
eructat	a breaking out	hallux	great (big) toe	later	side
erysi	red	hem	blood	laxat	to loosen
erythr/o	red	hemat	blood	lei/o	smooth
esophag/e	esophagus	hemat/o	blood	lemma	rind, sheath, husk
esophag/o	esophagus	hem/o	blood	lent	lens
esthesi/o	feeling	hemorrh	vein liable to bleed	lept	seizure
estr/o	mad desire	hepat	liver	letharg	drowsiness
eti/o	cause	hepat/o	liver	leuk	white
eunia	a bed	herni/o	hernia	leuk/o	white
excret	sifted out	hidr	sweat	levat	lifter
		hirsut	hairy	libr/i	balance
f(erat)	to bear	hist/o	tissue	lingu	tongue
fasc	a band (fascia)	hol/o	whole	lip	fat
fasci/o	a band (fascia)	horizont	horizon	lipid	fat
femor	femur	humer	humerus	lip/o	fat
fenestrat	window	hydr	water	lith	stone
fibr	fibrous tissue, fiber	hymen	hymen	lith/o	stone
fibrillat	fibrils (small fibers)	hypn	sleep	lob	lobe
fibrin/o	fiber	hyster	womb, uterus	lob/o	lobe
fibr/o	fiber	hyster/o	womb, uterus	lobul	small lobe
fibul	fibula			locat	to place
filtrat	to strain through	icter	jaundice	log	study
fixat	fastened	ile	ileum	log/o	word
flex	to bend	ile/o	ileum	lopec	fox mange
fluor/o	fluorescence	ili	ilium	lord	bending
foc	focus	ili/o	ilium	lucent	to shine
follicul	little bag	illus	foot	lumb	loin
format	a shaping	immun/o	safe, immunity	lumb/o	loin
fungat	mushroom, fungus	infarct	infarct (necrosis of an area)	lump	lump
fus	to pour	infect	infection	lun	moon
		infer/i	below	lymph	lymph, clear fluid
galact/o	milk	inguin	groin	lymph/o	lymph, clear fluid
ganglion	knot	insul	insulin		
gastr	stomach	insulin/o	insulin	malign	bad kind
gastr/o	stomach	integument	covering	mamm/o	breast
gen	formation, produce	intern	within	mandibul	lower jawbone
gene	formation, produce	ionizat	ion (going)	man/o	thin
genet	formation, produce	ion/o	ion	mast	breast
genital	belonging to birth	iont/o	ion	masticat	to chew
gen/o	kind	irid	iris	mast/o	breast
ger	old age	irid/o	iris	maxill	jawbone
gest	to carry	isch	to hold back	maxilla	jaw
gester	to bear	ischi	ischium	maxim	greatest
gigant	giant	is/o	equal	meat	passage
gingiv	gums			meat/o	passage
glandul	little acorn	jaund	yellow	med	middle
gli	glue			medi	toward the middle
gli/o	glue	kal	potassium	medull	marrow
glob	globe	kary/o	cell's nucleus	medull/o	marrow
globin	globule	kel	tumor	melan	black
globul	globe	kerat	cornea	melan/o	black
glomerul	glomerulus, little ball	kerat/o	horn, cornea	men	month
glomerul/o	glomerulus, little ball	keton	ketone	mening	membrane (meninges)
gloss/o	tongue	kil/o	a thousand	mening/i	membrane
gluc/o	sweet, sugar	kinet	motion	mening/o	membrane
glyc	sweet, sugar	kyph	a hump	menise	crescent
glyc/o	glucose, sweet, sugar			men/o	month
glycos	sweet, sugar	labi	lip	ment	mind
gonad	seed	labyrinth	maze	mes	middle
goni/o	angle	labyrinth/o	maze	mes/o	middle

mester	month	orth	straight	physi/o	nature
metr	to measure, womb, uterus	orth/o	straight	pil/o	hair
metr/i	womb, uterus	oscill	to swing	pine	pine cone
micturit	to urinate	oscill/o	to swing	pineal	pineal body
miliar	millet (tiny)	oste	bone	pin/o	to drink
minim	least	oste/o	bone	pituitar	phlegm
mi/o	less, smaller	ot	ear	plak	plate
mit	thread	ot/o	ear	plasma	a thing formed, plasma
mitr	mitral valve	ovar	ovary	plast	a developing
mnes	memory	ovul	ovary	pleur	pleura
mucos	mucus	ovulat	ovary	pleura	pleura
mucus	mucus	ox	oxygen	pleur/o	pleura
muscul	muscle	ox/i	oxygen	plicat	to fold
muscul/o	muscle	oxy	sour, sharp, acid	pneum/o	lung, air
muta	to change			pneumon	lung
mutat	to change	pachy	thick	poiet	formation
my	muscle	pancreat	pancreas	poli/o	gray
myc	fungus	paque	dark	pollex	thumb
myc/o	fungus	palat/o	palate	por	a passage
mydriat	dilation, widen	palliat	cloaked	porphyr	purple
myel	bone marrow, spinal cord	pallid/o	globus, pallidus	poster/i	behind, toward the back
myel/o	marrow	palm	palm	prand/i	meal
my/o	muscle	palpitat	throbbing	presby	old
my/os	muscle	papill	papilla	press	to press
myring	drum membrane	para	to bear	proct	anus, rectum
myring/o	drum membrane	paralyt	to disable, paralysis	proct/o	anus, rectum
myx	mucus	partum	labor	prolif	fruitful
		parturit	in labor	prophylact	guarding
narc/o	numbness	patell	kneecap, patella	prostat	prostate
nas/o	nose	path	disease	prosth/e	an addition
nat	birth	path/o	disease	prot/e	first
nat/o	birth	pause	cessation	proxim	near the point of origin
necr	death	pector	chest	prurit	itching
necr/o	death	pectorat	breast	psych	mind
nephr	kidney	ped	foot, child	psych/o	mind
nephr/o	kidney	ped/i	foot, child	pudend	external genitals
neur	nerve	pedicul	a louse	pulm/o	lung
neur/i	nerve	pelv/i	pelvis	pulmon	lung
neur/o	nerve	pen	penis	pulmonar	lung
neutr/o	neither	penile	penis	pupill	pupil
nid	nest	pept	to digest	purpur	purple
noct	night	perine	perineum	py	pus
nom	law	periton/e	peritoneum	pyel	renal pelvis
norm	rule	phac	lens	pyel/o	renal pelvis
nucl	nucleus	phac/o	lens	pylor	pylorus, gate keeper
nucle	kernel, nucleus	phag	to eat, engulf	py/o	pus
nyctal	blind	phag/o	to eat, engulf	pyret	fever
nystagm	to nod	phak	lentil, lens	pyr/o	heat, fire
		phalang/e	closely knit row		
occlus	to shut up	pharyng/o	pharynx	rach	spine
ocul	eye	pharyng	pharynx	rachi	spine
odont	tooth	phas	speech	radi	radius
olecran	elbow	phen/o	to show	rad/i	radiating out from a center
onc/o	tumor	phe/o	dusky	radiat	radiant
onych	nail	phim	a muzzle	radic/o	spinal nerve root
onych/o	nail	phleb	vein	radicul	spinal nerve root
o/o	ovum, egg	phleb/o	vein	radi/o	ray
oophor	ovary	phon	voice	rect/o	rectum
ophthalm	eye	phone	voice	relaxat	to loosen
ophthalm/o	eye	phon/o	sound	remiss	remit
opt	eye	phor	carrying	ren	kidney
opt/o	eye	phos	light	ren/o	kidney
or	mouth	phot/o	light	respirat	breathing
orch	testicle	phragm	partition	reticul/o	net
orchid	testicle	phragmat/o	partition	retin	retina
orchid/o	testicle	phras	speech		
organ	organ	physic	nature		

retin/o	retina	stern	sternum	trop	turning
rhabd/o	rod	stern/o	sternum	troph	a turning
rheumat	discharge	sterol	solid (fat)	tubercul	a little swelling
rheumat/o	discharge	steth	chest	tuss	cough
rhin/o	nose	steth/o	chest	tympan	ear drum
rhonch	snore	stigmat	point	tympan/o	drum
rhytid/o	wrinkle	stom	mouth		
roent	roentgen	stomat	mouth	uln	ulna, elbow
rotat	to turn	strabism	a squinting	uln/o	ulna, elbow
rrhyth	rhythm	strict	to draw, to bind	umbilic	navel
rrhythm	rhythm	superfic/i	near the surface	ungu	nail
rube/o	red	super/i	upper	ur	urine
		suppress	suppress	ure	urinate
sacr	sacrum	surrog	substituted	urea	urea
salping	tube, fallopian tube	sympath	sympathy	uret	urine
salping/o	tube, fallopian tube	synov	joint fluid	ureter	ureter
salpinx	tube, fallopian tube	syst	contraction	ureter/o	ureter
sarc	flesh	system	a composite whole	urethr	urethra
sarc/o	flesh	systol	contraction	urethr/o	urethra
scapul	shoulder blade			urin	urine
scler	hardening	tel	end, distant	urinat	urine
scler/o	hardening, sclera	tele	distant	urin/o	urine
scoli	curvature	tempor	temples	ur/o	urine
scoli/o	curvature	tend/o	tendon	uter	uterus
scop	to examine	tendin	tendon	uter/o	uterus
seb/o	oil	ten/o	tendon	uve	uvea
secund	second	tenon	tendon		
semin	seed	tenos	tendon	vagin	vagina
seminat	seed	tens	tension	vag/o	vagus, wandering
senile	old	tentori	tentorium, tent	varic/o	twisted vein
senil	old	terat	monster	vas	vessel
sept	putrefaction	testicul	testicle	vascul	small vessel
septic	putrefying	test/o	testicle	vas/o	vessel
ser (a)	whey	thalass	sea	vector	a carrier
ser/o	whey, serum	thel/i	nipple	ven	vein
sert	to gain	therm	hot, heat	venere	sexual intercourse
sexu	sex	therm/o	hot, heat	ven/i	vein
sial	saliva	thorac	chest	ven/o	vein
sial/o	salivary	thorac/o	chest	ventilat	to air
sider/o	iron	thorax	chest	ventr	near or on the belly side of the body
sigmoid	sigmoid	thromb	clot		
sigmoid/o	sigmoid	thromb/o	clot	ventricul	ventricle
sin/o	a curve	thym	thymus, mind, emotion	ventricul/o	little belly
sinus	a hollow curve	thyr	thyroid, shield	vermi	worm
situ	place	thyr/o	thyroid, shield	vers	turning
som	body	thyrox	thyroid, shield	vertebr	vertebra
somat	body	tibi	tibia	vertebr/o	vertebra
somat/o	body	tinnit	a jingling	vesic	bladder
somn	sleep	toc	birth	vesicul	vesicle
son	sound	tom/o	to cut	vir	virus (poison)
son/o	sound	ton	tone, tension	viril	masculine
spadias	a rent, an opening	ton/o	tone	viscer	body organs
spastic	convulsive	tonsill	tonsil, almond	volt	volt
sperm	seed (sperm)	topic	place	volunt	will
spermi	seed (sperm)	top/o	place	volvul	to roll
spermat	seed (sperm)	tors	twisted	vuls	to pull
spermat/o	seed (sperm)	tort/i	twisted		
sphygm/o	pulse	tox	poison	watt	watt
spin	spine, a thorn	toxic	poison		
spir/o	breath	trach/e	trachea	xanth/o	yellow
splen/o	spleen	trache/o	trachea	xen	foreign material
spondyl	vertebra	tract	to draw	xer	dry
spondyl/o	vertebra	trephinat	a bore	xer/o	dry
staped	stirrup	trich	hair	xiph	sword
steat	fat	trich/o	hair		
sten	narrowing	trigon	trigone	zo/o	animal
ster	solid	trism	grating	zoon	life

-able	capable	-grade	a step	-penia	lack of, deficiency
-ac	pertaining to	-graft	pencil, grafting knife	-pepsia	to digest
-ad	pertaining to	-gram	a weight, mark, record	-pexy	surgical fixation
-age	related to	-graph	to write, record	-phagia	to eat
-al	pertaining to	-graphy	recording	-phasia	to speak
-algesia	pain			-pheresis	removal
-algia	pain	-hexia	condition	-phil	attraction
-ant	forming			-philia	attraction
-ar	pertaining to	-ia	condition	-phobia	fear
-ary	pertaining to	-iasis	condition	-phoresis	to carry
-ase	enzyme	-ic	pertaining to	-phragm	a fence
-asthenia	weakness	-ide	having a particular	-phraxis	to obstruct
-ate	use, action		quality	-phylaxis	protection
-ate (d)	use, action	-in	chemical, pertaining to	-physis	growth
		-ine	pertaining to	-plakia	plate
-betes	to go	-ing	quality of	-plasia	formation, produce
-blast	immature cell, germ cell	-ion	process	-plasm	a thing formed, plasma
-body	body	-ism	condition	-plasty	surgical repair
		-ist	one who specializes, agent	-plegia	stroke, paralysis
-cele	hernia, tumor, swelling	-itis	inflammation	-pnea	breathing
-centesis	surgical puncture	-ity	condition	-poiesis	formation
-ceps	head	-ive	nature of, quality of	-praxia	action
-cide	to kill			-ptosis	prolapse, drooping
-clasia	a breaking	-kinesia	motion	-ptysis	to spit, spitting
-clave	a key	-kinesis	motion	-puncture	to pierce
-cle	small				
-clysis	injection	-lalia	to talk	-rrhage	to burst forth, bursting forth
-cope	strike	-lemma	a sheath, rind	-rrhagia	to burst forth, bursting forth
-crit	to separate	-lepsy	seizure	-rrhaphy	suture
-culture	cultivation	-lexia	diction	-rrhea	flow, discharge
-cusis	hearing	-liter	liter	-rrhexis	rupture
-cuspid	point	-lith	stone		
-cyesis	pregnancy	-logy	study of	-scope	instrument
-cyst	bladder	-lymph	clear fluid	-scopy	to view, examine
-cyte	cell	-lysis	destruction, to separate	-sepsis	decay
				-sis	condition
-derma	skin	-malacia	softening	-some	body
-dermis	skin	-mania	madness	-spasm	tension, spasm, contraction
-desis	binding	-megaly	enlargement, large	-stalsis	contraction
-dipsia	thirst	-meter	instrument to measure	-stasis	control, stopping
-drome	a course	-metry	measurement	-staxis	dripping, trickling
-dynia	pain	-mnesia	memory	-sthenia	strength
		-morph	form, shape	-stomy	new opening
-ectasia	dilatation			-systole	contraction
-ectasis	dilatation, distention	-noia	mind		
-ectasy	dilation			-taxia	order
-ectomy	surgical excision	-oid	resemble	-therapy	treatment
-edema	swelling	-ole	opening	-thermy	heat
-emesis	vomiting	-oma	tumor	-tic	pertaining to
-emia	blood condition	-omion	shoulder	-tome	instrument to cut
-er	relating to, one who	-on	pertaining to	-tomy	incision
-ergy	work	-one	hormone	-tone	tension
-esthesia	feeling	-opia	eye, vision	-tripsy	crushing
		-opsia	eye, vision	-troph (y)	nourishment, development
-form	shape	-opsy	to view	-trophy	nourishment, development
-fuge	to flee	-or	one who, a doer	-type	type
		-ory	like, resemble		
-gen	formation, produce	-orexia	appetite	-um	tissue
-genes	produce	-ose	like	-ure	process
-genesis	formation, produce	-osis	condition	-uria	urine
-genic	formation, produce	-ous	pertaining to	-us	pertaining to
-glia	glue				
-globin	protein	-paresis	weakness	-y	condition, pertaining to, process
-gnosis	knowledge	-pathy	disease		

Glossary

Number in parentheses ( ) indicates chapter.

accounting The system of reporting the financial results of a business through analysis, statement, or summary about financial matters. (13)

accounts payable The amounts owed to others for equipment and services that have not yet been paid. (14)

accounts receivable Accounts of money owed. (13, 14)

accreditation The process in which an institution (school) voluntarily completes an extensive self-study after which an accrediting association visits the school to verify the self-study statements. (1)

acquired immune deficiency syndrome (AIDS) A series of illnesses that occur as a result of infection by the human immunodeficiency virus (HIV), which causes the immune system to break down. (2)

active listening Paying attention to a speaker completely, concentrating on the verbal message, observing for nonverbal cues, and offering a response. (4)

active record A record of a patient who has been seen in the past few years and are currently being treated, usually from one to five years. (12)

active voice The subject of the sentence performs the action. (10)

acute condition An illness or injury that a patient suddenly experiences and requires treatment but may not be life threatening. (8)

age analysis The procedure for determining how long an account has been past due, and then instituting the necessary collection procedures. (13)

aggressive The practice of imposing a point of view on others or trying to manipulate others. (4)

alphabetic filling The most common system for filing records in a physician's office, based on placing files in an A to Z order. (12)

American Association of Medical Assistants (AAMA) The professional association for medical assistants that oversees program accreditation, graduate certification, and provides a forum for issues of concern to the physician. (1)

American Banker's Association (ABA) number A bank number printed on a check that originates and identifies the bank and location of the bank from which a check is written. (14)

American Disabilities Act (ADA) Legislation to protect the rights of the disabled regarding access to employment, public buildings, transportation, housing, schools, and health care facilities. (9)

American Medical Technologists (AMT) A professional association that provides oversight for the registration and testing of medical technologists. This association, in cooperation with the AMT Institute for Education (AMTIE) has developed a continuing education (CE) program and recording system. (1)

anesthesia The absence of partial or complete sensation. (2)

answering service A telephone response service that can be in effect to relieve staff at designated times. (6)

anthrax A deadly infectious disease caused by Bacillus anthracisis. Humans contract the disease from infected animal hair, hides, or waste. (2)

archive The storage of items, such as files or records for future reference or back up, usually placed in a storage container or facility and kept for a determined number of years. (8)

assertive The practice of making a point in a positive manner by standing firm, making decisions based on principles or values, and trusting ones own ideas or instincts in the situation. (4)

assessment An evaluation to determine a patient's medical problem. (4)

assignment of benefits A patient's written authorization giving the insurance company the right to pay the provider of services directly for billed charges. (13, 16)

attitude Opinion that develops from one's value system. (4)

audit Examination of all financial statements for accuracy. (14)

auditory By hearing. (4)

automated assistance program An automated telephone system that allows for separating callers to the appropriate people through a series of questions. (6)

bacteria Microorganisms that are capable of causing disease. (2)

bandwidth The number of bits processed in a computer at one time to represent and address. (11)

behavior The actions others see. (4)

benefit period The period of time that payments for Medicare inpatient hospital benefits are available. (15, 16)

bias An unfair preference or dislike of something that prevents an impartial opinion of someone or something. (4)

biohazard Biological substances, such as medical waste and samples of a virus or bacterium, that pose a threat to human beings and are potentially infectious. (5)

block A style or format of letter writing that is spaced with all lines, from the date through the signature line, flush with the left margin. There is a space separating each paragraph and between inside address, salutation, body, and close. (10)

body mechanics Coordination of body alignment, balance, and movement. (5)

bookkeeping The process of managing the accounts for a business, which is a continual process and should be done on a daily basis. (13)

breach of confidentiality Failure to keep something confidential. When patient information is released to others without authorization from the patient. (16)

breach of contract The failure by either party in a valid contract to comply with the terms of the agreement. (3)

cadaver A dead human body used to study the human anatomy. (2)

caduceus The recognized symbol for medicine depicts a healing staff with two snakes coiled around the staff. (2)

caller ID A telephone function that allows the telephone owners to know who is calling each time the telephone rings. (6)

canceled check A deposited check that has been processed and paid out to creditors by the bank. (14)

capital equipment Items that require a large dollar amount to purchase (generally over $500) and have a relatively long life. (9)

cash disbursement Payments made to creditors. (14)

central processing unit (CPU) The brain of the computer or main memory that executes the specific set of instructions. (11)

certification The issuance by an official body or professional organization of a certificate and credentials to one who has met the educational and experience standards of that organization. (1, 2)

Certified Medical Assistant (CMA) A multiskilled health care professional who assists providers in an allied health care setting and who has met the standards of the AAMA by achieving a satisfactory test result and is validated every five years, either by earning continuing education units (CEUs) or through reexamination. (1)

character The sum of the values, attitudes, and behaviors a person exhibits. (4)

claim A written and documented request for reimbursement for an eligible expense to the insurance company in a correct and timely manner. (15)

clarity In reference to your speaking voice, the quality or state of being understandable. (6)

clock speed The measurement of how many instructions per second the computer's processor can execute and is represented in MHz. (11)

closed record A record of a patient who has actively terminated his or her contact with the physician. The files are kept in storage for legal reasons. (12)

closed-panel HMO A clinic that is owned by the HMO and the physicians are employees of the HMO. (15)

close-ended question Question that can be answered with a yes or a no reply. (4)

collating Collecting into one file all records, test results, and information pertaining to a patient who is scheduled to be seen by the physician. It also refers to organizing the sub-group information (for example, laboratory and x-ray results) in records for the day's appointments as well as when filing. (7)

colleague A fellow member of a profession. (18)

computer A programmable machine, or system of hardware that responds to a specific set of instructions and

performs a list of instructions in programmed language called software. (11)

condescending Behavior that adopts a superior attitude and acting as though one is better than someone else. (4)

conference call Three or more parties at different locations from each other may speak with one another on the telephone at the same time. (6)

confidentiality Safeguarding a patient's confidences, particularly information in the medical record regarding family history, past or current diseases or illnesses, test results, and medications is vital to the patient and health care professional relationship. (1)

continuing education units (CEUs) Credit awarded for additional course work beyond certification, a unit of training or education is granted for each clock hour. The American Association of Medical Assistants requires 60 CEUs over a five-year period to maintain certification. (1)

contributory negligence The patient's contribution to the injury, which if proven, would release the physician as the direct cause. (3)

co-payment (copay) A designated amount of money that is required by a patient/member of some medical insurance plans to pay for medical services or medication, usually at the time of service. (7)

credit An addition of funds to an account. (14)

crossover claim A patient claim that is eligible for both Medicare and Medicaid. It is also called Medi/Medi. (15)

culture The values, beliefs, attitudes, views, and customs shared by a group of people and passed on through the generations. (4)

Current Procedural Terminology (CPT) A manual that provides procedure and service codes. (17)

cycle time The length of time the average patient spends in the medical office. (8, 9)

debit A charge against an account. (14)

deductible A sum of money that must be paid by the patient before the insurance plan pays benefits for services rendered. (15)

defamation of character A scandalous statement about someone that can injure the person's reputation. Defamation can result even when the statement is true. (3)

defensive behavior A reaction to a perceived threat that is usually unconscious. (4)

demographic Information or data relating to descriptive information such as age, gender, ethnic background, education, and Social Security number. (7)

deposit Money (cash and check payments) placed into a bank account. (14)

Diagnostic Related Groups (DRGs) A Medicare hospital payment system, which classifies each Medicare patient according to his or her illness. (2)

discretion The ability to make decisions responsibly, is tactful in communicating with others, and is able to be fair and be familiar with policies and regulations. (1)

discriminatory Prejudicial. (18)

double booking Scheduling two patients to be seen during the same time slot without allowing for any additional time in the schedule. (8)

electronic medical record (EMR) Electronic medical documentation relating to the patient. (12)

embezzlement The taking of funds by a breach of trust. (14)

empathy The ability to be sensitive to or understand the feelings of another individual and identify with what he or she is experiencing without necessarily experiencing the same thing. To have some insight or understanding of the pain or distress a patient is feeling and act in a kindly way that expresses sensitivity to the patient's feelings. (1, 4)

enunciation In reference to your speaking voice, the clear articulation and pronouncement of words. (6)

ergonomics Scientific information and data regarding human body mechanics used to design objects and overall environments for human use. (5)

established patient Any patient who has been previously seen by the physician and has an existing medical record/chart in the physician's practice. (8)

ethnicity A classification of people based on national origin. (4)

ethnocentric Belief that one's own cultural background is better than any other. (4)

Evaluation and Management (E/M) A classification of services in the CPT manual that includes codes for office visits, consultations, the physician's component for emergency services, and inpatient hospital care, etc. (17)

exclusive provider organization (EPO) A managed care system that allows the patient to only select from a defined panel of providers, who are reimbursed on a modified fee-for-service method. (15)

externship The experience that is required in which students work without payment in a physician's office, clinic, or hospital setting for 160 to 190 hours over several weeks during the final stage of their training. (1)

facsimile (fax) An electronically transmitted document containing print text and graphic information. (7)

fee schedule A list of the amount to be paid by an insurance company for each procedure or service, determined by a claims administrator and applied to claims subject to the fee schedule of a provider's managed care contract. (15)

feedback Any response to a communication. (4)

floppy disk A small flexible, magnetic disk in a rigid plastic case that stores data on and retrieves data by a computer. (11)

gender bias Indicating either male or female role by the language or image used. (10)

grievance Complaint. (18)

gross annual wage An individual's yearly work earnings before taxes and any withholdings are taken out. (14)

Ground Fault Circuit Interrupter (GFCI) An outlet designed to protect people from severe or fatal electric shocks. (5)

group practice Physicians who participate in a practice with other physicians to share the workload and expenses. (1)

guardian ad litem An adult who will act in the court on behalf of a minor. (Latin) (3)

Health Insurance Portability and Accountability Act (HIPAA) A federal act designed to improve portability and continuity of health insurance coverage. (4)

health maintenance organization (HMO) A managed care plan in which a range of health care services are made available to plan members for a predetermined fee (the capitation rate) per member, by a limited group of providers (such as physicians and hospitals). (15)

hierarchy A ranked order. (4)

holistic Viewing the overall situation such as the human body as a whole organism. (4)

homophones Words in the English language that have similar pronunciations but very different meanings and spellings. (10)

hospice A facility that provides an interdisciplinary program of care and supportive services for terminally ill patients and their families. (2, 4)

immunology The study of immunity or the resistance to or protection from disease. (2)

inactive record A medical record of a patient who has not been seen by the physician within the time period determined by office policy. The patient has not received a formal notification that the physician has terminated care. These files are maintained but generally kept in a separate storage file cabinet. They may return when a medical problem develops. (12)

incident report A formal written description of any unusual occurrence or accident in the medical setting. (5)

inflection In reference to your speaking voice, the pitch in your voice and the way words and phrases are uttered. (6)

informed consent Permission or approval given by a patient who is informed by the physician about the possible consequences of both having and not having certain procedures and treatment. (3)

integrated delivery system (IDS) An organization of provider sites, such as ambulatory centers, clinics, or hospitals, with a contracted relationship that offer services to subscribers. (15)

integrity Adherence to a code of values, honesty, dependability, and dedicated to high standards. To do what is expected, when it is expected, for the simple reason that it is expected. (1)

International Classification of Diseases, Ninth Revision Clinical Modification (ICD-9-CM) The accurate diagnostic numeric and alphanumeric code listing for patient diagnoses and identification on the medical insurance claim forms used for the insurance billing process. (17)

International Classification of Diseases, Tenth Revision (ICD-10) Diagnosis codes that contain increased specificity and include newly discovered or diagnosed diseases. (17)

Internet A computer network made up of thousands of interfacing networks worldwide. (11)

Internet service provider (ISP) A commercial service that provides access to the Internet. (11)

inventory A detailed master list that maintains all of the physical assets or capital equipment in an office. (9)

kilobyte (K or Kb) The measurement of a computer's memory or storage. Each kilobyte is 1,000 bytes (or characters) of information. (11)

kinesthetic Involving movement. (4)

ledger card A record of the charges, adjustments, payments, and current balance for the patient. (13)

licensure Granting of a license and authorization to practice one's profession. (2)

living will A document that allows patients to request that life-sustaining treatments and nutritional support not be used to prolong their life. This document gives patients the legal right to direct the type of care they wish to receive when their death is imminent and provides protection for physicians and hospitals when they follow the patient's wishes. (3)

Magnetic Ink Character Recognition (MICR) A system of combining characters and numbers on checks and deposit slips that is read by high-speed machinery, increasing the speed and accuracy of processing bank statements and check sorting. (14)

main memory The CPU of a computer acts as a traffic controller, directing the computer's activities and sending electronic signals to the right place at the right time. (11)

mass storage device Component of a computer that can retain large amounts of data, such as disk drives or zip drives. (11)

Material Safety Data Sheet (MSDS) Written or printed material information sheet for products and materials that contain a hazardous chemical. MSDS offers basic information needed to ensure the safety and health of the user at all stages of its manufacture, storage, use, and disposal. (5)

matrix Periods of time blocked out on the daily schedule when an appointment is unavailable. (8)

medical emergency A patient condition that may be life threatening if not treated. (7)

medical foundation A nonprofit integrated delivery system (IDS), which is an organization of provider sites (e.g. ambulatory centers, clinics, or hospitals) with a contracted relationship that offer services to subscribers. (15)

medical privilege A physician is given rights to practice medicine in a particular hospital or other health care facility. (2)

medical record All medical documentation relating to the patient including past patient history information, current diagnosis and treatment, and correspondence relating to the patient. (12)

megahertz (MHz) The measurement used for the time it takes for electronic signals to come and go. (11)

memory Part of a computer that provides storage for data and programs. (11)

microbe A one-celled form of life, such as bacteria. (2)

microfiche Sheets of microfilm. (12)

microfilm Miniaturized photographs of records. (12)

microorganism A minute living organism. (2)

microprocessor The heart of the CPU that performs the basic operations of a computer. (11)

modified block A (standard) style letter that has the date, complimentary closing, and the signature line beginning at the center and moving toward the right margin. All other lines are flush with the left margin. (10)

modified wave scheduling A flexible scheduling system built on the hour as the base of each block of time. (8)

modifier A two-digit code with preceding hyphen that clarifies a procedure in the CPT manual. (17)

monitor The display screen that allows the user to observe that the computer does what it was directed to do. (11)

morale The positive or negative state of mind (feeling of well-being) for employees with relationship to their work or work environment. (9)

morbidity rate The rate of disease and illness within a certain population. (2)

mouse A pointing and selecting device that gives the user control of the computer. (11)

National Committee for Quality Assurance (NCQA) An association that evaluates the quality of health plans in order to help consumers and employers make more informed decisions about their health care. (5)

negotiable instrument An instrument that actualizes or permits the transfer of money to another person, for example: a check. (14)

nonparticipating provider A physician or medical facility that bills the patient and the patient is expected to pay the charges for services. (16)

nonverbal communication Information conveyed through the language of gesture and actions including body language instead of using words. (4)

no-show A patient that does not keep his or her appointment and does not call to cancel the appointment. (7)

numerical filing A patient identification system that assigns a number to each patient's medical record, which is filed numerically. This system is used in hospitals and many larger clinics. (12)

Occupational Safety and Hazard Administration (OSHA) A governmental agency responsible for the safety of all employees of companies operating in the United States. (5)

office flow The organization of an office environment that lends itself easily to teamwork, time management, organized and efficient office equipment usage, and patient flow. (9)

open-ended question A question that requires more than a yes or no response. (4)

open-panel HMO A health care provider that is not employed by the HMO and does not belong to a medical group owned or managed by the HMO. (15)

osteopath A medical professional that places great emphasis on the relationship between the musculoskeletal systems and the organs of the body. The skill of manipulation therapy is learned in schools of osteopathy. (2)

overbooking Scheduling more than one patient in the same time slot. Also referred to as double or triple booking. (7)

pandemic An outbreak of a disease that infects many people in different countries at the same time such as the bubonic plague. (2)

participating provider A physician or medical facility that will accept the insurance company's allowed amount as payment in full (less patient co-payments) for services rendered. (16)

passive listening Simply listening to someone without having to reply such as when listening as a member of an audience. (4)

passive voice The subject of a sentence receives the action. (10)

pasteurization The process during which substances, such as milk and cheese, are heated to a certain temperature to eliminate bacteria. (2)

payee A person or company named as the receiving party to whom the amount on a check is payable. (14)

payer A person signing a check to release money. (14)

pitch In reference to your speaking voice, the loudness of your voice. (6)

point-of-service plan (POS) A flexible health care plan that allows patients to choose using the panel of providers within the HMO network or to utilize the services of non-HMO providers. (15)

post Enter amounts onto a record. (13)

practice of medicine Diagnosing and prescribing treatment or medication. (3)

preauthorization Prior approval from a health care plan administrator to receive reimbursement for surgery and other procedures to be performed. (15, 16)

preferred provider organization (PPO) A health care plan that stipulates that the patient must use a medical provider (physician or hospital) who is under contract with the insurer for an agreed-on-fee. (15)

prejudice An opinion form based on incorrect or irrational facts. (4)

premium A monthly fee paid by the insured for specific medical insurance coverage. (15)

prepaid plan A group of physicians or other health care providers who have a contractual agreement to provide services to subscribers on a negotiated fee-for-service or capitated basis (also called managed care plan). (15)

primary care physician (PCP) A physician who is part of a managed care plan that provides all primary health care services to members of the plan. Generally an internist, family practitioner, gynecologist, or pediatrician is a primary care physician. (15)

principal diagnosis A diagnosis of a particular condition that a patient sought care for on a particular date. It is used when performing coding in the hospital setting and when a final diagnosis was unable to be determined without further patient follow-up. (17)

printer A device to output information from a computer onto paper or a hardcopy. (11)

probationary period A trial period to observe a new employee at work and to determine if the new employee is suited to the position for which he or she was hired. (18)

problem oriented medical record (POMR) A system used for charting medical records. (12)

procedural coding The process of transferring a narrative description of procedures into numbers. (17)

professional courtesy (PC) A consideration of service offered by a physician to other physicians, family members, and indigent patients. Conditions must fall within federal guidelines, and be recorded in the patient's record. (13)

proofreading Reviewing and checking a written document or material for errors in content and typing. (10)

proximate cause Natural continuous sequence of events, without any intervening cause, which produces an injury. In a legal case of negligence, the defendant's acts (or failure to act) that directly cause an injury. (3)

quality assurance (QA) Gathering and evaluating information about services provided as well as the results achieved and comparing this information with an accepted standard. (5)

queue A waiting line. (6)

random-access memory (RAM) The highest amount of memory measured in the number of kilobytes that a computer can hold all at once. (11)

rapport An environment of cooperation. (4)

read-only memory (ROM) Storage of information that is not actively being used by the computer at that moment. (11)

real time Refers to automatically placing the appointment, patient needs, and information within the appropriate areas of a computer appointment program versus a manual system. (8)

reasonable person standard Exercising the ordinary standard of care and the type of care that a "reasonable" person would use in a similar circumstance. (3)

receptionist The staff employee in an office that greets and assists incoming patients and performs duties that make the office run smoothly and efficiently; often a medical assistant. (7)

reconciliation The agreement of the figures on the bank statement with the records maintained in the medical office and the adjustment of banking records. (14)

redundant Repetition of the same statement over again. (10)

referral Paperwork for the insurance company that is required from the primary care physician to send a patient to see a medical specialist for treatment. (6, 15)

Registered Medical Assistant (RMA) A medical assistant who meets the eligibility requirements and who can prove his or her competency to perform entry-level skills through written examination. The RMA is awarded to candidates who pass the AMT certification examination. A multiskilled health care professional assists providers in an allied health setting. (1)

registration A health care professional on record as part of an organization or association in a specific health care field that administers examinations and maintains a list of qualified individuals. (2)

res ipsa loquitur A doctrine meaning, "the thing speaks for itself," applies to the law of negligence. It refers to the breach (neglect) of duty that is so obvious that it does not need further explanation or "it speaks for itself." (Latin) (3)

respondeat superior A term meaning, "Let the master answer." It refers to the employer or physician who is liable for the negligent actions of anyone working for him or her. In some states, both the physician and the employee may be liable. (Latin) (3)

risk management Planning and implementing strategies for reducing the physician's risk of lawsuit in the medical setting. (4)

scheduling system A system that facilitates the coordination of appropriate time segments for staff, patients, and the practice's available equipment to provide efficient services. (8)

self-referral A health insurance enrollee chooses to see an out-of-network provider without authorization. (15)

seniority A status gained by being the individual who worked for an employer for the longest amount of time. (18)

signee The person who signs a check or document. (14)

software A set or sets of programmed language that gives instructions for a computer to process and perform. (11)

solo practice A physician who practices alone. (1)

solvent A company or practice capable of paying its bills and salaries. (18)

source oriented medical record Various medical reports that are filed in the medical records with tabs that label the source, such as laboratory, x-ray, consultation, and special study. (12)

specific time The time allocated on the schedule to each patient depending upon the purpose of the office visit or the type of examination or testing that is to be done. (8)

standard of care The level of knowledge, skill, and care a medical practitioner must provide to all patients for the same care that would commonly be provided by other similar medical care professionals under the same circumstances in the same locality. (3)

statute of limitations The maximum period of time during which a patient can take legal actions. (3, 13)

stem cell An undifferentiated cell that can give rise to other cells of the same type or from which specialized cells can develop. (2)

stereotyping Negative generalities concerning specific characteristics of a group that are applied unfairly to an entire population. (4)

stop-payment order An order issued by the payer, to suspend payment on a check not allowing the bank to disburse the funds. (14)

subjective, objective, assessment, and plan (SOAP) A system used for charting medical records. (12)

subscriber The person, also known as a member, who holds an insurance policy (that may include family members) providing medical coverage in return for a fixed monthly fee. (13, 15)

superbill (charge/encounter slip) The document generated by the medical office of services for billing and insurance processing and used as a charge slip, statement, and insurance reporting form. (13, 16)

surgical scheduler The person in the surgery department who sets up and maintains the schedule for surgery and procedures. (8)

symbol Icon or sign used in the CPT manual to distinguish changes or instructions to be used when coding. (17)

sympathy Feeling sorry or pity for a patient. (4)

tax withholding Money or amount of salary that is withheld from an employee's payroll check by the employer for the purposes of paying governmental taxes. (14)

telephone triage The telephone screening process for determining the order to take patients' calls according to the seriousness of their condition. (6)

Telnet (Telnet Protocol) Facilitates login to a computer host to execute commands. (11)

terminal digit filing A medical filing system based on the last digits of the ID number, which evenly distributes files within the entire filing system eliminating the need for frequent re-shifting of files. (12)

thesaurus A reference book that provides synonyms or similar meaning words. (10)

third-party check A check written by a party unknown to you. (14)

third-party payer A person or party other than the patient, such as an insurance company, who assumes responsibility for paying the patient's bill. (13)

tickler file A small file box organized into the dates that a reminder postcard should be mailed. (8)

time patterns Matrixing off time within an appointment schedule for catch-up time or non-scheduled appointments. (8)

triage The process of sorting or grouping patients according to the seriousness of their condition. (8)

Truth in Lending Act (formerly the Consumer Protection Act of 1968) A federal law affecting credit that was enacted to protect the consumer. (13)

universal serial bus (USB) A small portable storage device that can hold up to 4Gs of data, also known as jump drive, thumb drive, or flash drive. (11)

Usenet (Network News Transfer Protocol or NNTP) Distributes Usenet news articles derived from topical discussions on newsgroups. (11)

usual, customary, and reasonable (UCR) The fee charged for medical services that is determined by the physician or the practice's partners as a result of taking into consideration the time and services involved as well as the prevailing rate fee in the community. (13)

value A set of standards a person uses to measure the worth or importance of someone or something. (4)

vendor Supplier of office supplies and equipment. (9)

verbal communication A wide range of words and sounds or tone of voice that a person uses to convey vastly different meanings. (4)

visual By seeing (4)

voice messaging system A system for messages (voice mail) to be left or recorded when the medical assistant is unavailable to answer the telephone. (6)

warrant A statement issued to indicate that a debt should be paid, but not actually a negotiable check. (14)

warranty A guarantee in writing from the manufacturer that the product will perform correctly under normal conditions of use. (9)

wave scheduling A scheduling system that is set to begin and end each hour on time. Each hour is divided into equal segments of time depending on how many patients can be seen within an hour. It provides built-in flexibility to accommodate unforeseen situations, such as patients who require more time with the physician, a late arriving patient, or the patient who fails to keep an appointment (no-show). (8)

World Health Organization (WHO) A specialized health agency of the United Nations. (17)

World Wide Web (WWW) A system of Internet servers. (11)

Index

A

Abandonment, 46
Abbreviations. *See also* Medical
  terminology
  improving patient knowledge of, 77
  two-letter, United States and territories,
    185–187
  use of accepted medical, 183
Abuse, reports of, 53t
Accounting systems, 235–237
  accounts payable, 236–237
  accounts receivable, 236, 237
  computerized, 243
  patient accounts, 236
Accounts payable, 236–237
  use of online banking for, 248
Accounts receivable, 236, 252
  aging, 233
  control, 241–242, 243f
  insurance, 236
  procedure to perform accounts receivable,
    237
  terms related to, 236
Accreditation, 5
Accrediting Bureau of Health Education
  Schools (ABHES), 5, 9
Accrediting Commission of Career Schools
  and Colleges of Technology (ACCSCT), 5
Acquired immune deficiency syndrome
  (AIDS), 22, 82
Active listening, 72
Active records, 212
Active voice, 174
Activities of daily living (ADL), 35
Acute conditions, 151
  examples of, 153t
Adjustment, 236
Administrative area, of medical office, 160
Administrative law, 44, 45
Aggressive behavior, 75
  comparison of assertive and, 75t
Allergies, to scents, 131
Allergy and immunology, 27
Alphabetic filing system, 213–216
  key to, 215
  procedure for filing record in, 216
  rules for, 214t
Alpha-Z system (Smead Manufacturing
  Company), 217, 218t
American Association of Medical Assistants
  (AAMA), 4, 9–10
  Code of Ethics, 57, 59
  Creed of, 57
  DACUM philosophy (1979), 7
  Role Delineation Study (1997), 7
American Banker's Association (ABA), 249
American Board of Medical Specialties
  (ABMS), 23
American Board of Radiology, 29
American Cancer Society, 135
American Diabetic Association, 135
American Disabilities Act (ADA), 160
American Heart Association, 135
American Hospital Association, 58, 87
American Medical Association (AMA), 106
  essential of quality care, 106
  ethical behavior, according to, 57

handling of unethical behavior by, 57
  Principles of Medical Ethics, 57, 58
American Medical Technologists (AMT), 10
American Occupational Therapy Association
  (AOTA), 35
American Red Cross, 21
American Society of Clinical Pathologists
  (ASCP), 37
Ames Color File System, 217
AMT Institute for Education (AMTIE), 10
Anesthesia, 20
Anesthesiology, 27
Anesthetics, 19
Answering service, 124
  checking, before opening office, 132
Anthrax, 19
Application programs, computer, 197
Appointment books, 147–148
  archiving, 148
Appointment cards, 150–151
Appointment scheduling, 144–155
  advance booking, 150–151
  appointment books, 147–148
  appointment cards, 150–151
  building free time block into, 152–153
  double booking patients, 145
  for established patients, 154–155
  exceptions, 151–153
  follow-up, 151
  by grouping procedures, 145
  for hospital admission, 151
    patient information to be supplied
      when setting up, 152t
  inpatient surgical procedures, 153
  legal and ethical issues related to, 148
  methods, comparison of, 146t
  missed appointments and delays, 149–150
  modified wave scheduling, 145
  for new patients, 154
  for nonpatients, 155
  open office hours system, 145
  patient no-shows, 138, 150
  patient referrals, 151
  patient scheduling process, 148–151
  procedure for, 150
  scheduling outpatient procedures,
    151, 153
  scheduling surgery, 151
  specified time scheduling, 144
  systems, 146–148
  telephone and e-mail, 153–154
  time estimates for specific office
    procedures, 149t
  wave scheduling, 145
Archives, 148
Arraignment, 52
Assertive behavior, 75
  comparison of aggressive and, 75t
  guidelines, 76
  techniques, 75–76
Assessment, patient, 72
Assignment of benefits, 291
Assignment of benefits form, 231
Assisted-living facility, 33
Associate practice, 27
Attitudes, 66
  conveying positive, 71
Audiograms, 81

Audiologists, 81
Audiometric testing, 81
Auditory learners, 68
Audits, 265
Authoritarian leaders, 322
Automated assistance program, 122–123
Autopsies, 19
AZT, 22

B

Bacteria, 17, 19
Bacteriology, 19–20
Balance, 236
Bandwidth, 195
Bank drafts, 251
Banking
  accepting cash, 257
  bill paying, 254–255
  cash disbursement, 258
  checks, 249–254
  deposits, 256–257
  function of, 248
  hold on accounts, 258
  legal and ethical issues related to, 260
  online, 248
  procedures, saving documentation relating
    to, 259–260
  statements, 258–259
  types of bank accounts, 248
Bankruptcy, 234
Bank statements
  credits and debits on, 258
  procedure for reconciling, 259
  reconciliation of, 258–259
Barnard, Christian, 22
Barton, Clara, 21
Bathrooms, medical office, 163
Battery, 49
Behavior, 66
  assertive versus aggressive, 75
  defensive, 77
  exhibiting negative, 68
  patterns, dealing with wide scope of, 83
Benefit period, 270, 286
Better Business Bureau, 235
Bias, 79–80
Billing, 229–231
  computerized, 230–231
  credit policy, 231–232
  ledger cards, 229–230
  manual, 230
  methods, 229
  period: frequency, 231
  superbill/encounter form, 229
  third-party payers and minors, 231
Bill paying, 254–255
Biohazards. *See also* Hazardous medical
  waste
  definition of, 98
Biomedical equipment technician, 38
Births, reports of, 53t
Black death, 17
Black plague, 17
Blackwell, Elizabeth, 21
Blindness, 82
Block letter style format, 180–181, 182f
Bloodborne Pathogens Standards, 100–101

I

ICD-9-CM (International Classification
of Diseases, Ninth Clinical Modification)
abbreviations, symbols, and other
conventions, 303
coding
procedure for, 305
steps in, 302–303
E-code section of, 304f
formats and conventions of, 302
publishing of, 300
special codes in, 303
understanding, 300, 302
ICD-10 (International Classification
of Diseases, Tenth Revision), 303
Illness. *See also* Diseases
differing cultural views regarding, 78
link between stress and, 67–68
Immunization, for health care employees,
220
Immunology, 19–20, 27
advances in, 20–21
Inactive records, 213
Incident report, 104–105
example of typical, 105f
Incident reports, 219–220
Individual practice association (IPA), 272
Infectious waste, 100
Informed consent, 49–51
definition of, 49
document, sample of, 50f
exceptions to doctrine of, 50
forms, 211–212
medical assistants and, 55–56
Injuries, reportable, 53t
Ink-jet printers, 197
Input devices, computer, 195
Inside address, in correspondence, 178
Instant message format, 188
Insurance. *See also* Health insurance
accounts receivable, 236
billing, 229
claims. *See* Claims
long-term care, 276
major medical, 276
malpractice, 48
Insurance cards, 135
Insurance coding, 300. *See also*
ICD-9-CM (International Classification
of Diseases, Ninth Clinical Modification)
code linkage, 312
compliance, 312
history of, 300
procedure coding, 303
procedure for assigning a CPT code, 310
Insurance fraud, 308
Medicare definition of, 308, 311
prevention and detection, compliance
guidance for, 311–312
reporting suspected, 312
tips, 311
Integrated delivery system (IDS), 273
Integrated provider organization (IPO), 273
Integrity, of medical assistants, 7–8, 23
Intentional torts, 44t, 45
Intermediate-care facility (ICF), 32–33
Internal medicine, 28
Internal Revenue Service, 262
International Classification of Diseases (ICD),
243, 300. *See also* ICD-10; ICD-9-CM
International health and medical insurance,
276
International List of Causes of Death, 300
Internet, 199
advertising staff positions on, 324–325
building medical practice Web site on, 335
services on, 201

Internet service provider (ISP), 201
Internists, 27, 28
Interoffice memoranda, 181
Interpersonal dynamics, 66–68
Interview process, 325–326
Inventory
equipment, record of, 166t
list of sample drugs, maintaining, 167
order form, sample, 167f
supply control, 166–167

J

Janssen, Zacharias, 17
Jehovah's Witnesses, 51
Jenner, Edward, 18
Job applicants
checking references of, 326
hiring of, 326
interview process for, 325–326
learning important information about,
325
prohibitions against asking discriminatory
questions of, 325
testing thinking abilities of, 326
Joint Commission on the Accreditation of
Health Care Organizations (JCAHO), 31,
220
Joint Review Committee for Ophthalmic
Medical Personnel, 5

K

Keyboard, computer, 196–197
ergonomics and, 202
Kinesthetic learners, 68
Koch, Robert, 19
Kübler-Ross, Elisabeth, 82

L

Laboratory technicians, 37
Laennec, Rene, 18
Laptop computers, 194
Laser printers, 197
Law. *See also* Minors
civil law, 44–45
classification of, 44–46
confidentiality and, 49
criminal law, 44
governing collections, 47t
vaccines required by, 53t
Leading questions, 74
Learning styles, 68
Ledger cards, 229–230, 238, 240, 240f
Leeuwenhoek, Anton van, 17
Legal and ethical issues
computerized data, 199
dealing with insurance, 276, 295
employer responsibilities according
to OSHA guidelines, 100
federal coding regulations, 312
financial information regarding patients,
232
for medical assistants, 6
medical records confidentiality, 222
monitoring of dated material, 172
for office managers, 328
overseeing physician re-registrations and
renewals, 25
patient communication and, 77
patient safety during office visits, 138
performing banking procedures, 260
relating to scheduling process, 148
reporting of equipment defects, 166
understanding of ethical standards, 56
when speaking with patients over
telephone, 117

Legal terminology, understanding, 319
Letter writing, 172–181
active versus passive voice, 174, 174t
avoiding personal pronoun *I*, 174
business letters, 178–179
capitalization rules, 177
for collections, 234
composition, 174
error correction in office correspondence,
177–178
form letters, 179–180
gender bias, removing, 173
inflated phrases versus concise terms,
174t
letter styles, 180–181
parts of speech, 177
plurals, 176–177
repetition and redundancy in, 174
requesting payment, 172
sentence and paragraph length, 173
spelling, 176t
technical terminology, 172–173
two-page letters, 179
use of numbers in, 177, 177t
word choice, 172
Liability, preventing, 54–56
Libel, 49
Licensed practical nurse (LPN), 35, 87
Licensed vocational nurse (LVN), 35
Licensure, 24–25
endorsement, 25
examination for, 24–25
for health care professionals, 33
medical assistants and, 55
reciprocity, 25
revocation, 44
suspension or revocation, 25
Lifespan considerations, 9
appropriate appearance, 132
checks written by agents, 253
child proof and kid friendly medical
offices, 161
computer preparedness for older
employees, 230
computers and computer terminology,
201
confusion associated with filing claims,
294
dealing with elderly patients, 71, 105f
easing patient waiting time, 155
Medicare patients, 275
superbill questions, 300
when handling pediatric cases, 121
Life stages, 66–67, 67t
Limited checks, 251
Listening skills, 72–73
active listening, 72
guidelines for, 73
passive listening, 72
procedure for effective, 73
Litigation
appropriate documentation, to avoid, 89
avoiding, 54
use of medical records in, 52
Living will, 51
Long, Crawford, 20
Long distance calls, 123
being aware of time zones when
placing, 123
conference calls, 123
making, 123
Long-term care institutions, 32–33
assisted-living facility, 33
extended-care facility (ECF), 33
intermediate-care facility (ICF), 32–33
skilled nursing facility (SNF), 32
Long-term care insurance, 276
Loyalty, to employer, 87

M

Magnetic Ink Character Recognition (MICR), 249–250

Mail
certificate of mailing, 186
certified, 186
classifications of, 185–187, 186t
handling tips, 187
insurance, 186
postal money orders, 187
procedure for opening daily, 188
recall, 187
registered, 187
returned, 187
size requirements for, 187
special delivery, 186
special handling, 186
special postal services, 186–187
stationery and envelopes, 183t
tracing lost, 187
ZIP codes, 185

Main memory, computer, 195
Major medical insurance, 276
Malpractice, 48. *See also* Negligence
Malpractice insurance, 48

Managed care
advantages and disadvantages of, 271
claim forms, 286
exclusive provider organizations (EPOs), 273
health maintenance organizations (HMOs), 271–272
managed care organizations (MCOs), 270–273
preferred provider organizations (PPOs), 272–273
systems, history of, 271

Managed care organizations (MCOs), 270–273
Management service organization (MSO), 273

Marketing
assessing target market, 334
customer service, 335
free, and public relations, 335
medical practices, 333–335
Web sites, 335

Maslow, Abraham, 66–67
Mass storage devices, computer, 194
Material Safety Data Sheet (MSDS), 98
example of, 99f
Matrix, forming, 148–149
Mature minor, 51
M code, 303
Mechanical safety, 98
Medicaid, 32, 275
claim forms, 286

Medical assistants
administrative responsibilities, 6
assisting with medical meetings and speaking engagements, 332–333
certification, 55
characteristics of good, 7–9
clinical responsibilities, 7
confidentiality/privacy and, 55
cultural considerations for. *See* Cultural considerations
documentation, 55
drug regulations, 55
education and training for, 4–5
externship requirement for, 5. *See also* Externship
informed consent and, 55–56
job opportunities, 10–11
in health care departments and specialties, 11t
in inpatient and ambulatory settings, 11t

knowledge of entire medical office necessary for, 161
legal and ethical issues for. *See* Legal and ethical issues
letter writing by. *See* Letter writing
liability prevention role of, 54–56
licensing, 55
office management, 55
principles of medical ethics, 57
proofreading of correspondence by, 172
quality assurance role of, 108
responsibilities of, 5, 7
role of, 5–7
in role of receptionist. *See* Patient reception
safety and, 56
scope of practice issues dealt with by, 86–87
standard of care for, 58

Medical assisting
accreditation for programs in, 5
definition of, 4
history of, 4
professional organizations, 9–10. *See also specific organizations*

Medical care, quality, 105–106
defined by AMA, 106

Medical emergencies. *See also* Emergencies
in reception area, 130, 137–138

Medical ethics, 56–57
AMA Principles of, 57
ethical standards and behavior, 56–57

Medical insurance claims. *See* Claims; Health insurance claim forms
Medical laboratories, 37
Medical laboratory technician (MLT), 37

Medical offices
accounts payable expenditures in, 236–237
administrative responsibilities, 6
bathrooms, 163
care and maintenance of equipment in, 131
categories of files in, 212–213
closing, 138, 139
compliance plans, 311–312
creating sense of affiliation to, 321–322
defining goals of, with physician, 331
documentation needed by, 46
equipment, 163–165
ergonomics in, 105, 202
examination rooms, 136–137, 162–163
facilities planning, 160
housekeeping procedures, 163
importance of procedures manual to, 332
layout, 160–161
lost and found, 130–131
maintaining solvency of, 318
managing clinical aspect of, 318
medical meetings and speaking engagements, 332–333
no-show patients, 138, 150
office flow, 161
opening, 132
procedure for, 133
petty cash, 260
posting of payment policies, 228
procedure and policy manual, 86
reception area, 130, 137–138, 161–162
recurring monthly expenses of, 255
reference materials, 183
security, 102, 104–105
supplies, 166–167
telephones in. *See* Medical office telephones
typical layout, 161f
uses of computers in. *See also* Computers

Medical office telephones, 114–125
answering, 114–115
business telephone systems, 115–116

making calls, 115
things to avoid when placing callers on hold, 116
transferring calls, 116
using hold function, 115–116
and cultural considerations, 121
handling difficult calls, 122
handling emergency calls, 125
long distance calls, 123–124
making reminder calls and doing callbacks, 118
message taking, 116–118
caller ID, 117
call forwarding, 117
privacy manager, 117
procedure for, 117
speakerphones and headsets, 117–118
voice messaging system, 116
pagers and cell phones, 118
prescription refill requests, 121
taking message for, 122
for scheduling appointments, 153–154
screening calls, 118
telephone techniques, 114–118
telephone triage, 121–122
typical incoming calls, 119–121
from nonpatients, 120–121
from patients, 119–120
using answering service, 124
using telephone directory, 122–123

Medical Patients Rights Act, 59
Medical practice acts, 24–25
licensure, 24–25
registration, 25
suspension or revocation of medical licenses, 25

Medical practices, 10
marketing and customer service, 333–335
types of, 26–27
associate practice, 27
group practice, 10, 27
partnership, 27
professional corporation, 27
sole proprietorship, 27
solo practice, 10, 26–27
use of professional advertising service by, 333
ways to promote, 335

Medical practitioners, 23–24
medical privileges of, 32
title of doctor, 23
designations and initials for, 24t
others with, 23–24

Medical privileges, 32

Medical records, 208
access to, 221
collating, 132
procedure for, 133
computerized, 198–199
consultation report, 212
diagnosis and treatment plan, 212
discharge summary, 212
disclosure without consent, 221
electronic and computerized, 210
electronic signatures, 201–202
family and medical history, 211
fax transmission of, 132
HIPAA guidelines for area containing, 161
informed consent forms, 211–212
as legal documents, 209
operative report, 212
ownership of, 222–223
pathology report, 212
patient correspondence and follow-up care, 212
patient registration form, 211
physical examination results, 211

procedure for adding or changing items on, 210
procedure to organize a patient medical record, 213
professionalism when handling, 291
radiology report, 212
from referred physicians or hospital visits, 211
reflecting all services and care in, 311
release form for, 221f
releasing, 221
retention and destruction of, 223
specially protected medical information, 221
storing, 221
test results, 211
transcription of, 222
types of, 208–210
types of forms and reports, 210–212
use of, in litigation, 52
Medical records technician, 37
Medical social workers, 36–37
Medical specialties, 27–29
allergy and immunology, 27
anesthesiology, 27
cardiology, 27
dermatology, 27–28
emergency medicine, 28
family practice, 28
geriatric medicine, 28
gynecology, 29
hematology, 28
internal medicine, 28
nephrology, 28
neurology, 28
nuclear medicine, 28
obstetrics, 29
oncology, 28
ophthalmology, 29
orthopedics, 29
otorhinolaryngology, 29
pathology, 29
pediatrics, 29
physical medicine, 29
psychiatry, 29
radiology, 29
rehabilitative medicine, 29
rheumatology, 29
Medical technologist (MT), 37
Medical terminology. See also Abbreviations
common misspellings of, 176t
and corresponding synonyms, 173t
patients and use of, 77
use of correct, 172–173
Medical transcription, 38, 222
career opportunities, 223
equipment, 164
sound-alike words, 222
Medical transcriptionists, 222
physically challenged, 164
Medicare, 32, 274–275
billing, use of CMS-1500 for, 300
claim forms, 286
coding and reimbursement, 300
coverage in hospice setting, 33
definition of insurance fraud, 308, 311
taxes, 262
Medicare Catastrophic Coverage Act, 300
Medications, preparing, 55
Medicine
during the 18th century, 17–18
during the 19th century, 18–20
during the 20th century, 20–21
computer use in, 194
contributions of ancient civilizations to, 16
early, 16–18
firsts in, 22
frontiers of, 22–23

health care costs and payments, 25–26
history of early, 16–23
medical and surgical specialties, 27–30
medical practice acts, 24–25
medical practitioners, 23–24
modern, and the future, 21–23
remedies used in early, 16
types of medical practices, 26
women in, 21
MedLearn, 229
Megahertz (MHz), 195
Memory, computer, 194, 195
Memos, 181
Mentally/emotionally impaired patients, 82–84
Microfiche, 208
Microfilm, 208
Microorganisms, 17
diseases caused by, 19
Microprocessors, 195
Middle digit filing system, 216
Military benefits, 275
claim forms, 286
Minors. See also Children
billing, 231
emancipated, 51
lawsuits on behalf of, 48
legal implications when treating, 51
mature, 51
rights of, 51
Misdemeanor, 44
Mistakes, admitting and correcting, 54
Modified block style format, 181, 182f
with indented paragraphs, 182f
Modified wave scheduling, 145
Money orders, 251
Monitor, computer, 195
ergonomics and, 202
Morbidity rates, 20
Mouse, computer, 197
Multicultural issues, 77–80
bias, prejudice, and stereotyping, 79–80
culture, 78–79
language, 77–78

N

Name pins/tags, receptionist, 131
National Archives and Records Administration (NARA), 281
National Board of Respiratory Therapy, 35
National Certification Agency for Medical Laboratory Personnel, 37
National Childhood Vaccine Injury Act (1960), 53t
National Committee for Quality Assurance (NCQA), 108
National Council Licensure Examination (NCLEX), 35
National Federation of Licensed Practical Nurses, 35
National Health Care Skills Standards (NHCSS), 34
Neglect of duty, 45
Negligence. See also Malpractice
four Ds of, 45
res ipsa loquitur, 48
Negotiable instruments, 249
Nephrologists, 29
Nephrology, 28
Neurology, 28
Nightingale, Florence, 21
Non-English speaking patients, 77–78
disadvantages of, 84
Nonparticipating providers, 294
Nonverbal communication, 70, 72
use of, with non-English speaking patients, 77–78

Norton, William, 20
No-shows, 138, 150
Nuclear medicine, 28
Numbers, in correspondence, 177, 177t
Numerical filing system, 215–217
middle digit filing, 216
serial numbering, 216
straight numerical filing, 215
terminal digit filing, 215
unit numbering, 216
Nurses, 34–35
Nursing homes, 32–33

O

Obstetrics, 29
Occupational Safety and Hazard Administration (OSHA), 220
authority and responsibilities of, 96
Bloodborne Pathogens Standards, 100–101
Exposure Control Plan, 100–101
guidelines for using personal protective equipment and clothing, 101
Hazardous Communications section regarding chemical hazards, 98
housekeeping procedures, 102
Occupational therapist (OT), 35
Office flow, 161
Office for Civil Rights (OCR), 220
Office management, 38
clinical office management, 318
communication, 319
creating team atmosphere, 323–324
employee records, 318
facility and equipment management, 318
financial management, 318
legal concepts, 319
medical assistants and, 55
personnel responsibilities, 318
scheduling, 318
systems approach to, 318–319
Office managers, 38. See also Personnel management
alerting physician to patient no-shows, 138
effective use of performance evaluation by, 328–329
establishment of priority list by, 331
general duties, 319–322
hiring of new staff members by, 324
importance of time management for, 330–331
as integral part of team, 323
leadership styles, 322–323
monthly planning, 320
motivation of employees by, 321–322
orientation and training methods of effective, 326
responsibilities to employee and physician/employer, 319t
skills observed in good, 319
staff meetings, 320
use of personnel policy manual by, 331–332
Office procedures manual, 332
contents of, 333t
functions of, 332
Office security, 102, 104–105
Once-a-month billing, 231
Oncology, 28
Online banking, 248
Open-ended questions, 73
Open-panel HMO, 272
Operative report, 212
Ophthalmology, 29
Optical Character Recognition (OCR), 185
Organ donations, 52